Understanding Parkinson's Disease

Understanding Parkinson's Disease

Edited by Helena Shelton

hayle medical

New York

Hayle Medical,
750 Third Avenue, 9th Floor,
New York, NY 10017, USA

Visit us on the World Wide Web at:
www.haylemedical.com

ISBN: 978-1-63241-672-8

The publisher's policy is to use permanent paper from mills that operate a sustainable forestry policy. Furthermore, the publisher ensures that the text paper and cover boards used have met acceptable environmental accreditation standards.

Printed in China.

Cataloging-in-Publication Data

Understanding Parkinson's disease / edited by Helena Shelton.
p. cm.
Includes bibliographical references and index.
ISBN 978-1-63241-672-8
1. Parkinson's disease. 2. Brain--Diseases. I. Shelton, Helena.
RC382 .U57 2019
616.833--dc23

Table of Contents

Preface

Parkinson's disease is a degenerative disease affecting the central nervous system, which affects the motor system. At the onset of the disease, symptoms such as rigidity, difficulty in walking, shaking and slowness of movement appears. Difficulties in thinking and behavioral changes may also occur. In the advanced stages of the disease, dementia sets in. The cause of Parkinson's disease is not completely understood, but it is believed that it may occur due to genetic and environmental factors. The motor symptoms of the disease can be attributed to the death of cells in the substantia nigra. The diagnosis of Parkinson's disease is based on a clinical examination of symptoms. In the initial stages, antiparkinson medication levodopa and dopamine agonists are prescribed. However with the progression of the disease and with the continued loss of neurons, these medications are rendered ineffective. Surgeries aimed at deep brain stimulation can also be performed in severe cases. This book explores the clinical aspects of Parkinson's disease in the modern day scenario. It strives to provide a fair idea about the symptoms and complications of Parkinson's disease and its medical care and management strategies. It will serve as a valuable source of reference for graduate and post-graduate students.

The information shared in this book is based on empirical researches made by veterans in this field of study. The elaborative information provided in this book will help the readers further their scope of knowledge leading to advancements in this field.

Finally, I would like to thank my fellow researchers who gave constructive feedback and my family members who supported me at every step of my research.

Editor

1

Differential Diagnosis of Parkinson Disease, Essential Tremor, and Enhanced Physiological Tremor with the Tremor Analysis of EMG

Jie Zhang,[1] Yan Xing,[1] Xiuli Ma,[1] and Liqun Feng[2]

[1]*Aviation General Hospital, China Medical University, Beijing 10023, China*
[2]*Anzhen Hospital, Capital Medical University, Beijing 10029, China*

Correspondence should be addressed to Jie Zhang; drzhangjie361@126.com

Academic Editor: Xiaoxing Xiong

We investigate the differential diagnostic value of tremor analysis of EMG on Parkinson's disease (PD), essential tremor (ET), and enhanced physiological tremor (EPT). Clinical data from 25 patients with PD, 20 patients with ET, and 20 patients with EPT were collected. The tremor frequency and muscle contraction pattern of the resting, posture, and 500 g and 1000 g overload were recorded. The frequency of PD tremor was 4–6 Hz, and the frequency of ET was also in this range; the frequency of EPT is 6–12 hz having some overlap with PD. The muscle contraction patterns of the ET and EPT group were mainly synchronous contraction, and the muscle contraction mode of the PD group was mainly alternating contraction. Having tremor latency from rest to postural position and having changes in tremor amplitude after mental concentration in PD might distinguish ET. Tremor analysis of EMG was able to distinguish PD from ET and EPT by varying the tremor frequency and muscle contraction pattern. It can also differentiate between PD and ET by the latency and concentration effect and ET and EPT by weight load effect.

1. Introduction

Parkinson's disease tremor is a common type of tremor. In addition to the clinical manifestations, the tremor of Parkinson's disease is lack of relative objective diagnostic basis. The diagnosis of PD and its differentiation from other types of tremor such as ET and EPT are frequently difficult [1]. Especially in early disease stages it remains problematic because tremor in PD may occur not only at rest, but also at posture and/or during action. On the other hand, tremor at rest is not pathognomonic for PD [2], for it has been observed in ET [3]. It is also difficult to differentiate mild ET from EPT. One study suggested that about 50% of clinical diagnoses of ET are incorrect [4]. The early misdiagnosis rate of Parkinson's disease that only displays the tremor was 25% [5]. It is necessary to identify the ET and PD. Because of the different prognosis of the three kinds of diseases, it is urgent to use a kind of examination method to identify the early stage of PD and ET and EPT. The purpose of this study was to investigate the value of the tremor analysis of EMG in the differential diagnosis of PD and ET as well as EPT.

2. Clinical Data and Methods

2.1. Clinical Data. Clinical data were collected from January 2015 to November 2015 in Aviation General Hospital neurology department with tremor as the main manifestation of Parkinson's disease in 25 patients (PD group). There were 13 males and 12 females, aged 45 to 76 years with an average age of 64.1 years. Duration of PD ranges from 6 months to 4 years with an average of 2.7 years. At the same time, 20 patients with ET were selected (ET group). Tremor is the only clinical manifestation. There were 9 males and 11 females, aged 39 to 82 years. Duration of ET ranges from 2 to 10 years with an average age of 60 years, with an average of 6.2 years. 20 patients were with EPT tremor (EPT group). There were 12 males and 8 females, with the age of 28–74 years and average 51 years. Duration of EPT ranges from 0.3 to 2 years with an average of 0.9 years.

2.2. Methods. The Medelec Synergy EMG machine of Oxford company was used in this study with 4 EMG surface electrodes and 1 pressure accelerator [6]. The surface electrodes

Table 1: Tremor frequency, latency, concentration effect, and synchronous EMG of Parkinson's disease, essential tremor, and enhanced physiological tremor.

	Resting (Hz)	Posture (Hz)	Loaded 500 g (Hz)	Loaded 1000 g (Hz)	Latency	Concentration effect	Synchronous EMG
ET ($n = 20$)	5.38 ± 1.23	7.32 ± 2.63	6.46 ± 2.04	6.31 ± 1.36	0%	0%	80%
PD ($n = 25$)	4.52 ± 0.43	4.94 ± 0.66	5.17 ± 0.62	4.71 ± 0.96	80%	100%	20%
EPT ($n = 20$)	8.48 ± 4.41	12.6 ± 4.52	7.47 ± 2.81	9.3 ± 1.26	0%	0%	85%

At rest, PD versus EPT $P < 0.05$; postural ET and PD versus EPT $P < 0.01$; ET and PD versus EPT $P < 0.05$ when loading 1000 g; PD versus ET; EPT $P < 0.05$ with mental activity and latency; PD versus EPT $P < 0.05$ with synchronous EMG.

were applied to the muscles of the flexor carpi ulnaris and the extensor carpi ulnaris, respectively. The electrode was fixed at the distal side of the third metacarpal bone in the same hand. The frequency and amplitude of patients' tremor were recorded when they were in the sitting position at rest (put relaxed hand on thighs), in posture position (double forearm straight forward), and in forearm loaded by 500 g and 1000 g, respectively. Each recording last for 30 s. Patients were observed if they had tremor immediately from static to postural changes to determine whether tremor had latency and were asked to continuously calculate the subtraction "100-7" when postural tremor occurred in order to determine whether mental activity had an effect on tremor.

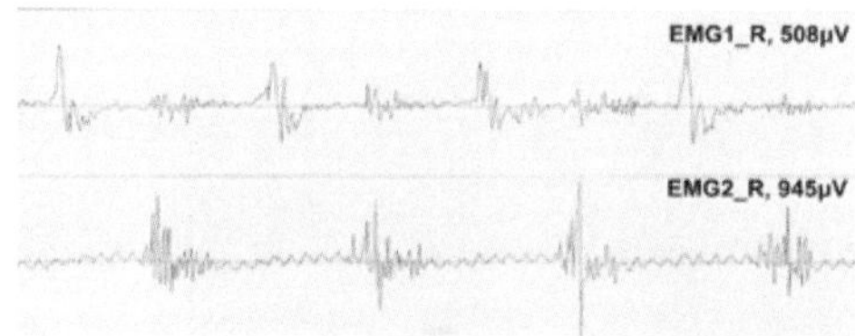

Figure 1: Patterns of muscle contraction in Parkinson's disease tremor.

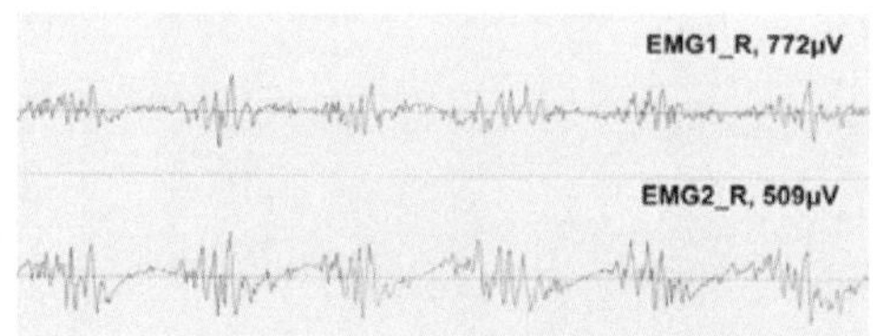

Figure 2: Patterns of muscle contraction in essential tremor.

2.2.1. Data Analysis. Internationally recognized tremor analysis software (TRAS system) was used for the analysis of the EMG activity data and tremor frequency. The frequency range of tremor was between 1 and 30 Hz. Tremulous energy is recorded as amplitude and simultaneous recording of EMG activity associated with tremor.

2.2.2. Statistic Treatment. SPSS 16 software was used to analyze the data. The data were expressed as mean ± standard deviation ($\chi \pm$ s), and the t-test was used. $P < 0.05$ was statistically significant.

3. Result

In 20 patients with ET, there were 6 patients with static tremor by naked eye. In 25 patients with PD, there were 9 patients with visible postural tremor; there was 1 patient with visible static tremor in EPT. However, there was a significant increase in ET, PD, and EPT by tremor analysis of EMG, shown in 10 cases, 15 cases, 5 cases, respectively. In PD group, the tremor frequency at rest, posture, and weights 500 g and 1000 g was at about 4–6 Hz. The tremor frequency of ET patients at rest, posture, and weight was about 5–8 Hz. The frequency of EPT was increased to 6–12 Hz. The frequency of EPT was significantly reduced by weight load effect, and the reduction was about 50%. There was no significant difference between the tremor frequency at rest and after loading between PD group and ET group ($P > 0.05$). The tremor frequency of PD group was significantly different from that of EPT for several conditions, including rest, posture, and weight bearing 1000 g ($P < 0.05$ or $P < 0.01$) (Table 1). These results implied that it was difficult to distinguish between PD and ET only through the tremor frequency at rest condition. The main difference between the two groups was that the main tremor muscle contraction pattern of PD was as the main alternative (Figure 1), but ET was for synchronization (Figure 2) and the different changes about concentration effect and latency. Compared with the ET and EPT groups, postural tremor in PD patients was significantly delayed, and mental activity significantly increased the amplitude of PD tremor.

4. Discussion

As a common clinical manifestation, tremor can be divided into static tremor, postural tremor, intention tremor, and so on. The common types of tremor mainly include Parkinson's disease tremor and essential tremor. Traditionally, PD is equal to resting tremor, and ET is postural tremor, which is quite one-sided [7]. Parkinson's disease tremor is relatively poor because of its relatively poor prognosis. It is easy to be confused because of some similarities to ET and EPT.

Although patients with Parkinson's disease display tremor, rigidity, bradykinesia, postural abnormalities, and other typical clinical manifestations, still many patients were with atypical clinical manifestations or showed only a symptom. The diagnosis of PD and its differentiation from other types of tremor such as ET and EPT are frequently difficult. Especially in early disease stages it remains problematic. Postural tremor may be the isolated or predominant symptom in early stages of PD, in which rest tremor, bradykinesia, rigidity, and postural stability may be slight or inexistent [8].

Now, the differential diagnoses of PD, ET, and EPT are still mostly based on clinical phenomena. The accurate diagnosis of tremor is of fundamental importance to both patients and clinicians because assessment of prognosis and treatment selection depend on tremor type. It is crucial to the success of therapeutic trials [8].

We found that PD and ET were difficult to distinguish in tremor frequency, and there was a superposition of the tremor frequency, the frequency of PD tremor was 4–6 Hz, and the frequency of ET was also in this range; the frequency of EPT is 6–12 hz having some overlap with PD. We found that although the frequency of PD tremor and ET tremor is difficult to identify, ET has more postural tremor. If static tremor is present, static tremor frequency was generally less than the frequency of postural tremor 1.5–2 hz [8]. Our study found that the difference between the two was 1.8 Hz, also in line with foreign literature reports. And we found no delay of postural tremor from resting to lifting upper limb in ET, and PD had obvious delay. For PD patients, the two muscles of the forearm mainly displayed alternating contraction but synchronous contractions were mostly observed in ET patients. However, ET muscle contraction was mainly synchronous contraction, and alternating contraction was rare. Most of the PD and ET could be identified by the combination of different patterns of muscle contraction. But some scholars believe that the pattern of muscle contraction can show different burst at different times by long-term recording [9]. We found that if there was postural tremor in PD patients, most would have increased tremor amplitude during mental activity. The reason is unknown, but whether this phenomenon is principle similar to Jendrassik manoeuvre in the tendon reflex needs further investigation.

The origin of the tremor of PD is located in the globus pallidus; some scholars believe that the subthalamic nucleus hyperexcitability leads to increased number of cells in the posterior part of the globus pallidus [10]. ET is probably caused by abnormal reticular formation or abnormal nuclear motion in the central nervous system. At present, the pathogenesis of the two diseases is different to extent. A recent comprehensive review suggests that the relative risk of patient with ET to develop PD is 2–4 times higher than in the general population [11]. Of course, in addition to electrophysiology, we also need to ask about family history and so on. One approach may be to use the term essential tremor only as a transitional node in the deep phenotyping of tremor disorders based on historical, phenomenological, and neurophysiological features to facilitate its etiologic diagnosis or serve for future gene and biomarker-discovery efforts [12].

But both PD and ET can show static and postural tremor; only one of them shows one main manifestation, and the frequency of tremor of the two diseases is similar. The tremor analysis of EMG finding more static or postural tremor than by naked eyes may indicate that these two diseases are probably homologous; just resting tremor was activated in PD but was suppressed in ET.

In the early stages of PD, in this study, we find that tremor frequency is stable in patients with central oscillator, such as PD and ET, but unstable in EPT. We can differentiate PD and ET by the latency and concentration effect and ET and EPT by weight load effect. Neurophysiologic tests may help in cases of coexistence of postural and rest tremor. We think some neurophysiologic criteria for the diagnosis of PD are useful: (1) there is rhythmic burst of rest tremor on EMG, (2) tremor frequency is stable at 4–6 Hz; (3) if postural tremor exists, there is tremor latency from rest to postural position; (4) changes of the dominant frequency peak are less than or equal to 1 hz after the weight load test; (5) there are changes in tremor amplitude after mental concentration. EMG tremor analysis can be used to identify Parkinson's disease and essential tremor and enhanced physiological tremor. The method is based on accelerometer and surface electromyography (EMG) electrodes. It is readily available, noninvasive, and cost-efficient diagnostic tool. But due to the small sample statistics, further large sample is needed for further research, and future research work will be further observed after treatment of PD and idiopathic tremor, strengthen the change frequency and patterns of muscle physiological tremor, and be combined with clinical assessment scale.

5. Conclusion

Tremor analysis of EMG is suitable for clinical use. It was able to distinguish PD from ET and EPT by varying the tremor frequency and muscle contraction pattern. It can also differentiate PD and ET by the latency and concentration effect and ET and EPT by weight load effect. As a noninvasive, sensitive, and repeated examination technique, it is believed that tremor analysis of EMG should have wider application prospects and research prospects in clinical practice.

References

[1] E. D. Louis and S. L. Pullman, "Comparison of clinical vs. electrophysiological methods of diagnosing of essential tremor," *Movement Disorders*, vol. 16, no. 4, pp. 668–673, 2001.

[2] H. Reichmann, "Clinical criteria for the diagnosis of Parkinson's disease," *Neurodegenerative Diseases*, vol. 7, no. 7, pp. 284–290, 2010.

[3] L. J. Findley and M. A. Gresty, "Tremor and rhythmical involuntary movements in Parkinsons diease," in *Movement Disorders*, L. J. Finfley and R. Capildeo, Eds., pp. 295–302, Macmillan, London,UK, 1984.

[4] K. P. Bhatia, A. Schrag, A. Muenchau, N. p. Quinn, and C. D. Marsden, "Overdiagnosis of essential tremor," *Lancet*, vol. 353, no. 9163, pp. 1498-1499, 1999.

[5] A. M. Woods, *Differentiation of Parkinson's Tremor from Essential Tremor using Action Tremor Analysis*, University of Otago, Dunedin, New Zealand, 2012.

[6] M. Lauk, J. Timmer, C. H. Lücking, J. Honerkamp, and G. Deuschl, "A software for recording and analysis of human tremor," *Computer Methods and Programs in Biomedicine*, vol. 60, no. 1, pp. 65–77, 1999.

[7] O. Cohen, S. Pullman, E. Jurewicz, D. Watner, and E. D. Louis, "Rest tremor in patients with essential tremor: Prevalence, clinical correlates, and electrophysiologic characteristics," *Archives of Neurology*, vol. 60, no. 3, pp. 405–410, 2003.

[8] A. Gironell, J. Kulisevsky, B. Pascual-Sedano, and M. Barbanoj, "Routine neurophysiologic tremor analysis as a diagnostic tool for essential tremor: A prospective study," *Journal of Clinical Neurophysiology*, vol. 21, no. 6, pp. 446–450, 2004.

[9] A. Boose, S. Spieker, C. Jentgens, and J. Dichgans, "Wrist tremor: Investigation of agonist-antagonist interaction by means of long-term EMG recording and cross-spectral analysis," *Electroencephalography and Clinical Neurophysiology - Electromyography and Motor Control*, vol. 101, no. 4, pp. 355–363, 1996.

[10] W. D. Hutchison, A. M. Lozano, R. R. Tasker, A. E. Lang, and J. O. Dostrovsky, "Identification and characterization of neurons with tremor-frequency activity in human globus pallidus," *Experimental Brain Research*, vol. 113, no. 3, pp. 557–563, 1997.

[11] G. Kuhlenbäumer, F. Hopfner, and G. Deuschl, "Genetics of essential tremor: meta-analysis and review," *Neurology*, vol. 82, no. 11, pp. 176–178, 2014.

[12] A. J. Espay, A. E. Lang, R. Erro et al., "Essential pitfalls in "essential" tremor," *Movement Disorders*, vol. 32, no. 3, pp. 325–331, 2017.

2

Mitochondrial Serine Protease HTRA2 p.G399S in a Female with Di George Syndrome and Parkinson's Disease

Stefano Gambardella,[1] Rosangela Ferese,[1] Simona Scala,[1] Stefania Carboni,[2] Francesca Biagioni,[1] Giardina Emiliano,[2,3] Stefania Zampatti,[1,2] Nicola Modugno,[1] Francesco Fabbiano,[1] Francesco Fornai,[1,4] Diego Centonze,[1] and Stefano Ruggieri[1]

[1]*IRCCS Neuromed, Pozzilli, Italy*
[2]*Molecular Genetics Laboratory UILDM, Santa Lucia Foundation, Rome, Italy*
[3]*Department of Biomedicine and Prevention, University of Rome "Tor Vergata", Rome, Italy*
[4]*Department of Translational Research and New Technologies in Medicine and Surgery, University of Pisa, Pisa, Italy*

Correspondence should be addressed to Stefano Gambardella; stefano.gambardella@neuromed.it

Academic Editor: Jan Aasly

Deletion at 22q11.2 responsible for Di George syndrome (DGs) is a risk factor for early-onset Parkinson's disease (EOPD). To date, all patients reported with 22q11.2 deletions and parkinsonian features are negative for a family history of PD, and possible mutations in PD-related genes were not properly evaluated. The goal of this paper was to identify variants in PD genes that could contribute, together with 22q11.2 del, to the onset of parkinsonian features in patients affected by Di George syndrome. To this aim, sequencing analysis of 4800 genes including 17 PD-related genes was performed in a patient affected by DGs and EOPD. The analysis identified mutation p.Gly399Ser in *OMI/HTRA2* (PARK13). To date, the mechanism that links DGs with parkinsonian features is poorly understood. The identification of a mutation in a PARK gene suggests that variants in PD-related genes, or in genes still not associated with PD, could contribute, together with deletion at 22q11.2, to the EOPD in patients affected by DGs. Further genetic analyses in a large number of patients are strongly required to understand this mechanism and to establish the pathogenetic role of p.Gly399Ser in *OMI/HTRA2*.

1. Introduction

The 22q11.2 deletion syndrome (22qDS), also known as Di George syndrome (DGs), is a multisystem disorder caused by a chromosomal microdeletion most commonly involving a 3 Mb segment on the long arm of chromosome 22. The hallmark features of the syndrome consist of typical facial appearance, velopharyngeal failure, conotruncal heart disease, parathyroid and immune dysfunction, developmental delays, and learning difficulties. Late-onset complications, including recurrent seizures and schizophrenia, are common [1]. In a considerable amount of patients carrying 22qDS, early-onset, nonfamilial Parkinson's disease (EOPD) is described which represents the focus of the present report.

Parkinson's disease (PD) is a neurodegenerative movement disorder characterized by tremor, muscle rigidity, bradykinesia, gait disturbances, and a variety of nonmotor symptoms. The life-time risk for developing PD is 1-2% [2]. PD typically occurs late in life, but 4% of cases has an onset before the age of 50 [3].

Early neurological reports described the occurrence of movement disorders in 22qDS, which were already evident in childhood and adolescence [4]. These extrapyramidal motor symptoms were initially interpreted as a consequence of antipsychotic medication [5]. The idea that parkinsonian symptoms in 22qD patients occur specifically as the consequence of nigrostriatal degeneration has been proposed years later when two 22qDS patients without antipsychotic medications were found to develop EOPD (age < 45 years) [6].

Nonetheless, the association between 22qDS and PD remained at the anecdotal level. Later on, a case-control study confirmed a high prevalence of PD in 22qDS patients. Very recently, a large study including more than 9,000 PD patients indicates that 22q11.2 deletions lead to 20-fold increased risk to develop EOPD [7]. This report, despite highlighting a strong epidemiological evidence, it does not provide a genetic investigation of PD-related genes apart from the 22q11.2 mutation. Moreover previous studies analyzing a few patients, report only very few or no genetic analysis related to PD [8, 9].

In an effort to correlate at the molecular level the clinical association between DGs and EOPD, in the present study, we report a detailed genetic study carried out by analyzing the clinical exome including 18 PD-related genes in a woman with a clinical diagnosis of DGs confirmed by the presence of a 22q deletion.

2. Materials and Methods

Genomic DNA was isolated from peripheral blood leukocytes according to standard procedures. Clinical exome sequencing considering 4800 human genes including 18 genes related to Parkinson's disease (PARK1: *SNCA*; PARK2: *PRKN*; PARK3: *SPR*; PARK4: *SNCA* Dup/Del; PARK5: *UCHL1*; PARK6: *PINK1*; PARK7: *DJ1*; PARK8: *LRRK2*; PARK9: *ATP13A2*; PARK10: *ELAVL4*; PARK11: *GIGYF2*; PARK12: *TAF1*; PARK13: *HTRA2*; PARK14: *PLA2G6*; PARK15: *FBXO7*; PARK16: *ADORA1*; PARK17: *VPS35*; PARK18: *EIF4GI*) (TruSight One Sequencing Panels, Illumina) were performed on MiSeq platform (Illumina). Variant Studio was used for annotation and characterization of variants. The manual examination and visualization of the sequence data were performed by the Integrative Genomics Viewer v.2.3, while selection of potentially pathogenetic variant by Tgex software (LifeMap Sciences). Mutations were resequenced by Sanger sequencing (ABI 3130xl Genetic Analyzer, Applied Biosystems).

3. Results

The woman reported in the present study had a clinical diagnosis of DGs confirmed by the presence of a 22q deletion. Specifically, dysmorphological features were recorded (hypertelorism, low-set ears, abnormal folded pinna, short philtrum, micrognathia, and hypoacousia). The mother and her 9-year-old son were also affected by DGs.

She came to our hospital in 2011, when she was 35 years old, due to the onset of extrapyramidal tremor of the left hand which was a slight progressive start up at 12 months before hospital admission. This symptom further progressed to impair fine motor control which deteriorated up to a loss of dexterity in the left hand. She had a hypomimic face and suppressed blinking. She was bradykinetic, and swinging while walking was reduced much more in the left than the right side. She suffered from muscle rigidity which was prevalent in the upper left limb.

SPECT scan using the radioisotope [123I]-beta-CIT showed a decreased dopamine (DA) uptake bilaterally in the putamen (Figure 1(a)). Magnetic resonance imaging (MRI) scan showed a normal profile with aspecific gliotic microvascular outbreaks in subcortical white matter of front-insular hemispheres (Figure 1(b)).

IQ evaluation revealed a value under the mean. In fact, the WAIS-R (Wechsler Adult Intelligence Scale-Revised; Wechsler, 1981) revealed (i) verbal IQ: 72/100, (ii) performance IQ: 70/100, (iii) total IQ: 70/100 points (Wechsler and Ogdon, 1981); the MMPI (Minnesota Multiphasic Personality Inventory) showed Pd score: 73/100 and Pa: 75/100. Laboratory exams revealed hypocalcemia (7.3 mg/dl), hyperprolactinemia (she was under oral estroprogestinic anticontraceptive therapy), mild hypercholesterolemia (209 mg/dl), and increased ESR (65 mm). The clinical and ultrasonographic cardiological evaluation revealed a mild tricuspid and mitral valves regurgitation with 66% ejection fraction. Audiometry was normal.

In 2013, [^{18}F] DOPA PET scan revealed decreased uptake in the right putamen. The UPDRS-III scored 57 and 27 before and after levodopa administration, respectively, and 21 following apomorphine.

In 2015, neuropsychological evaluation confirmed previous results both at WAIS-R and at MMPI. Hypocalcemia was still present. After administration of 250 mg of levodopa and 25 mg of carbidopa, the patients showed dyskinesia and dystonia at the left lower arm.

At this time, molecular genetic evaluation was carried out. Clinical exome sequencing identified the mutation p.Gly399Ser (c.1195G>A, NM_013247.4) in *OMI/HTRA2* (OMIM #606441), recently designated as Parkinson disease-13 locus (PARK13). No mutations in other PD-related genes was identified (Table 1). This variant was detected also in the mother, who did not show either movement disorder or other neurological deficit.

4. Discussion

To date, less than 20 patients carrying 22q11.2 deletions and PD have been reported worldwide [6–10]. Unfortunately, in all of them, a whole genetic analysis for PD is missing despite all patients reporting EOPD symptoms (age at onset ranging between 39 and 48 years) [10]. Most of them were treated with dopamine replacement therapy (L-DOPA), with some initial improvement in motor symptoms quickly followed by motor fluctuations and dyskinesia [8–10]. Psychotic symptoms are frequent with anxiety and depressed mood up to suicide attempts. Degeneration of the nigrostriatal dopamine system has been reported in vivo by presynaptic dopamine imaging, and it is confirmed at brain autopsy showing PD neuropathology which was suggested to be quite reminiscent of LRRK2-associated PD [10, 11].

To date, all patients carrying concomitantly 22q11.2 deletions and parkinsonian features were negative for a family history of PD and any known pathogenic PD-related mutations. However, the latter were poorly investigated. This is the first report of a 22q11.2 patient affected by PD where a dedicated next generation sequencing analysis for PD genes was carried out. This extensive approach allowed detecting a specific mutation affecting a gene known to be involved in PD.

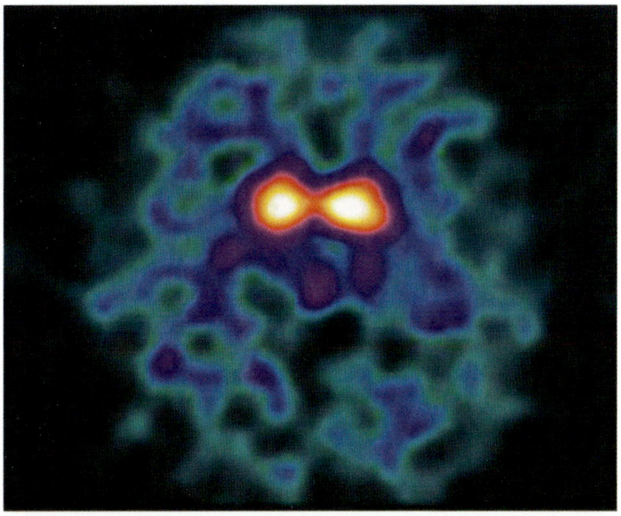

(a)

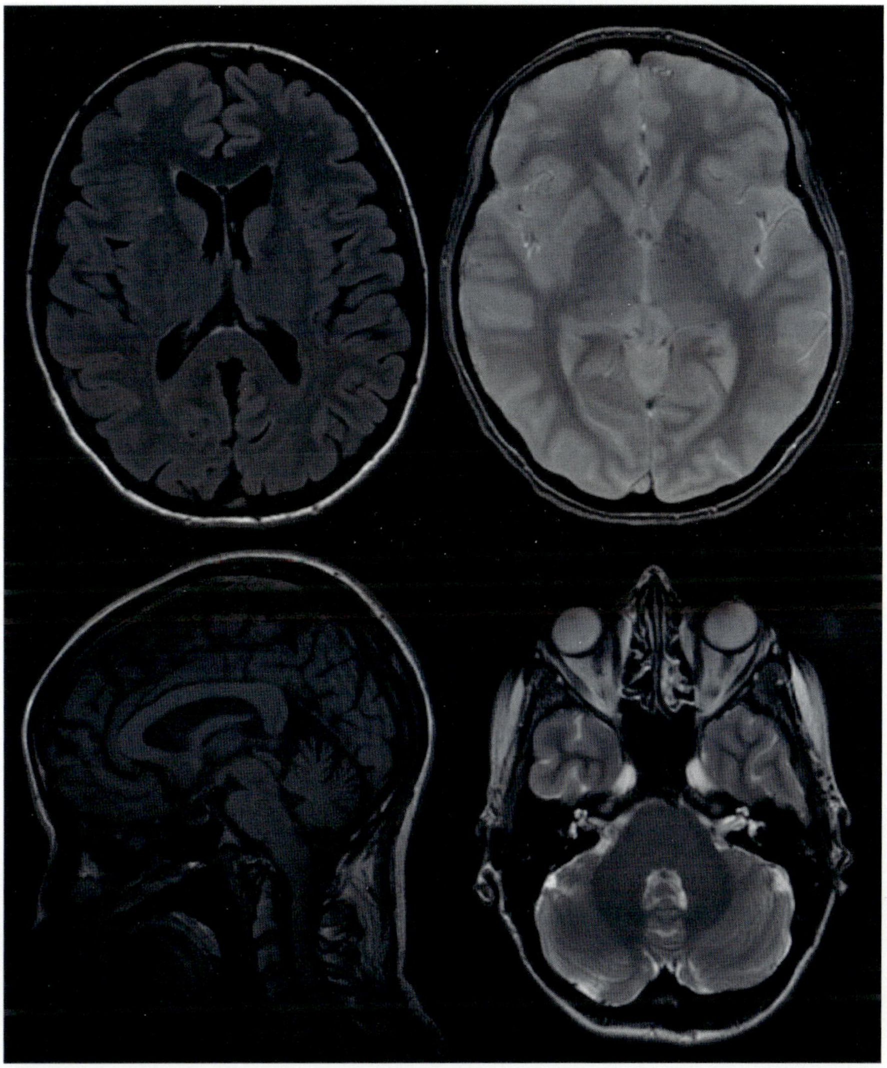

(b)

Figure 1: DaTSCAN and magnetic resonance imaging. (a) DaTSCAN image showing a reduced tracer uptake in both striatal regions, especially on the right side. (b) Magnetic resonance imaging (MRI) scan showed a normal profile with aspecific gliotic microvascular outbreaks in subcortical white matter of front-insular hemispheres. Axial Flair MRI scan shows aspecific gliotic microvascular outbreaks in subcortical white matter of front-insular hemispheres; Axial GRE MRI scan shows normal putamina bilaterally in absence of degeneration signs or deposits; sagittal-T1 MRI scan shows normal midbrain; axial-T2 MRI scan shows normal cerebellum.

TABLE 1: List of sequence variants identified.

Locus	Gene	Genotype	HGVSc	HGVSp	SIFT	PolyPhen	Class	Criteria	dbSNP ID
PARK8	LRRK2	hom	NM_198578.3:c.149G>A	NP_940980.3: p.Arg50His	Tolerated (0.61)	Benign (0)	1	BA1	rs2256408
		het	NM_198578.3:c.2857T>C	NM_198578.3: c.2857T>C (p.=)			1	BA1	rs7966550
		het	NM_198578.3:c.7155A>G	NM_198578.3: c.7155A>G (p.=)			1	BA1	rs33962975
		het	NM_198578.3:c.7190T>C	NP_940980.3: p.Met2397Thr	Tolerated (0.71)	Benign (0.001)	1	BA1	rs3761863
PAKK2	PRKN	het	NM_004562.2:c.1138G>C	NP_004553.2: p.Val380Leu	Tolerated (0.83)	Benign (0.001)	1	BA1	rs1801582
PARK17	VPS35	hom	NM_018206.4:c.1938C>T	NM_018206.4: c.1938C>T (p.=)			1	BA1	rs168745
PARK6	PINK1	het	NM_032409.2:c.189C>T	NM_032409.2: c.189C>T (p.=)			1	BA1	rs45530340
		hom	NM_032409.2:c.388-7A>G				1	BA1	rs2298298
		hom	NM_032409.2:c.960-5G>A				1	BA1	rs3131713
PARK9	ATP13A2	hom	NM_022089.2:c.3516G>A	NM_022089.2: c.3516G>A (p.=)			1	BA1	rs3170740
		hom	NM_022089.2:c.3192C>T	NM_022089.2: c.3192C>T (p.=)			1	BA1	rs9435659
		hom	NM_022089.2:c.2970G>A	NM_022089.2: c.2970G>A (p.=)			1	BA1	rs761421
		hom	NM_022089.2:c.2637C>T	NM_022089.2: c.2637C>T (p.=)			1	BA1	rs9435662
		hom	NM_022089.2:c.1815C>T	NM_022089.2: c.1815C>T (p.=)			1	BA1	rs2076603
PARK15	FBXO7	hom	NM_012179.3: c.122+272T>G				1	BA1	rs8137714
		hom	NM_012179.3:c.345G>A	NP_036311.3: p.Met115Ile	Tolerated (0.19)	Benign (0)	1	BA1	rs11107
		het	NM_012179.3:c.540A>G	NM_012179.3: c.540A>G (p.=)			1	BA1	rs41311141
		hom	NM_012179.3:c.949C>T	NM_012179.3: c.949C>T (p.=)			1	BA1	rs9726
SLC52A3	hom	NM_033409.3: c.1233T>C	NM_033409.3: c.1233T>C (p.=)				1	BA1	rs910857
		hom	NM_033409.3:c.765C>T	NM_033409.3: c.765C>T (p.=)			1	BA1	rs3746805
		het	NM_033409.3:c.321C>T	NM_033409.3: c.321C>T (p.=)			1	BA1	rs3746808
PARK10	ELOVL4	het	NM_022726.3:c.895A>G	NP_073563.1: p.Met299Val	Tolerated (0.92)	Benign (0)	1	BA1	rs3812153
PARK11	GIGYF2	hom	NM_001103147.1:c.3003A>G	NM_001103147.1: c.3003A>G (p.=)			1	BA1	rs3816334
		hom	NM_001103147.1: c.3524-9G>A				1	BA1	rs2305137
		hom	NM_001103147.1: c.3693_3695delACA	NP_001096617.1: p.Gln1232del			1	BA1	rs10555297
PARK13	HTRA2	het	NM_013247.4:c.1195G>A	NP_037379.1: p.Gly399Ser	Deleterious (0.04)	Probably damaging (0.924)	4	PS3, PP3, PP5	rs72470545
PARK18	EIF4G1	hom	NM_001194947.1:c.502A>G	NP_001181876.1: p.Thr168Ala	Tolerated (0.81)	Benign (0)	1	BA1	rs13319149
		hom	NM_001194947.1:c.1315A>G	NP_001181876.1: p.Met439Val	Tolerated (0.36)	Benign (0)	1	BA1	rs2178403
		hom	NM_001194947.1: c.3974+9A>C				1	BA1	rs939317

For each variant, the following are reported: locus, gene, genotype detected, HGVS nomenclature (coding and protein, resp., HGVSc and HGVSp), SIFT and PolyPhen prediction (if available), and SNP ID. Furthermore, variants has been classified according to ACMG guidelines in five classes according to Richards et al. [24]. Class and criteria are listed in dedicated columns (BA1: stand-alone evidence of benign impact; PS3: criteria number 3 of strong evidence of pathogenicity; PP3 and PP5: criteria numbers 3 and 5, respectively, of supporting evidence of pathogenicity) [24].

The PARK13 locus, OMI/HTRA2 (OMIM #606441), encodes a serine-protease with proapoptotic activity and a mitochondrial targeting sequence placed at its N-terminal region. Despite the existing controversial data [12–21], several findings suggest a potential link between *OMI/HTRA2* and PD [12, 13]. In fact, *Omi/HtrA2* knockout or transgenic mice possess a phenotype either reminiscent of PD or motor neuron disease, respectively. Remarkably, in vitro Omi/HtrA2 interacts with PINK1 which is known to sense and regulate mitochondrial alteration and removal [14–17].

Based on these intriguing links between *Omi/HtrA2* and PD, *Omi/HtrA2* was recently designated as *Parkinson disease-13* locus (*PARK13*). Mutations in *OMI/HTRA2* were associated with both PD and essential tremor, and these data are strengthened by the presence of Omi/Htra2 in Lewy bodies in brains of idiopathic PD patients [12, 18]. In particular, the variant p.G399S leads to mitochondrial dysfunction, altered mitochondrial morphology, and decreased protease activity.

Thus, the pathological role of p.G399S in PD still has to be fully understood concerning its pathogenicity and penetrance. We suggest that, in patients with 22qdel, this variant increases the risk to develop EOPD. In fact, variants that confer an improved or decreased risk to PD and variants with a reduced penetrance are a common feature of neurodegenerative disorders, including several PD loci (e.g., *LRRK2*, *SNCA*, and *VPS35*) [22].

This is compatible with the presence of the p.G399S variant in the proband's mother, who did not show either movement disorder or other neurological deficit. The genetic test in the son of the proband is mandatory to improve our knowledge on the penetrance of this mutation. Unfortunately, the mother did not give her permission to perform genetic analysis on her 9-year-old son.

Moreover, the genetic analysis performed has been focused only on PD-related genes, not considering the potential role of variants in other genes not related with parkinsonian phenotype. Therefore, this does not imply that p.G399S is responsible for the parkinsonian phenotype as a single mutation or in a complex genetic network.

Anyway, this novel finding suggests that 22q deletion is not the unique PD-related genetic alterations in patients carrying 22q11.2 deletions and PD, opening new avenues on potential associations between 22qdel patients and other genetic variants.

5. Conclusions

In this report, a mechanism that links DGs with parkinsonian features is proposed. In fact, to improve our knowledge about the role of concomitant mutations in patients with 22q11.2 deletions and EOPD, molecular testing considering all known PD-related genes is mandatory, which should now be included on the first rank PARK13 analysis.

This could help to decipher whether the 22q11.2 deletion links various neuropsychiatric disorders including schizophrenia. At the same time, a wide PD genes screening is expected to predict whether a single molecular mechanism links 22q11.2 deletion to PARK13 to produce a final common pathway or whether genetic defects other than PARK13 may be involved, alone or in combination with PARK13, to DGs phenotypes when coexisiting with 22q11.2 deletions [23].

At this time, clinicians should be alerted about the chance to detect 22q11.2 deletions in patients with early-onset PD or possessing clinical features which are typically associated with the chromosome 22q11.2 deletion syndrome or both. Patients known to carry a 22q11.2 deletion should be monitored for the development of parkinsonian symptoms.

Authors' Contributions

Stefano Gambardella, Stefano Ruggieri, and Francesco Fornai were involved in the conception of the research project. Diego Centonze, Nicola Modugno, and Francesco Fabbiano organized the clinical data. Rosangela Ferese and Simona Scala were responsible for the next-generation sequencing design. Stefania Carboni and Emiliano Giardina performed the next-generation sequencing analysis. Francesca Biagioni did Sanger sequencing. Stefania Zampatti did genetic counseling. Stefano Gambardella and Francesco Fornai wrote the first draft. Diego Centonze and Stefano Ruggieri reviewed and gave critiques.

References

[1] D. M. McDonald-McGinn and K. E. Sullivan, "Chromosome 22q11.2 deletion syndrome (DiGeorge syndrome/velocardiofacial syndrome)," *Medicine*, vol. 90, no. 1, pp. 1–18, 2011.

[2] A. Elbaz, J. H. Bower, D. M. Maraganore et al., "Risk tables for parkinsonism and Parkinson's disease," *Journal of Clinical Epidemiology*, vol. 55, no. 1, pp. 25–31, 2002.

[3] S. K. Van Den Eeden, C. M. Tanner, A. L. Bernstein et al., "Incidence of Parkinson's disease: variation by age, gender, and race/ethnicity," *American Journal of Epidemiology*, vol. 157, no. 11, pp. 1015–1022, 2003.

[4] A. Swillen, K. Devriendt, E. Legius et al., "The behavioural phenotype in velo-cardio-facial syndrome (VCFS): from infancy to adolescence," *Genetic Counseling*, vol. 10, pp. 79–88, 1999.

[5] L. E. Krahn, D. M. Maraganore, and V. V. Michels, "Childhood-onset schizophrenia associated with parkinsonism in a patient with a microdeletion of chromosome 22," *Mayo Clinic Proceedings*, vol. 73, no. 10, pp. 956–959, 1998.

[6] C. Zaleski, A. S. Bassett, K. Tam et al., "The co-occurrence of early onset Parkinson disease and 22q11.2 deletion syndrome," *American Journal of Medical Genetics Part A*, vol. 149A, no. 3, pp. 525–528, 2009.

[7] K. Y. Mok, U. Sheerin, J. Simón-Sánchez et al., "Deletions at 22q11.2 in idiopathic Parkinson's disease: a combined analysis of genome-wide association data," *The Lancet Neurology*, vol. 15, no. 6, pp. 585–596, 2016.

[8] R. Pollard, M. Hannan, J. Tanabe et al., "Early-onset Parkinson disease leading to diagnosis of 22q11.2 deletion syndrome," *Parkinsonism and Related Disorders*, vol. 25, pp. 110-111, 2016.

[9] A. F. Rehman, R. Dhamija, E. S. Williams et al., "22q11.2 deletion syndrome presenting with early-onset Parkinson's disease," *Movement Disorders*, vol. 30, no. 9, pp. 1289-1290, 2015.

[10] N. J. Butcher, T. R. Kiehl, L. N. Hazrati et al., "Association between early-onset Parkinson disease and 22q11.2 deletion

syndrome: identification of a novel genetic form of Parkinson disease and its clinical implications," *JAMA Neurology*, vol. 70, no. 11, pp. 1359–1366, 2013.

[11] S. Gambardella, R. Ferese, F. Biagioni et al., "The monoamine brainstem reticular formation as a paradigm for re-defining various phenotypes of Parkinson's disease owing genetic and anatomical specificity," *Frontiers in Cellular Neuroscience*, vol. 11, p. 102, 2017.

[12] K. M. Strauss, L. M. Martins, H. Plun-Favreau et al., "Loss of function mutations in the gene encoding Omi/HtrA2 in Parkinson's disease," *Human Molecular Genetics*, vol. 14, no. 15, pp. 2099–2111, 2005.

[13] V. Bogaerts, K. Nuytemans, J. Reumers et al., "Genetic variability in the mitochondrial serine protease HTRA2 contributes to risk for Parkinson disease," *Human Mutation*, vol. 29, no. 6, pp. 832–840, 2008.

[14] L. M. Martins, A. Morrison, K. Klupsch et al., "Neuroprotective role of the reaper-related serine protease HtrA2/Omi revealed by targeted deletion in mice," *Molecular and Cellular Biology*, vol. 24, no. 22, pp. 9848–9862, 2004.

[15] J. M. Jones, P. Datta, S. M. Srinivasula et al., "Loss of Omi mitochondrial protease activity causes the neuromuscular disorder of mnd2 mutant mice," *Nature*, vol. 425, no. 6959, pp. 721–727, 2003.

[16] K. S. Patil, I. Basak, S. Lee et al., "PARK13 regulates PINK1 and subcellular relocation patterns under oxidative stress in neurons," *Journal of Neuroscience Research*, vol. 92, no. 9, pp. 1167–1177, 2014.

[17] H. Plun-Favreau, K. Klupsch, N. Moisoi et al., "The mitochondrial protease HtrA2 is regulated by Parkinson's disease-associated kinase PINK1," *Nature Cell Biology*, vol. 9, no. 11, pp. 1243–1252, 2007.

[18] H. Unal Gulsuner, S. Gulsuner, F. N. Mercan et al., "Mitochondrial serine protease HTRA2 p.G399S in a kindred with essential tremor and Parkinson disease," *Proceedings of the National Academy of Sciences*, vol. 23, no. 111, pp. 18285–18290, 2014.

[19] O. A. Ross, A. I. Soto, C. Vilariño-Güell et al., "Genetic variation of Omi/HtrA2 and Parkinson's disease," *Parkinsonism and Related Disorders*, vol. 14, no. 7, pp. 539–543, 2008.

[20] J. Simón-Sánchez and A. B. Singleton, "Sequencing analysis of OMI/HTRA2 shows previously reported pathogenic mutations in neurologically normal controls," *Human Molecular Genetics*, vol. 1, no. 17, pp. 1988–1993, 2008.

[21] R. Krüger, M. Sharma, O. Riess et al., "A large-scale genetic association study to evaluate the contribution of Omi/HtrA2 (PARK13) to Parkinson's disease," *Neurobiology of Aging*, vol. 32, no. 3, p. 548.e9-18, 2011.

[22] S. Gambardella, F. Biagioni, R. Ferese et al., "Vacuolar protein sorting genes in Parkinson's disease: a re-appraisal of mutations detection rate and neurobiology of disease," *Frontiers in Neuroscience*, vol. 24, no. 10, p. 532, 2016.

[23] A. S. Bassett and E. W. Chow, "Schizophrenia and 22q11.2 deletion syndrome," *Current Psychiatry Reports*, vol. 10, no. 2, pp. 148–157, 2008.

[24] S. Richards, N. Aziz, S. Bale et al., "Standards and guidelines for the interpretation of sequence variants: a joint consensus recommendation of the American College of Medical Genetics and Genomics and the Association for Molecular Pathology," *Genetics in Medicine*, vol. 17, no. 5, pp. 405–424, 2015.

3

Stress Management Training (SMT) Improves Coping of Tremor-Boosting Psychosocial Stressors and Depression in Patients with Parkinson's Disease: A Controlled Prospective Study

C. Buhmann,[1] D. Jungnickel,[2] and E. Lehmann[1]

[1]*Department of Neurology, University Medical Center Hamburg-Eppendorf, Martinistrasse 52, 20246 Hamburg, Germany*
[2]*Department of Social Sciences, University of Hamburg, Allende-Platz 1, 20146 Hamburg, Germany*

Correspondence should be addressed to C. Buhmann; buhmann@uke.uni-hamburg.de

Academic Editor: Karsten Witt

Background. Stress reduction and relaxation exercises are therapeutically suggested to patients with Parkinson's disease (PD) and tremor, but data regarding efficacy or preferential methods are missing. *Objective.* To investigate the effect of a standardized stress management training (SMT) according to Kaluza on coping with tremor-boosting psychosocial stress factors. *Methods.* 8-week SMT was applied to 82 PD patients with tremor and 30 controls. Changes in stress-associated factors were measured applying four scales: Kaluza's "warning signs for stress" and "stress-amplifying thoughts" and Beck Depression Inventory (BDI) and quality of life (PDQ-8). Short-term outcome (8 weeks) was evaluated in both groups, and long-term outcome (3–6 months) was evaluated only in PD patients. *Results.* At baseline, PDQ-8 was worse in PD patients compared to controls. PD patients improved significantly regarding short- and long-term outcome scores of "warning signs for stress," "stress-amplifying thoughts," and BDI scores, independently of disease severity or duration. Younger and male PD patients showed the best benefit. Controls improved comparably to PD patients but significantly only with respect to "stress-amplifying thoughts." Retrospectively, 88% (29/33) of PD patients were rated SMT as helpful 12–18 months later. Self-practicing SMT exercises correlated significantly with subjectively better coping with tremor-related daily impairment and subjective short-term and long-term tremor reduction. *Conclusion.* SMT should be a part of therapy of PD patients with tremor.

1. Introduction

Tremor is a frequent symptom in Parkinson's disease (PD) and affects the majority of patients already as an early motor sign [1]. Although medication generally improves tremor in PD to more than 50% [2], a relevant proportion of patients remain disabled by their tremor. In these patients, tremor is not only functional hindering but also clearly visible as a disease symptom. This can lead to real or felt social stigmatization, anxiety, depression, or social isolation [3, 4] and reduced quality of life [5].

Although there are limited data of clinical studies confirming stress-induced tremor in PD [6], it is clinically well known and has been described early in the literature that tremor in patients with PD increases when stress factors or emotional involvement is present [7, 8]. Hereby, the increase of adrenergic activation is supposed to play a key role [9, 10]. In daily clinical practice, patients are suggested to use relaxation techniques to reduce tension and stress levels to improve frequency, intensity, or coping of existing tremor. However, there is lack of clinical data on whether relaxation training really can improve coping with tremor and/or reduce tremor in PD. Relaxation techniques seem to be of different effect [11], but there are no controlled data on which kind of relaxation training might be most effective.

For healthy subjects, it has been shown that stress management programs imparting relaxation skills improve coping of general stress-related tension and stress-related situations [12–15].

Participation in the cognitive-behavioural stress management training (SMT) according to Kaluza [16, 17] has been proven to be efficient for coping of all-day stressors with a change in problem awareness and improvement of emotional and physical well-being [18] based on improved active and cognitive coping strategies and decreased subjective appraisals of interpersonal stressors [19]. SMT was effective not only in healthy subjects but also in patients with chronic diseases other than PD [20]. Furthermore, long-term effects of SMT have been demonstrated for healthy subjects with ongoing improved active coping strategies, less resigned-avoidant tendencies, and improved psychological mood status [21] 6 months after intervention.

In this study, we primarily aimed to evaluate whether participation for 8 weeks in SMT [16, 17] leads to improvement of tremor-boosting stressors, expressed more specifically as warning signs for stress and stress-amplifying thoughts and reflected more generally as depression and quality of life. Secondarily, we assessed the influence of patient characteristics on SMT outcome measurements and evaluated the subjective benefit of SMT in PD patients on coping of tremor-related daily impairment.

We hypothesized a beneficial effect of SMT on stress levels and coping of tremor in PD patients.

2. Methods

2.1. Study Design. In this monocentric, controlled, and prospective interventional study, 82 PD patients with tremor and 30 controls underwent stress management training as group therapy with 6–8 participants for 2 hours per week for 8 weeks. The influence of the training was evaluated based on the questionnaire at baseline, as short-term outcome at the end of the course after 8 weeks, and as long-term outcome after 3–6 months. In a pilot study with participants from different social demographic sectors, intelligibility of the questionnaire had been evaluated and considered for the final version. Non-PD subjects served as controls for estimation of baseline stress levels in PD patients prior to SMT. Although we primarily did not aim for group comparison, we also analyzed whether SMT had differential effects in PD patients compared to controls after the end of SMT. The course and the evaluation were realized from 2013 until 2016 within the facilities of the University Medical Center Hamburg-Eppendorf (UKE).

First, we assessed as the primary aim prospectively the influence of the stress management training (SMT) as described by Kaluza [16] and specified later [17] on levels of warning signs for stress and stress-amplifying thoughts on depression according to Beck Depression Inventory (BDI) [22, 23] and on quality of life (QoL) according to PDQ-8 [24]. Second, we evaluated the influence of age, gender, disease severity [25], and disease duration on outcome parameters. Subsequently, we retrospectively assessed the influence of the training on self-estimation of tremor-related daily impairment and tremor intensity in a follow-up investigation during a normal clinical consultation 12–18 months after the end of SMT using a 5-point Likert's scale.

Questionnaires had to be completed under identical conditions for each participant prompt and without interruption in presence of the course teacher (EL). Contact with a third party was not allowed. In case of questions for a better understanding or other needs for support to complete the questionnaire, participants were allowed to ask the instruction teacher. Completion of the questionnaire took an average of 1 to 1.5 hours. After completion of the questionnaires, data were pseudonymized for analysis.

2.2. Ethics. Written informed consent was obtained from every participant. The research protocol considered the Good Clinical Practice (GOP) criteria, followed the recommendations of the Declaration of Helsinki (7th revision, 64th meeting, Fortaleza, Brazil), and was approved by the Ethics Committee of the Hamburg Medical Council (votum PV 4886).

2.3. Patients and Controls. Patients were recruited in the movement disorder outpatient clinic of the University Medical Center Hamburg-Eppendorf. PD diagnosis according to UK Brain Bank criteria [26] was confirmed by a movement disorder specialist (CB). Patients who reported to be psychologically impaired due to tremor (independently of tremor severity) or patients with an objective (physician-assessed) functional tremor-related impairment (such as problems with writing or dexterity) were consecutively asked to take part in the stress management training and enrolled if agreed to take part in the study.

Controls were not allowed to have any present or history of neurological or psychiatric disease or any other relevant acute or chronic disease and were recruited from the familiar or social surrounding of the PD patients or the working staff of the hospital. Subjects with known severe psychosocial impairment interfering with participation in a group therapy were excluded. Furthermore, subjects with relevant cognitive impairment were excluded because they potentially would not have been able to fulfill demands of the course. We chose an MMSE $\leq$ 20/30 points as cutoff because Folstein et al. found MMSE values of 20 or less only in patients with dementia [27].

2.4. Interventional Training Course (Stress Management Training (SMT)). The cognitive-behavioural stress management training (SMT) according to Kaluza [16, 17] was applied to course participants under supervision of a certificated psychologist (EL). The SMT consists of different modules aiming to cope with and reduce stress levels: 4 training modules and 5 supplemental modules supporting activation of positive resources. Training modules consist of (i) relaxation training such as progressive muscle relaxation according to Jacobsen [28] (modified version according to [29]) or autogenic training, (ii) cognition training to detect and modify personal stress triggers or boosters [17], (iii) structured problem-solving training to detect, accept, and modify stress situations, and (iv) enjoyment training for recreation and enjoyment [30, 31]. Supplemental modules included stress management instruments such as physical activity, social support, definition of aims, time management, and emergency strategies.

All patients completed the four training modules and were advised to choose one supplemental module.

2.5. Questionnaire-Based Assessment. Two dimensions of psychosocial stress factors according to Kaluza, i.e., "levels of warning signs for stress" and "stress-amplifying thoughts," and depression and quality of life were assessed.

2.5.1. Psychosocial Stress Factors according to Kaluza. The total score of *warning signs for stress* ranges from 0 to 70 points and is based on 35 symptoms/characteristic in the 4 categories "physical warning signs" (14 questions), "emotional warning signs" (6 questions), "cognitive warning signs" (6 questions), and "behavioural warning signs" (9 questions). Each symptom was self-rated by the patient to be present "barely or not at all" (score 0), "slight" (score 1), or "severe" (score 2). For individual diagnostics, outcome is divided into 3 categories. 0 to 10 points correspond with relative good health stability. In these subjects, relaxing training likely will have a prevention character; 11–20 points indicate that chain reactions of physical and mental stress reactions do take place already. The start of increasing personal competences in stress management is suggested in time; 21 points or more indicate that the subject is already deeply involved into the vicious circle of tension, emotional burden, and health dysfunction. Here, the subject should do something against his/her stress, and it is strictly suggested that the subject has to ensure to get more calmness, rest, and capability [17]. Table 1(A) shows the 35 questions of warning signs in the 4 categories.

The total score of *stress-amplifying thoughts* ranges from 0 to 50 points and is based on the 5 categories "be perfect," "be popular," "be strong," "be on your guard," and "I cannot." Each category consists of 5 attributes. Presence of each attribute was rated by the patient to be either 0 ("never"), 1 ("sometimes"), or 2 ("frequent"). The higher the value is, the more the stress-amplifying thoughts in the subdomain or in total the subject has. Table 1(B) shows the 25 questions of stress-amplifying thoughts in the 5 categories.

2.5.2. Depression and Quality of Life. To evaluate depression, Beck Depression Inventory (BDI) [22, 23] was used. To assess quality of life (QoL), PDQ-8 [24] was used.

2.6. Statistics. Analysis was done using SPSS 6.1.3 (1995) for Microsoft Windows. Power analysis was performed using G*Power [32] and revealed a sample size of $n = 80$ based on an alpha-failure of 1%, a test power of 90%, and expecting average effects of $d = 0.35$ (absolute).

As known for the PDQ-8, where the 8 items were summed together and transformed onto a score from 0 to 100, scales according to Kaluza (warning signs for stress and stress-amplifying thoughts) and BDI values were converted to POMP scores also for comparison purposes with the range from 0 to 100% [33].

For longitudinal assessment, treatment effects on different scales for the intervention group were calculated using Student's paired t-test for dependent groups by calculating the differences in test scores from short term (8 weeks) and long term (3–6 months) versus baseline, respectively. Positive values of calculated differences indicate worsening, and negative values indicate improvement for all applied scales.

Between-group differences of outcome parameters were calculated using Student's t-test for independent groups and due to a high number of single subitem comparisons ($n = 126$) applied only for items with Cohen's d value >0.25. Data of all applied total scores (BDI, PDQ-8, "warning signs of stress," and "stress-amplifying thoughts") were normally distributed (Kolmogorov–Smirnov's goodness-of-fit test).

The chi-squared test and Pearson's R test were used to assess the influence of disease severity and disease duration on outcome measurements.

Point-biserial correlations were applied to evaluate potential patient characteristic immanent bias influencing the drop-out rate at long-term evaluation.

3. Results

Eighty-two patients with PD and 30 controls completed the stress management training (SMT). Short-term data of prospective outcome measurements were complete at the end of the course after 8 weeks in 82 PD patients (100%) and 27 controls (90%). 3 controls terminated SMT prematurely (2 due to lack of time and 1 reported discomfort in a group with PD patients). Long-term outcome measurement data were complete for the study follow-up examination 3–6 months after the end of the course in 49 PD patients (59.8%; missing subjects could not have been reached or motivated for the follow-up investigation). The drop-out rate was not influenced by age, gender, BDI score, or PDQ-8 score (the range of 2-tailed tested correlations was −0.212 to +0.146 with all correlations being insignificant).

Furthermore, retrospective subsequent outcome data of 33 PD patients (40.2%) could have been obtained at a normal scheduled clinical follow-up consultation to assess the effect of SMT and ongoing self-practice of exercises 12–18 months after the end of SMT. Patients with available long-term data did not differ regarding age, gender, BDI score, and PDQ-8 score from patients without reported long-term data (59.8%). Long-term outcome of controls was not assessed as controls primarily were included to estimate the global level of tremor-boosting psychosocial stress factors in PD patients.

3.1. Characteristics of Participants. Parkinson's disease patients were in average 6.4 years older than controls and had a highly significant worse quality of life (25.82 [16.35] vs. 5.77 [9.41]; $p < 0.0001$; d values of all PDQ-8 subitems ranged from 0.81 to 1.33) [34]. No significant differences were seen regarding gender or for the aspects depression (total BDI score), warning signs for stress, or stress-amplifying thoughts (total scores and all single items) between PD patients and controls prior to SMT (Cohen's

Table 1: Psychosocial stress factors according to Kaluza.

(A) Warning signs for stress	
The following aspects can be signs of excessive demand. Which of them did you self-percept within the last week?	
Physical warning signs	Palpitation; tight feelings in the breast; difficulty breathing; difficulty falling asleep; chronic fatigue; indigestion; stomach pain; anorexia; sexual dysfunction; muscle tension; headache; back pain; cold feet/hands; severe sweating
Emotional warning signs	Nervousness/inner restlessness; irritability/anger feelings; fear emotions/fear of failure; dissatisfaction/unbalance; listlessness (including sexual); inner emptiness/"burned out"
Cognitive warning signs	Constantly circling thoughts/musing; concentration disorders; emptiness in the head/"black out"; daydreams; nightmares; loss of power/high frequency of mistakes
Behavioural warning signs	Aggressive behaviour against others/"to fly off the handle"; finger thrumming/to shuffle one's feet/trembling/to gnash one's teeth; speak too fast/stuttering; interrupt someone/inability to listen to someone; irregular eating; consuming of alcohol or drugs for calming; not cultivating private contacts/"to let contacts slide"; smoking more than intended; doing less sport and exercise than desired
(B) Stress-amplifying thoughts	
	Personal stress enhancer profile
I cannot	I cannot stand it; I will fail; I can never make it; I cannot stand the pressure (fear, pain, etc.); problems and difficulties simply are terrible
Be on your guard	It is horrible if something is not running as I want; it is important that I have everything under control; in decisions I must be 100% sure; I always have to think about what could happen; it is terrible if I do not know what is coming towards me
Be strong	I like to do everything myself; strong people need no help; when I rely on others I'm abandoned; without me nothing works; it is terrible to depend on others
Be popular	I do not want to disappoint others; it is terrible when others are evil to me; I want to get along well with all others; It's bad when others criticize me; it is important that everyone likes me
Be perfect	It is not acceptable if I am not able to cope with a job or meet a deadline; I always have to be available for my company; there is nothing worse than making mistakes; there must be 100% reliability on me; I always have to make everything right

Part A shows the 35 questions of warning signs for stress in the 4 categories according to Kaluza [17]. The total score ranges from 0 to 70 points, and each symptom was self-rated by the patient to be present "barely or not at all" (score 0), "slight" (score 1), or "severe" (score 2). The higher the value is, the more the warning signs for stress in the subdomain or in total the subject has. Part B shows the 25 questions of stress-amplifying thoughts in the 5 categories according to Kaluza [17]. The total score ranges from 0 to 50 points, and presence of each attribute was rated by the patient to be either "never" (score 0), "sometimes" (score 1), or "frequently" (score 2). The higher the value is, the more the stress-amplifying thoughts in the subdomain or in total the subject has.

d values ranged from −0.28 to 0.31). However, 2 of 21 subitems of the BDI (worthlessness [*d* value 0.45] and loss of energy [*d* value 0.40]) were different between groups at baseline (Table 2).

Within the PD patient group, genders did not differ significantly regarding any outcome measurement parameter at baseline, but women with PD tended to be more depressive than men (BDI score 21.78 [11.3] vs. 17.09 [11.5]; $p = 0.070$). Disease severity (H&Y) categorized into mild (H&Y stage 1), moderate (H&Y stage 2), and severe (H&Y stages 3 and 4) did not differ significantly between genders (χ^2 (2,$N = 82$) = 5.05; $p = 0.080$). However, while percentage of patients with H&Y stage 2 was almost identical in both genders (55.3% and 56.1%), men were by trend more severely diseased than women with H&Y stage ≥3 in 34% vs. 17%. H&Y stage 4 was only seen in 2 patients (1 male/1 female). It is worth to note that disease severity (H&Y) was not dependent on disease duration (χ^2 (2,$N = 79$) = 3.59; $p = 0.464$).

3.2. Effect of Stress Management Training (SMT) on Psychosocial Stress Factors according to Kaluza in PD Patients and Controls. SMT significantly improved coping of stress expressed as reduced warning signs of stress and stress-amplifying thoughts as short-term outcome and long-term outcome in PD patients. In controls, significant improvement of stress-amplifying thoughts was obtained as short-term outcome.

PD patients and controls did not differ significantly regarding the magnitude of improvement of any psychosocial stress factor at the end of SMT after 8 weeks (Figure 1).

Figure 2 shows an overview, and Tables 3 and 4 show detailed results of outcomes with respect to all total scores and subscales. Subscales of the applied German BDI score [23] were translated into English by the authors.

3.2.1. Short-Term Outcome at the End of the Course after 8 Weeks. In PD patients, SMT improved total mean [±SD] of global scores for warning signs of stress (−5.66 [11.50]; $p < 0.0001$) with all 4 single warning signs (physical, emotional, cognitive, and behavioural) found significantly better at the end of training. Thereby, improvement of emotional stress was most prominent with 28.6%.

Furthermore, total mean [±SD] of stress-amplifying thoughts improved (−6.00 [17.19]; $p = 0.003$) with 3 of 5 single stress-amplifying thoughts ("be popular," "be on guard," and "I cannot") getting better. Thereby, the stress factor "to be popular" improved the most with reduction of this demand of 24.0%.

In controls, SMT did not improve total mean of global scores for warning signs of stress significantly.

Table 2: Characteristics of participants at baseline prior to SMT.

	PD (n = 82)	CON (n = 30)	p value	Test
Age [SD]	66.3 [8.16]	59.9 [15.8]	0.041	t-test
Males (%)	39 (47.6 %)	12 (40 %)	0.48	Phi 0.067
BDI score [SD]	19.55 [11.72]	17.09 [10.99]	0.319	t-test
PDQ-8 [SD]	25.82 [16.35]	5.77 (n = 24) [9.41]	<0.0001*	t-test
Warning signs for stress [SD]	29.13 (n = 80) [17.51]	29.31 (n = 29) [16.70]	0.961	t-test
Stress-amplifying thoughts [SD]	39.36 (n = 81) [22.72]	39.52 (n = 29) [18.73]	0.973	t-test
Disease duration (months) [SD]	5.96 (n = 79) [0.51], range 1–23	NA	NA	
Disease severity (Hoehn and Yahr) [SD]	2.15 (n = 79) [0.08], range 1–4	NA	NA	

Data are shown as means with standard deviation [SD]. Significantly different frequencies between groups as detected in an unpaired 2-tailed t-test with $p < 0.05$ are labeled with an asterisk. "BDI": Beck Depression Inventory [22, 23]; "PDQ-8": Parkinson's Disease Questionnaire with 8 questions [24].

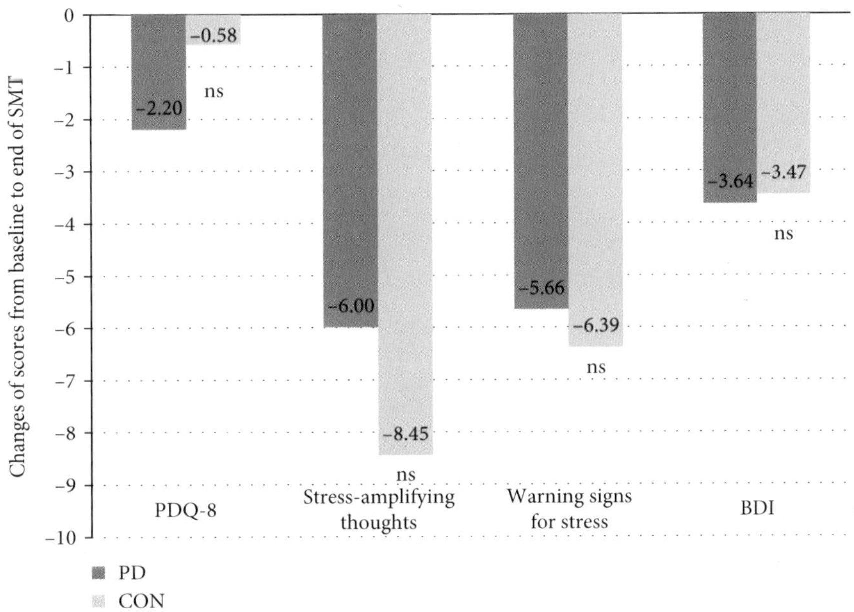

Figure 1: Comparison of changes in psychosocial stress factors according to Kaluza, severity of depression (BDI), and quality of life (PDQ-8) in PD patients and controls after 8 weeks of SMT. The short-term changes in psychosocial stress factors according to Kaluza (warning signs for stress and stress-amplifying thoughts), severity of depression according to Beck Depression Inventory (BDI), and quality of life (PDQ-8) of PD patients and controls from baseline (black bars) at the beginning of stress management training (SMT) to the end of SMT after 8 weeks (light grey bars) are shown. Differences in scale values refer to scales transformed to a score from 0 to 100 points (0–100%) for comparison purposes after conversion to POMP scores [33]. PD = patients with Parkinson's disease; CON = healthy controls.

However, 1 of 4 single warning signs (emotional warning) was found to be 34.1% better at the end of the training (p = 0.014).

SMT improved short-term total mean [±SD] outcome of stress-amplifying thoughts (−8.45 [11.87]; p = 0.003) in controls with 4 of 5 single aspects ("be perfect," "be popular", "be on guard" and "I cannot") getting better and best improvement for the item "be popular" with 26.1%.

3.2.2. Long-Term Outcome at Follow-Up after 3 to 6 Months. In PD patients, SMT improved total mean [±SD] of global scores for warning signs of stress (−4.86 [11.98]; p = 0.008), including 2 of 4 single warning signs (emotional and cognitive). It is worth to note that improvement of emotional stress compared to baseline was maintained on the high level with 30.2%.

Total mean [±SD] of stress-amplifying thoughts improved (−7.71 [16.52]; p = 0.002), including 2 of 5 single stress-amplifying thoughts ("be popular" and "I cannot"). Thereby, the burden to think "I cannot" even improved from 22.8% after the end of the course to 39.0% in the long term 3–6 months later.

3.3. Effect of Stress Management Training (SMT) on Depression and Quality of Life in PD Patients and Controls. SMT significantly improved depression assessed as the short-term and long-term BDI outcome in PD patients. Improvement of the BDI score did not reach significance after the end of SMT in controls, although magnitude of improvement was comparable in both PD patients and controls (Figure 1). Quality of life was by trend better directly after the end of SMT in PD patients (PDQ-8 sum score −2.20 [11.14];

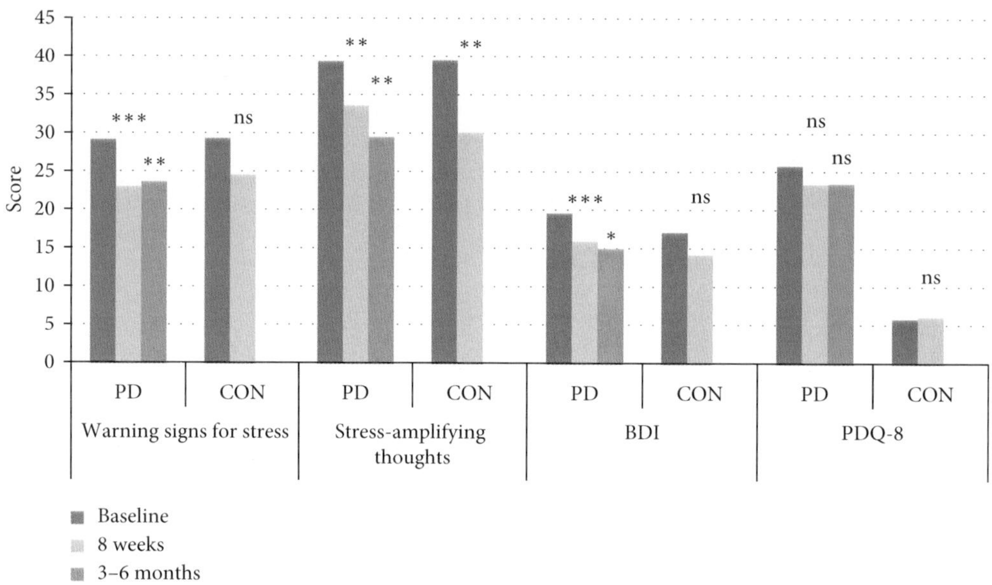

FIGURE 2: Psychosocial stress factors according to Kaluza, severity of depression (BDI), and quality of life (PDQ-8) of PD patients and controls before and after SMT. Psychosocial stress factors according to Kaluza (warning signs for stress and stress-amplifying thoughts), severity of depression according to Beck Depression Inventory (BDI), and quality of life (PDQ-8) of PD patients and controls at baseline (black bars) at the beginning of stress management training (SMT) and as short-term outcome directly at the end of SMT after 8 weeks (light grey bars) are shown. Outcome of PD patients additionally is shown as long-term outcome 3–6 months after completing SMT (dark grey bars). All scales are summed together and transformed to a score from 0 to 100 points (0–100%) for comparison purposes after conversion to POMP scores [33]. Significantly different scores between baseline and short-term outcome (8 weeks) and baseline and long-term outcome (3–6 months) are labeled with an asterisk with $^{*}p < 0.05$, $^{**}p < 0.01$, and $^{***}p < 0.001$. PD = patients with Parkinson's disease; CON = healthy controls.

$p = 0.082$) but without reaching statistical significance for both short- and long-term outcomes.

3.3.1. Short-Term Outcome at the End of the Course after 8 Weeks. In PD patients, SMT improved total mean [±SD] of the BDI score (−3.64 [8.26]; $p < 0.0001$). Amongst the 21 subscales of the BDI scale, 8 significantly improved (Table 3). Hereby, "attachment disorder" ($p < 0.0001$), "feeling of guilt" ($p = 0.003$), and "indecisiveness" ($p = 0.010$) were improved most markedly with 36.3%, 49.2%, and 29.0%, respectively.

In controls, no significant change in the total mean BDI score was seen. However, 2 of 21 subscales improved significantly (change in "sleep disturbance" ($p = 0.006$) and "attachment disorder" ($p = 0.036$), with 36.3% and 40.0%, respectively; Table 3).

3.3.2. Long-Term Outcome at Follow-Up after 3 to 6 Months. In PD patients, SMT improved outcome of total mean [±SD] of the BDI score (−3.21 [8.77]; $p = 0.014$). Thereby, the 3 subitems "feeling inadequate/inferior" ($p = 0.049$), "attachment disorder" ($p = 0.31$), and "suicidal contents" ($p = 0.10$) improved about 65.7%, 20.0%, and 62.2%, respectively.

3.4. Influence of Age, Gender, Disease Severity, and Disease Duration on the Efficacy of the Stress Management Training (SMT) on Psychosocial Stress Factors in PD Patients. With higher age, efficacy of SMT on reduction of depression was lower in the short-term ($r = 0.30$; $p < 0.01$) and long-term ($r = 0.29$; $p < 0.01$) follow-up. Age did not influence any other measured outcome parameter. Despite that, subjective efficiency of SMT was rated higher in the younger patient ($r = -0.35$; $p < 0.01$).

In men, benefit of SMT on long-term outcome of BDI (categorized into better, unchanged, and worse) was better than that in women (χ^2 $(2, N = 82) = 11.83$ ($p = 0.003$) and $r = 0.33$ ($p = 0.003$)). Gender had no influence on short-term or long-term outcomes for warning signs of stress, stress-amplifying thoughts, or quality of life.

Neither disease severity nor disease duration had any influence on short- or long-term outcomes of any measured coping factors after SMT.

3.5. Subjective Benefit of SMT in PD Patients on Coping of Tremor-Related Daily Impairment in General and in Relation to Tremor Reduction and Self-Exercising. Twelve to 18 months after finishing SMT, patients were asked during a regular consultation how they retrospectively rate the SMT regarding a general benefit on coping tremor-related daily impairment (yes/no) and the effect on subjective tremor reduction in daily life at the end of the course (8 weeks) and 3–6 months after SMT and whether they self-practiced the SMT at home beyond 3 months after the end of the course (yes/no).

Answers could have been obtained from 40% of PD patients (33/82). 87.9% (29/33) rated the SMT as beneficial in general for coping with tremor in daily life, independently of

Table 3: Beck Depression Inventory (BDI).

Scale with subitems	PD patients ($n = 82$)																			Controls ($n = 30$)										
	Baseline			Short term (8 weeks)			Long term (3–6 months)			Short-term mean (8 weeks) – baseline mean (paired 2-tailed t-test)					Long-term mean (3–6 months) – baseline mean (paired 2-tailed t-test)					Baseline			Short term (8 weeks)			Short-term mean (8 weeks) – baseline mean (paired 2-tailed t-test)				
	n	Mean	SD	n	Mean	SD	n	Mean	SD	Diff.	t value	df	$p(t)$	Sig.	Diff.	t value	df	$p(t)$	Sig.	n	Mean	SD	n	Mean	SD	Diff.	t value	df	$p(t)$	Sig.
Sadness/unhappiness	82	14.63	25.17	81	8.23	17.90	48	12.50	23.44	−6.58	−2.49	80	0.015	*	−1.39	−0.35	47	0.728		30	14.44	18.94	27	12.35	22.92	−2.47	−0.63	26	0.537	
Pessimism/ hopelessness	82	16.67	31.54	81	14.40	31.15	48	16.67	33.69	−2.47	−0.70	80	0.489		−4.17	−0.68	47	0.503		30	7.78	18.94	27	7.41	21.35	−1.23	−0.24	26	0.802	
Feeling inadequate/ inferior	82	10.57	20.87	80	5.42	15.41	48	4.86	15.36	−5.42	−2.40	79	0.019	*	−6.94	−2.02	47	0.049	*	30	8.89	17.36	27	8.64	19.81	0.00				
Inability to enjoy	82	27.24	19.69	81	17.28	17.57	49	19.73	17.90	−9.88	−4.29	80	0.000	***	−5.44	−2.22	48	0.031	*	30	27.78	19.74	27	18.52	23.27	−11.11	−2.21	26	0.036	*
Conscious guilt	82	14.23	22.24	81	7.41	14.91	48	8.33	16.13	−7.00	−3.01	80	0.003	**	−2.08	−0.68	47	0.497		30	18.89	22.63	27	13.58	16.69	−6.17	−1.55	26	0.134	
Self-punishment	82	8.54	18.00	81	7.00	13.66	48	3.47	10.29	−1.65	−0.78	80	0.436		−2.08	−1.00	47	0.322		30	5.55	15.37	26	1.28	6.54	−5.13	−1.69	25	0.103	
Self-denial/dislike	82	11.79	19.86	81	7.41	17.48	48	5.56	14.31	−4.53	−2.36	80	0.021	*	−4.17	−1.63	47	0.110		30	7.73	14.34	26	8.97	17.78	1.28	0.33	25	0.746	
Self-accusation	82	18.70	30.13	81	16.05	27.44	48	7.64	14.16	−2.88	−0.84	80	0.403		−6.25	−1.77	47	0.083		30	13.33	24.13	26	11.54	18.72	2.56	0.70	25	0.490	
Suicidal contents	82	8.94	15.76	81	5.76	12.68	48	2.78	9.31	−3.29	−2.37	80	0.020	*	−5.56	−2.69	47	0.010	**	30	5.56	15.37	26	3.85	10.86	−2.56	−0.81	25	0.425	
Frequency of crying	82	19.51	28.18	81	14.40	24.69	48	11.11	23.15	−5.35	−1.53	80	0.129		−7.64	−1.56	47	0.125		30	14.44	27.24	26	8.97	22.23	−7.69	−1.66	25	0.110	
Irritability	82	26.02	27.23	80	26.67	32.87	48	15.97	26.62	.42	0.10	79	0.917		−7.64	−1.38	47	0.175		30	27.78	31.66	27	18.52	23.27	−9.88	−1.69	26	0.103	
Indifference to other people	82	11.79	20.54	81	9.05	18.27	49	10.88	17.20	−2.88	−1.09	80	0.277		−0.68	−0.22	48	0.830		30	12.22	20.50	27	11.11	20.67	−2.47	−0.53	26	0.602	
Indecisiveness	82	25.20	23.75	82	17.89	19.73	49	21.09	21.18	−7.32	−2.64	81	0.010	**	−2.72	−0.94	48	0.351		30	21.11	20.50	26	17.95	19.39	−6.41	−1.55	25	0.134	
Reduced physical appearance	82	29.27	31.60	81	25.93	30.28	48	20.83	30.46	−3.70	−1.05	80	0.295		−3.47	−0.71	47	0.481		30	15.56	27.31	27	13.58	24.91	−1.23	−0.23	26	0.823	
Loss of drive/ workableness	82	32.11	26.94	81	24.69	23.44	49	27.21	24.22	−7.82	−2.56	80	0.012	*	−0.68	−0.18	48	0.855		30	22.22	18.22	27	27.16	22.72	4.94	1.16	26	0.256	
Sleep disturbances	82	41.46	32.53	81	36.21	29.91	49	36.05	29.53	−5.76	−1.67	80	0.099		−5.44	−1.43	48	0.159		30	47.78	33.54	27	33.33	30.66	−17.28	−3.02	26	0.006	**
Fatigability/tiredness	82	31.71	20.89	82	29.27	13.24	49	28.57	15.21	−2.44	−0.97	81	0.333		−2.72	−0.81	48	0.420		30	28.89	25.87	26	21.79	18.72	−7.69	−1.24	25	0.228	
Loss of appetite	82	8.13	15.33	80	8.75	18.18	48	6.94	15.31	.42	0.23	79	0.820		−1.39	−0.47	47	0.642		30	8.89	19.44	26	7.69	17.15	−2.56	−1.00	25	0.327	
Loss of weight	82	1.63	11.60	81	0.82	7.41	48	0.69	4.81	−.82	−0.53	80	0.596		−2.08	−0.90	47	0.371		30	0.00	0.00	26	0.00	0.00	0.00				
Somatic preoccupation	82	22.76	22.15	81	27.57	24.03	48	27.08	23.48	4.53	1.44	80	0.153		7.64	1.91	47	0.062		30	21.11	22.29	27	17.28	25.10	−2.47	−0.46	26	0.646	
Loss of libido	82	29.67	37.04	82	27.64	35.06	49	29.93	36.80	−2.03	−0.62	81	0.545		−2.72	−0.66	48	0.511		30	28.89	33.60	27	37.04	37.36	4.94	0.60	27	0.566	
Ø Beck Depression Score	82	19.55	11.72	82	15.91	10.81	49	15.00	10.32	−3.64	−3.99	81	0.000	***	−3.21	−2.52	48	0.014	*	30	17.09	10.99	27	14.17	10.08	−3.47	−1.61	27	0.119	

$^{*}p < 0.05$; $^{**}p < 0.01$; $^{***}p < 0.001$.

TABLE 4: PDQ-8, stress-amplifying thoughts, and warning signs for stress.

Scales with subitems	PD patients ($n = 82$)																				Controls ($n = 30$)									
	Baseline			Short term (8 weeks)			Long term (3–6 months)			Short-term mean (8 weeks) − baseline mean (paired 2-tailed t-test)					Long-term mean (3–6 months) − baseline mean (paired 2-tailed t-test)					Baseline			Short term (8 weeks)			Short-term mean (8 weeks) − baseline mean (paired 2-tailed t-test)				
	n	Mean	SD	n	Mean	SD	n	Mean	SD	Diff.	t value	df	$p(t)$	Sig.	Diff.	t value	df	$p(t)$	Sig.	n	Mean	SD	n	Mean	SD	Diff.	t value	df	$p(t)$	Sig.
Mobility	82	22.56	20.75	80	20.97	21.18	48	22.57	21.69	−1.32	−0.86	78	0.392		−0.75	−0.42	47	0.676		24	4.75	8.65	19	5.85	10.39	0.46	0.57	17	0.579	
Activities of daily living	82	21.34	18.14	80	21.25	18.09	48	20.66	18.77	0.00					0.78	0.44	47	0.659		24	2.43	11.05	19	3.29	13.36	0.23	1.00	17	0.331	
Emotional well-being	82	30.44	23.21	80	26.56	18.79	48	27.26	19.01	−3.65	−2.02	79	0.046	*	−4.60	−2.00	47	0.051		24	6.60	11.32	19	9.21	16.23	1.62	0.72	17	0.484	
Stigma	82	24.01	23.40	80	20.08	17.78	48	16.93	16.46	−3.36	−1.68	79	0.097		−3.26	−1.18	47	0.242		24	4.69	10.14	19	4.61	12.65	−0.69	−0.46	17	0.651	
Social support	82	15.96	20.12	80	14.37	19.67	48	15.28	19.25	−1.67	−0.92	79	0.359		−0.69	−.23	47	0.816		24	1.39	5.31	19	1.75	5.94	0.00				
Cognition	82	33.92	22.29	80	31.41	19.84	48	29.69	19.01	−2.27	−1.16	79	0.251		−2.21	−0.81	47	0.421		24	11.72	19.79	19	11.18	16.35	−2.08	−1.06	17	0.302	
Communication	82	24.29	20.46	80	22.08	19.08	48	21.18	18.11	−1.88	−0.96	79	0.341		−2.78	−1.03	47	0.307		24	2.78	9.73	19	3.51	9.34	0.00				
Bodily discomfort	82	34.04	25.97	80	30.42	22.15	48	33.85	21.91	−3.44	−1.42	79	0.159		0.00					24	11.81	21.41	19	9.21	16.41	−4.17	−1.84	17	0.083	
Ø PDQ-8 score	82	25.82	16.35	80	23.39	14.03	48	23.43	13.30	−2.20	−1.76	79	0.082		−1.69	−1.18	47	0.244		24	5.77	9.41	19	6.08	10.27	−0.58	−1.42	17	0.174	
Be perfect	82	36.83	29.48	79	34.30	26.97	48	25.83	24.91	−1.90	−0.65	78	0.515		−6.88	−1.82	47	0.074		30	37.00	29.84	22	27.73	31.91	−6.36	−2.19	21	0.040	*
Be popular	82	46.46	27.23	79	34.94	25.86	48	32.08	26.65	−11.14	−4.38	78	0.000	***	−13.13	−3.89	47	0.000	***	30	47.00	27.18	22	30.00	29.44	−12.27	−2.69	21	0.014	*
Be strong	82	39.27	22.98	79	34.94	20.99	48	36.04	19.76	−3.92	−1.85	78	0.068		−0.21	−0.09	47	0.929		30	38.00	17.30	22	35.45	15.95	−4.55	−1.52	21	0.144	
Be on your guard	82	47.44	27.79	79	40.51	27.87	48	36.25	24.20	−6.33	−2.53	78	0.013	*	−6.88	−1.79	47	0.081		30	46.67	23.24	22	34.55	24.83	−11.36	−2.49	21	0.021	*
I cannot	81	29.38	25.07	79	23.29	23.68	48	17.29	17.95	−6.71	−3.27	78	0.002	**	−11.46	−4.10	47	0.000	***	29	31.03	22.57	22	22.73	23.54	−7.73	−2.51	21	0.020	*
Ø Stress-amplifying thoughts	81	39.36	22.72	79	33.59	21.62	48	29.50	18.49	−6.00	−3.10	78	0.003	**	−7.71	−3.23	47	0.002	**	29	39.52	18.73	22	30.09	22.06	−8.45	−3.34	21	0.003	**
Physical warnings	80	31.79	19.38	80	26.43	16.29	48	27.98	16.93	−4.95	−3.27	77	0.002	**	−3.34	−1.76	46	0.084		29	28.69	16.41	22	24.84	14.31	−4.55	−1.17	21	0.255	
Emotional warnings	81	35.80	25.29	80	25.10	24.82	48	25.69	23.50	−10.23	−4.61	78	0.000	***	−10.82	−3.42	46	0.001	**	30	43.06	28.03	21	28.97	24.24	−14.68	−2.68	20	0.014	**
Cognitive warnings	81	29.84	24.15	80	23.13	21.46	48	21.18	16.84	−6.12	−3.19	78	0.002	**	−7.98	−3.06	46	0.004	**	30	30.83	23.48	22	28.03	22.94	−5.30	−1.17	21	0.256	
Warnings in behaviour	81	19.68	14.52	80	16.25	11.88	48	17.13	14.17	−3.23	−2.31	78	0.024	*	−1.18	−0.56	46	0.579		30	22.41	17.11	22	17.93	13.82	−4.80	−1.21	21	0.241	
Ø Warning signs for stress	80	29.13	17.51	80	23.02	15.47	48	23.63	14.75	−5.66	−4.35	77	0.000	***	−4.86	−2.78	46	0.008	**	29	29.31	16.70	21	24.56	13.12	−6.39	−1.74	20	0.098	

*$p < 0.05$; **$p < 0.01$; ***$p < 0.001$.

gender. General benefit of SMT on life was more reported by patients who self-practiced exercises at home (χ^2 (1,N = 26 (reduced N according to missing data)) = 5.52; $p = 0.019$; and $r = 0.461$; $p = 0.018$) and who reported subjective reduction of tremor at the end of the SMT course (χ^2 (1,N = 32) = 5.88; $p = 0.015$; and $r = 0.429$; $p = 0.015$). Ongoing home exercising correlated with tremor reduction 4 weeks (χ^2 (1,N = 25) = 4.57; $p = 0.033$; and $r = 0.428$; $p = 0.033$) and >3 months (χ^2 (1,N = 24) = 10.15; $p = 0.0014$; and $r = 0.650$; $p = 0.0006$) after SMT.

4. Discussion

It is well known that tremor in patients with PD increases with stress factors or emotions. The objective of this study was to evaluate prospectively the effect of the structured educational stress management training (SMT) that teaches techniques for physical and mental stress reduction on coping of tremor-boosting psychosocial stressors according to Kaluza, depression, and quality of life in PD patients with tremor. We did not aim to evaluate the effect of SMT on objectively measured tremor or to compare SMT effects between PD patients and controls. Controls served as an indicator for baseline stress levels in PD patients prior to SMT and were used to assess whether SMT might be especially effective in PD patients with tremor compared to other subjects.

We showed that SMT reduces tremor-boosting psychosocial stressors such as warning signs of stress and stress-amplifying thoughts as well as depression independently of disease severity and disease duration in the short-term (8 weeks) and long-term (3–6 months) follow-up in PD patients.

Both PD patients and controls benefit comparably from SMT after 8 weeks of training. While improvement of stress-amplifying thoughts was significant in both subject groups, improvement of warning signs of stress and depression reached statistical significance only in the PD group. Within the PD group, improvement of depression was better in younger patients and in men. The majority of patients rated SMT retrospectively as beneficial for coping tremor-related daily impairment and self-practicing of SMT exercises at home correlated with subjective tremor reduction.

Emotional stress increases tremor in PD patients [7], and cognitive stress recently has been found to even reduce the levodopa effect [35]. Therefore, it is reasonable that physicians advise their patients to learn and practice relaxation techniques such as progressive muscle relaxation or autogenic training. However, data are lacking on which technique might be preferential to improve tremor intensity or coping with tremor [11].

Our results first support that applying relaxation techniques indeed is meaningful to compensate with tremor-related stress and second suggest that SMT according to Kaluza [16, 17] is helpful for PD patients with tremor. SMT offers a broad approach of stress reduction techniques to improve relaxation, cognitive behavioural aspects, problem solving, and enjoyment. In contrast to other stress management programs, SMT according to Kaluza does not only focus on assessment of negative health conditions such as anxiety or depression but also considers outcome measurements of positive aspects such as awareness of stressors, emotional well-being, and subjective changes of burden or coping strategies [36], which are primary measures for health promotion. The training has been proven to increase active and cognitive coping strategies, to improve mood states, and to decrease subjective appraisals of interpersonal stressors in the family and at work in a study with 99 healthy subjects [19]. PD patients with tremor suffer even more from psychosocial stressors due to their physical dysfunction and visible impairment [3, 4]. As a vicious circle, increased stress and emotional involvement increase tremor, and vice versa [7]. As a result, it is rather the acute stressful situation such as searching for coins in the purse at the supermarket cash desk or eating in a nonfamiliar society that triggers tremor than a general increased stress level. Most PD patients report that they have much less tremor in their familiar setting. This is supported by our results showing comparable baseline psychosocial stress levels between PD patients and controls and a comparable improvement after SMT. It is worth to note that controls were subjects without history of any relevant disease but not necessarily individuals without elevated stress levels and/or mild depressive symptoms. In contrast to PD patients, controls indeed had a mean baseline BDI score (17 points) still in the range defined as normal and below the mean cutoff defined to express mild depression in the original work of Beck [37]. However, especially standard deviation of 11 points and suggested lower BDI screening cutoffs for mild depression in a general population (e.g., 12/13 points) [38] indicate that some controls exhibited depressive symptoms. Part of controls was related to PD patients, which might trigger depressive symptoms [39].

Nevertheless, QoL in PD patients was worse compared to that in controls prior to and at the end of SMT, indicating additional other problems than tremor in PD patients.

In PD patients, improvement of self-perception of stressors and warning signs for stress and development of stress management strategies are meaningful to break the vicious cycle in tremor-boosting situations. In accordance, SMT especially decreased the items "emotional stress" and the stressful thoughts to "be popular" and "I cannot" in PD patients. These aspects are crucial to keep calm in stressful situations. The results indicate that patients acquired better self-confidence with less negative disease-related emotional involvement. Additionally, as other relaxation trainings, SMT offers PD patients a possibility for a general improvement of the well-being, and participation in the course was rated to be beneficial and pleasant by most of the patients.

Although patients' motivation for change and their perceived self-efficacy are not well studied to date [40], we demonstrated that PD patients were able and willing to learn stress management techniques for 2 hours weekly over 8 weeks and accept SMT as chance to lower disease-related stress factors and symptoms. In accordance, none of the PD patients finished SMT prematurely (in contrast to controls). Improvement of psychosocial stressors persisted at least up to 3–6 months after SMT, suggesting long-term coping with stressors is possible. However, ongoing self-exercising seems to be necessary to maintain improved stress management strategies in PD patients. This probably differs in healthy subjects, where maintained active and distancing cognitive coping, compensation strategies, less resignative-avoidant tendencies, and improved psychological mood states have been found 6 months after termination of SMT in the majority of participants as compared to a noninterventional control group [21]. This difference likely is PD immanent. As known for other nonmedical interventions with demand of regular physical activity, treatment effects in PD patients are vanishing after stopping active intervention [41]. It has been shown that PD patients perform better with coaching [41], and it is a particular challenge to motivate the patients to self-exercise at home. This assumingly is related to the high prevalence of dysexecutive function independent of dementia [42], apathy [43], fatigue [44], and depression [45] in PD patients.

We suggest that a stress management programme or course should become a brick in the multimodal landscape of activating therapies in treatment of PD patients with tremor. Based on former results of SMT in healthy subjects and patients with chronic diseases [19, 20, 36] as well as on findings in the present study, we recommend SMT as a suitable technique that should be offered by a psychologist or a certified trainer qualified for prevention stress management. We furthermore propose to monitor therapeutic effects applying both stress scales of Kaluza, which have been developed to assess psychosocial aspects. Meanwhile, SMT is part of our therapeutic landscape for PD patients and supported by almost all public health insurances in Germany, who reimburse 80% of the costs and appreciate SMT as a tremor prevention course. However, SMT might be beneficial also in PD patients without tremor. It has been shown that autogenic training, when used as an adjunct to physiotherapy, is more effective than physiotherapy alone in improving motor performances assessed as the UPDRS motor score in PD patients [46]. Relaxation-guided imagery techniques reduced not only tremor [11] but also motor fluctuations in PD [47].

We also found a positive short- and long-term effect of SMT on depression in PD patients. This might be related to less emotional involvement and better coping of tremor. Appropriately, subitems of the BDI improved significantly, which could be related to tremor-associated social stigmatization and isolation, such as feeling inadequate/inferior or self-denial/dislike. However, SMT includes aspects of a cognitive-behaviour therapy (CBT) that has been shown to be effective in a small case series of three depressed PD patients [48] and is an established, evidence-based therapy of depression in other populations [49]. In line, BDI scores improved comparably in controls as short-term outcome. Furthermore, it cannot be excluded that depression improved due to the attention of the therapist or a secure feeling within the group. Of note, depression improved especially in younger and male patients, indicating that also men accept this kind of "psychological" SMT.

Quality of life assessed with the PDQ-8 score was not significantly changed after participation in SMT. However, total PDQ-8 consists of several aspects that cannot be aimed to improve by SMT such as mobility, concentration, communication, or pain. Despite that, there was a trend to an improvement ($p = 0.082$) of total PDQ-8 as a consequence of improvements of the subscales "emotional well-being" (significant; $p = 0.046$) and "stigma" (by trend; $p = 0.097$), supporting efficacy of SMT on depression and coping of tremor.

4.1. Study Limitations. Short-term outcome results after 8 weeks of SMT are based on a 100% participation rate in PD patients and 90% in controls. Long-term outcome results 3–6 weeks after SMT were available in only 60% of PD patients and so have to be interpreted with caution.

Both Kaluza's scales to measure psychosocial stressors have not been validated in a validation study. However, both scales have been proven to be sufficient in clinical daily practice, indicating a reliable content validity. Furthermore, 2-factor analysis revealed both a high reliability (Cronbach's alpha coefficient of around 0.90 for homogeneity) and a high factorial validity (for all 9 subscales (4 warning signs + 5 stress-amplifying thoughts)) at baseline with an explained variance of 76% for the two factors of both applied psychosocial scales, suggesting applied questionnaires to be sufficient, reliable, and valid.

The study is not appropriate to evaluate the effect of SMT on tremor severity or frequency. Instead, we assessed as additionally subsequent outcome parameter the efficacy of SMT on tremor coping and self-estimation of tremor severity in daily life. These data were acquired retrospectively and unsystematically during a normal consultation 12 to 18 months after finishing SMT. This implies risk for a recall bias, and only 40% of PD patients participating in SMT could be reached for this assessment.

So these results can only indicate that ongoing self-practice of relaxation techniques is helpful to maintain acquired improved coping with psychosocial stress factors and to perceive tremor as less severe. Prospective further studies should confirm this impression.

To cover the important aspect of quality of life (QoL), we evaluated the effect of SMT on PDQ-8. This instrument has been designed for use in PD patients but not in healthy controls or non-PD populations. Therefore, the significant and high difference of QoL between PD patients and controls found prior to and at the end of SMT might be biased by applying the score also in non-PD subjects. However, due to the enormous difference in PDQ-8 values between groups, it is likely that PD patients indeed have a worse QoL. However, better (but not significantly different) improvement of QoL after SMT compared to controls might be related to the higher scores at baseline in PD patients.

4.2. Study Strengths. We demonstrated efficacy of a defined SMT on improvement of physical and mental stressors and depression in a controlled and prospective study in a large group of 82 PD patients with tremor as short-term and long-term outcomes. Intensity of the training course was high with a total of 16 hours, and techniques were taught by a specialized psychologist. To our knowledge, a comparable study concept of applying any stress reduction technique in patients with PD has not been reported so far.

In conclusion, stress management training can help patients to cope with tremor and is suggested as part of the therapeutic concept in PD patients with tremor.

Authors' Contributions

EL, DJ, and CB drafted/revised the manuscript for content, including medical writing for content, was responsible for the study concept or design, and performed analysis or interpretation of data. EL and CB acquired the data. DJ and CB performed statistical analysis. CB supervised or coordinated the study.

Acknowledgments

C. Buhmann has been supported by funding from the Georg & Jürgen Rickertsen Stiftung Hamburg and received travel funding from Abbvie and Desitin and received honoraria as speaker and/or scientific advisory board member from Desitin, GE Healthcare, TEVA, UCB, and Zambon.

References

[1] C. R. Baumann, "Epidemiology, diagnosis and differential diagnosis in Parkinson's disease tremor," *Parkinsonism & Related Disorders*, vol. 18, no. 1, pp. S90–S92, 2012.

[2] G. Deuschl, "New treatment options for tremors," *New England Journal of Medicine*, vol. 342, no. 7, pp. 505–507, 2000.

[3] S. K. Lageman, T. V. Cash, and M. N. Mickens, "Patient-reported needs, non-motor symptoms, and quality of life in essential tremor and Parkinson's disease," *Tremor and Other Hyperkinetic Movements*, vol. 4, p. 240, 2014.

[4] R. D. Salazar, A. M. Le, S. Neargarder, and A. Cronin-Golomb, "The impact of motor symptoms on self-reported anxiety in Parkinson's disease," *Parkinsonism & Related Disorders*, vol. 38, pp. 26–30, 2017.

[5] A. Dural, M. B. Atay, C. Akbostanci, and A. Kucukdeveci, "Impairment, disability, and life satisfaction in Parkinson's disease," *Disability and Rehabilitation*, vol. 25, no. 7, pp. 318–323, 2003.

[6] H. J. Lee, W. W. Lee, S. K. Kim et al., "Tremor frequency characteristics in Parkinson's disease under resting-state and stress-state conditions," *Journal of the Neurological Sciences*, vol. 362, pp. 272–277, 2016.

[7] C. D. Marsden and D. A. Owen, "Mechanisms underlying emotional variation in parkinsonian tremor," *Neurology*, vol. 17, no. 7, pp. 711–715, 1967.

[8] J. Raethjen, K. Austermann, K. Witt, K. E. Zeuner, F. Papengut, and G. Deuschl, "Provocation of Parkinsonian tremor," *Movement Disorders*, vol. 23, no. 7, pp. 1019–1023, 2008.

[9] T. H. Foley, C. D. Marsden, and D. A. Owen, "Evidence for a direct peripheral effect of adrenaline on physiological tremor in man," *Journal of Physiology*, vol. 189, no. 2, pp. 65P-66P, 1967.

[10] C. D. Marsden, T. H. Foley, D. A. Owen, and R. G. McAllister, "Peripheral beta-adrenergic receptors concerned with tremor," *Clinical Science*, vol. 33, no. 1, pp. 53–65, 1967.

[11] I. Schlesinger, O. Benyakov, I. Erikh, S. Suraiya, and Y. Schiller, "Parkinson's disease tremor is diminished with relaxation guided imagery," *Movement Disorders*, vol. 24, no. 14, pp. 2059–2062, 2009.

[12] A. Chiesa and A. Serretti, "Mindfulness-based stress reduction for stress management in healthy people: a review and meta-analysis," *Journal of Alternative and Complementary Medicine*, vol. 15, no. 5, pp. 593–600, 2009.

[13] J. J. van der Klink, R. W. Blonk, A. H. Schene, and F. J. van Dijk, "The benefits of interventions for work-related stress," *American Journal of Public Health*, vol. 91, no. 2, pp. 270–276, 2001.

[14] K. M. Richardson and H. R. Rothstein, "Effects of occupational stress management intervention programs: a meta-analysis," *Journal of Occupational Health Psychology*, vol. 13, no. 1, pp. 69–93, 2008.

[15] M. Dharmawardene, J. Givens, A. Wachholtz, S. Makowski, and J. Tjia, "A systematic review and meta-analysis of meditative interventions for informal caregivers and health professionals," *BMJ Supportive & Palliative Care*, vol. 6, no. 2, pp. 160–169, 2016.

[16] G. Kaluza, *Gelassen und sicher im Streß: Psychologisches Programm zur Gesundheitsförderung*, Springer, Heidelberg, Germany, 1996.

[17] G. Kaluza, *Stressbewältigung: Trainingsmanual zur Psychologischen Gesundheitsförderung*, Springer, Berlin, Germany, 2004.

[18] G. Kaluza, "Belastungsbewältigung und Gesundheit," *Zeitschrift für Medizinische Psychologie*, vol. 5, pp. 147–155, 1996.

[19] G. Kaluza, "Effekte eines kognitiv-behavioralen Streßbewältigungstrainings auf Belastungen, Bewältigung und (Wohl-)Befinden—eine randomisierte, kontrollierte prospektive Interventionsstudie in der primären Prävention," *Zeitschrift für Klinische Psychologie*, vol. 27, no. 4, pp. 234–243, 1998.

[20] G. Kaluza, E. Krane, H. Klus, and M. Pilz-Oertel, "Salutogenese in der praxis: indikations-übergreifendes, ressourcenorientiertes Gesundheitstraining für chronisch kranke Menschen—interventionskonzept und Evaluation," *Praxis der Klinischen Verhaltensmedizin und Rehabilitation*, vol. 58, pp. 148–155, 2002.

[21] G. Kaluza, "Sind die Effekte eines primäpräventiven Stressbewältigungstrainings von Dauer? Eine randomisierte, kontrollierte Follow-up-Studie," *Zeitschrift für Gesundheitspsychologie*, vol. 7, no. 2, pp. 88–95, 1999.

[22] A. T. Beck, J. Rush, B. F. Shaw, and G. Emery, *Cognitive Therapy of Depression*, Guilford Press, New York, NY, USA, 1979.

[23] A. T. Beck, *Kognitive Therapie der Depression*, M. Hautzinger, Ed., vol. 3, Beltz/PVU, Weinheim, Germany, 2004.

[24] C. Jenkinson, R. Fitzpatrick, V. Peto, R. Greenhall, and R. Iansek, "The PDQ-8: development and validation of a short-form Parkinson's disease questionnaire," *Psychology and Health*, vol. 12, no. 6, pp. 805–814, 1997.

[25] M. M. Hoehn and M. D. Yahr, "Parkinsonism: onset, progression and mortality," *Neurology*, vol. 17, no. 5, pp. 427–442, 1967.
[26] A. J. Hughes, S. E. Daniel, L. Kilford, and A. J. Lees, "Accuracy of clinical diagnosis of idiopathic Parkinson's disease: a clinico-pathological study of 100 cases," *Journal of Neurology, Neurosurgery, and Psychiatry*, vol. 55, no. 3, pp. 181–184, 1992.
[27] M. F. Folstein, S. E. Folstein, and P. R. McHugh, "Mini-mental state". A practical method for grading the cognitive state of patients for the clinician," *Journal of Psychiatric Research*, vol. 12, no. 3, pp. 189–198, 1975.
[28] F. Kohl, ""Die Progressive Muskelrelaxation" nach Jacobson—methodischer Ansatz, konzeptionelle Entwicklungen und Grundzüge der gegenwärtigen Anwendungspraxis," *Krankenhauspsychiatrie*, vol. 8, pp. 189–193, 1998.
[29] D. A. Bernstein, T. D. Borkovec, and Entspannungstraining, *Handbuch der Progressiven Muskelentspannung*, Pfeiffer Verlag, München, Germany, 1997.
[30] R. Lutz and E. Koppenhöfer, "Kleine Schule des Genießens," in *Genuß und Genießen*, R. Lutz, Ed., pp. 112–125, Beltz, Weinheim, Germany, 1983.
[31] R. Lutz, "Genußtraining," in *Verhaltenstherapie: Techniken und Einzelverfahren*, M. Linden and M. Hautzinger, Eds., pp. 155–159, Springer, Berlin, Germany, 1993.
[32] F. Faul, E. Erdfelder, A. G. Lang, and A. Buchner, "G∗Power 3: a flexible statistical power analysis program for the social, behavioral, and biomedical sciences," *Behavior Research Methods*, vol. 39, no. 2, pp. 175–191, 2007.
[33] P. Cohen, J. Cohen, L. S. Aiken, and S. G. West, "The problem of units and the circumstance for POMP," *Multivariate Behavioral Research*, vol. 34, no. 3, pp. 315–346, 1999.
[34] J. Cohen, *Statistical Power Analysis for the Behavioral Science*, Academic Press, Cambridge, MA, USA, 1988.
[35] H. Zach, M. F. Dirkx, J. W. Pasman, B. R. Bloem, and R. C. Helmich, "Cognitive stress reduces the effect of levodopa on Parkinson's resting tremor," *CNS Neuroscience & Therapeutics*, vol. 23, no. 3, pp. 209–215, 2017.
[36] G. Kaluza, "Evaluation von Streßbewältigungstrainings in der primären Prävention—eine Mata-Analyse (quasi-)experimentieller Feldstudien," *Zeitschrift für Gesundheitspsychologie*, vol. 5, pp. 149–169, 1997.
[37] A. T. Beck, D. H. M. M. Ward, J. Mock, and J. Erbaugh, "An inventory for measuring depression," *Archives Of General Psychiatry*, vol. 4, no. 6, pp. 561–571, 1961.
[38] L. Lasa, J. L. Ayuso-Mateos, J. L. Vazquez-Barquero, F. J. Diez-Manrique, and C. F. Dowrick, "The use of the Beck Depression Inventory to screen for depression in the general population: a preliminary analysis," *Journal of Affective Disorders*, vol. 57, no. 1–3, pp. 261–265, 2000.
[39] J. Sanyal, S. Das, E. Ghosh, T. K. Banerjee, L. V. Bhaskar, and V. R. Rao, "Burden among Parkinson's disease care givers for a community based study from India," *Journal of the Neurological Sciences*, vol. 358, no. 1-2, pp. 276–281, 2015.
[40] T. Zimmermann, E. Puschmann, S. Porzelt et al., "Promoting self-management in primary care—the association of motivation for change, self-efficacy and psychological distress prior to the onset of intervention," *Psychiatrische Praxis*, vol. 42, no. 1, pp. S44–S48, 2015.
[41] B. R. Bloem, N. M. de Vries, and G. Ebersbach, "Nonpharmacological treatments for patients with Parkinson's disease," *Movement Disorders*, vol. 30, no. 11, pp. 1504–1520, 2015.
[42] L. Brennan, K. M. Devlin, S. X. Xie et al., "Neuropsychological subgroups in non-demented Parkinson's disease: a latent class analysis," *Journal of Parkinson's Disease*, vol. 7, no. 2, pp. 385–395, 2017.
[43] M. G. den Brok, J. W. van Dalen, W. A. van Gool, E. P. Moll van Charante, R. M. de Bie, and E. Richard, "Apathy in Parkinson's disease: a systematic review and meta-analysis," *Movement Disorders*, vol. 30, no. 6, pp. 759–769, 2015.
[44] P. Barone, A. Antonini, C. Colosimo et al., "The PRIAMO study: a multicenter assessment of nonmotor symptoms and their impact on quality of life in Parkinson's disease," *Movement Disorders*, vol. 24, no. 11, pp. 1641–1649, 2009.
[45] O. Riedel, J. Klotsche, A. Spottke et al., "Frequency of dementia, depression, and other neuropsychiatric symptoms in 1,449 outpatients with Parkinson's disease," *Journal of Neurology*, vol. 257, no. 7, pp. 1073–1082, 2010.
[46] M. S. Ajimsha, N. A. Majeed, E. Chinnavan, and R. P. Thulasyammal, "Effectiveness of autogenic training in improving motor performances in Parkinson's disease," *Complementary Therapies in Medicine*, vol. 22, no. 3, pp. 419–425, 2014.
[47] I. Schlesinger, O. Benyakov, I. Erikh, and M. Nassar, "Relaxation guided imagery reduces motor fluctuations in Parkinson's disease," *Journal of Parkinson's Disease*, vol. 4, no. 3, pp. 431–436, 2014.
[48] R. D. Dobkin, L. A. Allen, and M. Menza, "A cognitive-behavioral treatment package for depression in Parkinson's disease," *Psychosomatics*, vol. 47, no. 3, pp. 259–263, 2006.
[49] M. Floyd, F. Scogin, N. L. McKendree-Smith, D. L. Floyd, and P. D. Rokke, "Cognitive therapy for depression: a comparison of individual psychotherapy and bibliotherapy for depressed older adults," *Behavior Modification*, vol. 28, no. 2, pp. 297–318, 2004.

4

Median and Ulnar Neuropathy Assessment in Parkinson's Disease regarding Symptom Severity and Asymmetry

Nilgul Yardimci,[1] Ozlem Cemeroglu,[2] Eda Ozturk,[3] Gülsüm Gürlü,[4] Esra Şahin,[4] Saliha Bozkurt,[4] Tugba Cengiz,[5] Gulderen Karali,[5] Hasim Cakirbay,[2] and Atilla İlhan[6]

[1]*Neurology Department, Minasera Aldan Hospital, Ahmet Taner Kislali Mah. 2741, Street No. 2 Cayyolu, Ankara, Turkey*
[2]*Physical Medicine and Rehabilitation Department, Medical Park Ankara Hospital, Kentkoop Mah., Kentkoop Parkici Yolu, Yenimahalle, Ankara, Turkey*
[3]*Biostatistics Department, Medicine Faculty, Hacettepe University, Hacettepe Mah., 06230 Ankara, Turkey*
[4]*Physical Medicine and Rehabilitation Department, Medicine Faculty, Turgut Ozal University, Alparslan Turkes Cad. No. 57, Emek, 06510 Ankara, Turkey*
[5]*Neurology Department, Medicine Faculty, Turgut Ozal University, Alparslan Turkes Cad. No. 57, Emek, 06510 Ankara, Turkey*
[6]*Neurology Department, Medicine Faculty, Gazi University, Emniyet, Yenimahalle, 06560 Ankara, Turkey*

Correspondence should be addressed to Nilgul Yardimci; ntuncel@yahoo.com

Academic Editor: Jan Aasly

Background. While increasing evidence suggests comorbidity of peripheral neuropathy (PNP) and Parkinson's disease (PD), the pathogenesis of PNP in PD is still a debate. The aim of this article is to search the core PD symptoms such as rigidity and tremor as contributing factors to mononeuropathy development while emphasizing each individual patient's asymmetric symptom severity. *Methods.* We studied 62 wrists and 62 elbows of 31 patients (mean age 66.48 ± 10.67) and 64 wrists and 64 elbows of 32 age-gender matched healthy controls (mean age 62.03 ± 10.40, $p = 0.145$). The Hoehn and Yahr disability scale and Unified Parkinson's Disease Rated Scale were used to determine the severity of the disease. *Results.* According to electrodiagnostic criteria, we confirmed median neuropathy in 16.12% (bilateral in two-thirds of the patients) and ulnar neuropathy in 3.22% of the PD group. While mean age ($p = 0.003$), age at PD onset ($p = 0.019$), and H&Y scores ($p = 0.016$) were significant, tremor and rigidity scores were not. The comparison of the mean indices of electrophysiologic parameters indicated subclinical median and ulnar nerve demyelination both at the wrist and at the elbow in the patient groups where a longer disease duration and mild tremor and rigidity scores are prominent, remarkably. *Conclusion.* A disease related peripheral neurodegeneration beyond symptom severity occurs in PD.

1. Introduction

Parkinson's disease (PD) is the second most common neurodegenerative disorder, characterised by tremor, rigidity, bradykinesia, and postural instability associated with degeneration of dopaminergic neurons in the substantia nigra pars compacta and the presence of eosinophilic intracytoplasmic inclusions [1].

Identifying comorbid conditions in addition to the core PD symptoms may increase satisfaction from traditional therapies by maximizing the health status of the patient. In accordance with this, the possible relationship between PD and peripheral neuropathy (PN) has begun receiving attention. Although the pathogenic mechanism remains unclear, some studies suggest PN as a neurodegenerative process involving both central and peripheral nervous systems [2]. It is still a debate whether PN in PD should be accepted as an acquired neuropathy due to long-term levodopa intake or as an intrinsic neuropathy developed by neurodegeneration involving the peripheral nervous system in PD pathophysiology.

Although by advancing therapeutic options more successful symptom control has been provided in PD patients today, rigidity and tremor still remain the challenging motor symptoms of the disease. Besides being one of the cardinal symptoms of PD, the characteristic rest tremor seen as "pill-rolling" action of the hands has been also accused of being the trigger of the carpal tunnel syndrome because of causing repetitive trauma to the median nerve [3, 4]. Striatal hand and foot deformities occur in varying degrees associated with the disease severity and may cause functional disability also. The pathogenesis of striatal deformities involves decreased striatal dopamine, dystonia, and parkinsonian rigidity [5]. The classical position of the elbow in accordance with the striatal deformities of the PD which is superimposed with tremor has not been searched as the potential risk for ulnar neuropathy before [6].

In this study, we aimed to search if the severity of clinical symptoms such as tremor and rigidity affects neuronal transmission and contributes to entrapment neuropathy evolution in PD. In regard to this, we also investigated if each patient's initial and latter affected extremities which demonstrate varying symptom severity during the progressive disease course differ electrophysiologically. These hypotheses are being searched for the first time in the literature and aim to call attention to peripheral neuropathy while planning therapeutic options in each individual PD patient.

2. Patients and Methods

2.1. Parkinson's Disease Group. Patients were recruited from the Neurology Outpatient Unit in the Department of Neurology, Turgut Ozal University Faculty of Medicine. Consecutive patients who attended the clinic were examined by a neurologist and those who fulfilled the study criteria were entered in the study. 40 patients were enrolled in the study. Among these patients, 1 was excluded from the study because of previous left elbow fracture, 3 had diabetes mellitus, and 5 had polyneuropathy. Totally, 62 elbows and 62 wrists of 31 patients with PD diagnosed by means of the United Kingdom Parkinson's Disease Society Brain Bank Clinical Diagnosis Criteria [7] [18 women (58.1%) and 13 men (41.9%)] with an age range of 45–83 years (mean age, 66.48 ± 10.67 years) were included in the study. Exclusion criteria included coexistence of any systemic disease known to cause median or ulnar neuropathy such as diabetes mellitus, chronic renal failure, hypothyroidism, rheumatoid arthritis, cervical radiculopathy, and trauma. All patients were examined in the "on" condition. The Hoehn and Yahr (H&Y) disability scale [8] and Unified Parkinson's Disease Rated Scale (UPDRS) [9] were used to assess the severity of the disease. The patients were not symptomatic regarding pain or numbness suggesting nerve entrapment in the territory of a root or nerve.

Firstly, the patients were examined for existence of any median or ulnar neuropathy according to the electrophysiologically diagnostic criteria based on control data performed in our laboratory.

In elderly subjects such as our study population, subclinical neuropathy is common and might increase the frequency of mononeuropathy. We compared the means of electrophysiological indices of the patients and the controls for any statistically significant difference also.

As known, PD symptoms begin unilateral initially and in the following years the initial affected extremities demonstrate more severe symptoms when compared with the latter affected ones. Keeping this rule in mind, we compared the initial and latter affected sides of each patient electrophysiologically in regard to tremor and rigidity severity.

Later, each patient was categorized as mild or severe according to the H&Y scores, tremor and rigidity severity, and disease duration. These groups electrophysiologic parameters were compared statistically.

2.2. Comparison Group. 64 elbows and 64 wrists of 32 healthy controls [22 women (68.8%) and 10 men (31.3%)] with an age range of 46–87 years (mean age, 62.03±10.40, $p = 0.145$) who had no disease known to cause median or ulnar neuropathy, no history of frequent, repetitive use of the hand, wrist, or elbow, and no trauma or any other condition affecting peripheral neural transmission and whose neurologic examination was normal were included in the study. The subjects were volunteers from the community matched by age and sex with the PD patients. Any subject with electrophysiological pathology was excluded from the study.

Informed consent was obtained from all individual participants included in the study and the study was approved by Turgut Ozal University Medicine Faculty Ethical Committee.

2.3. Electrophysiological Evaluation. Sensory nerve conduction velocity (SNCV) and motor nerve conduction velocity (MNCV) were measured with a Medelec Synergy Electromyography instrument (Oxford Instruments Medical, Inc., UK) in an air-conditioned room at 23°C to 25°C. Limb temperature was maintained above 32°C using a warm compress if needed during the nerve conduction studies. Median and ulnar nerve conduction studies were performed bilaterally in all patients and control groups using the standard techniques of supramaximal percutaneous stimulation [10].

The EMG criteria for diagnosis of median neuropathy include prolonged distal motor latencies of the median nerve greater than 4.2 m/s, a decrease in sensory conduction velocity below 41 m/s for digit-wrist segment, 5 mV for amplitude of muscle action potential, and 10 mV for amplitude of sensory nerve action potential [11].

The EMG criteria for diagnosis of ulnar neuropathy include prolonged motor nerve conduction velocity (NCV) from above elbow (AE) to below elbow (BE) of less than 40 m/s and an AE to BE segment greater than 10 m/s slower than BE to wrist (W) segment which suggests conduction block or temporal dispersion indicative of focal demyelination.

2.4. Statistical Analysis. For continuous variables, results were presented as mean ± standard deviation or median (minimum, maximum). Categorical variables were presented by frequency and percentage. Comparisons between two categorical variables were performed using the chi-square analysis. Kruskal-Wallis test or one-way ANOVA (analysis of variance) were used for comparison of more than two independent samples followed by the Bonferroni-adjusted Mann–Whitney U test or Tukey test when appropriate. All

TABLE 1: The clinical characteristics of the patients and the control group.

Variables	PD group (n = 31)	Control group (n = 32)	p
Gender (F/M)	18/13	22/10	
Age (year)	65.93 ± 10.58	62.03 ± 10.40	0.145
Age at onset (year)	59.48 ± 10.68		
PD duration (year)	6.45 ± 4.35		
Hoehn and Yahr stage	2.73 ± 0.94		
UPDRS part III score	21.86 ± 8.90		
Parkinson disease questionnaire	64.63 ± 24.09		

TABLE 2: Demographic and clinical characteristics of PD patients with median neuropathy versus without median neuropathy.

Variables	Median neuropathy (+)	Median neuropathy (−)	p
Mean age	77.00 ± 2.60	63.28 ± 10.03	**0.003**
PD duration (year)	8.50 ± 4.18	5.96 ± 4.33	0.205
Age at PD onset	68.50 ± 3.83	57.32 ± 10.70	**0.019**
Tremor score	1.83 ± 0.75	1.45 ± 0.97	0.390
Rigidity score	2.50 ± 0.54	1.79 ± 0.83	0.059
UPDRS part III score	30.66 ± 12.61	19.66 ± 6.33	**0.005**
Hoehn and Yahr stage	3.50 ± 1.04	2.54 ± 0.83	**0.023**
PDQ[a]	85.33 ± 15.43	59.45 ± 23.24	**0.016**

[a]Parkinson's disease questionnaire.

analyses were performed using IBM SPSS Statistics 21 (IBM, Armonk, NY USA). All tests were two-sided and a p value of less than 0.05 was considered to be statistically significant.

3. Results

All patients were receiving levodopa and/or dopaminergic agonist and were examined during "on" condition. The clinical characteristics of the study population are summarized in Table 1.

According to diagnostic electrophysiologic criteria, 10 wrists (16.12%) in 6 patients were diagnosed as having definite median neuropathy and 2 elbows (3.22%) in 2 patients were diagnosed as having ulnar neuropathy. The electrophysiologic parameters of the healthy control group were in normal limits. The clinical characteristics of the patients with median neuropathy are listed in Table 2. Median neuropathy was diagnosed as bilateral in 4 patients and unilateral in 2 patients. Among the patients with median neuropathy, mean age (p = 0.003), age at Parkinson disease onset (p = 0.019), UPDRS III motor score (p = 0.005), Hoehn and Yahr stage (p = 0.023), and Parkinson disease questionnaire scores (p = 0.016) were statistically significantly higher. Tremor (p = 0.390) and rigidity (p = 0.059) scores which we were particularly interested in were not significantly different.

As the ulnar neuropathy in this study was observed in 2 patients representing 3.2% of the study population, we did not mention the patient details in Table 2 but preferred to explain them as follows: the first patient was a 75-year-old male with a 2-year duration of disease scored as 2 according to H&Y stage with mild tremor and rigidity scores and the second patient was a 64-year-old female with a 10-year duration of disease scored as 4 according to H&Y stage with severe tremor and rigidity.

The comparison of the means of electrophysiological indices on the left and right sides between controls and the patients is shown in Table 3. While right and left median nerve sensorial velocities at the wrist were decreased, right and left median nerve motor latencies were prolonged statistically significantly indicating demyelination. There was a significant decrease in the right median nerve motor amplitude whereas the decrease in the left median nerve motor amplitude did not reach statistically significant levels. It might be suggested that there was a possible median nerve axonal deterioration also. While there was a significant decrease in the left ulnar nerve sensorial velocity at the wrist, the decrease in the right ulnar nerve did not reach significant level. The prolongation of the right and left ulnar nerves' motor latencies were significant. These findings suggested ulnar nerve demyelination at the wrist when compared with the age-gender matched controls. The reduction in the left ulnar nerve motor velocity at the elbow level was significantly decreased while the reduction in the right was not significant. These results suggested a tendency to ulnar nerve entrapment at the elbow in the patient group.

In concordance with our hypothesis that more severe tremor and rigidity might worsen neuronal transmission, we compared each patient's median and ulnar nerve electrophysiologic parameters between the initial and latter affected extremities (Table 4). All parameters regarding ulnar and median nerves were studied and mean indices were compared with each other. No significant difference was found but if we could have learned the time span between the first and second affected sides of the body for each patient accurately and categorized it as years, the results might have been more objective.

Later, each patient was categorized as mild or severe according to the mentioned criteria; Mild H&Y group (stage I-II) consisted of 14 patients (45.16%) with an age range of 45–76 years (mean age 63.15 ± 10.51) and the severe H&Y group (stage III-IV) consisted of 17 patients (54.83%) with an age range of 47–82 years (mean age 69.63 ± 9.75, p = 0.084). In our study, mean of the disease duration was calculated as 6 years statistically, and mild group suffering from the disease for 6 years or less consisted of 17 patients (54.83%) with an age range of 45–78 years (mean age 63.72 ± 10.63) and the severe group with more than 6 years of the disease consisted of 14 patients (45.16%) with an age range of 47–83 years (mean age 69.80 ± 10.06, p = 0.104); mild tremor group (score 0-1-2) consisted of 21 patients (67.74%) with an age range of 45–79 years (mean age 65.68 ± 10.39) and the severe tremor group (score 3-4) consisted of 10 patients (32.25%) with an age range of 56–83 years (mean age 71.71 ± 9.77, p = 0.180); mild rigidity group (score 0-1-2) consisted of 20 patients (64.51%) with an age range of 45–79 years (mean age 65.25 ± 10.27) and

TABLE 3: The mean indices of electrophysiologic parameters between PD patients and controls.

	PD patients	Controls	p
Rmediandigit2velocity (s)	51.15 (41.10–60)	53.30 (40–64.90)	**0.049**
Lmediandigit2velocity (s)	51.10 (30–58.50)	52.20 (40–61.50)	**0.020**
Rulnardigit5wristvelocity (s)	53.70 (42.30–59.60)	55 (42.30–64.70)	0.250
Lulnardigit5wristvelocity (s)	53.03 ± 5.05	55.74 ± 4.93	**0.037**
RmedianAPBwristlatency (m)	3.63 ± 1.09	3.10 ± 0.42	**0.015**
RmedianAPBwristamp (m)	6.25 ± 2.53	7.52 ± 2.02	**0.033**
RmedianAPBelbowlatency (m)	7.36 ± 0.69	6.86 ± 0.81	**0.011**
RmedianAPBelbowampl (m)	5.68 ± 2.08	7.08 ± 2.06	**0.011**
RmedianAPBelbowvelocity (m)	57.52 ± 5.32	61.80 ± 8.19	**0.019**
LmedianAPBwristlatency (m)	3.35 (2.75–7.75)	3.00 (2.25–3.90)	**<0.001**
LmedianAPBwristampl (m)	6.37 ± 2.50	7.25 ± 2.16	0.145
LmedianAPBelbowlatency (m)	7.47 ± 1.16	6.76 ± 0.59	**0.004**
LmedianAPBelbowampl (m)	5.88 ± 2.21	6.64 ± 2.06	0.228
LmedianAPBelbowvelocity (m)	57.80 (44–184)	62.90 (51.70–73.30)	0.091
RulnarADMwristlatency (m)	2.55 (2.05–3.20)	2.35 (1.85–3.50)	**0.023**
RulnarADMwristampl (m)	9.31 ± 1.39	9.66 ± 1.52	0.351
RulnarADMb.elbowvelocity (m)	60.30 (50.50–78.80)	62 (51.10–94.10)	0.176
RulnarADMa.elbowvelocity (m)	58.50 ± 1.28	58.77 ± 1.60	0.148
LulnarADMwristlatency (m)	2.60 (2.15–4)	2.35 (2–3.30)	**0.011**
LulnarADMwristampl (m)	10.10 (6.10–89)	10 (6.40–14.30)	0.607
LulnarADMb.elbowvelocity (m)	58.30 (41.20–77.20)	63 (55.80–83)	**0.002**
LulnarADMa.elbowvelocity (m)	53.80 (35.90–73.70)	57.10 (41.90–80)	**0.017**

(s): sensorial; (m): motor; R: right; L: left; ampl: amplitude; APB: abductor pollicis brevis; ADM: adductor digiti minimi; a: after; b: below.

TABLE 4: Correspondence of mean indices of electrophysiologic parameters between initial and later symptomatic sides in PD patients.

	Initial symptomatic side	Later symptomatic side	p
mediandigit2latency (s)	2.76 ± 0.08	2.53 ± 0.42	0.523
mediandigit2velocity (s)	51.41 ± 3.89	49.50 ± 6.15	0.082
mediandigit2peakampl (s)	37.36 ± 16.38	35.16 ± 18.86	0.457
ulnardigit5wristlatency (s)	2.11 ± 0.23	2.13 ± 0.23	0.528
ulnardigit5wristvelocity (s)	53.55 ± 4.58	52.83 ± 4.65	0.295
ulnardigit5wristpeakampl (s)	29.18 ± 14.93	29.83 ± 14.40	0.777
ulnarlatency (m)	2.22 ± 0.32	2.22 ± 0.21	0.971
ulnarpeakampl (m)	23.79 ± 15.84	20.20 ± 14.28	0.052
medianlatency (m)	2.54 ± 0.29	2.53 ± 0.26	0.927
medianpeakampl (m)	20.11 ± 12.30	18.26 ± 11.70	0.289
medianAPBwristlatency (m)	3.63 ± 1.12	3.73 ± 1.11	0.475
medianAPBwristamp (m)	6.61 ± 2.52	6.00 ± 2.51	0.257
medianAPBelbowlatency (m)	7.32 ± 0.70	7.53 ± 1.17	0.636
medianAPBelbowampl (m)	6.05 ± 2.04	5.49 ± 2.24	0.406
medianAPBelbowvelocity (m)	57.66 ± 5.21	62.24 ± 23.79	0.252
ulnarADMwristlatency (m)	2.62 ± 0.32	2.61 ± 0.41	0.884
ulnarADMwristampl (m)	9.44 ± 1.73	12.44 ± 14.58	0.288
ulnarADMb.elbowlatency (m)	6.41 ± 0.65	6.42 ± 0.83	0.83
ulnarADMb.elbowampl (m)	8.83 ± 1.58	8.88 ± 1.88	0.882
ulnarADMb.elbowvelocity (m)	59.81 ± 6.51	59.46 ± 7.65	0.756
ulnarADMa.elbowlatency (m)	7.85 ± 0.80	7.88 ± 1	0.823
ulnarADMa.elbowampl (m)	8.52 ± 1.53	8.51 ± 1.84	0.982
ulnarADMa.elbowvelocity (m)	54.85 ± 5.97	55.24 ± 7.15	0.79

(s): sensorial; (m): motor; ampl: amplitude; APB: abductor pollicis brevis; ADM: adductor digiti minimi; b: before; a: after.

TABLE 5: The statistical comparison of mean indices of median and ulnar nerve electrophysiologic parameters at the wrist level between mild and severe patient groups and controls.

Variables	Disease duration (years)		Hoehn & Yahr score		Rigidity		Tremor	
	Shorter than 6 years	Longer than 6 years	Mild	Severe	Mild	Severe	Mild	Severe
m-dml								
R	NS	0.002	0.041	NS	0.007	NS	0.003	0.003
L	NS	0.001	0.002	0.002	0.001	0.001	0.002	NS
m-amp								
R	NS	NS	NS	0.041	NS	NS	NS	NS
L	NS	NS	NS	NS	NS	NS	NS	NS
m-ncv								
R	NS	NS	NS	0.035	NS	NS	NS	NS
L	NS	NS	NS	NS	NS	NS	NS	NS
u-dml								
R	NS	0.037	NS	NS	NS	0.049	NS	NS
L	NS	0.008	NS	0.025	0.034	NS	NS	0.011
u-amp								
R	0.031	0.031	NS	NS	NS	NS	NS	NS
L	NS	NS	NS	NS	NS	NS	NS	NS
u-ncv								
R	NS	NS	NS	NS	NS	NS	NS	NS
L	NS	NS	NS	NS	NS	NS	NS	NS

m: median; dml: distal motor latency; amp: amplitude; ncv: nerve conduction velocity; u: ulnar; NS: not significant; R: right; L: left.

the severe group consisted of 11 patients (35.48%) with an age range of 56–83 years (mean age 72.25 ± 9.55, $p = 0.100$). Each group was studied electrophysiologically.

In our study population, the statistical evaluation of the median of the duration of the disease as years was calculated as "6" years. The median and ulnar motor latencies at the wrist of the patients who had been suffering from the disease for more than 6 years were found to be significantly prolonged bilaterally.

According to the Hoehn and Yahr scores, bilateral median nerve motor latencies were found to be prolonged at the wrist significantly in the mild group (Table 5) suggesting a tendency to demyelination.

According to the rigidity and tremor scores, bilateral median nerve motor latencies at the wrist were found to be prolonged (Table 5) only in the mild group but not in the severe group.

There was no significant difference in ulnar nerve electrophysiologic parameters at the elbow level in the patient group neither regarding initial and latter affected sides nor regarding mild and severe groups and disease duration.

4. Discussion

In our study, we found the frequency of CTS as 16.12% is significantly prominent in older and more severe patients. A remarkable result was that CTS was bilateral among the two-thirds of the patients. As the prevalence of CTS in the general population has been reported to be 125 to 220 per 100000 [12], ratios mentioned above were significantly higher, calling attention to median neuropathy in PD. Similarly, Yucel et al. [4] found frequency of CTS as 24.4% electrophysiologically in their study where they reported a larger median nerve cross-sectional area sonographically in the severe PD patients. The anatomical site, wrist, was also evaluated in PD patients sonographically by Yang et al. [3] and median nerve cross-sectional area indicating median nerve swelling with edema was found to be larger ($p < 0.05$) in concordance with tremor severity due to the cumulative injury. In our study, although CTS was more prominent in patients suffering more severe disease, tremor and rigidity were not found to be contributing factors to median neuropathy evolution.

Rigidity, defined as a hypertonic state with increased resistance within the range of movement about a joint [13], may lead to tendon contractures and atrophy [14] and trigger the characteristic limb posture called striatal deformity accompanied by flexion at the elbow, ulnar deviation at the wrist, flexion at the metacarpophalangeal joints, and extension at the interphalangeal joints in varying severity [8]. Moreover, repetitive movement of the elbow superimposed by rest tremor at the wrist causes a narrowing of the tunnel and constriction of the nerve initiating a cycle of inflammation and oedema and increases the strain. The cubital tunnel cross-sectional area narrows by up to 55% as intraneural pressures increase up to 20-fold [15]. We confirmed ulnar neuropathy electrophysiologically as 3.22% in PD group whereas the incidence of the ulnar neuropathy (cubital tunnel syndrome) in the general population has been reported as 24.7 per 100.000 [16]. However, we did not find any association between neither rigidity and tremor severity nor H&Y scores and disease duration and ulnar neuropathy existence.

Our study's patient population (mean age 65.93 ± 10.58) and age-gender matched control group (mean age 62.03 ± 10.40, $p = 0.145$) consisted of elderly patients. We compared the mean indices of electrophysiologic parameters among each group for any subclinical involvement. Axonal degeneration causes decreased amplitude values whereas loose myelin causes prolonged distal motor latency and decreased sensorial nerve conduction velocities electrophysiologically in the peripheral nerves [17]. In regard to this, in the patient group, we evaluated significant median and ulnar demyelination at the wrist bilaterally and a tendency to ulnar nerve entrapment at the elbow being significant at the left and probable at the right. Advancing age factor in the development of entrapment neuropathy was excluded in the study population ($p = 0.145$). We call attention to the tendency of median and ulnar neuropathy in the PD group.

In our study, there was a relationship between median and ulnar nerve demyelination with both mild tremor and rigidity groups and mild H&Y group. As Parkinson's disease is progressive, mild symptomatology in the abovementioned groups confirms that these patients are at the early stages of the disease. Evidence suggests that peripheral nervous system involvement, sometimes occurring before clinical diagnosis, might be discussed as an intrinsic peripheral neuropathy before spreading of neurodegeneration to the central nervous system (CNS) [2]. Lewy body inclusions have been reported to be present both in the basal ganglia and in the peripheral nervous system [2]. Moreover, neuronal loss due to alpha-synuclein deposition, impaired axonal transport, and mitochondrial dysfunction causing neuronal death in the brain is being discussed as pathomechanisms of the neurodegenerative process in PD [2]. Doppler et al. [18] found alpha-synuclein deposition in cutaneous nerves of PD patients and speculated that both retrograde axonal degeneration due to impaired axonal transport and anterograde degeneration due to sensory neuronal cell death may lead to peripheral neuropathy and suggested that skin biopsy might be a useful diagnostic test for PD. Wang et al. [19] reported alpha-synuclein deposits in skin nerve fibers and suggested the possibility of a disease related peripheral neurodegeneration in PD.

Our results indicating no association with tremor and rigidity severity and mononeuropathy evolution are in accordance with the findings that in each individual PD patient suffering from different tremor and rigidity severity asymmetrically no difference was found in median and ulnar nerve neural transmission electrophysiologically. By this way, we excluded the extrinsic factors such as levodopa medication and intrinsic factors such as disease duration in each patient and had the opportunity to focus on symptom severity and asymmetry only.

In chronic demyelinating neuropathies, neuropathic tremor was reported in antagonist muscle pairs with a frequency of 3 to 6 Hz [20] which is similar to rest tremor. It has been proposed that distortion of the peripheral sensory input and feedback to the CNS, as the result of demyelination, leads to mismatch in spindle and tendon organ afferents and errors in the timing of muscle activity generated within the CNS [20, 21]. The tremor is most dominant in the upper extremities. As evaluated in our study, the demyelination of median and ulnar nerves especially at the wrist level might be an additive factor for tremor generation in the hands.

We observed median and ulnar demyelination at the wrist level in patients suffering from the disease for a longer period. The patients with a longer disease duration were not older than the ones with a shorter disease period ($p = 0.104$). In our study population, the mean of disease duration was calculated as 6 years statistically. In the literature, peripheral neuropathy with the advanced disease is mostly related with cumulative levodopa intake [2]. Chronic levodopa intake has been reported to increase homocysteine and reduce vit B12 serum levels suggesting a pharmacotoxic cause due to interactions of levodopa metabolism with the methylation pathways of vit B12. While polyneuropathy occurs mostly gradually and in subclinical form in patients on oral levodopa therapy, more severe acute/subacute forms were reported with enteral levodopa usage [2]. The question that is longer disease duration prone to polyneuropathy related to cumulative levodopa intake or is there a critic period when intrinsic factors contribute to polyneuropathy is open to discussion.

This study had some limitations. First, it will be necessary to validate these findings in a larger cohort. Second, as per this study, we aimed to evaluate if symptom severity has an additive effect on mononeuropathy generation; we did not focus on cumulative levodopa intake; and total time levodopa has been used.

In conclusion, this is the first study investigating symptom severity regarding tremor and rigidity as a potential risk for mononeuropathy generation in each individual patient. Although our results did not support the hypothesis that severity of rigidity and tremor might contribute to mononeuropathy evolution, we draw attention to disease related intrinsic factors in peripheral neurodegeneration. As PD has been proven to be a systemic disease not only related to CNS, future large-scale longitudinal studies focusing on pathophysiology of peripheral neurodegeneration in PD will provide a better understanding of the disease and will guide the clinician while applying patient specific therapeutic options in PD.

Competing Interests

The authors declare that there is no conflict of interests regarding the publication of this paper.

Acknowledgments

The authors wish to thank Dr. Zubeyde Ayturk and Dr. Onur Serdar Gencler for excellent technical assistance.

References

[1] A. J. Lees, J. Hardy, and T. Revesz, "Parkinson's disease," *The Lancet*, vol. 373, no. 9680, pp. 2055–2066, 2009.

[2] G. Cossu and M. Melis, "The peripheral nerve involvement in Parkinson Disease: a multifaceted phenomenon," *Parkinsonism & Related Disorders*, vol. 25, pp. 17–20, 2016.

[3] S. N. Yang, H. J. Kang, J. S. Yoon, S. J. Won, W.-K. Seo, and S. B. Koh, "Is median nerve enlargement at the wrist associated with tremor in Parkinson disease?" *Journal of Ultrasound in Medicine*, vol. 33, no. 12, pp. 2079–2083, 2014.

[4] A. Yucel, O. Yilmaz, S. Babaoglu, M. Acar, and B. Degirmenci, "Sonographic findings of the median nerve and prevalence of carpal tunnel syndrome in patients with Parkinson's disease," *European Journal of Radiology*, vol. 67, no. 3, pp. 546–550, 2008, Erratum to *European Journal of Radiology*, vol. 68, no. 3, pp. 499–502, 2008.

[5] P. Gortvai, "Deformities of the hands and feet in Parkinsonism and their reversibility by operation," *Journal of Neurology, Neurosurgery, and Psychiatry*, vol. 26, pp. 33–36, 1963.

[6] G. Mengi-Ozsarac, "Carpal tunnel syndrome in Parkinsons disease," *European Journal of Radiology*, vol. 67, article 550, 2008.

[7] A. J. Hughes, S. E. Daniel, L. Kilford, and A. J. Lees, "Accuracy of clinical diagnosis of idiopathic Parkinson's disease: a clinico-pathological study of 100 cases," *Journal of Neurology Neurosurgery and Psychiatry*, vol. 55, no. 3, pp. 181–184, 1992.

[8] M. M. Hoehn and M. D. Yahr, "Parkinsonism: onset, progression, and mortality," *Neurology*, vol. 17, no. 5, pp. 427–442, 1967.

[9] Movement Disorder Society Task Force on Rating Scales for Parkinson's Disease, "The unified Parkinson's disease rating scale (UPDRS): status and recommendations," *Movement Disorders*, vol. 18, pp. 738–750, 2003.

[10] C. K. Jablecki, M. T. Andary, M. K. Floeter et al., "Practice parameter: electrodiagnostic studies in carpal tunnel syndrome," *Neurology*, vol. 58, no. 11, pp. 1589–1592, 2002.

[11] C. K. Jablecki, M. T. Andary, M. K. Floeter et al., "Practice Parameter: electrodiagnostic studies in carpal tunnel syndrome. Report of the American Association of Electrodiagnostic Medicine, American Academy of Neurology and the American Academy of Physical Medicine and Rehabilitation," *Neurology*, vol. 58, pp. 1589–1592, 2002.

[12] D. M. Dawson, "Entrapment neuropathies of the upper extremities," *The New England Journal of Medicine*, vol. 329, no. 27, pp. 2013–2018, 1993.

[13] G. Deuschl, P. Bain, and M. Brin, "Consensus statement of the Movement Disorder Society on Tremor. Ad Hoc Scientific Committee," *Movement Disorders*, vol. 13, supplement 3, pp. 2–23, 1998.

[14] D. Riley, A. E. Lang, R. D. G. Blair, A. Birnbaum, and B. Reid, "Frozen shoulder and other shoulder disturbances in Parkinson's disease," *Journal of Neurology Neurosurgery and Psychiatry*, vol. 52, no. 1, pp. 63–66, 1989.

[15] C.-O. Werner, P. Ohlin, and D. Elmqvist, "Pressures recorded in ulnar neuropathy," *Acta Orthopaedica*, vol. 56, no. 5, pp. 404–406, 1985.

[16] R. M. van Rijn, B. M. A. Huisstede, B. W. Koes, and A. Burdorf, "Associations between work-related factors and specific disorders at the elbow: a systematic literature review," *Rheumatology*, vol. 48, no. 5, pp. 528–536, 2009.

[17] D. Rempel, L. Dahlin, and G. Lundborg, "Pathophysiology of nerve compression syndromes: response of peripheral nerves to loading," *The Journal of Bone & Joint Surgery—American Volume*, vol. 81, no. 11, pp. 1600–1610, 1999.

[18] K. Doppler, S. Ebert, N. Üçeyler et al., "Cutaneous neuropathy in Parkinson's disease: a window into brain pathology," *Acta Neuropathologica*, vol. 128, no. 1, pp. 99–109, 2014.

[19] N. Wang, C. H. Gibbons, J. Lafo, and B. S. R. Freeman, "α-synuclein in cutaneous autonomic nerves," *Neurology*, vol. 81, no. 18, pp. 1604–1610, 2013.

[20] P. G. Bain, T. C. Britton, I. H. Jenkins et al., "Tremor associated with benign IgM paraproteinaemic neuropathy," *Brain*, vol. 119, no. 3, pp. 789–799, 1996.

[21] I. S. Smith, "The natural history of chronic demyelinating neuropathy associated with benign IgM paraproteinaemia: a clinical and neurophysiological study," *Brain*, vol. 117, no. 5, pp. 949–957, 1994.

5

Deep Brain Stimulation in Parkinson's Disease: New and Emerging Targets for Refractory Motor and Nonmotor Symptoms

Dustin Anderson, Grayson Beecher, and Fang Ba

Department of Medicine, University of Alberta, Edmonton, AB, Canada T6G 2G3

Correspondence should be addressed to Fang Ba; fb@ualberta.ca

Academic Editor: Aparna Wagle Shukla

Parkinson's disease (PD) is a progressive neurodegenerative condition characterized by bradykinesia, tremor, rigidity, and postural instability (PI), in addition to numerous nonmotor manifestations. Many pharmacological therapies now exist to successfully treat PD motor symptoms; however, as the disease progresses, it often becomes challenging to treat with medications alone. Deep brain stimulation (DBS) has become a crucial player in PD treatment, particularly for patients who have disabling motor complications from medical treatment. Well-established DBS targets include the subthalamic nucleus (STN), the globus pallidus pars interna (GPi), and to a lesser degree the ventral intermediate nucleus (VIM) of the thalamus. Studies of alternative DBS targets for PD are ongoing, the majority of which have shown some clinical benefit; however, more carefully designed and controlled studies are needed. In the present review, we discuss the role of these new and emerging DBS targets in treating refractory axial motor symptoms and other motor and nonmotor symptoms (NMS).

1. Introduction

Parkinson's disease (PD) is a common neurodegenerative condition. Many successful pharmacological therapies and strategies have been developed to treat both the motor and nonmotor manifestations of PD; however, as PD progresses it often becomes intractably difficult to treat, typically as a result of motor complications related to treatment. Since the seminal study by Benabid et al. targeting the ventral intermediate nucleus (VIM) of the thalamus [1], deep brain stimulation (DBS) has emerged as a key player in the treatment of PD. Multiple randomized controlled studies have demonstrated subthalamic nucleus- (STN-) and globus pallidus interna- (GPi-) DBS to be superior to medical treatment alone in treating a number of the cardinal symptoms and motor complications from therapy [1–3]. The benefit of DBS on axial symptoms is less clear. Several reports have indicated improvement of posture, gait, and balance control after STN- or GPi-DBS, when these symptoms were responsive to levodopa treatment before DBS surgery [4–9]; however, the benefit on postural instability (PI) and gait is not sustained [4]. Moreover, it has been noted that a significant number of patients report postoperative worsening of gait, despite concurrent improvement in motor scores and global outcomes after bilateral STN-DBS. Further, fall risk has been demonstrated to increase and levodopa-resistant freezing of gait (FoG) persists or worsens [10–16]. The axial domains of speech [17–19] and swallowing [20, 21] have also shown to be impacted by DBS. To complicate matters further, stimulation parameters (i.e., high frequency stimulation) can also lead to adverse axial effects in patients. These disparities in outcome have fueled the exploration for novel DBS targets that may prove beneficial at treating the axial motor symptoms of PD. In addition to refractory axial motor symptoms, it is clear that nonmotor symptoms (NMS) can also become particularly troublesome [22], as PD progresses and increases in severity. NMS have a significant impact on prognosis and quality of life [23], again highlighting the need for alternative DBS targets that will have therapeutic benefit not only for refractory motor symptoms, but for NMS in PD as well.

In the present review, we discuss new and emerging DBS targets currently being investigated for the treatment of refractory motor symptoms and NMS in PD. These targets include the pedunculopontine nucleus (PPN), the caudal zona incerta (ZI), the substantia nigra (SN) pars reticulate (SNr) (Figure 1), the motor cortex, and other less explored targets.

2. New and Emerging DBS Targets for Refractory Motor Symptoms

2.1. Refractory Tremor. For tremor-dominant PD, where severe and disabling tremor is refractory to treatment, VIM-DBS has been shown to suppress tremor effectively. In addition, STN- and GPi-DBS both provide sustained benefit for PD resting tremor. For severe tremor and coexisting essential tremor, DBS leads implanted in the posterior aspect of the GPi or STN (i.e., ZI region bordering the STN) appear to be of benefit [23].

2.1.1. Caudal Zona Incerta. The ZI is a small heterogeneous cellular nucleus that lies within the anatomical location termed the posterior subthalamic area (PSA) [24, 25]. The borders of the PSA include the posterior border of the STN anteriorly, the dorsal SN inferiorly, the ventral thalamic nuclei superiorly, the anterolateral red nucleus posteromedially, the medial lemniscus posteriorly, and the internal capsule laterally [24, 25]. The rostral ZI lies along the dorsal and medial STN, while the caudal ZI (cZI) is located posteromedially to the STN [26] (Figure 1(b)). Various functions of the ZI have been postulated throughout the literature; however, it is commonly held that the ZI plays a role in visceral function, arousal, attention, and posture and locomotion, with the cZI mediating the latter [26]. The cZI has widespread afferent and efferent projections amongst the cerebral cortex, diencephalon, brainstem, cerebellum, and spinal cord, the majority of which are GABAergic [26]. While its circuitry remains complex and poorly understood, it is postulated that the cZI may act as an integrator within and between the basal ganglia-thalamocortical loop and the cerebellothalamocortical loop, assisting in the synchronization of oscillatory neuronal firing in both of these pathways [27]. Abnormalities in oscillatory neuronal synchronization that are generated along either of these loops or at the level of the cZI are thought to play a major role in the generation of tremor [24, 25, 27].

The benefit of cZI-DBS for tremor control has been well established in studies investigating its role in essential tremor [28]. In PD, the majority of information that has been gleaned regarding the cZI has come from lesional studies. It has previously been shown that subthalamotomy including the region of the ZI can lead to clinical improvement in PD [29]. Subsequent work focusing on the ZI and the cZI has led to significant discoveries regarding the promise of this structure as a DBS target in PD [24, 25]. The relevance of the cZI as a DBS target in PD was brought to the forefront by Plaha et al., in their study comparing motor outcomes amongst three DBS targets: the cZI, the posterodorsal STN, and dorsomedial/medial STN [30]. When compared to STN stimulation, unilateral cZI stimulation with mean frequency of 150 Hz led to greater improvement in tremor control and overall Unified Parkinson's Disease Rating Scale (UPDRS) motor scores.

A subsequent longitudinal, observational study by Plaha et al. again demonstrated the utility of cZI-DBS (bilateral, 145 Hz) in reducing parkinsonian tremor, as well as a variety of other tremor types, including cerebellar outflow, essential, and dystonic tremor at 12 months of follow-up [27]. Recent work by Blomstedt et al., in an open labeled study with 18 months of follow-up [23–25], echoed the results of Plaha et al. [27], demonstrating the benefit of unilateral cZI-DBS with mean frequency of 160 Hz in the treatment of contralateral, severe parkinsonian tremor. The benefit on rigidity and bradykinesia was not as profound as in STN-DBS; however, a number of studies have suggested that cZI-DBS has a lower incidence of speech deterioration and is associated with better neuropsychological outcomes [27, 31]. That being said, cZI-DBS is not as well established as STN- or GPi-DBS in PD. Further larger scale studies are required to guide future target selection.

2.1.2. Centromedian and Parafascicular Nuclei. The centromedian and parafascicular nuclei (CMPf) (Figure 1(c)) are the two main constituents of the intralaminar nucleus of the thalamus and have several connections within the basal ganglia, with projections to the STN, substantia nigra (SN), and GPi [32]. It has been postulated that CMPf-DBS affects other thalamic components [ventralis oralis anterior (VOA) and VIM] whose role in tremor control has been well established [33, 34].

Interest in the CMPf as a DBS target resurfaced following the observation by Krauss et al. that stimulation of CMPf appeared to abolish resting tremor in 1 patient and involuntary choreoathetotic and dyskinetic movements in 2 others [35]. In subsequent reports, it was observed that CMPf stimulation, independent of STN stimulation, led to reduction of tremor-related muscle activity in 2 patients with PD [36, 37]. Additionally, they demonstrated better tremor control compared with STN-DBS alone. Mazzone et al. [38] demonstrated that combination of CMPf- and GPi-DBS reduced UPDRS III scores by 49.9%, a value significantly different when compared to CMPf or GPi stimulation alone. Unfortunately, tremor control was not specified within the study. Further studies should help clarify whether CMPf stimulation is superior to VIM-DBS for tremor control in PD.

2.2. Refractory Axial Motor Symptoms-Gait and Balance. FoG, in addition to other gait disturbances such as decreased stride length and gait variability, is associated with increased fall risk in patients with PD [50]. These symptoms are typically refractory to therapy, including STN- and GPi-DBS [51, 52], and are thus a significant source of morbidity in PD [53]. The pathophysiology and neuropathological substrates underlying FoG remain largely unknown. FoG may be due to a failure to adequately scale amplitudes for the intended movement [54] and/or defective motor programming by the supplementary motor area (SMA) and its maintenance by the basal ganglia, leading to a mismatch between intention and automation [54].

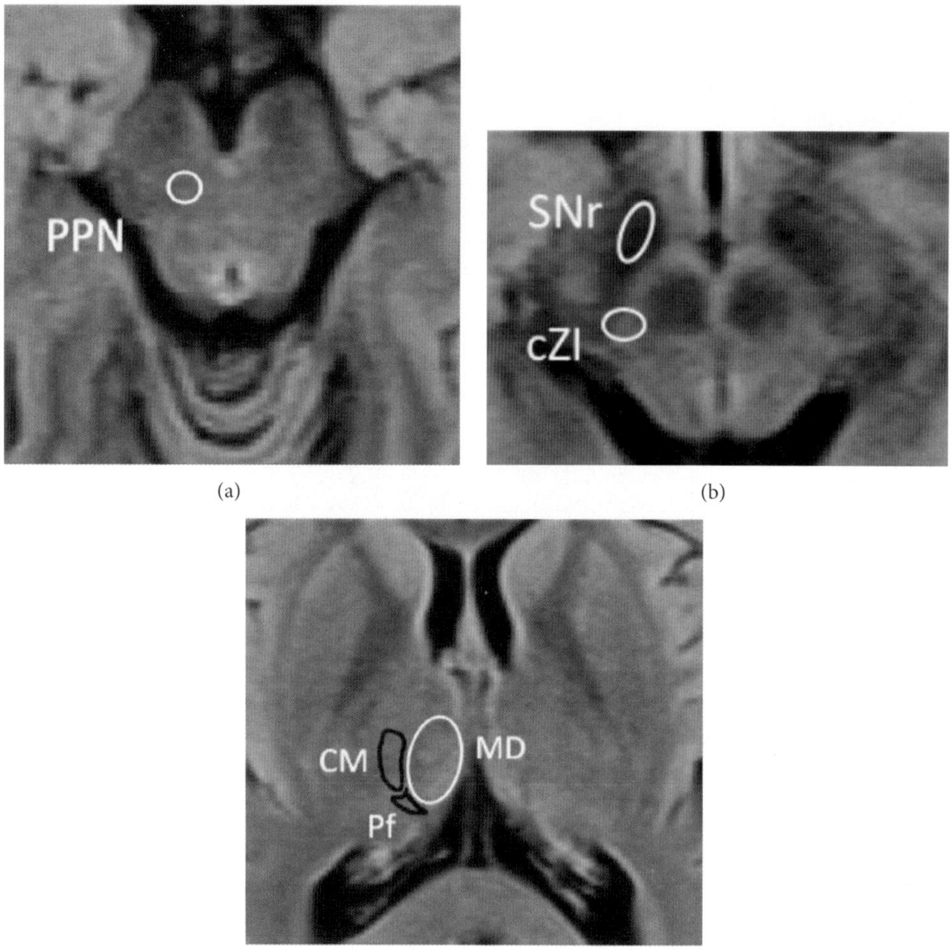

FIGURE 1: Axial MRI imaging at the level of the midbrain and thalamus, demonstrating the anatomical locations of DBS targets described in the review. CMPf, centromedian-parafascicular nuclear complex; cZI, caudal zona incerta; PPN, pedunculopontine nucleus; SNr, substantia nigra pars reticulata.

2.2.1. Pedunculopontine Nucleus. The mesencephalic locomotor region (MLR) appears critical for normal gait function [61]. The PPN is a key component of the MLR [62] (Figure 1(a)). Widespread projections involving the PPN include direct glutamatergic inputs from the motor cortex and GABAergic inputs from SNr, GPi, STN, and deep nuclei of the cerebellum. Ascending efferent projections target GPi, SN pars compacta [63], and thalamus. Descending efferent projections target pontine and medullary reticular formations, as well as spinal cord structures vital to the control of muscle tone and locomotion. The PPN appears to play a key role in the initiation, acceleration, deceleration, and termination of locomotion through connections to the basal ganglia and higher cortical regions [61]. PPN neuronal loss is evident in PD [64]. Ways to modulate PPN connectivity and activity have proven elusive. Acetylcholinesterase inhibitors may affect the PPN but effects are likely modest.

Jenkinson et al. were the first group to demonstrate the efficacy of PPN-DBS, in a 1-methyl-4-phenyl-1,2,3,6-tetrahydropyridine- (MPTP-) exposed macaque [65]. Following MPTP exposure, unilateral PPN stimulation was equivalent to levodopa in improving motor activity scores [65]. In 2005, 2 case studies were the first to establish the safety and efficacy of PPN-DBS in humans [39, 40] (Table 1), demonstrating improvements in UPDRS motor scores. Subsequently, a study by Plaha and Gill was the first to show the role of PPN-DBS in improving gait dysfunction and PI in PD [40]. Multiple open labeled PPN-DBS studies have demonstrated clinical improvement in patients with PD, although results have been variable [41, 42, 45, 47] (Table 1). Additional open labeled studies from Thevathasan et al. [45, 46, 66, 67] demonstrated that PPN stimulation (20–35 Hz) improved frequency of falls in PD patients with severe FoG and PI during the "on" state [45]. One study showed improvement in gait and falls questionnaire score but not UPDRS III score in 5 patients with PD implanted with bilateral PPN electrodes [46]. The first double-blinded assessment of PPN-DBS was performed by Ferraye and colleagues [43], demonstrating improvement in FoG but not PI or overall UPDRS scores. The lack of improvement in global motor function and axial symptoms, other than FoG, was in opposition to previous studies (Table 1) [39–41, 46, 48]. Moro

Table 1: Summary of studies on PD patients implanted with PPN-DBS for gait and balance impairment.

Study	Number of Patients	Inclusion criteria	Study design	Stimulation target	Stimulation parameters	Outcomes	Adverse events	Comments
Mazzone et al. [39]	2	FoG	Open label	Bilateral PPN	Bipolar; 10 Hz	Intraoperative improvement of UPDRS III score	NR	First human study to demonstrate the potential efficacy of PPN-DBS in PD
Plaha and Gill [40]	2	FoG, PI, and frequent falls	Open label	Bilateral PPN	Bipolar; 20–25 Hz	UPDRS improved by 53%; UPDRS III by 57%	Certain stimulation frequencies can exacerbate gait	Short follow-up, 42 days for patient 1 and 16 days for patient 2
Stefani et al. [41]	6	FoG, 3 had "on" FoG, UPDRS-III > 70, and levodopa-induced dyskinesias	Open label	Bilateral STN and PPN	Bipolar; 25 Hz at PPN	PPN stimulation showed more benefit on posture and gait items compared to STN stimulation; UPDRS III improved by 32%; axial symptoms (UPDRS 27–30) by 60%	Paresthesia	Total length of study was 6 months; noted decline in motor benefit; trend of improved UPDRS scores with both STN and PPN stimulation
Strafella et al. [42]	1	Advanced PD, FoG, PI	Open label	Unilateral PPN	70 Hz	UPDRS improved by 19%, mainly in relation to gait, tremor, and bradykinesia	NR	PET studies showed increased rCBF in different subcortical areas, most notably in the thalamus bilaterally
Ferraye et al. [43]	6	Severe FoG unresponsive to levodopa and STN stimulation	Double-blinded assessment	Bilateral STN and PPN	Bipolar; 15–25 Hz	Only FoG showed clear improvement; gait and PI scores did not improve; falls unrelated to FoG were unchanged in 5/6	Seizure in 1 patient; stimulation frequency dependent oscillopsia; paresthesias; limb myoclonus	The total length of the study was 1 year; objective improvement of FoG in 2 patients
Moro et al. [44]	6	Age < 70, severe "off" FoG and PI; no dementia	Double-blinded assessment	Unilateral PPN	Bipolar; chronic stimulation frequency of 67 Hz	Improvement in UPDRS item 13 (falling) by 75% at 3 and 12 months	Stimulation frequency dependent oscillopsia and paresthesias	First double-blinded study to investigate unilateral PPN stimulation; total study length was 1 year
Thevathasan et al. [45]	11	Severe FoG and PI, in addition to falls both in the "on" and "off" states	Open label	Bilateral PPN in 8 patients, bilateral PPN and ZI in 2 patients, and unilateral PPN and bilateral ZI in 1 patient	Bipolar; 20–35 Hz	Improvement in frequency of falls and gait	NR	Follow-up 3–38 months
Thevathasan et al. [46]	5	Severe FoG and PI, in addition to falls persisting in the "on" state	Open label	Bilateral PPN	Monopolar; 35 Hz; PPN target more caudal than previous	Improvement in all by FoG and falls questionnaire at 3 months and 2 years	Stimulation frequency dependent decline in motor function and gait; oscillopsia	Total study length was 2 years; assessments at 3 months and 2 years
Khan et al. [47]	7	PD patients with severe FoG, PI, falls during "on" and "off" states	Open label	Bilateral PPN, in combination with cZi stimulation	Bipolar; 60 Hz (PPN)	Improvement in UPDRS III score (18.8%) and axial symptoms score (26.3%)	Akinesia in 2 patients	Follow-up 12 months; similar benefit with ZI stimulation versus ZI and PPN "on"

Table 1: Continued.

Study	Number of Patients	Inclusion criteria	Study design	Stimulation target	Stimulation parameters	Outcomes	Adverse events	Comments
Thevathasan et al. [48]	7	PI, severe FoG, and falls during "on" state	Open label	5 bilateral and 2 unilateral	Bipolar; 35 Hz	Improvement in freezing of gait questionnaire, turn task duration, and cadence	NR	First study to directly compare unilateral versus bilateral stimulation; less robust result in unilateral PPN
Mazzone et al. [49]	28	24 patients had PD and 4 had PSP	Open label	Both bilateral (6) and unilateral (22) PPN	Bipolar; unilateral (40 Hz) and bilateral (25 Hz)	Improvement in UPDRS III score in "off" medication and "on" stimulation	None	The largest and longest study of PPN DBS to date with a mean follow-up of 3.8 years; included patients from prior studies

FoG, freezing of gait; NR, not reported; PD, Parkinson's disease; PET, positron emission tomography; PI, postural instability; PPN, pedunculopontine nucleus; PSP, progressive supranuclear palsy; rCBF, regional cerebral; STN, subthalamic nucleus; UPDRS, United Parkinson Disease Rating Scale; ZI, zona incerta.

et al. were the first to investigate the role of unilateral\PPN-DBS in a double-blinded study of 6 patients with PD [44]. At study end period (1 year), UPDRS item 13 (falling) showed 75% improvement, with no statistically significant changes in other motor domains. Furthermore, bilateral stimulation proved more effective than unilateral stimulation [48].

The largest study with the longest follow-up of PPN-DBS in PD was reported by Mazzone et al. [49, 68, 69]. A total of 24 patients with PD and 4 with progressive supranuclear palsy (PSP) [49] were followed for a mean follow-up of 3.8 years. At study end period, they demonstrated an improvement in UPDRS III scores and in axial symptoms (UPDRS items 27–30) (off levodopa therapy); however, no difference was detected between the "on" medication and "off" stimulation state and the "off" medication and "on" stimulation state.

Connectivity to and from the MLR/PPN appears critical for normal gait function and is likely a factor in FoG as well. Structural deficits in connectivity are evident between the basal ganglia and PPN, in addition to other tracts in patients with FoG [70, 71]. Functional connectivity studies suggest that FoG patients may have significantly stronger connectivity between the PPN and supplementary motor area (SMA) [70], possibly reflecting maladaptive compensatory mechanisms. The integrity of these tracts has not been studied in patients who have undergone PPN-DBS. The variability of this deficit in structural and functional connectivity to and from the PPN may at least partially explain the variable results within the literature. In addition, the PPN tends to be spatially diffuse in humans and microelectrode recording is not helpful intraoperatively, thus making precise lead placement difficult and potentially contributing to further variability from study to study.

The experience and results with PPN-DBS are in their infancy. More precise targeting strategies with improved technology (i.e., improved imaging and programming) are required. It remains to be seen whether PPN-DBS should be an adjunct target to STN- or GPi-DBS for better overall motor control.

2.2.2. Combined Pedunculopontine Nucleus and Caudal Zona Incerta Stimulation. Khan et al. investigated the effects of bilateral PPN-DBS and caudal cZI-DBS in a blinded study of 7 patients with PD [47]. The authors demonstrated an 18.8% improvement in UPDRS III score and a 26.3% improvement in axial symptoms (items 27–30 on UPDRS III) of levodopa therapy. However, the same subscore was only significantly reduced in the "on" medication state when the PPN and cZI were stimulated in concert. This study suggested that, with these stimulation parameters, PPN stimulation alone was insufficient in improving "on" medication and resistant axial symptoms and that costimulation of cZI could provide an additive, beneficial role.

2.2.3. Substantia Nigra Pars Reticulata. The SN is a dense, laterally oriented collection of dopaminergic and GABAergic neurons located within the ventral midbrain, just dorsal to the corticospinal and corticobulbar tracts, ventral to the red nuclei, and lateral to the ventral tegmental area [72]. Its 2 components, the SNr and SNc [63], have traditionally been considered the major output and input nuclei, respectively, of the basal ganglia. While there is fair overlap, the SNr lies ventrally and laterally to the SNc in the midbrain [73]. In the classically held framework of basal ganglia circuitry, facilitation of movement was felt to be achieved through activation of a direct pathway from striatum to output nuclei (SNr and GPi), while inhibition of movement occurred through excitation of an indirect pathway (through globus pallidus externus and STN) [72]; however, recent advances in modeling of striatonigral-thalamocortical pathways have made it clear that while the classical model of basal ganglia circuitry provides a solid foundation for the understanding of its complex interconnections, it hardly captures its complete intricacies [72].

The SNr is another key player in the MLR, via its significant efferent GABAergic input to the PPN [74]. Efferents from the lateral SNr to the PPN are felt to modulate postural tone, while its medial efferents projecting to the cuneiform nucleus of the MLR influence locomotion [74]. It may not then be surprising that axial motor symptomatology, including gait impairment and PI, in patients with PD has shown favorable response to SNr stimulation in the literature [55–57, 75] (Table 2). Significant improvements in UPDRS III axial motor subscores and braking capacity, but not in distal motor symptoms (segmental akinesia, limb rigidity, and tremor), have been observed previously with SNr-DBS [55]. In contrast, one of the more recent double-blind, cross-over, randomized controlled trials with combined STN and SNr stimulation did show significant improvement in FoG, but not in other axial symptoms when compared to STN-DBS alone [56]. With SNr-DBS, one should be cautious about the possibility of worsening akinesia, as increased immobility and recurrent falls were reported in 1 patient in the same study during the last week of follow-up under combined STN and SNr stimulation [56].

While some benefit from SN stimulation has been reported, significant and variable impacts on mood and behavior can occur, likely owing to its limbic projections [76, 77]. Reports of acute depression [78, 79], hypomania [77], and mania [76, 80] secondary to high frequency SN stimulation are evident in the literature. While it is difficult to rule out STN participation in the provocation of mood symptoms, it is clear that stimulation of more ventrally placed leads within the SN and likely the SNr can preferentially elicit these symptoms.

2.2.4. Motor Cortex. Extradural motor cortex stimulation (EMCS) has been studied as another treatment modality in PD, particularly for those patients with advanced PD who are poor surgical candidates [81–86]. The primary motor cortex is a key component of corticobasal ganglia loops and thus forms a potential therapeutic target in PD [87]. Tremor and rigidity in PD can be suppressed by EMCS [58, 88], and benefit has been seen in advanced PD [82, 83]. Since initial reports, numerous studies have investigated the role of EMCS for the treatment of advanced PD, with variable results [58–60, 84, 86, 89–91] (Table 2).

Table 2: Summary of studies on PD patients implanted with novel DBS targets (SNr, motor cortex, CMPf) for gait and balance impairment.

Study	Study subjects/inclusion criteria	Study design	Effect on FoG/PI/falls	Motor effects	Comments
			SNr		
Chastan et al. [55]	7 patients with levodopa and STN-DBS. At least one contact of each electrode was located within the SNr	Open label	Significant improvements in UPDRS III axial motor subscores and in braking capacity	No improvement in motor symptoms (segmental akinesia, limb rigidity, and tremor)	No specific criteria for axial involvement
Weiss et al. [56]	12 patients, with combined STN and SNr stimulation; axial UPDRS ≥ 12; advance PD patients with gait/balance impairment; refractory to medical treatment	Double-blind, cross-over, randomized controlled trial	With combined STN and SNr stimulation improvement in FoG at the 3-week follow-up	No global effect on axial motor domains; no benefit for segmental motor functions	Immediate assessment and 3-week follow-up; long term effects unclear
Brosius et al. [57]	1 patient with advance PD, severe FoG; unilateral STN/SNr stimulation	Case report	Significantly improved FoG in a patient with advanced PD, using interleaving setting		Contralateral STN, the more severe side with STN/SNr
			Motor cortex		
Pagni et al. [58]	41 patients with advanced PD; not DBS candidates, Hoehn-Yahr III–V; unilateral lead over hand area of motor cortex	Open label	Improvement in standing, gait, and motor performance; significant improvement in UPDRS axial scores	Improved "off" medication UPDRS-III; not significant for "on" medication score	Sustained improvement of quality of life measures through 3-year follow-up
Cilia et al. [59]	5 patients with advanced PD	Open label	Subjective improvement of axial symptomatology	No quantifiable clinical benefit at 6 months	Small sample size; subjective improvement only
Fasano et al. [60]	1 patient with severe PD who was unable to stand from sitting without assistance	Case report	Able to stand without assistance, with improvement in both axial akinesia and walking		Case report; short lasting benefit (5 months)
			CMPf		
Mazzone et al. [38]	6 PD patients with disabling FoG, with GPi and CMPf-DBS	Open label	CMPf activation was more efficacious on freezing of gait	A significant amelioration of UPDRS scores was achieved	Small sample size; observation of CMPf stimulation alone may not control PD motor symptoms adequately

CMPf, centromedian-parafascicular nuclear complex; FoG, freezing of gait; GPi, globus pallidus, internal segment; PD, Parkinson disease; PI, postural instability; SNr, substantia nigra pars reticulata; STN, subthalamic nucleus; UPDRS, United Parkinson Disease Rating Scale.

The largest study of EMCS in 41 patients with advanced PD (not eligible for DBS) showed improvement in standing, gait, and motor performance [58], though these results were not supported by other studies [59, 60, 91]. Additional studies have shown that EMCS improved quality of life parameters and modestly reduced levodopa dose but did not improve UPDRS III scores or axial symptoms [90, 92].

2.2.5. Centromedian and Parafascicular Nuclei. A single study demonstrated that CMPf stimulation alone led to significantly reduced FoG, where GPi stimulation alone did not [38]; however, this study had a sample size of only 6 patients. The authors further observed that CMPf stimulation alone may not control PD motor symptoms adequately. This observation raised the possibility of multiple-target stimulation strategy to optimize axial symptoms and overall motor control in PD.

2.3. Refractory Axial Symptoms-Speech and Swallowing. To date, no convincing evidence has demonstrated improvements in speech or swallowing in PD with STN- or GPi-DBS. Speech and swallowing can worsen with DBS surgery or programming. Research on the impact of cZI-DBS on associated motor symptomatology in PD has also taken place. Particular focus in the literature has been given to the effects of cZI-DBS on speech and its related domains. Stimulation of cZI was shown to have a deleterious effect on voice intensity when compared to STN-DBS [93], while articulatory precision of speech also worsens in patients receiving cZI-DBS [94]. Significant impairment in verbal fluency is also observed in the immediate postoperative period; however, this deficit does not maintain significance in the long term [95]. Speech intelligibility has been demonstrated to be significantly reduced in cZI-DBS patients speaking from a read-speech passage [96]; however, this effect was not reproduced when evaluated from spontaneous speech at 1 year postoperatively, suggesting that the impact of cZI-DBS on speech intelligibility may have initially been overstated [97]. While STN-DBS has beneficial effects on pitch variability and range, cZI-DBS displayed no such benefit in a small study of 16 patients with 1-year follow-up [98]. The effect of cZI-DBS on swallowing dysfunction has also been evaluated in 2 longitudinal, prospective studies of 8 and 9 patients [99, 100]. Both studies demonstrated that cZI-DBS did not have a clinically significant impact on either swallowing function or self-reported swallowing-specific quality of life at 1 year postoperatively. Further studies should help clarify the effect of cZI-DBS on both speech and swallowing dysfunction. In 1 study of EMCS in advanced PD, Pagni et al. demonstrated improved speech and swallowing in patients who are not DBS candidates [58].

Speech and swallowing symptoms following DBS have yet to be defined within the current literature. Methodology in assessing the symptoms varies from study to study. Severity of dysarthria/dysphagia preoperatively, duration and severity of disease, and positioning of the electrode(s) are all critical contributing factors in speech outcomes. Large-scale studies and systemic analyses are required.

3. Nonmotor Symptoms of PD

NMS are debilitating in PD. Robust evidence is lacking for STN- and GPi-DBS in treating NMS. A number of reports have demonstrated that PPN-DBS is capable of modulating the NMS of PD, including cognition, sleep, and attention [101–103]. The cognitive benefit of PPN-DBS has been reported in a small number of uncontrolled studies, with bilateral PPN stimulation reducing reaction time when assessing executive function and working memory and improving delayed recall and verbal fluency [101, 102]. It has been postulated that the cognitive improvement in these domains might be mediated via activation of ascending cholinergic neurons to the thalamic CMPf, subsequently leading to widespread activation via intralaminar thalamic nuclei. Indeed, functional imaging via positron emission tomography has shown an increase in fluorodeoxyglucose uptake in prefrontal areas, suggesting a modulation of thalamic metabolism after PPN-DBS [104]. Romigi was the first to identify the role of PPN-DBS in sleep, demonstrating that bilateral PPN stimulation resulted in increased rapid eye movement (REM) sleep in patients with PD [105]. Similarly, Lim et al. showed that unilateral PPN-DBS in 3 PD patients and 2 PSP patients resulted in increased nocturnal REM sleep [106]. In a subsequent study by the same group, the authors noted that bilateral, low-frequency stimulation of the PPN resulted in improved attention in 2 patients with PD [107]. No other studies to date have investigated the role of PPN-DBS in attention.

DBS targets involved in memory circuits have garnered interest in recent years. To date, only 1 human study of DBS with bilateral STN and nucleus basalis of Meynert (NBM) stimulation in PD dementia (PDD) has evaluated the potential for cognitive and/or memory improvement [108]. In this study, STN-DBS alone yielded significant improvements in motor functioning, but not in memory or cognition. The addition of NBM stimulation to STN stimulation produced significant improvements in memory and cognitive functioning, manifested as improved performance on the Rey Auditory Verbal Learning Task, Trail-Making Test A, and the Clock Drawing Test.

4. Discussion

A multitude of new developments have been made in the area of alternative DBS targets in PD treatment over the last two decades. Research has focused on novel DBS targets, with the aim of relieving motor symptoms and NMS that are usually refractory to dopaminergic agents and traditional STN-, GPi-, and VIM-DBS.

Stimulation of the cZI has shown promise in alleviating severe parkinsonian tremor, amongst other types, and its costimulation with PPN could provide an additive benefit on axial symptoms and PI. cZI stimulation is relatively new in its conception and additional studies are required to further evaluate its possible deleterious effects on speech, particularly voice intensity and articulatory precision.

Studies investigating axial motor symptomatology and PI with PPN stimulation have yielded mixed results. From a technical aspect, considerable variability exists amongst stimulation parameters in PPN-DBS studies (Table 1) and may account for the variable degrees of success in relieving axial motor symptoms. Additionally, the PPN tends to be spatially diffuse in humans and electrophysiological recording intraoperatively is not as helpful [109] as that of the STN, GPi, or VIM. The connectivity deficit of the PPN should also be taken into account with invasive procedures like DBS. White matter tract integrity may prove fruitful with respect to patient selection. With regard to study design, a PD population with clear dopamine-resistant gait and balance deficits should be chosen. Moreover, whether or not study subjects have concurrent STN- or GPi-DBS should be considered and studied systemically to verify the therapeutic benefit of PPN stimulation. As indicated in Table 1, few studies have been randomized and double-blinded. High quality randomized studies with standardized outcomes are needed.

The SNr represents an area of great importance in the complex hierarchy of basal ganglia circuitry and studies evaluating its potential as a DBS target have yielded mixed results. While some studies of SNr-DBS have shown improvement in axial motor symptoms, the incidence of acute mania, hypomania, and depression suggests that its utility as a target in alleviating PD symptoms may be limited by these adverse changes.

EMCS and CMPf-DBS provide some benefit in PD symptomatology. However, evidence is not conclusive for either target to be superior to STN or GPi in motor control.

NMS symptoms are disabling in PD patients. Although there is some evidence that PPN-DBS improves NMS, data are as of yet too limited to consider PPN-DBS as a therapeutic option for this domain of symptomatology. PPN-DBS may prove to be a safer target in the cognitive domain, particularly when considering the possible impact of STN- and GPi-DBS on cognition.

5. Conclusions

The future of DBS in PD appears promising. The field has advanced significantly with a number of new targets to address the refractory symptoms of PD. Amongst the studies investigating these novel targets, the large majority are open-label and are not powerful enough to determine true therapeutic benefit. Future, large-scale randomized studies focusing on identifying ideal candidates, optimal targets, and stimulation parameters would certainly be of utility in triggering the DBS community to perform more robust comparisons across studies.

Abbreviations

cZI: Caudal zona incerta
CMPf: Centromedian-parafascicular nuclear complex
DBS: Deep brain stimulation
EMCS: Extradural motor cortex stimulation
FoG: Freezing of gait
GPi: Globus pallidus pars interna
MLR: Mesencephalic locomotor region
MPTP: 1-Methyl-4-phenyl-1,2,3,6-tetrahydropyridine
NBM: Nucleus basalis of Meynert
NMS: Nonmotor symptoms
PD: Parkinson's disease
PI: Postural instability
PPN: Pedunculopontine nucleus
PSA: Posterior subthalamic area
PSP: Progressive supranuclear palsy
REM: Rapid eye movement
SMA: Supplementary motor area
SN: Substantia nigra
SNc: Substantia nigra pars compacta
SNr: Substantia nigra pars reticulata
STN: Subthalamic nucleus
UPDRS: Unified Parkinson's Disease Rating Scale
VIM: Ventral intermediate nucleus
VOA: Ventralis oralis anterior
ZI: Zona incerta.

Authors' Contributions

Dustin Anderson and Grayson Beecher contributed equally to this work.

References

[1] A. L. Benabid, P. Pollak, A. Louveau, S. Henry, and J. De Rougemont, "Combined (thalamotomy and stimulation) stereotactic surgery of the vim thalamic nucleus for bilateral parkinson disease," *Stereotactic and Functional Neurosurgery*, vol. 50, no. 1-6, pp. 344–346, 1987.

[2] A. Fasano, L. M. Romito, A. Daniele et al., "Motor and cognitive outcome in patients with Parkinson's disease 8 years after subthalamic implants," *Brain*, vol. 133, no. 9, pp. 2664–2676, 2010.

[3] M. G. Rizzone, A. Fasano, A. Daniele et al., "Long-term outcome of subthalamic nucleus DBS in Parkinson's disease: from the advanced phase towards the late stage of the disease?" *Parkinsonism and Related Disorders*, vol. 20, no. 4, pp. 376–381, 2014.

[4] A. Castrioto, A. M. Lozano, Y.-Y. Poon, A. E. Lang, M. Fallis, and E. Moro, "Ten-year outcome of subthalamic stimulation in Parkinson disease: A blinded evaluation," *Archives of Neurology*, vol. 68, no. 12, pp. 1550–1556, 2011.

[5] G. Cossu and M. Pau, "Subthalamic nucleus stimulation and gait in Parkinson's Disease: a not always fruitful relationship," *Gait Posture*, vol. 52, pp. 205–210, 2017.

[6] G. Guzzi, "Critical reappraisal of DBS targeting for movement disorders," *Journal of Neurosurgical Sciences*, vol. 60, no. 2, pp. 181–188, 2016.

[7] A. Collomb-Clerc and M.-L. Welter, "Effects of deep brain stimulation on balance and gait in patients with Parkinson's disease: a systematic neurophysiological review," *Neurophysiologie Clinique*, vol. 45, no. 4-5, pp. 371–388, 2015.

[8] M. S. Okun, "Subthalamic deep brain stimulation with a constant-current device in Parkinson's disease: an open-label

randomised controlled trial," *Lancet Neurol*, vol. 11, no. 2, pp. 140–149, 2012.

[9] M. C. Rodriguez-Oroz, J. A. Obeso, A. E. Lang et al., "Bilateral deep brain stimulation in Parkinson's disease: A multicentre study with 4 years follow-up," *Brain*, vol. 128, no. 10, pp. 2240–2249, 2005.

[10] K. A. Follett, "Pallidal versus subthalamic deep-brain stimulation for Parkinson's disease," *New England Journal of Medicine*, vol. 362, no. 22, pp. 2077–2091.

[11] B. F. L. van Nuenen, R. A. J. Esselink, M. Munneke, J. D. Speelman, T. van Laar, and B. R. Bloem, "Postoperative gait deterioration after bilateral subthalamic nucleus stimulation in Parkinson's disease," *Movement Disorders*, vol. 23, no. 16, pp. 2404–2406, 2008.

[12] M. U. Ferraye, B. Debû, V. Fraix et al., "Effects of subthalamic nucleus stimulation and levodopa on freezing of gait in Parkinson disease," *Neurology*, vol. 70, no. 16, pp. 1431–1437, 2008.

[13] M. E. McNeely and G. M. Earhart, "Medication and subthalamic nucleus deep brain stimulation similarly improve balance and complex gait in Parkinson disease," *Parkinsonism and Related Disorders*, vol. 19, no. 1, pp. 86–91, 2013.

[14] P. Crenna, I. Carpinella, M. Rabuffetti et al., "Impact of subthalamic nucleus stimulation on the initiation of gait in Parkinson's disease," *Experimental Brain Research*, vol. 172, no. 4, pp. 519–532, 2006.

[15] H. Stolze, S. Klebe, M. Poepping et al., "Effects of bilateral subthalamic nucleus stimulation on parkinsonian gait," *Neurology*, vol. 57, no. 1, pp. 144–146, 2001.

[16] F. Xu et al., "Deep brain stimulation of pallidal versus subthalamic for patients with Parkinson's disease: a meta-analysis of controlled clinical trials," *Neuropsychiatr Dis Treat*, vol. 12, pp. 1435–1444, 2016.

[17] S. Alomar, N. K. King, J. Tam, A. A. Bari, C. Hamani, and A. M. Lozano, "Speech and language adverse effects after thalamotomy and deep brain stimulation in patients with movement disorders: A meta-analysis," *Movement Disorders*, vol. 32, no. 1, pp. 53–63, 2017.

[18] D. Aldridge, D. Theodoros, A. Angwin, and A. P. Vogel, "Speech outcomes in parkinson's disease after subthalamic nucleus deep brain stimulation: a systematic review," *Parkinsonism and Related Disorders*, vol. 33, pp. 3–11, 2016.

[19] G. Deuschl, J. Herzog, G. Kleiner-Fisman et al., "Deep brain stimulation: postoperative issues," *Movement Disorders*, vol. 21, 14, pp. S219–S237, 2006.

[20] M. S. Troche, A. E. Brandimore, K. D. Foote, and M. S. Okun, "Swallowing and deep brain stimulation in parkinson's disease: a systematic review," *Parkinsonism and Related Disorders*, vol. 19, no. 9, pp. 783–788, 2013.

[21] L. W. J. Baijens and R. Speyer, "Effects of therapy for dysphagia in parkinson's disease: Systematic review," *Dysphagia*, vol. 24, no. 1, pp. 91–102, 2009.

[22] M. A. Hely, W. G. J. Reid, M. A. Adena, G. M. Halliday, and J. G. L. Morris, "The Sydney multicenter study of parkinson's disease: the inevitability of dementia at 20 years," *Movement Disorders*, vol. 23, no. 6, pp. 837–844, 2008.

[23] P. Blomstedt, A. Fytagoridis, M. Åström, J. Linder, L. Forsgren, and M. I. Hariz, "Unilateral caudal zona incerta deep brain stimulation for parkinsonian tremor," *Parkinsonism and Related Disorders*, vol. 18, no. 10, pp. 1062–1066, 2012.

[24] P. Blomstedt, A. Fytagoridis, and S. Tisch, "Deep brain stimulation of the posterior subthalamic area in the treatment of tremor," *Acta Neurochirurgica*, vol. 151, no. 1, pp. 31–36, 2009.

[25] P. Blomstedt, U. Sandvik, A. Fytagoridis, and S. Tisch, "The posterior subthalamic area in the treatment of movement disorders: past, present, and future," *Neurosurgery*, vol. 64, no. 6, pp. 1029–1038, 2009.

[26] J. Mitrofanis, "Some certainty for the "zone of uncertainty"? exploring the function of the zona incerta," *Neuroscience*, vol. 130, no. 1, pp. 1–15, 2005.

[27] P. Plaha, S. Khan, and S. S. Gill, "Bilateral stimulation of the caudal zona incerta nucleus for tremor control," *Journal of Neurology, Neurosurgery and Psychiatry*, vol. 79, no. 5, pp. 504–513, 2008.

[28] A. Chopra, B. T. Klassen, and M. Stead, "Current clinical application of deep-brain stimulation for essential tremor," *Neuropsychiatric Disease and Treatment*, vol. 9, pp. 1859–1865, 2013.

[29] N. K. Patel, P. Heywood, K. O'Sullivan, R. McCarter, S. Love, and S. S. Gill, "Unilateral subthalamotomy in the treatment of parkinson's disease," *Brain*, vol. 126, no. 5, pp. 1136–1145, 2003.

[30] P. Plaha, Y. Ben-Shlomo, N. K. Patel, and S. S. Gill, "Stimulation of the caudal zona incerta is superior to stimulation of the subthalamic nucleus in improving contralateral parkinsonism," *Brain*, vol. 129, no. 7, pp. 1732–1747, 2006.

[31] A. M. Burrows, P. D. Ravin, P. Novak et al., "Limbic and motor function comparison of deep brain stimulation of the zona incerta and subthalamic nucleus," *Operative Neurosurgery*, vol. 70, 1, pp. 125–130, 2012.

[32] E. E. Benarroch, "The midline and intralaminar thalamic nuclei: anatomic and functional specificity and implications in neurologic disease," *Neurology*, vol. 71, no. 12, pp. 948-949, 2008.

[33] K. D. Foote, P. Seignourel, H. H. Fernandez et al., "Dual electrode thalamic deep brain stimulation for the treatment of posttraumatic and multiple sclerosis tremor," *Neurosurgery*, vol. 58, no. 2, pp. S-280–S-285, 2006.

[34] G. Broggi, C. Giorgi, and D. Servello, "Stereotactic neurosurgery in the treatment of tremor," *Acta Neurochir Suppl (Wien)*, vol. 39, pp. 73–76, 1987.

[35] J. K. Krauss et al., "Deep brain stimulation of the centre median-parafascicular complex in patients with movement disorders," *Journal of Neurology, Neurosurgery & Psychiatry*, vol. 72, no. 4, pp. 546–548, 2002.

[36] A. Stefani, A. Peppe, and M. Pierantozzi, "Multi-target strategy for Parkinsonian patients: the role of deep brain stimulation in the centromedian-parafascicularis complex," *Brain Research Bulletin*, vol. 78, no. 2-3, pp. 113–118, 2009.

[37] A. Peppe, A. Gasbarra, A. Stefani et al., "Deep brain stimulation of CM/PF of thalamus could be the new elective target for tremor in advanced parkinson's disease?" *Parkinsonism and Related Disorders*, vol. 14, no. 6, pp. 501–504, 2008.

[38] P. Mazzone, F. Stocchi, S. Galati et al., "Bilateral implantation of centromedian-parafascicularis complex and GPi: a new combination of unconventional targets for deep brain stimulation in severe parkinson disease," *Neuromodulation*, vol. 9, no. 3, pp. 221–228, 2006.

[39] P. Mazzone, A. Lozano, P. Stanzione et al., "Implantation of human pedunculopontine nucleus: a safe and clinically relevant target in parkinson's disease," *NeuroReport*, vol. 16, no. 17, pp. 1877–1881, 2005.

[40] P. Plaha and S. S. Gill, "Bilateral deep brain stimulation of the pedunculopontine nucleus for parkinson's disease," *NeuroReport*, vol. 16, no. 17, pp. 1883–1887, 2005.

[41] A. Stefani, A. M. Lozano, A. Peppe et al., "Bilateral deep brain stimulation of the pedunculopontine and subthalamic nuclei in severe parkinson's disease," *Brain*, vol. 130, part 6, pp. 1596–1607, 2007.

[42] A. P. Strafella, A. M. Lozano, B. Ballanger, Y.-Y. Poon, A. E. Lang, and E. Moro, "rCBF changes associated with PPN stimulation in a patient with parkinson's disease: A PET study," *Movement Disorders*, vol. 23, no. 7, pp. 1051–1054, 2008.

[43] M. U. Ferraye, B. Debû, and V. Fraix, "Effects of pedunculopontine nucleus area stimulation on gait disorders in parkinson's disease," *Brain*, vol. 133, part 1, pp. 205–214, 2010.

[44] E. Moro, C. Hamani, Y.-Y. Poon et al., "Unilateral pedunculopontine stimulation improves falls in parkinson's disease," *Brain*, vol. 133, no. 1, pp. 215–224, 2010.

[45] W. Thevathasan, P. A. Silburn, and H. Brooker, "The impact of low-frequency stimulation of the pedunculopontine nucleus region on reaction time in parkinsonism," *Journal of Neurology, Neurosurgery and Psychiatry*, vol. 81, no. 10, pp. 1099–1104, 2010.

[46] W. Thevathasan, T. J. Coyne, J. A. Hyam et al., "Pedunculopontine nucleus stimulation improves gait freezing in parkinson disease," *Neurosurgery*, vol. 69, no. 6, pp. 1248–1253, 2011.

[47] S. Khan, L. Mooney, P. Plaha et al., "Outcomes from stimulation of the caudal zona incerta and pedunculopontine nucleus in patients with parkinson's disease," *British Journal of Neurosurgery*, vol. 25, no. 2, pp. 273–280, 2011.

[48] W. Thevathasan, A. Pogosyan, J. A. Hyam et al., "Alpha oscillations in the pedunculopontine nucleus correlate with gait performance in parkinsonism," *Brain*, vol. 135, no. 1, pp. 148–160, 2012.

[49] P. Mazzone, S. Sposato, A. Insola, and E. Scarnati, "The clinical effects of deep brain stimulation of the pedunculopontine tegmental nucleus in movement disorders may not be related to the anatomical target, leads location, and setup of electrical stimulation," *Neurosurgery*, vol. 73, no. 5, pp. 894–906, 2013.

[50] Y. Okuma, "Freezing of gait and falls in parkinson's disease," *Journal of Parkinson's Disease*, vol. 4, no. 2, pp. 255–260, 2014.

[51] S. Perez-Lloret, L. Negre-Pages, P. Damier et al., "Prevalence, determinants, and effect on quality of life of freezing of gait in Parkinson disease," *The JAMA Neurology*, vol. 71, no. 7, pp. 884–890, 2014.

[52] C. A. Z. Coste, "Detection of freezing of gait in Parkinson disease: preliminary results," *Sensors (Basel, Switzerland)*, vol. 14, no. 4, pp. 6819–6827, 2014.

[53] J. D. Schaafsma, Y. Balash, T. Gurevich, A. L. Bartels, J. M. Hausdorff, and N. Giladi, "Characterization of freezing of gait subtypes and the response of each to levodopa in Parkinson's disease," *European Journal of Neurology*, vol. 10, no. 4, pp. 391–398, 2003.

[54] R. Chee, A. Murphy, M. Danoudis, N. Georgiou-Karistianis, and R. Iansek, "Gait freezing in parkinson's disease and the stride length sequence effect interaction," *Brain*, vol. 132, no. 8, pp. 2151–2160, 2009.

[55] N. Chastan, G. W. M. Westby, J. Yelnik et al., "Effects of nigral stimulation on locomotion and postural stability in patients with parkinson's disease," *Brain*, vol. 132, no. 1, pp. 172–184, 2009.

[56] D. Weiss, M. Walach, C. Meisner et al., "Nigral stimulation for resistant axial motor impairment in parkinson's disease?a randomized controlled trial," *Brain*, vol. 136, no. 7, pp. 2098–2108, 2013.

[57] S. N. Brosius, C. L. Gonzalez, J. Shuresh, and H. C. Walker, "Reversible improvement in severe freezing of gait from parkinson's disease with unilateral interleaved subthalamic brain stimulation," *Parkinsonism and Related Disorders*, vol. 21, no. 12, pp. 1469-1470, 2015.

[58] C. A. Pagni et al., "Results by motor cortex stimulation in treatment of focal dystonia, parkinson's disease and post-ictal spasticity. The experience of the italian study group of the italian neurosurgical society," *Acta Neurochir Suppl*, vol. 101, pp. 13–21, 2008.

[59] R. Cilia, A. Landi, F. Vergani, E. Sganzerla, G. Pezzoli, and A. Antonini, "Extradural motor cortex stimulation in parkinson's sisease," *Movement Disorders*, vol. 22, no. 1, pp. 111–114, 2007.

[60] A. Fasano, C. Piano, C. De Simone et al., "High frequency extradural motor cortex stimulation transiently improves axial symptoms in a patient with parkinson's disease," *Movement Disorders*, vol. 23, no. 13, pp. 1916–1919, 2008.

[61] M. S. Lee, J. O. Rinne, and C. D. Marsden, "The pedunculopontine nucleus: its role in the genesis of movement disorders.," *Yonsei Medical Journal*, vol. 41, no. 2, pp. 167–184, 2000.

[62] T. L. Tattersall, P. G. Stratton, T. J. Coyne et al., "Imagined gait modulates neuronal network dynamics in the human pedunculopontine nucleus," *Nature Neuroscience*, vol. 17, no. 3, pp. 449–454, 2014.

[63] I. Guella et al., "Alpha-synuclein genetic variability: a biomarker for dementia in parkinson disease," *Ann Neurol*, vol. 79, no. 6, pp. 991–999, 2016.

[64] J. O. Rinne, S. Y. Ma, M. S. Lee, Y. Collan, and M. Röyttä, "Loss of cholinergic neurons in the pedunculopontine nucleus in parkinson's disease is related to disability of the patients," *Parkinsonism and Related Disorders*, vol. 14, no. 7, pp. 553–557, 2008.

[65] N. Jenkinson, D. Nandi, R. C. Miall, J. F. Stein, and T. Z. Aziz, "Pedunculopontine nucleus stimulation improves akinesia in a Parkinsonian monkey," *NeuroReport*, vol. 15, no. 17, pp. 2621–2624, 2004.

[66] W. Thevathasan, M. H. Cole, C. L. Graepel et al., "A spatiotemporal analysis of gait freezing and the impact of pedunculopontine nucleus stimulation," *Brain*, vol. 135, no. 5, pp. 1446–1454, 2012.

[67] W. Thevathasan, A. Pogosyan, J. A. Hyam et al., "A block to pre-prepared movement in gait freezing, relieved by pedunculopontine nucleus stimulation," *Brain*, vol. 134, no. 7, pp. 2085–2095, 2011.

[68] P. Mazzone, S. Sposato, A. Insola, V. Dilazzaro, and E. Scarnati, "Stereotactic surgery of nucleus tegmenti pedunculopontini," *British Journal of Neurosurgery*, vol. 22, no. 1, pp. S33–S40, 2008.

[69] P. Mazzone, S. Sposato, A. Insola, and E. Scarnati, "The deep brain stimulation of the pedunculopontine tegmental nucleus: towards a new stereotactic neurosurgery," *Journal of Neural Transmission*, vol. 118, no. 10, pp. 1431–1451, 2011.

[70] B. W. Fling, R. G. Cohen, M. Mancini et al., "Functional reorganization of the locomotor network in parkinson patients with freezing of gait," *PLoS ONE*, vol. 9, no. 6, Article ID e100291, 2014.

[71] S. Vercruysse, I. Leunissen, G. Vervoort, W. Vandenberghe, S. Swinnen, and A. Nieuwboer, "Microstructural changes in white matter associated with freezing of gait in parkinson's disease," *Movement Disorders*, vol. 30, no. 4, pp. 567–576, 2015.

[72] L. Yetnikoff, H. N. Lavezzi, R. A. Reichard, and D. S. Zahm, "An update on the connections of the ventral mesencephalic dopaminergic complex," *Neuroscience*, vol. 282, pp. 23–48, 2014.

[73] S. N. Haber, "The place of dopamine in the cortico-basal ganglia circuit," *Neuroscience*, vol. 282, pp. 248–257, 2014.

[74] K. Takakusaki, R. Chiba, T. Nozu, and T. Okumura, "Brainstem control of locomotion and muscle tone with special reference to the role of the mesopontine tegmentum and medullary reticulospinal systems," *Journal of Neural Transmission*, vol. 123, no. 7, pp. 695–729, 2016.

[75] D. Weiss, R. Klotz, R. B. Govindan et al., "Subthalamic stimulation modulates cortical motor network activity and synchronization in parkinson's disease," *Brain*, vol. 138, no. 3, pp. 679–693, 2015.

[76] M. Ulla, S. Thobois, J.-J. Lemaire et al., "Manic behaviour induced by deep-brain stimulation in parkinson's disease: evidence of substantia nigra implication?" *Journal of Neurology, Neurosurgery and Psychiatry*, vol. 77, no. 12, pp. 1363–1366, 2006.

[77] M. Ulla, S. Thobois, P.-M. Llorca et al., "Contact-dependent reproducible hypomania induced by deep brain stimulation in Parkinson's disease: clinical, anatomical, and functional imaging study," *Journal of Neurology, Neurosurgery and Psychiatry*, vol. 82, no. 6, pp. 607–614, 2011.

[78] B.-P. Bejjani, P. Damier, I. Arnulf et al., "Transient acute depression induced by high-frequency deep-brain stimulation," *The New England Journal of Medicine*, vol. 340, no. 19, pp. 1476–1480, 1999.

[79] P. Blomstedt, M. I. Hariz, A. Lees et al., "Acute severe depression induced by intraoperative stimulation of the substantia nigra: a case report," *Parkinsonism & Related Disorders*, vol. 14, no. 3, pp. 253–256, 2008.

[80] J. Kulisevsky, M. L. Berthier, A. Gironell, B. Pascual-Sedano, J. Molet, and P. Parés, "Mania following deep brain stimulation for parkinson's disease," *Neurology*, vol. 59, no. 9, pp. 1421–1424, 2002.

[81] E. Benvenuti, F. Cecchi, A. Colombini, and G. Gori, "Extradural motor cortex stimulation as a method to treat advanced parkinson's disease: New perspective in geriatric medicine," *Aging Clinical and Experimental Research*, vol. 18, no. 4, pp. 347-348, 2006.

[82] S. Canavero and R. Paolotti, "Extradural motor cortex stimulation for advanced Parkinson's disease: case report," *Movement Disorders*, vol. 15, no. 1, pp. 169–171, 2000.

[83] S. Canavero, R. Paolotti, V. Bonicalzi et al., "Extradural motor cortex stimulation for advanced parkinson disease: report of two cases," *Journal of Neurosurgery*, vol. 97, no. 5, pp. 1208–1211, 2002.

[84] B. Cioni, "Motor cortex stimulation for parkinson's disease," *Acta Neurochir Suppl*, vol. 97, no. 2, pp. 233–238, 2007.

[85] C. A. Pagni et al., "Extradural motor cortex stimulation (EMCS) for parkinson's disease. history and first results by the study group of the Italian neurosurgical society," *Acta Neurochir Suppl*, vol. 93, pp. 113–119, 2005.

[86] C. A. Pagni, S. Zeme, F. Zenga, and R. M. Villani, "Further experience with extradural motor cortex stimulation for treatment of advanced parkinson's disease: report of 3 new cases," *Journal of Neurosurgical Sciences*, vol. 47, no. 4, pp. 189–193, 2003.

[87] R. L. Albin, A. B. Young, and J. B. Penney, "The functional anatomy of disorders of the basal ganglia," *Trends in Neurosciences*, vol. 18, no. 2, pp. 63-64, 1995.

[88] C. N. Woolsey, T. C. Erickson, and W. E. Gilson, "Localization in somatic sensory and motor areas of human cerebral cortex as determined by direct recording of evoked potentials and electrical stimulation.," *Journal of Neurosurgery*, vol. 51, no. 4, pp. 476–506, 1979.

[89] J. E. Arle, D. Apetauerova, J. Zani et al., "Motor cortex stimulation in patients with Parkinson disease: 12-Month follow-up in 4 patients," *Journal of Neurosurgery*, vol. 109, no. 1, pp. 133–139, 2008.

[90] J. C. Gutiérrez, F. J. Seijo, M. A. Á. Vega, F. F. González, B. L. Aragoneses, and M. Blázquez, "Therapeutic extradural cortical stimulation for parkinson's disease: report of six cases and review of the literature," *Clinical Neurology and Neurosurgery*, vol. 111, no. 8, pp. 703–707, 2009.

[91] E. Moro, J. M. Schwalb, P. Piboolnurak et al., "Unilateral subdural motor cortex stimulation improves essential tremor but not parkinson's disease," *Brain*, vol. 134, no. 7, pp. 2096–2105, 2011.

[92] A. R. Bentivoglio, A. Fasano, C. Piano et al., "Unilateral extradural motor cortex stimulation is safe and improves parkinson disease at 1 year," *Neurosurgery*, vol. 71, no. 4, pp. 815–825, 2012.

[93] S. Lundgren, T. Saeys, F. Karlsson et al., "Deep brain stimulation of caudal zona incerta and subthalamic nucleus in patients with parkinson's disease: effects on voice intensity," *Parkinson's Disease*, Article ID 658956, 2011.

[94] E. Eklund, J. Qvist, L. Sandström, F. Viklund, J. Van Doorn, and F. Karlsson, "Perceived articulatory precision in patients with parkinson's disease after deep brain stimulation of subthalamic nucleus and caudal zona incerta," *Clinical Linguistics and Phonetics*, vol. 29, no. 2, pp. 150–166, 2015.

[95] A. Fytagoridis, R. L. Sjöberg, M. Åström, A. Fredricks, L. Nyberg, and P. Blomstedt, "Effects of deep brain stimulation in the caudal zona incerta on verbal fluency," *Stereotactic and Functional Neurosurgery*, vol. 91, no. 1, pp. 24–29, 2013.

[96] L. Johansson, S. Möller, K. Olofsson et al., "Word-level intelligibility after caudal zona incerta stimulation for parkinson's disease," *Acta Neurologica Scandinavica*, vol. 130, no. 1, pp. 27–33, 2014.

[97] L. Sandström, P. Hägglund, L. Johansson, P. Blomstedt, and F. Karlsson, "Speech intelligibility in parkinson's disease patients with zona incerta deep brain stimulation," *Brain and Behavior*, vol. 5, no. 10, 2015.

[98] F. Karlsson, K. Olofsson, P. Blomstedt, J. Linder, and J. van Doorn, "Pitch variability in patients with parkinson's disease: effects of deep brain stimulation of caudal zona incerta and subthalamic nucleus," *Journal of Speech, Language, and Hearing Research*, vol. 56, no. 1, pp. 150–158, 2013.

[99] S. Sundstedt et al., "Swallowing quality of life after zona incerta deep brain stimulation," *Ann Otol Rhinol Laryngol*, vol. 126, no. 2, pp. 110–116, 2017.

[100] S. Sundstedt, K. Olofsson, J. van Doorn, J. Linder, E. Nordh, and P. Blomstedt, "Swallowing function in parkinson's patients following Zona Incerta deep brain stimulation," *Acta Neurologica Scandinavica*, vol. 126, no. 5, pp. 350–356, 2012.

[101] S. Alessandro, R. Ceravolo, L. Brusa et al., "Non-motor functions in parkinsonian patients implanted in the pedunculopontine nucleus: Focus on sleep and cognitive domains," *Journal of the Neurological Sciences*, vol. 289, no. 1-2, pp. 44–48, 2010.

[102] A. Costa, G. A. Carlesimo, C. Caltagirone et al., "Effects of deep brain stimulation of the peduncolopontine area on working memory tasks in patients with parkinson's disease," *Parkinsonism and Related Disorders*, vol. 16, no. 1, pp. 64–67, 2010.

[103] H. Morita, C. J. Hass, E. Moro, A. Sudhyadhom, R. Kumar, and M. S. Okun, "Pedunculopontine nucleus stimulation: where are we now and what needs to be done to move the field forward?" *Frontiers in Neurology*, vol. 5, article no. 243, 2014.

[104] R. Ceravolo, L. Brusa, S. Galati et al., "Low frequency stimulation of the nucleus tegmenti pedunculopontini increases cortical metabolism in Parkinsonian patients," *European Journal of Neurology*, vol. 18, no. 6, pp. 842–849, 2011.

[105] A. Romigi, "Pedunculopontine nucleus stimulation influences REM sleep in parkinson's disease," *European Journal of Neurology*, vol. 15, no. 7, pp. e64–e65, 2008.

[106] A. S. Lim, E. Moro, A. M. Lozano et al., "Selective enhancement of rapid eye movement sleep by deep brain stimulation of the human pons," *Annals of Neurology*, vol. 66, no. 1, pp. 110–114, 2009.

[107] I. Arnulf, M. Ferraye, V. Fraix et al., "Sleep induced by stimulation in the human pedunculopontine nucleus area," *Annals of Neurology*, vol. 67, no. 4, pp. 546–549, 2010.

[108] H. J. Freund et al., "Cognitive functions in a patient with Parkinson-dementia syndrome undergoing deep brain stimulation," *Arch Neurol*, vol. 66, no. 6, pp. 781–785, 2009.

[109] M. Weinberger, C. Hamani, W. D. Hutchison, E. Moro, A. M. Lozano, and J. O. Dostrovsky, "Pedunculopontine nucleus microelectrode recordings in movement disorder patients," *Experimental Brain Research*, vol. 188, no. 2, pp. 165–174, 2008.

6

The Level of Knowledge of Parkinson's Disease among Nonprofessional Caregivers in a Movement Disorders Center in Turkey

Murat Gultekin,[1] Ayse Caglar Sarılar,[1] Ayten Ekinci,[1] Gozde Erturk,[2] and Meral Mirza[1]

[1] *Department of Neurology, Erciyes University School of Medicine, Kayseri, Turkey*
[2] *Department of Biostatistics, Erciyes University School of Medicine, Kayseri, Turkey*

Correspondence should be addressed to Murat Gultekin; gultekin@erciyes.edu.tr

Academic Editor: Peter Hagell

Introduction. Only a few studies have been conducted to determine the level of knowledge among caregivers about Parkinson's disease (PD). The aim of the current study was to determine the knowledge of PD among caregivers at a movement disorder clinic in Turkey. *Methods.* We conducted a questionnaire based interview with the subjects in a tertiary care neurology facility in Turkey. The questions were divided into two parts covering the symptomatology and treatment of PD. A questionnaire consisting of 10 questions was applied to the subjects who had to mark the correct option in a stipulated time. *Results.* Eighty caregivers were included in the study. The caregivers' mean age was 47.94 years (SD = 12.40). There were 47 female caregivers (58.8%). The most well-known question was that the number of drugs given to the patient may vary with time (76.3%), whereas "the benefit noted in the patient's treatment decreases over time" was the least known question (11.3%). *Discussion.* This study is the first in our country and shows the necessity to increase the knowledge of PD among caregivers and the public. Education programs may have a positive role in imparting knowledge to the caregivers of PD patients.

1. Introduction

Parkinson's disease (PD) is a progressive neurodegenerative illness [1]. In the diverse treatment of chronic diseases, the training of the caregiver has an important role in the success of treatment [2, 3]. In progressive PD, in many areas such as the time when medicine is taken, determination of the duration of medicines, observation of the response to treatment, and monitoring the motor complications related to the disease and treatment, the contribution of the caregiver affects the patient directly.

There are very few studies about caregivers' level of information about PD [4]. In these studies, the caregivers' level of information about PD was found to be very low [5, 6]. Most caregivers mention that following the diagnosis of their relatives they have insufficient information [7]. The lack of general information of both patients with PD and their caregivers may cause communication problems among the doctor, patient, and the caregiver. This situation negatively affects the treatment of the disease and the daily life activities of the patient directly. There are no data on this subject in the literature in our country.

The purpose of this study is to measure the knowledge and attitude of caregivers of PD patients about Parkinson's disease. In this way, during the informing and training of caregivers of PD patients, what is significant and remarkable will be revealed.

2. Methods

2.1. Sample. The study included 80 volunteer caregivers of PD patients who were diagnosed according to the criteria of the United Kingdom Parkinson's Disease Brain Bank and followed up in Erciyes University Medical Faculty, at the Department of Neurology movement disorder clinic between January 2016 and April 2016. The exclusion criterion was determined as caregivers under 18 years of age. This study was approved by the Ethics Committee of Clinical

Research of Erciyes University on 18.12.2015 (with number 538). The data were obtained after giving information about the purpose of the study and with the written consent of the participants. The participants first of all filled in the demographic information form. Next, to determine the level of information of the caregivers about PD, a questionnaire was applied. The necessary information about the clinical status of the patient for the study was added by a neurologist with experience in movement disorders. The questions were answered by the participant caregivers by marking the correct answer in accordance with their own knowledge.

2.2. The Evaluation Tools Used

2.2.1. Demographic Information Form. In keeping with the purpose of the study, a form was applied by the researchers to the caregivers and patients; it meets the inclusion criteria of the study to determine information on age, gender, level of education, and other demographic information. With the current form, besides the demographic information, the degree of relationship of the caregivers to the patient, caregiving situation, the duration of PD, and the clinical staging information according to the of Hoehn-Yahr scale were asked and recorded.

2.2.2. Questionnaire Form. A questionnaire was applied to the caregivers of the PD patients to determine their information level about the treatment of disease. The questionnaire has ten questions of which eight are multiple choices and two are open ended. The questions were designed by the researchers after an analysis of the general literature.

2.3. Statistical Analysis. For the comparison of the categorical data in the study, the exact method of Pearson chi-square test statistics was used. In the comparison of two groups, in independent samples, the Student t-test was used. In the comparison of more than two groups, one-way variance analysis (ANOVA) was used. In multiple comparison tests (post hoc) Tukey HSD test statistics was used. The evaluation of the data distribution was checked with Shapiro-Wilks test statistics. The appropriate test statistics have been chosen and test statistic was made. The analyses of the data have been evaluated with SPSS 22 (IBM Corp; Armonk, NY, USA). The significance level has been accepted as $p > 0.05$.

3. Results

The study included 80 caregivers of PD patients. Forty-seven of these were female (58.8%) and the mean age of the caregivers was found as 47.94 years (SD = 12.40). It was observed that most of the caregivers were the spouses of the patients (43.8%) or their children (43.8%). Also 67.6% of the caregivers were retired or not working. It was also found that only 18.8% of the caregivers were university graduates. The mean duration of caregiving was 7.8 years and it was determined that most of them (67.5%) cared for the patients full time. At the same time, it was also determined that most of the caregivers (65%) did not have previous experience of caregiving. The demographic characteristics of the caregivers and patients with PD are summarized in Table 1.

Table 1: Demographic characteristics of the participants (caregivers and patients).

n = 80	Caregiver		Patients with PD	
	n	%	n	%
Gender				
Female	47	58.8	39	48.8
Male	33	41.3	41	51.3
Level of education				
Illiterate	4	5.0	19	23.8
Literate/elementary	39	48.8	41	51.3
Middle/high	22	27.6	14	17.5
University	15	18.8	6	7.5
Occupation				
Not working	39	48.8	40	50
Retired	15	18.8	40	50
Working	26	32.5		
Caregiving situation				
Rarely	14	17.5		
Mostly	12	15		
Full time	54	67.5		
Age [mean (SD)]	47.94 (12.40)		62.46 (10.19)	
Duration of illness [mean (SD)]	—		6.96 (5.69)	

Forty-seven (58.8%) of the patients were female. Nineteen (23.8%) of the patients were illiterate. The mean duration of the disease was found as 6.96 years (SD = 5.69). Of the patients, 53.7% said that they did not do any exercises. In addition, 21.2% of the patients said that they did not go for regular clinical checkups. Also, we found that there was no significant difference between the knowledge level and caregiving situation ($p = 0.339$).

The answer rates of the caregivers for the first 8 multiple choice questions in the questionnaire are shown in Table 2. Regarding this, the areas in which caregivers had the least information about PD are as follows: 11.3% of the caregivers answered that the current treatment is aimed at controlling the symptoms of the disease; 13.8% of the caregivers answered that the benefit of treatment can change over time; 16.3% of the caregivers answered that they only knew of oral treatment for PD. In addition, the question to which the caregivers answered as "I don't have an idea" is related to nonoral treatments for PD (52.5%). The best known treatment option is the possibility of changing the number of drugs used by the patient (76.3%).

With the correct answers to the questions, no significant difference was found among the stage of the disease, duration of the disease, and the level of education of caregivers. However, when the genders of the caregivers were checked, for only the first question (What is your opinion about the state of Parkinson disease?) was there a significant difference

TABLE 2: The frequencies of the answers in the questionnaire ($n = 80$).

Questions	Correct answer (%)	Wrong answer (%)	No idea (%)
(1) What is the state of Parkinson disease?	43 (53.8)	31 (38.8)	6 (7.5)
(2) Does the number of drugs change during treatment?	61 (76.3)	9 (11.3)	10 (12.5)
(3) Are there nonmotor symptoms in Parkinson disease?	44 (55)	27 (33.8)	9 (11.3)
(4) *Are there treatment choices other than oral?*	13 (16.3)	25 (31.3)	42 (52.5)
(5) *What is the purpose of the current treatment in Parkinson disease?*	9 (11.3)	63 (78.8)	8 (10)
(6) What is the effect of exercise in Parkinson disease?	54 (67.5)	7 (8.8)	19 (23.8)
(7) How often should the drugs be taken in Parkinson disease?	57 (71.3)	21 (26.3)	2 (2.5)
(8) *Does the benefit to the patient change over time?*	11 (13.8)	38 (47.5)	31 (38.8)

Lower frequencies for the correct answers are shown in darker print.

between the answers ($p = 0.023$). In this question, the progressive nature of Parkinson's disease was asked. Thirteen men answered correctly (30.2%) whereas 30 women (69.8%) answered correctly.

The last two questions were open ended. To the 9th question, namely, "How often should a patient with PD come to clinical checks?," 56.3% of the caregivers answered that patients should go to clinical checks at two-month periods and 21.2% of them said at four-month periods. However, 18.7% of the caregivers answered that patients should go to clinical checks if they have any complaints related to PD. This question was asked to determine patients who receive inadequate treatment and do not come to the clinic.

In the 10th question, the caregivers were asked to guess about the complaints of the patients, namely, "Could they guess that patients had PD before it was diagnosed?" According to this, before diagnosis, only 15% of the caregivers mentioned that their patients could have PD.

In addition to the questionnaire, caregivers were asked about their sources for information. Most of them named "doctor only" (61,3%) as their source. The Internet was referred to by 10%; other carers were referred to by 6.3% and books-brochures were referred to by 5%.

4. Discussion

In this study, we present our country's first data concerning the level of knowledge and perceptions of caregivers regarding PD. According to these data, it was determined that 65% of caregivers are not experienced or trained in providing care to PD patients or to those with a chronic disease. However, in spite of the progress in neurodegenerative diseases like PD, it was shown that caregivers do not have sufficient information about PD. Therefore, it is obvious that the patient treatment may be negatively affected. Our findings show a similarity with other studies on this subject [4, 8].

In a study conducted by Yadav et al. in India a multiple choice questionnaire comprising 10 questions was applied to caregivers. It was shown that participants are misinformed mostly in the following areas: biochemical abnormality in PD, stage in which patients are considered suitable for deep brain stimulation and the surgical treatment methods available in PD. In these matters, it was shown that caregivers are misinformed regarding the surgical methods available in PD [4]. In our data, the fact that caregivers believe that drugs can totally cure PD (78.8%) was the most widely found misunderstanding. This was followed, respectively, by the beliefs that the benefit of treatment will not change over time (47.5%) and that there are no equipment supported treatments for PD (31.3%).

There are different studies about caregivers' level of information about PD in the literature. Tan et al. conducted one study to show comparing knowledge of genetic testing in PD patients and caregivers in American and Asian population [5]. It was found that American PD patients had a higher level of knowledge of PD genetics than Asian PD patients. A greater number of American PD patients and caregivers reported a positive attitude towards the potential medical benefits of genetic testing compared to their Asian counterparts. Furthermore, Sakanaka et al. conducted a similar study to show knowledge of genetic PD patients and caregivers [6]. It was shown that only 51.6% of PD participants and 55.6% of caregivers knew that "scientists have identified genes associated with a higher risk of developing PD." Also, it was concluded that PD patients may benefit from education and genetic counseling on the implications of genetic testing.

For optimum daily living activities (DLA), patients with PD and their caregivers need to know about the disease and its treatment. In particular, this situation is essential in the middle and advanced stages of PD [9]. For example, some patients in this period may need nonoral treatments because of the limitation of their DLA due to motor complications. In fact, with equipment supported treatments, patients with PD and their caregivers' DLA can be significantly improved [10]. However, our data revealed that few caregivers (16.3%) have information about these treatments.

Although the caregivers in our working group were not trained, we observed that they answered correctly the questions about when medicines should be taken and the changes in the number of medicines. This is thought to be due to the patients' caregivers being well-informed (73.8%) and is thought to be linked to interviews with experts in the field. This situation may depend on interviews between caregivers and doctors in clinics and later may depend on the questionnaire. In our working group, the knowledge resource of PD is mostly "doctors" (61.3%) which verifies this situation.

More information about PD in printed and electronic media is needed and the establishment of clinics dedicated to movement disorders and centers of excellence with special education programs would go a long way in increasing the awareness and knowledge of PD among caregivers in our country. Furthermore, the practitioners should give sufficient time to caregivers and help in providing them with correct information by means of books, brochures, and websites.

Limitations of the Study. Because the number of caregivers is small and ours is a small scaled and local study, it may not reflect our data very strongly. Most of the questions in the questionnaire including subjects' knowledge about treatment reveal only one side of PD.

Strengths of the Study. Although our study is small scaled, because it reflects the first data in our country, it is considered as important. The information presented herein may help to fill the gap in caregivers' training.

5. Conclusion

Patient and caregiver education programs may have a positive role in imparting knowledge to PD patients and their caregivers. Studies are needed to understand the knowledge, attitude, and perceptions regarding Parkinson's disease among the general population.

References

[1] M. C. De Rijk, C. Tzourio, M. M. B. Breteler et al., "Prevalence of Parkinsonism and Parkinson's disease in Europe: the EUROPARKINSON collaborative study," *Journal of Neurology, Neurosurgery and Psychiatry*, vol. 62, no. 1, pp. 10–15, 1997.

[2] S. Sörensen, M. Pinquart, and P. Duberstein, "How effective are interventions with caregivers? an updated meta-analysis," *The Gerontologist*, vol. 42, no. 3, pp. 356–372, 2002.

[3] W. H. Oertel and H. Ellgring, "Parkinson's disease—medical education and psychosocial aspects," *Patient Education and Counseling*, vol. 26, no. 1-3, pp. 71–79, 1995.

[4] R. Yadav, G. Shukla, V. Goyal, S. Singh, and M. Behari, "Knowledge of Parkinson's disease among patients and caregivers attending movement disorder clinic at a tertiary care centre in north India," *Annals of Indian Academy of Neurology*, vol. 15, no. 4, pp. 294–296, 2012.

[5] E.-K. Tan, J. Lee, C. Hunter, L. Shinawi, S. Fook-Chong, and J. Jankovic, "Comparing knowledge and attitudes towards genetic testing in Parkinson's disease in an American and Asian population," *Journal of the Neurological Sciences*, vol. 252, no. 2, pp. 113–120, 2007.

[6] K. Sakanaka, C. H. Waters, O. A. Levy et al., "Knowledge of and interest in genetic results among Parkinson disease patients and caregivers," *Journal of Genetic Counseling*, vol. 23, no. 1, pp. 114–120, 2014.

[7] D. McLaughlin, F. Hasson, W. G. Kernohan et al., "Living and coping with Parkinson's disease: perceptions of informal carers," *Palliative Medicine*, vol. 25, no. 2, pp. 177–182, 2011.

[8] K. S. Lee, A. Merriman, A. Owen, B. Chew, and T. C. Tan, "The medical, social, and functional profile of Parkinson's disease patients," *Singapore Medical Journal*, vol. 35, no. 3, pp. 265–268, 1994.

[9] E. H. Tew, S. L. Naismith, M. Pereira, and S. J. G. Lewis, "Quality of life in Parkinson's disease caregivers: the contribution of personality traits," *BioMed Research International*, vol. 2013, Article ID 151872, 6 pages, 2013.

[10] S. B. Fowler, "Hope and a health-promoting lifestyle in persons with Parkinson's disease," *Journal of Neuroscience Nursing*, vol. 29, no. 2, pp. 111–116, 1997.

7

Deep Brain Stimulation of Hemiparkinsonian Rats with Unipolar and Bipolar Electrodes for up to 6 Weeks: Behavioral Testing of Freely Moving Animals

Kathrin Badstuebner,[1] Ulrike Gimsa,[2] Immo Weber,[1] Armin Tuchscherer,[3] and Jan Gimsa[4]

[1] *Department of Neurology, University of Rostock, Rostock, Germany*
[2] *Institute of Behavioural Physiology, Leibniz Institute for Farm Animal Biology, Dummerstorf, Germany*
[3] *Institute of Genetics and Biometry, Leibniz Institute for Farm Animal Biology, Dummerstorf, Germany*
[4] *Chair of Biophysics, University of Rostock, Rostock, Germany*

Correspondence should be addressed to Jan Gimsa; jan.gimsa@uni-rostock.de

Academic Editor: Raja Mehanna

Although the clinical use of deep brain stimulation (DBS) is increasing, its basic mechanisms of action are still poorly understood. Platinum/iridium electrodes were inserted into the subthalamic nucleus of rats with unilateral 6-OHDA-induced lesions of the medial forebrain bundle. Six behavioral parameters were compared with respect to their potential to detect DBS effects. Locomotor function was quantified by (i) apomorphine-induced rotation, (ii) initiation time, (iii) the number of adjusting steps in the stepping test, and (iv) the total migration distance in the open field test. Sensorimotor neglect and anxiety were quantified by (v) the retrieval bias in the corridor test and (vi) the ratio of migration distance in the center versus in the periphery in the open field test, respectively. In our setup, unipolar stimulation was found to be more efficient than bipolar stimulation for achieving beneficial long-term DBS effects. Performance in the apomorphine-induced rotation test showed no improvement after 6 weeks. DBS reduced the initiation time of the contralateral paw in the stepping test after 3 weeks of DBS followed by 3 weeks without DBS. Similarly, sensorimotor neglect was improved. The latter two parameters were found to be most appropriate for judging therapeutic DBS effects.

1. Introduction

Electrical stimulation of the brain is an emerging area for the treatment of a growing number of neurological and psychiatric diseases. Deep brain stimulation (DBS) is well established for the treatment of movement disorders, such as Parkinson's disease (PD) [1]. For patients in the advanced stages of PD, DBS of the *subthalamic nucleus* (STN) is highly effective in reversing motor deficits. In addition to locomotor and sensorimotor deficits, PD patients also suffer from emotional disturbances, namely, depression and anxiety. Anxiety may result not only from the impairment of motor function but also from dysfunction in the STN [2]. More recently, DBS has also been applied at earlier stages of PD [3]. Nevertheless, STN-DBS does not always improve symptoms, and it may actually worsen them [4]. However, only limited information is available on (i) the effects of DBS on cognitive and emotional traits; (ii) the efficiency of different stimulation modes, in particular unipolar versus bipolar stimulation; and (iii) the long-term sustainability of symptom alleviation after the cessation of DBS.

The STN is one of the most important target regions for high-frequency (approx. 130 Hz) DBS in patients, especially in patients in the advanced stages of PD who are refractory to conventional therapy [5, 6]. Historically, DBS was developed as a modification of ablative surgery, in which basal ganglia, such as the STN, were irreversibly destroyed as a final treatment option in late-stage PD [7]. During surgery, electric stimulation was used to guide neurosurgeons to the precise position of the lesions. The main advantages of DBS over surgical lesions are its reversibility and the ability to modulate the stimulation parameters [8]. It has been well documented that DBS of the STN may also improve the cardinal motor symptoms of PD in the long-term [9, 10].

Maesawa et al. [11] were the first to describe a DBS-related protection of dopaminergic neurons in the SNc by STN-DBS of 6-OHDA hemiparkinsonian rats. Later, Harnack et al. [12] described a preservation of approx. 50% of the dopaminergic nigral neurons in the SNc by STN-DBS compared to sham-stimulated and naïve rats. Spieles-Engemann et al. [13] demonstrated an increase in the levels of the brain-derived neurotrophic factor and Wu et al. [14] observed decreased apoptosis in the nigrostriatal system after STN-DBS of 6-OHDA-lesioned rats. Other authors have described the preservation of neurons or even neurogenesis by DBS in other brain regions [15, 16].

Clearly, more information is needed to explore the full therapeutic potential of DBS. For example, optimum target regions are not always known, and the basic mechanisms by which DBS acts are still poorly understood [17–22]. In addition, adverse side effects cannot always be avoided. Therefore, research on both the optimal DBS technique and its neurological mechanisms is needed. To allow for a comparison with the clinical situation, the availability of animal models for long-term examinations and behavioral testing is of the utmost importance. Many groups have reported results from animal models with external stimulators, although these used very short durations of DBS. In some cases, only anaesthetized animals were used. Long-term behavioral outcomes have not been sufficiently examined (for reviews see [23, 24]). Nevertheless, miniaturized mobile stimulators for the chronic instrumentation of freely moving mice or rats for up to five weeks have recently been developed by a few groups [11, 25–32], including our own [33]. Such animal models allow the testing of drug-induced or spontaneous behaviors as a way to quantify the effects of lesion-induced or DBS-induced changes in locomotor function and behavior.

In pioneering work on experimental DBS, stainless steel electrodes have been used to optimize the electrode position in the brain [34, 35]. However, stainless steel electrodes are obsolete and not ideal for current studies. Their use in long-term experiments is prevented because of corrosion and the detrimental effects this has on the surrounding brain tissue [36–38].

Here, we combined a revised version of our miniaturized constant-current-pulse generator [33] with new Pt/Ir electrodes to test the effects of different modes of STN-DBS on the behavioral performance of 6-OHDA-induced hemiparkinsonian rats [39]. Several tests have been developed for the detailed evaluation of spontaneous motor and sensorimotor function in rodents [40–42]. Here, we chose four different behavioral tests: (i) an apomorphine-induced rotation test [43, 44], (ii) the stepping test [45], (iii) the corridor test [46], and (iv) a modified version of the classical open field test [47]. From these tests, six quantitative parameters were determined to describe the effects of lesion- and DBS-induced changes in locomotor function, sensorimotor neglect, exploration, and anxiety-like behavior.

2. Materials and Methods

2.1. Animals. Male Wistar Han rats (240 g–260 g; Crl:WI(Han) Rattus norvegicus: RRID:RGD_2308816) were obtained from Charles River Laboratory (Sulzfeld, Germany) and housed under temperature-controlled conditions in a 12-h light-dark cycle with conventional rodent chow and water provided ad libitum. The study was carried out in accordance with the European Community Council directive 86/609/EEC for the care of laboratory animals and was approved by the local animal care committee (LALLF M-V/TSEM/7221.3-1.2-019/10).

2.2. Electrodes. Two types of microelectrodes were custom-made from round Pt/Ir alloy (Pt90/Ir10) wires, which were insulated with polyesterimide but left bare at the tips (Figure 1). The unipolar microelectrodes were purchased from Polyfil (Zug, Switzerland) and the bipolar microelectrodes were purchased from FHC (Bowdoin, ME, USA). Their distal ends were connected with biocompatible insulated wire. To avoid excessive heating from soldering, the cables were connected with conductive silver glue, covered by biocompatible heat-shrink tubing and sealed with biocompatible silicon glue (NuSil Technology, Carpinteria, USA). The unipolar electrodes were driven against a gold-wire counter electrode (length 30 mm, diameter 200 μm). The bipolar electrodes did not require the implantation of an additional counter electrode.

2.3. Surgery. The surgical procedures were performed using a stereotactic frame (Stoelting, Wood Dale, IL, USA). Rats were anesthetized by intraperitoneal injection of ketamine hydrochloride (10 mg per 100 g body weight, Ketanest S®, Pfizer, Karlsruhe, Germany) and xylazine (0.5 mg per 100 g body weight, Rompun®, Pfizer). During surgery, their eyes were protected from dehydration by Vidisic® (Bausch and Lomb, Berlin, Germany).

The skull was opened using a dental rose-head bur (Kaniedenta, Herford, Germany). To induce hemiparkinsonism, rats were lesioned with a unilateral injection of 6-OHDA into the right medial forebrain bundle. Twenty-four μg 6-OHDA dissolved in 4 μl 0.1 M citrate buffer were delivered over 4 min via a 5 μl Hamilton microsyringe. Sham-lesioned rats received 4 μl 0.1 M citrate buffer delivered in the same fashion. The stereotactic coordinates, relative to bregma, were anterior-posterior (AP: −2.3 mm), medial-lateral (ML: 1.5 mm), and dorsal-ventral (DV: −8.5 mm) ([48]; RRID:SCR_006369). After surgery, the wound was sutured and the animals received 0.1 ml novaminsulfone (Ratiopharm, Ulm, Germany) and 4 ml saline subcutaneously. To prevent hypothermia, a heat lamp was used until vital functions returned to normal. The success of the lesion procedure was evaluated with the apomorphine-induced rotation test 12–14 days after surgery.

Approximately 3 weeks after lesion induction, the electrodes were implanted with their stimulating tips localized in the STN. The tip coordinates, relative to bregma, were AP: −3.5 mm, ML: 2.4 mm, and DV: −7.6 mm ([48];

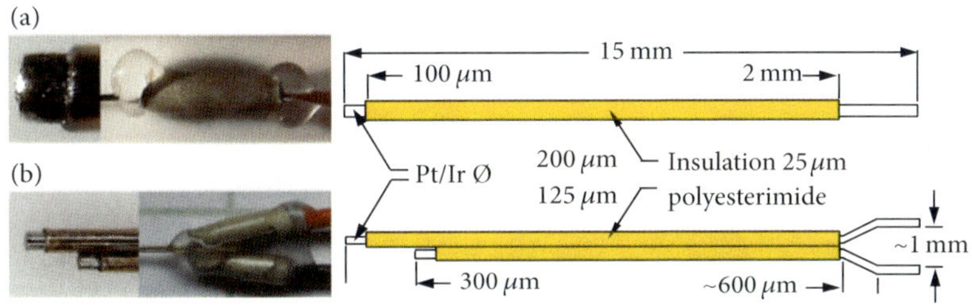

FIGURE 1: Photographs of tips (left), distal connections (center), and schematic drawings (right) of (a) the unipolar (200 μm wire diameter) and (b) the bipolar microelectrode (125 μm wire diameter). The electrode shafts were insulated with 25 μm polyesterimide. All electrode tips were bare for 100 μm.

RRID:SCR_006369). The shorter counter electrode tips of the bipolar electrodes were oriented so that they were lateral to the stimulating tip. The electrode shafts were fixed to the skull by an adhesive-glue bridge of dental acrylic resin (Pontiform automix 10 : 1, Müller & Weygandt GmbH, Büdingen) attached to an anchor screw fixed to the skull above the left hemisphere. Figure 2 illustrates the unipolar electrode orientation.

Following electrode implantation, the cables of the stimulating and the counter electrode contacts were implanted subcutaneously with a central dorsal outlet port (Figure 3(a)). After surgery, the rats were treated in the same manner as after the 6-OHDA injection. Rats were allowed to recover for eight days before stimulation started.

2.4. Chronic Instrumentation. One week after surgery, a plug connector (M52-040023V0545, Harwin Plc, Hampshire, UK) was crimped to the electrode cables (Figure 3(b)). The connector ensured flexibility in the use of commercial rat jackets (Lomir Biomedical, Quebec, Canada), which contained the stimulators and batteries in a custom-made fabric backpack (Figure 2(e)).

The setup allowed for the completely free movement of the animals over long periods of time. The stimulator plate was protected from mechanical strain and moisture by a custom-made polymethyl-methacrylate box and was connected to the external current-pulse battery. At the start of the stimulation, the electrode connector was plugged into the stimulator (Figure 2). The entire stimulator system was miniaturized and designed for minimum power consumption relative to our preliminary versions [33]. A separate long-lasting pulse-generator battery was inserted at the bottom of the DBS stimulator. Only the current-pulse battery (Figure 2(e)) had to be exchanged at 4 weeks.

The jacket and cables were checked daily to ensure the long-term effectiveness of the device. Cables that were torn off by the animal in exceptional cases were replaced immediately. The jackets had to be replaced every week because of wear. The stimulator signal was checked with an oscilloscope at the same time as the jackets were replaced. There has never been a problem with the batteries or the stimulator hardware.

2.5. Stimulation Conditions. The stimulator provided rectangular monophasic current pulses. Different treatment groups were stimulated for 3 days, 3 weeks, or 6 weeks. In all experiments, the stimulators were adjusted to a pulse width of 60 μsec with the negative pulse current of −200 μA applied to the stimulating unipolar electrode or to the proximal tip of the bipolar electrode. The pulse repetition frequency was 130 Hz. For sham-DBS controls, only bipolar electrodes were used because they induce more mechanical stress to the tissue during the surgical procedure.

2.6. Behavioral Tests. The effects of lesion- and DBS-induced changes in the animals' behavior were quantified using the drug-induced apomorphine-stimulated rotation test and three non-drug-induced tests (the stepping, corridor, and open field tests). Experiments were conducted at different times: (i) prior to lesion induction; (ii) 12–14 days after lesion or sham lesion induction; (iii) after 3 days of DBS or 3 days with the stimulator off (sham stimulation); (iv) after 3 weeks of DBS or 3 weeks with the stimulator off (sham stimulation); (v) ≥3 days after the cessation of DBS subsequent to 3 weeks of DBS; (vi) after 6 weeks of DBS; and (vii) 3 weeks after the cessation of DBS subsequent to 3 weeks of DBS. For details see Table 1 and Figure 4.

2.7. Apomorphine-Induced Rotation Test. For assessing drug-induced locomotor function, apomorphine (0.25 mg/kg body weight dissolved in saline) was injected subcutaneously. Rotation was quantified in a custom-made "rodent-rotometer" modified according to Ungerstedt and Arbuthnott [44]. The rate of pathological circling, in rotations per minute (rpm), contralateral to the 6-OHDA-lesion site was determined electronically over 40 min. Rotation counts of at least 2 rpm indicated successful lesions. Subsequently, animals were assigned to groups such that the groups were composed of rats that had approximately the same mean rotation values. The rotation tests were repeated after one day because the first apomorphine application did not usually result in the maximum response.

2.8. Stepping Test. The stepping test, which assesses forelimb akinesia, was essentially performed as described by Olsson et al. [45]. In brief, rats were set on a table and allowed to settle with all limbs on the table. The experimenter then lifted the lower body by grabbing the rat around neck and behind the forepaws in a way that only the forepaws were touching the

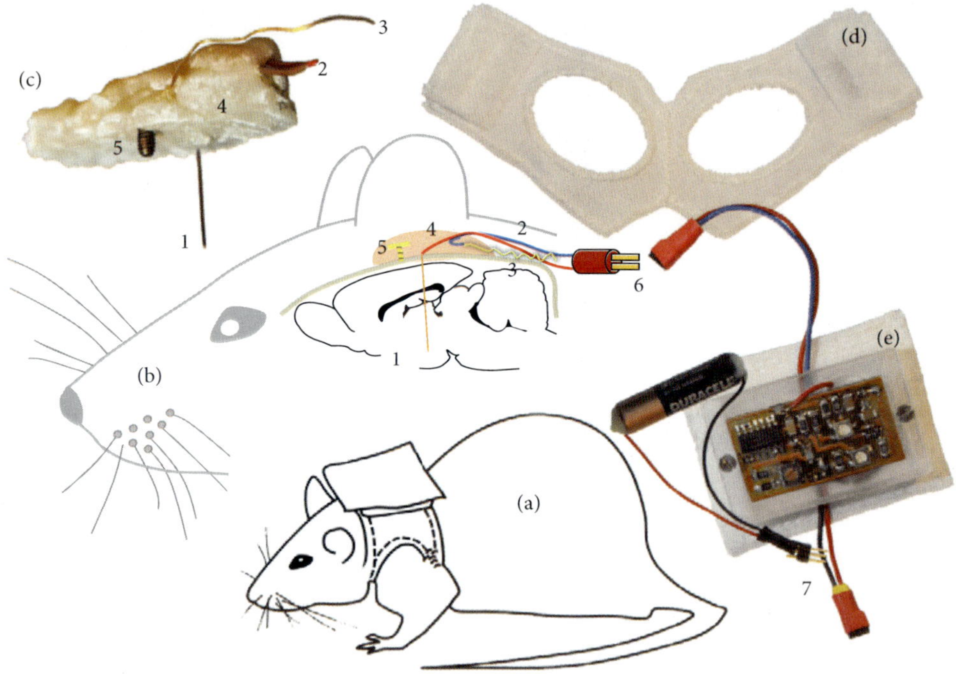

Figure 2: Schematic views of the unipolar DBS rat model. (a) Rat with stimulator in backpack; (b) sagittal view illustrating the locations of the implanted unipolar DBS electrode; (c) image of an explanted DBS mounting; (d) backpack vest with Velcro hooks; (e) stimulator in PMMA housing with pocket and current-pulse battery. 1: unipolar Pt/Ir electrode; 2: electrode cables; 3: gold-wire counter electrode; 4: biocompatible dental acrylic embedding all components; 5: anchor screw to fix the acrylic mounting to the skull; 6: electrode connector; 7: current-pulse battery connector.

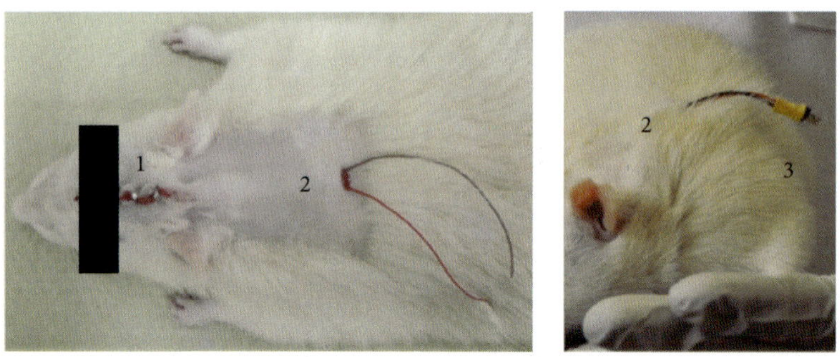

(a) (b)

Figure 3: (a) Details of the outlet port for the subcutaneous cables centered at the dorsum. (b) Rat with electrode connector one week after surgery. 1: suture clips; 2: dorsal cable outlet port; 3: crimped plug connector.

Table 1: Experimental design. The number of rats refers to the group sizes at the time of the apomorphine-induced rotation tests.

Group name	6-OHDA lesion	Electrode	DBS duration	Number of animals
Naive_3 d/3 w	–	—	—	10
Naive_sham_3 w	–	Bipolar	—	9
6-OHDA_sham_3 d/3 w	+	Bipolar	—	7
Sham_bi_3 d	Sham	Bipolar	3 days	9
Sham_bi_3 w	Sham	Bipolar	3 weeks	10
Sham_uni_6 w	Sham	Unipolar	6 weeks	7
6-OHDA_bi_3 d	+	Bipolar	3 days	7
6-OHDA_bi_3 w	+	Bipolar	3 weeks	5
6-OHDA_uni_3 d	+	Unipolar	3 days	13
6-OHDA_uni_3 w/3 w + 3 d off	+	Unipolar	3 weeks	11
6-OHDA_uni_6 w	+	Unipolar	6 weeks	7
6-OHDA_uni_3 w + 3 w off	+	Unipolar	3 weeks	8

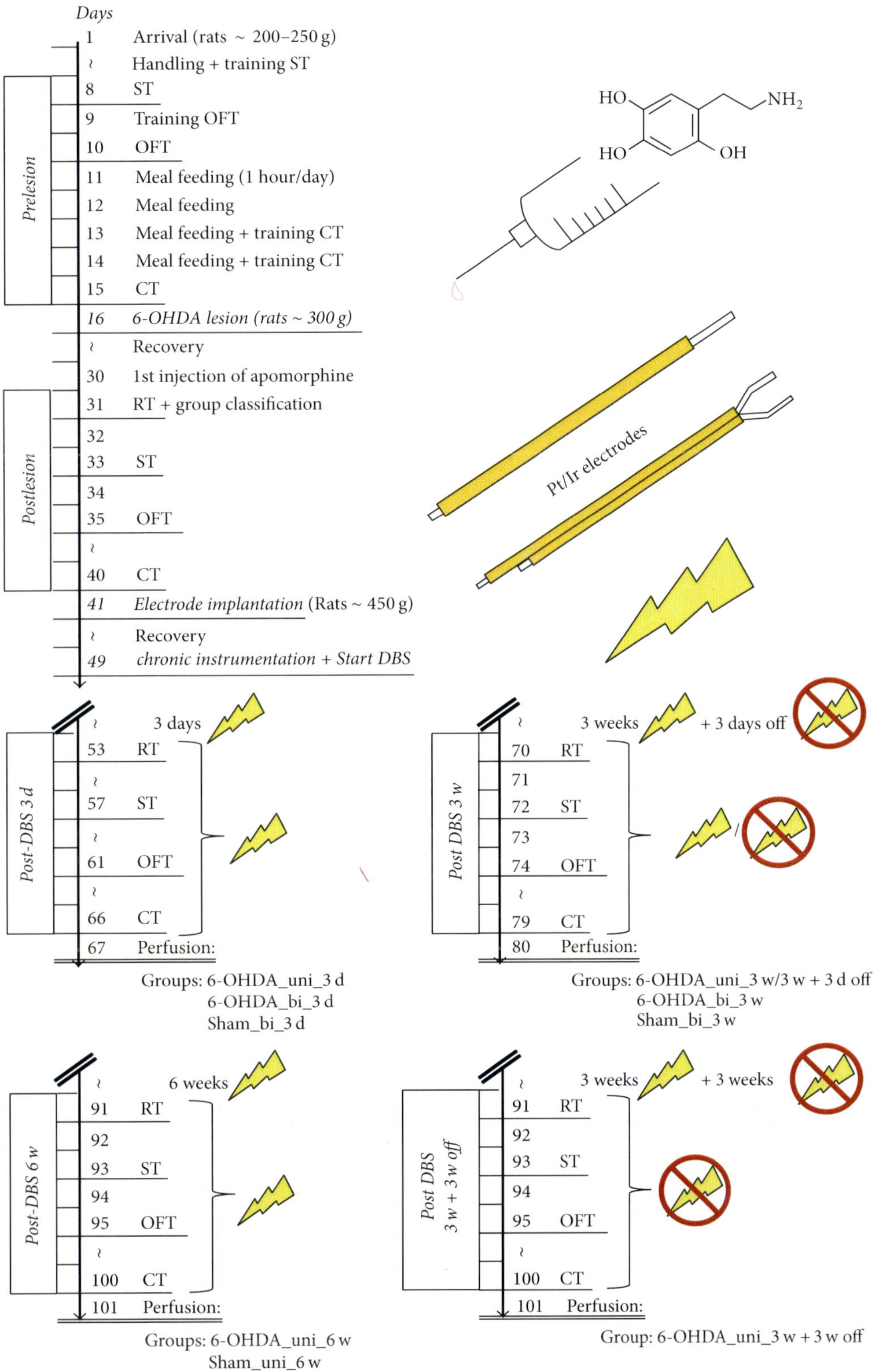

FIGURE 4: Schedules of the test procedures. RT, ST, OFT, and CT refer to the rotation, stepping, open field, and corridor tests, respectively.

table. Then, one forepaw was restrained, and the free forepaw, which was still touching the table, was moved sideways at a steady pace along the table surface in both directions at a rate of approximately 1 m per 5 s. The number of adjusting steps was counted manually for the movement of both forepaws in the forehand and backhand directions. For both directions, the contralateral bias was calculated as the percentage of steps of the contralateral paw with respect to the sum of the steps of both forepaws (50% was expected for control). In addition, the time needed for the initiation of the first adjusting step toward the rats' home cage was recorded for both forepaws. In the cases of an immediate response (i.e., when the initiation time was too short to be registered manually), the time was recorded as zero.

2.9. Corridor Test. To assess sensorimotor neglect, we used the corridor test [46]. A long narrow wooden corridor (240 cm long, 7 cm wide, and 23 cm high) was equipped with 14 equidistant pairs of adjacent pots (diameter: 1.2 cm) placed along both sides of the corridor. Each pot contained five sucrose reward tablets (5TUT; TestDiet®, USA). The clear plastic lid of the corridor allowed us to observe the rats during testing. Before the tests, rats were food-restricted with only 1 hour per day allowed for feeding ("meal feeding") for 4 days. Two tests were performed on two consecutive days under the same conditions. The trials started with placing the rat into one end of the corridor, where it was free to explore, turn around, and feed on pellets. One "retrieval" was counted when the animal poked its nose into a pot with sugar pellets, regardless of whether it actually retrieved or fed on any pellets. The exploration of each new pot was counted as an additional retrieval. To reduce exploration behavior of the corridor itself, rats were placed into an identical, empty corridor beforehand. The number of retrievals ipsilateral and contralateral to the side of the lesion were recorded manually over 5 min. The contralateral bias was expressed as the percentage of the retrievals made on the contralateral side relative to the total number of retrievals.

2.10. Open Field Test. Spontaneous mobility and anxiety were evaluated by placing the rats in a square open field arena (46 cm × 45 cm) inside an isolation box. The animals were kept in the dark in the examination room 1 h before the start of the test. The open field was illuminated by a white photo bulb providing 200 to 250 Lux. During testing, rats were monitored by a video camera. The open field was divided into a center area (22 cm × 22 cm) and a peripheral zone using the tracking software Ethovision XT (Noldus Information Technology, Leesburg, VA, USA; RRID:SCR_000441). This allowed for the automatic recording of the rat's movement in the two zones. Each rat was tested once for 10 minutes. After each session, the open field was cleaned to prevent odor from influencing the next animal's behavior. The total migration distances were taken as a measure of spontaneous mobility and the ratio of the migration distance within the center area to the total distance moved was interpreted as a measure of anxiety.

2.11. Statistics. Data analysis was conducted with the SAS software package, Version 9.4 for Windows (Copyright, SAS Institute Inc., Cary, NC, USA, RRID:SCR_008567). Descriptive statistics and tests for normality were calculated with the UNIVARIATE procedure using Base SAS software. Data that could be considered as approximately normal was analyzed by one-way repeated measurement ANOVA with the MIXED procedure of the SAS/STAT software module. The models for the investigated treatments contained the fixed factor "time" with different levels (prelesion, postlesion, 3 d, 3 w, 3 w + 3 d, and 6 w) for each treatment. Repeated measures on the same animal were taken into account in the REPEATED statement of the MIXED procedure using time as the repeated effect, the SUBJECT = animal option to define the blocks of the residual covariance matrix and the TYPE = CS option to define their covariance structure. Least-square means (LSM) and their standard errors (SE) were computed for each time level of each treatment and compared with the "postlesion"-LSM using the Dunnett-Hsu procedure (pairwise multiple comparisons with the control).

The investigated treatments for each time (prelesion, postlesion, 3 d, 3 w, 3 w + 3 d, and 6 w) were analyzed by one-way ANOVA with the MIXED procedure of the SAS/STAT software module. The models for the times contained the fixed factor treatment (see Table 1). LSM and their SE were computed for each treatment level of each time and were compared pairwise using the Tukey-Kramer procedure (pairwise multiple comparisons of all possible pairs). Effects and differences were considered significant for $p \leq 0.05$.

3. Results

3.1. Confirmation of Electrode Placement. The localization of electrode tips in the STN was evaluated by retrospective analyses of Nissl-stained cryosections of the STN of selected rats. It suggested a precise electrode placement in approximately 75% of the cases, analogous to the success rate of the lesion surgery (see below). A comprehensive histological evaluation is currently underway.

3.2. Locomotor Activity. The success of lesion induction was evaluated based on the apomorphine-induced rotation test results 12–14 days after surgery. The success rate (rpm $\geq$ 2) was approximately 75%, and the mortality rate was less than 10%. In the apomorphine-induced rotation test, reduced rotation was detected with DBS after 3 days and after 3 weeks. In these cases, unipolar stimulation was more effective than bipolar stimulation (Figure 5). However, after 6 weeks, pathological rotation was detected again, regardless of whether the DBS had been continued or discontinued after 3 weeks. As expected, no pathological rotation was detected in naïve or sham-lesioned rats.

Spontaneous locomotor activity was assessed based on the total migration distance in the open field test. 6-OHDA lesions reduced the total migration distance, whereas naïve rats showed a marginal increase in total distance with each trial, which can be explained by habituation to the open

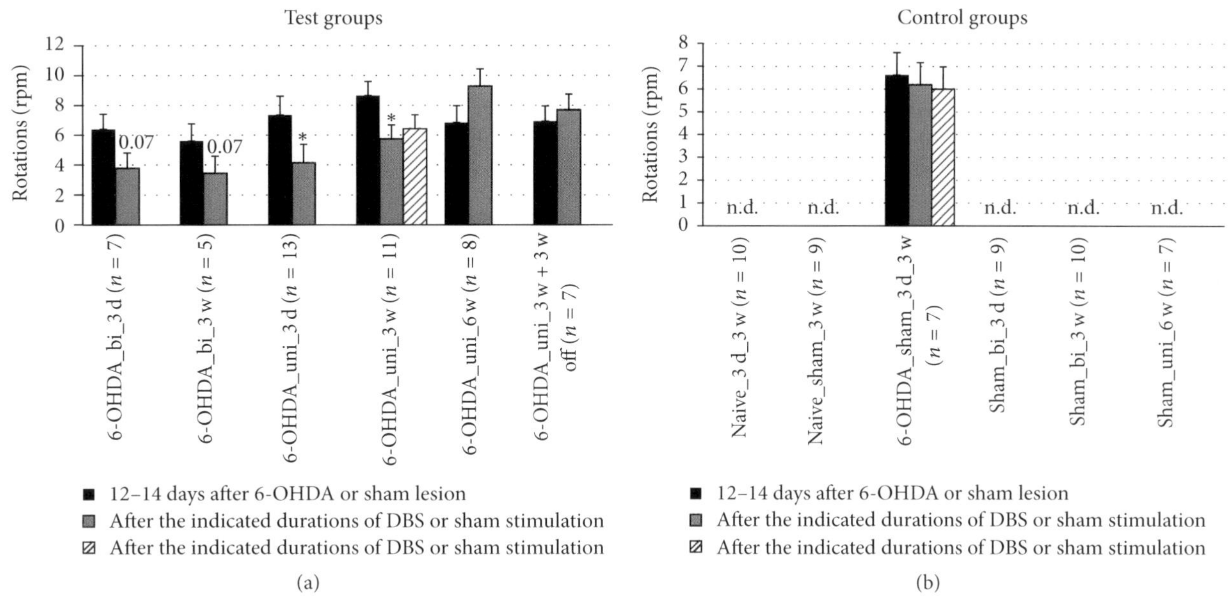

FIGURE 5: Short-term and long-term effects of DBS with uni- and bipolar electrodes on the apomorphine-induced rotation behavior of hemiparkinsonian rats. (a) and (b) refer to test groups and controls, respectively. Different column patterns indicate the different times of behavioral testing; black: 12–14 days after 6-OHDA or sham lesion; gray and hatched: after the durations of DBS or sham stimulation indicated in the group labels. For experimental details see Table 1. Significance levels are indicated with asterisks as follows: $^{*}p \leq 0.05$, b (borderline): $0.05 < p \leq 0.08$ according to one-way ANOVA. Asterisks refer to comparisons with corresponding black columns.

field with repeated exposure. In contrast, DBS reduced the total migration distance, in most of the groups. The total migration distance increased at 3 days after the cessation of DBS subsequent to 3 weeks of DBS with unipolar electrodes (Figure 11).

3.3. Akinesia. To assess the effects of the lesion-induced akinesia, the parameters "initiation time of paw movement" and "number of adjusting steps" were recorded in the stepping test. In rats receiving bipolar DBS, a significant reduction in the initiation time of contralateral forepaw stepping was observed after 3 days but not after 3 weeks of DBS (Figure 6). In long-term, unipolar DBS, significant improvements were found 3 weeks after the cessation of DBS subsequent to 3 weeks of DBS. A similar effect was observed after 6 weeks of continuous stimulation, although with borderline significance.

Unexpectedly, we observed an increase in the initiation time of ipsilateral forepaw stepping after 6-OHDA lesioning in one group and no beneficial effect of DBS in any of the groups. Moreover, we found an aggravating effect of DBS effect after 3 weeks that vanished 3 days after the cessation of DBS (Figure 7).

Impaired contralateral paw movement (contralateral bias) was determined based on the number of contralateral versus ipsilateral adjusting steps of the forepaws. A significant difference in the contralateral bias during forced sidestepping was found in only one case. The contralateral bias in the forehand direction worsened after 6 weeks of unipolar DBS (Figure 8). In the backhand direction, no significant effects of DBS were detected (Figure 9). Overall, the contralateral bias measured in the stepping test did not seem to be affected by DBS therapy (Table 2).

3.4. Sensorimotor Neglect. In the corridor test, DBS reduced the amount of sensorimotor neglect when applied by unipolar electrodes for 3 weeks (Figure 10). The beneficial effect persisted for at least 3 weeks after the cessation of DBS, although with borderline significance. Interestingly, 6 weeks of continuous DBS did not demonstrate the same beneficial effect, and DBS with bipolar electrodes did not show any significant beneficial effects.

3.5. Anxiety. The open field test provided information on locomotor activity and anxiety-like behavior. Although the total distance moved (Figure 11) was determined by both locomotor function and anxiety, the ratio of distances (central versus peripheral movement) predominantly reflects anxiety. In untreated naïve rats, the distance ratio generally increased with time, indicating a habituation effect, and sham DBS-treated naïve rats and DBS-treated sham-lesioned rats retained this behavior (Figure 12). However, the distance ratio significantly increased in the groups treated by DBS with unipolar electrodes after 3 or 6 weeks, but not after 3 days. In contrast, the distance ratio was increased in the groups treated by DBS with bipolar electrodes after 3 days, but not after 3 weeks. A minor increase ($p = 0.053$) in the distance ratio was also observed after 6 weeks of sham stimulation with unipolar electrodes.

Table 2 summarizes the test results for DBS-induced parameter changes.

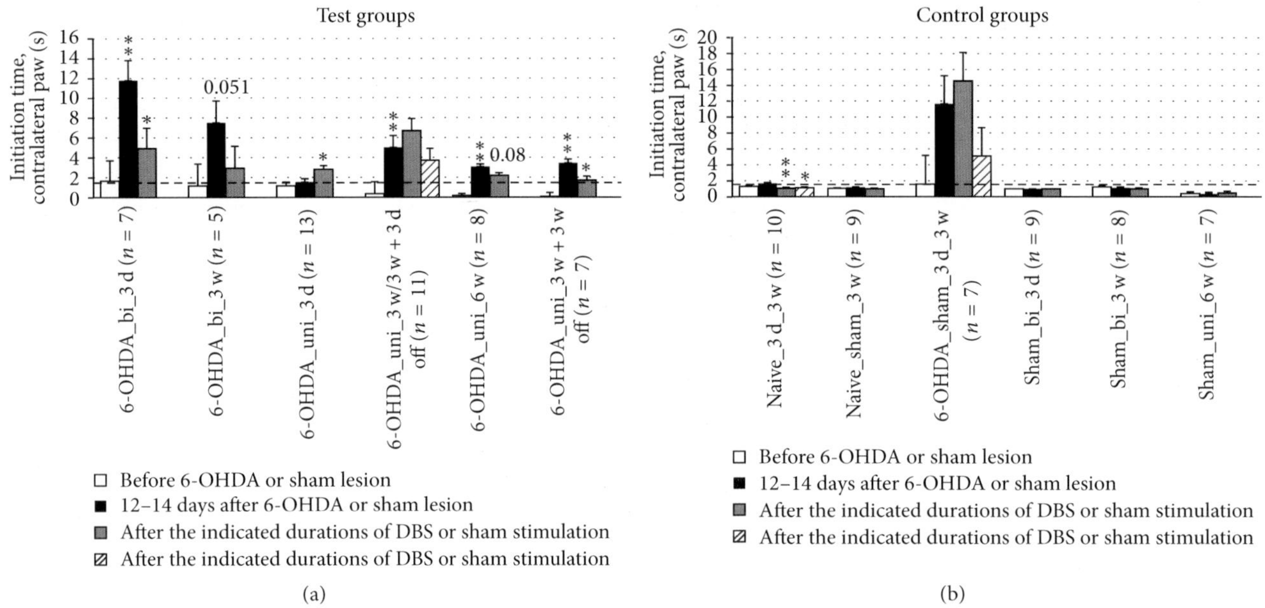

FIGURE 6: Short-term and long-term effects of DBS with uni- and bipolar electrodes on akinesia as measured by the initiation time of the first adjusting step of the contralateral forepaw in the stepping test. (a) and (b) refer to test groups and controls, respectively. The dashed line at 1 s allows for an easier comparison with Figure 7 and between (a) and (b). Different column patterns indicate different times of behavioral testing; white: before 6-OHDA or sham lesion; black: 12–14 days after 6-OHDA or sham lesion; gray and hatched: after the durations of DBS or sham stimulation indicated in the group labels. For experimental details see Table 1. Significance levels are indicated with asterisks as follows: $^{**}p \leq 0.01$, $^{*}p \leq 0.05$, b (borderline): $0.05 < p \leq 0.08$ according to one-way ANOVA. Asterisks above black columns refer to white columns; all others refer to black columns.

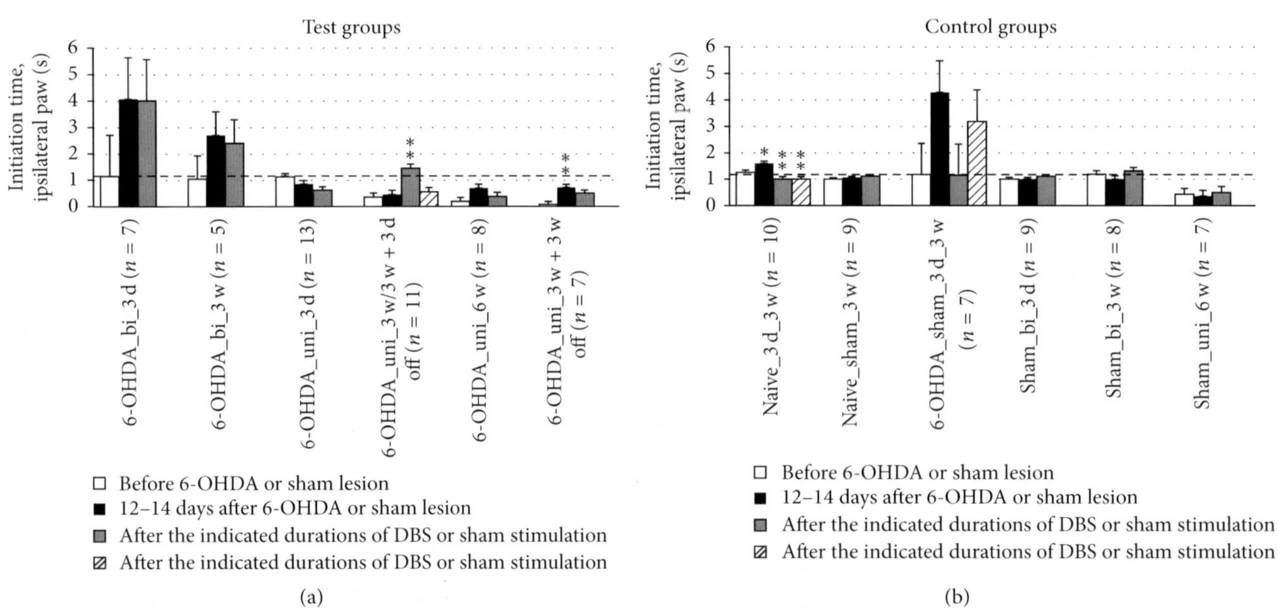

FIGURE 7: Short-term and long-term effects of DBS with uni- and bipolar electrodes on the akinesia of hemiparkinsonian rats as measured by the initiation time of the first adjusting step of the ipsilateral forepaw in the stepping test. (a) and (b) refer to test groups and controls, respectively. The dashed line at 1 s allows for an easier comparison with Figure 6 and between (a) and (b). Different column patterns indicate different times of behavioral testing; white: before 6-OHDA or sham lesion; black: 12–14 days after 6-OHDA or sham lesion; gray and hatched: after the durations of DBS or sham stimulation indicated in the group labels. For experimental details see Table 1. Significance levels are indicated with asterisks as follows: $^{**}p \leq 0.01$, $^{*}p \leq 0.05$, b (borderline): $0.05 < p \leq 0.08$ according to one-way ANOVA. Asterisks above black columns refer to white columns; all others refer to black columns.

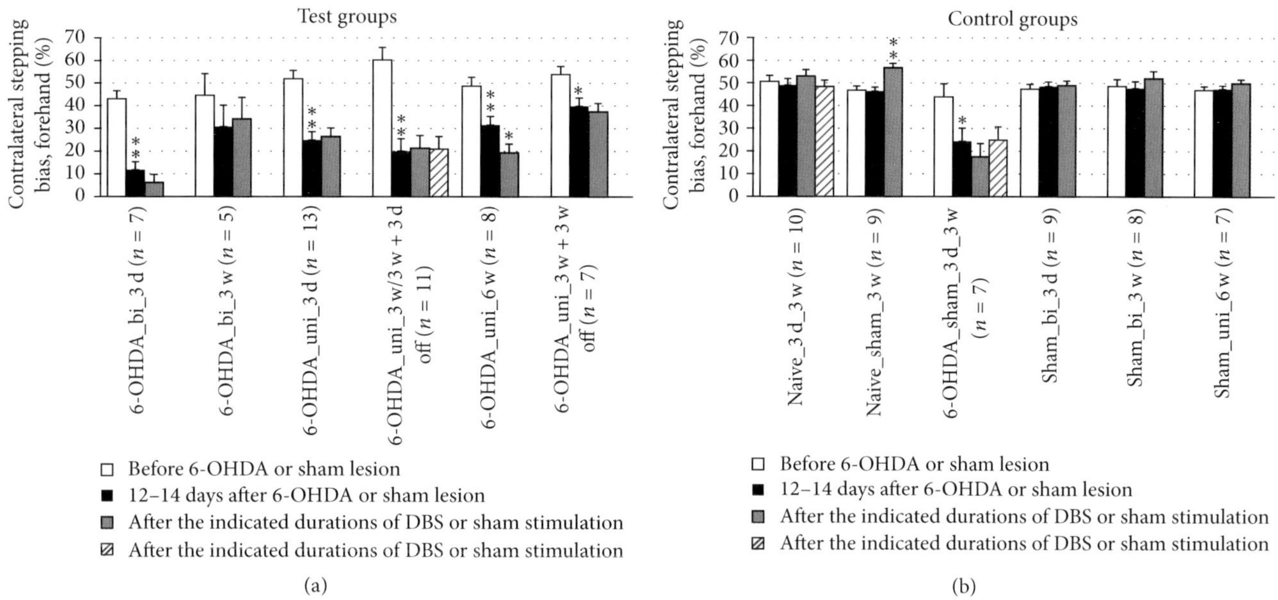

FIGURE 8: Short-term and long-term effects of DBS with uni- and bipolar electrodes on akinesia as measured by forced sidestepping of the forepaws in the forehand direction in the stepping tests. (a) and (b) refer to test groups and controls, respectively. Different column patterns indicate different times of behavioral testing; white: before 6-OHDA or sham lesion; black: 12–14 days after 6-OHDA or sham lesion; gray and hatched: after the durations of DBS or sham stimulation indicated in the group labels. For experimental details see Table 1. Significance levels are indicated with asterisks as follows: $^{**}p \leq 0.01$, $^{*}p \leq 0.05$, b (borderline): $0.05 < p \leq 0.08$ according to one-way ANOVA. Asterisks above black columns refer to white columns; all others refer to black columns.

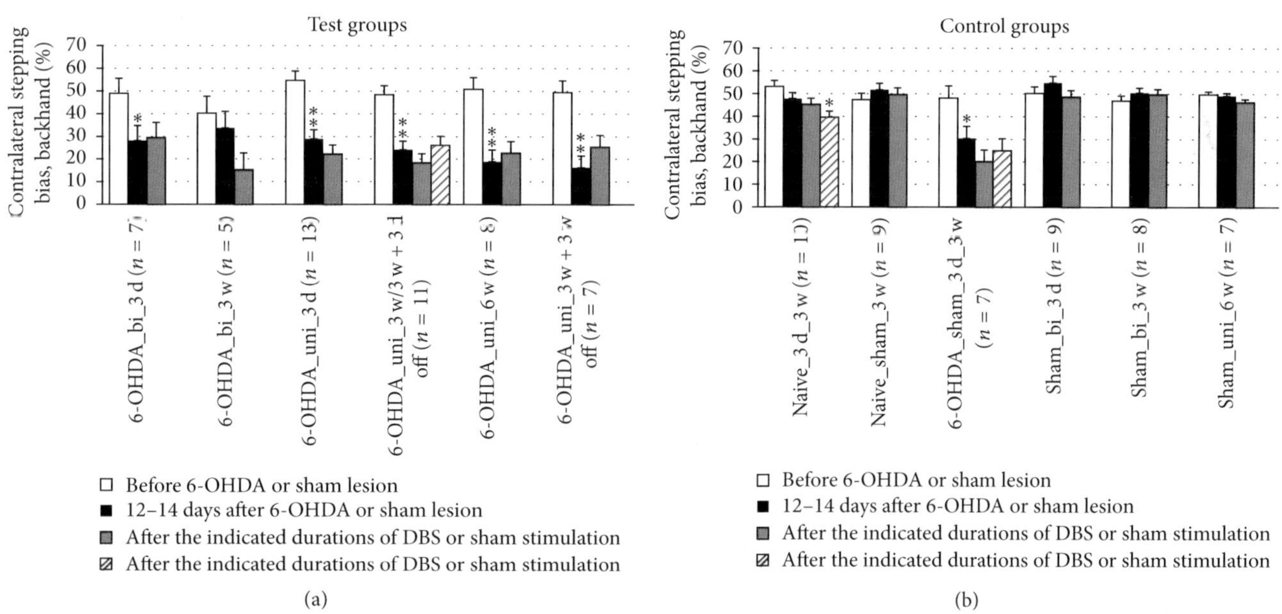

FIGURE 9: Short-term and long-term effects of DBS with uni- and bipolar electrodes on the akinesia of hemiparkinsonian rats as measured by forced sidestepping of the forepaws in the backhand direction in the stepping tests. (a) and (b) refer to test groups and controls, respectively. Different column patterns indicate different times of behavioral testing; white: before 6-OHDA or sham lesion; black: 12–14 days after 6-OHDA or sham lesion; gray and hatched: after the durations of DBS or sham stimulation indicated in the group labels. For experimental details see Table 1. Significance levels are indicated with asterisks as follows: $^{**}p \leq 0.01$, $^{*}p \leq 0.05$, b (borderline): $0.05 < p \leq 0.08$ according to one-way ANOVA. Asterisks above black columns refer to white columns; all others refer to black columns.

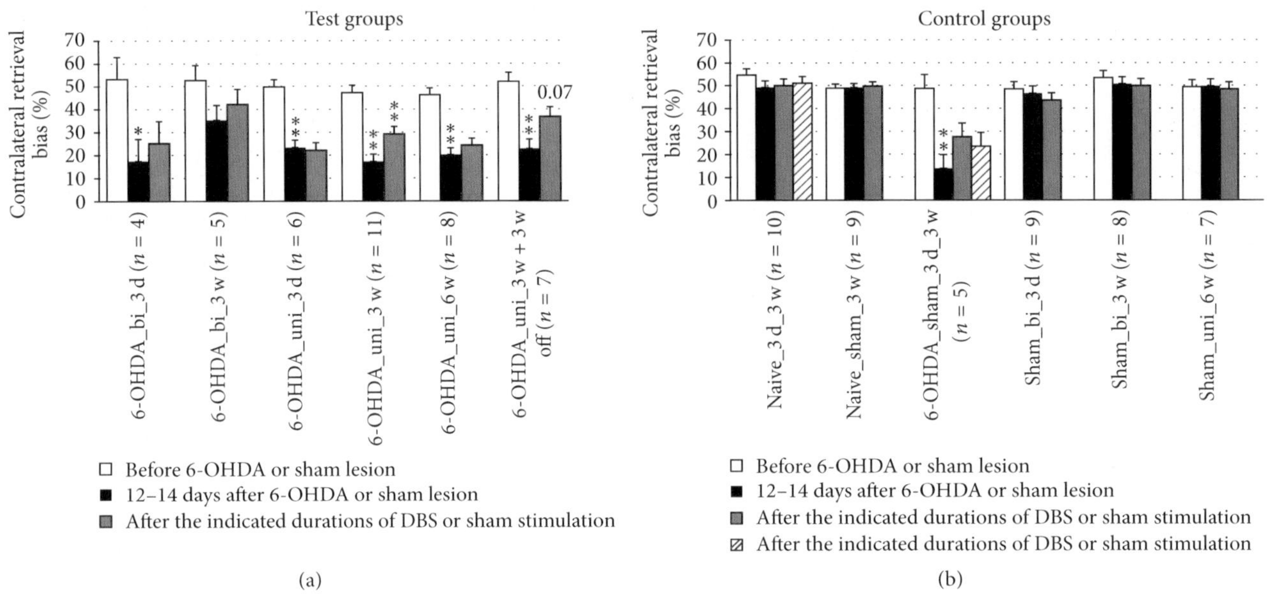

FIGURE 10: Short-term and long-term effects of DBS with uni- and bipolar electrodes on the sensorimotor neglect of hemiparkinsonian rats as measured by the corridor test. (a) and (b) refer to test groups and controls, respectively. Different column patterns indicate different times of behavioral testing; white: before 6-OHDA or sham lesion; black: 12–14 days after 6-OHDA or sham lesion; gray and hatched: after the durations of DBS or sham stimulation indicated in the group labels. For experimental details see Table 1. Significance levels are indicated with asterisks as follows: $^{**}p \leq 0.01$, $^{*}p \leq 0.05$, b (borderline): $0.05 < p \leq 0.08$ according to one-way ANOVA. Asterisks above black columns refer to white columns; all others refer to black columns.

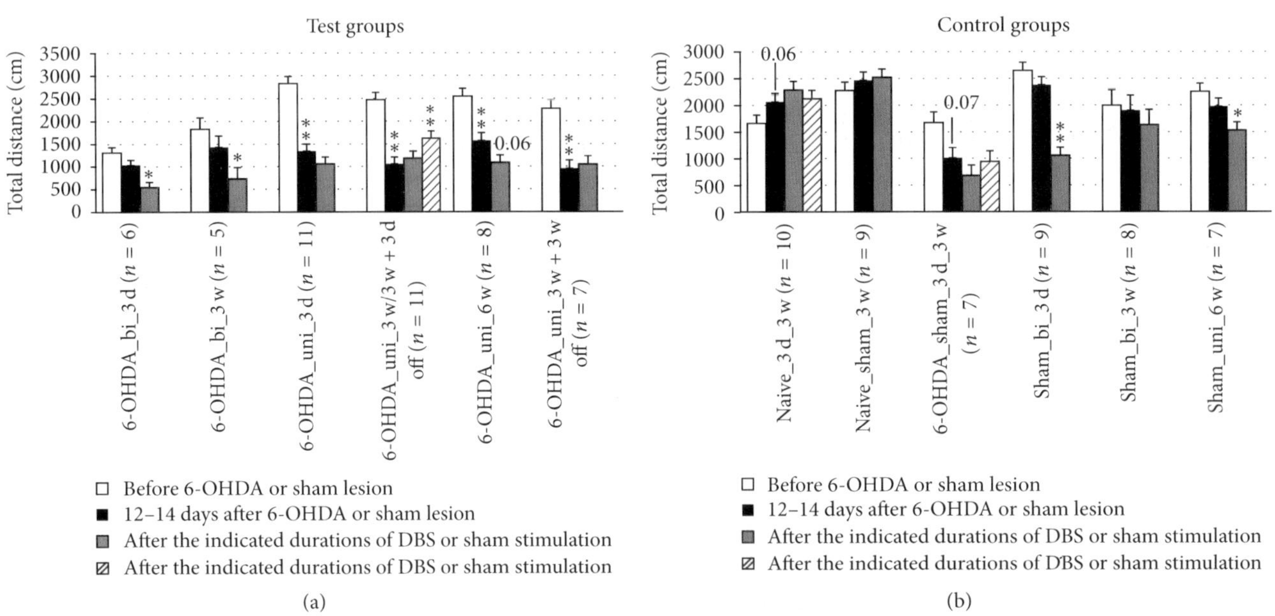

FIGURE 11: Short-term and long-term effects of DBS with uni- and bipolar electrodes on the locomotor activity of hemiparkinsonian rats as measured by the total migration distance in the open field. (a) and (b) refer to test groups and controls, respectively. Different column patterns indicate different times of behavioral testing; white: before 6-OHDA or sham lesion; black: 12–14 days after 6-OHDA or sham lesion; gray and hatched: after the durations of DBS or sham stimulation indicated in the group labels. For experimental details see Table 1. Significance levels are indicated with asterisks as follows: $^{**}p \leq 0.01$, $^{*}p \leq 0.05$, b (borderline): $0.05 < p \leq 0.08$ according to one-way ANOVA. Asterisks above black columns refer to white columns; all others refer to black columns.

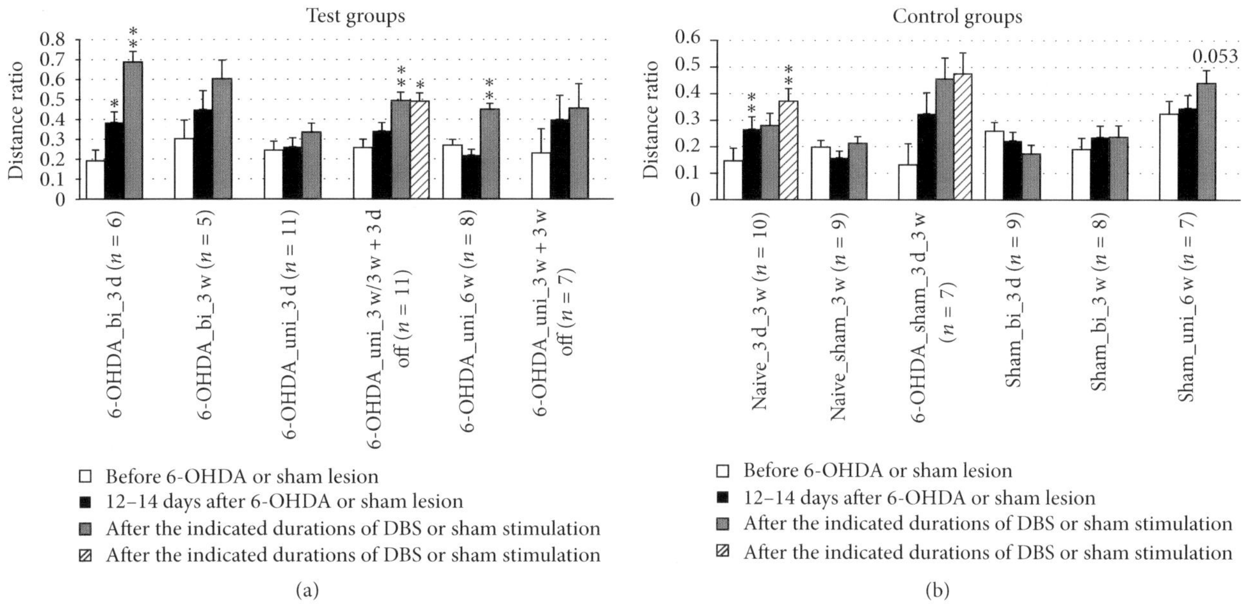

FIGURE 12: Short-term and long-term effects of DBS with uni- and bipolar electrodes on the anxiety-like behavior (b) of hemiparkinsonian rats as measured by the ratio: migration distance in the center/total migration in the open field. (a) and (b) refer to test groups and controls, respectively. Different column patterns indicate different times of behavioral testing; white: before 6-OHDA or sham lesion; black: 12–14 days after 6-OHDA or sham lesion; gray and hatched: after the durations of DBS or sham stimulation indicated in the group labels. For experimental details see Table 1. Significance levels are indicated with asterisks as follows: $^{**}p \leq 0.01$, $^{*}p \leq 0.05$, b (borderline): $0.05 < p \leq 0.08$ according to one-way ANOVA. Asterisks above black columns refer to white columns; all others refer to black columns.

TABLE 2: Summary of test results. The improvement and worsening of lesion-induced parkinsonian symptoms by DBS are marked by (+) and (−), respectively. Borderline changes ($0.05 < p \leq 0.08$) are marked by (b); parameters with no detectable DBS effects are marked (0); n.d. stands for "not determined." The results marked with an asterisk could not be interpreted in terms of the therapeutic DBS effects.

Group name	Rotation test	Stepping test initiation time	Stepping test contralateral bias		Corridor test	Open-field test	
		Contralateral paw	Forehand	Backhand		Total distance	Distance ratio*
6-OHDA_bi_3 d	b+	+	0	0	0	—	Up
6-OHDA_bi_3 w	b+	b+	0	0	0	—	0
6-OHDA_uni_ 3 d	+	b−	0	0	0	—	0
6 OHDA_uni_ 3 w	I	0	0	0	I	0	Up
6-OHDA_uni_ 3 w + 3 d off	0	0	0	0	n.d.	+	Up
6-OHDA_uni_ 6 w	0	b+	—	0	0	b−	Up
6-OHDA_uni_ 3 w + 3 w off	0	+	0	0	b+	0	0

4. Discussion

4.1. The Hemiparkinsonian Rat Model. The 6-OHDA-induced hemiparkinsonian rat model has been established for the study of therapeutic approaches for treating PD [11, 35, 49–51]. Although this model is known to reflect the major behavioral impairments that are characteristic of PD patients, animal studies are hampered by restrictions on free movement and/or invasive surgery and by short observation periods lasting from a few minutes [35, 49, 51–54] to a number of days [12, 24, 55–57]. To our knowledge, removable and reusable devices have been previously used by only Forni et al. [28].

Frequencies from 90 to 130 Hz are generally accepted as optimal to elicit the therapeutic effects of DBS in patients [52]. In this frequency range, the clinically observed benefits are maximal and a more normal activity pattern in the nuclei downstream is restored [22]. Recent findings in patients with advanced PD who became refractory to the common high-frequency stimulation have shown a restoration in the improvement of segmental and axial symptoms, gait disturbance, and levodopa-induced dyskinesia after the stimulation frequency was reduced to 60 Hz [58]. Here, we used a pulse frequency of 130 Hz in all experiments, even though this frequency was established for DBS in the much larger human brain.

In PD patients, unipolar stimulation is the preferred mode of DBS. So et al. [51] have also suggested using unipolar stimulation in the hemiparkinsonian rat model, although they did not find differences between the effects of uni- and bipolar stimulations in a drug-induced locomotor test. Our first experiments (up to 3 weeks) revealed greater beneficial effects with unipolar DBS than with bipolar DBS. For these reasons, only the unipolar experiments were extended out to 6 weeks (Figure 4).

4.2. The Outcome of the Different Behavioral Tests. To test the success of lesioning and test initial locomotor function, the classical drug-induced rotation assay was used. Pathological rotation is measured in response to the administration of either the dopamine (DA) receptor agonist apomorphine or the DA-releasing drug amphetamine [43, 44, 59, 60].

In partially lesioned animals, Hefti et al. [59] did not find apomorphine-induced rotation, whereas amphetamine induced a dose-dependent ipsilateral rotation. These authors observed a contralateral apomorphine-induced rotation only in severely lesioned animals, which is comparable to our results. These findings are in line with the results of Da Cunha et al. [60], who investigated the directions of rotation that were induced by either apomorphine or amphetamine in partially and severely lesioned animals. In severely 6-OHDA-lesioned mice, apomorphine-induced rotation was shown to be more informative than amphetamine-induced rotation in discriminating between the different degrees of lesions [61].

Interestingly, we found a reduction in apomorphine-induced rotation if DBS was applied for 3 days or 3 weeks in either the bipolar or unipolar modes, with the latter being more effective (Figure 5; Table 2). Apomorphine-induced rotation returned to pre-DBS levels after 6 weeks of continuous DBS or after 3 weeks of continuous DBS followed by 3 weeks without DBS. As discussed below, STN-DBS-induced therapeutic effects are not predicted to be reflected in the rate of apomorphine-induced rotation. Therefore, the reason for the reduction in apomorphine-induced rotation after 3 weeks of DBS was unclear. This effect was not surgery-induced because it did not occur in the 6-OHDA-lesioned sham-stimulated rats. Assuming that STN-DBS temporarily increases striatal DA turnover, as described by Meissner et al. [50], the hypersensitivity of DA receptors could be transiently reduced at a time scale of weeks. We assume that this effect was not permanent in our model because it is known that the dopaminergic neurons in the substantia nigra pars compacta (SNc) eventually degenerate leading to an almost complete lack of DA release in the striatum.

We believe that apomorphine-induced rotation is not an appropriate parameter for testing the beneficial effects of STN-DBS. Limitations of the apomorphine-induced rotation test have been previously demonstrated. Metz and Whishaw [62] have shown that the apomorphine-induced rotation rate did not correlate with spontaneous and skilled reaching or ladder rung walking tasks. In a study on apomorphine-induced rotation, Chang et al. [63] failed to demonstrate any effect of STN-DBS in 6-OHDA-induced hemiparkinsonian rats. They concluded that the apomorphine-induced imbalance of dopaminergic activation may not necessarily be improved by DBS. In contrast, STN-DBS has been shown to reduce or even reverse the direction of amphetamine-induced rotation in 6-OHDA-lesioned rats [11, 35, 49, 51]. Nevertheless, the amphetamine-induced rotation test has its limitations. Kirik et al. [64] showed that the test for the initiation time in stepping was a more sensitive metric than the amphetamine-induced rotation test. Because of these limitations, some authors have introduced new methods to evaluate the effect of DBS, such as an automated rotarod method for the drug-free quantitative evaluation of overall motor deficits [65].

Additionally, our results showing that a reduction of the initiation time of the contralateral forepaw was induced by DBS were not consistent with the results of the rotation test with unipolar stimulation. The shortest initiation times of the contralateral paw were observed 3 weeks after the cessation of DBS subsequent to 3 weeks of continuous DBS (Figure 6; Table 2). Our histological investigations showed that dopaminergic neurons were not regenerated in the substantia nigra (results not published). This suggests that the persistent DBS effects might be related to the neuronal plasticity in young rats. The increase of the initiation time of the ipsilateral paw after 6-OHDA lesion was much less than the increase on the contralateral side. However, this result did show that both hemispheres are affected by unilateral 6-OHDA lesion, as we have previously shown for the activation of astrocytes in the contralateral striatum after 6-OHDA lesion [66].

Locomotor activity changes detected in the open field test should be interpreted with caution as they may be influenced by various modifying factors, including habituation, the need for exploration, and anxiety effects. Indeed, we observed a habituation to the open field in naïve rats in both the total migration distance and in the anxiety parameter distance ratio. Lesions induced a reduction in locomotor activity, as measured by total migration distance. DBS induced a further decrease, even in sham-lesioned rats (Figure 11; Table 2). This additional decrease was reversed after the cessation of DBS and did not occur in sham-stimulated rats. We interpret the DBS-induced decrease in locomotor activity as a reduction in the health of the animals caused by the electrical stimulation. These results indicate that stimulation parameters have to be reconsidered in future experiments.

In PD patients, anxiety may result from not only the impairment of motor function but also dysfunction of the STN. Experiments with bilaterally STN-lesioned rats in the elevated plus maze test also suggest such a connection [67]. Here, we assessed anxiety-like behavior using the open field parameter "ratio of migration distance in the center to total migration." This parameter quantifies the balance between the need of the animal to explore their environment with the need to be cautious, which prevents them from exploring the unprotected center of a brightly lit open field box. In our setting, naïve rats became more curious and less anxious over time due to habituation. Likewise, the decrease in anxiety-like behavior by 6-OHDA-lesioned rats can be explained by habituation to the open field (Figure 12). Based on these results, the increasing distance ratio observed after DBS may not be an effect of DBS but rather an effect of habituation. In contrast, the distance ratio of sham-lesioned rats and sham-stimulated naïve rats (i.e., healthy rats with disconnected electrodes) remained at their initial levels. The reduced activity of the rats after electrode implantation suggests adverse effects of the surgery itself and a treatment-related reduction in the rats' health.

The corridor test was originally established to detect lateralized sensorimotor integration [61]. It has been successfully applied to demonstrate the feasibility of the thalamic center-median parafascicular nucleus as a target for DBS in 6-OHDA-lesioned rats [55, 68]. In our study, 3 weeks of STN-DBS with unipolar electrodes reduced sensorimotor neglect. After the cessation of DBS, this effect persisted with borderline significance for at least 3 more weeks (Figure 10). Six weeks of continuous DBS did not have the same beneficial effect.

These findings raise questions about whether different mechanisms are responsible for the observed effects of acute and chronic DBS, as well as about the persistent effects on locomotor and sensorimotor functions. One possible reason for these differences may be the development of an insensitivity toward DBS, reflecting changes in the basal ganglia network [22]. In addition, readjustment of the stimulation parameters may be necessary in chronic DBS, as is common in clinical practice, to compensate for the increasing impedance caused by the development of adventitia tissue at the electrode-tissue interface [69].

Here, we propose that tests of spontaneous locomotion, such as the stepping test, are more relevant for detecting the beneficial effects of DBS and provide different information than the apomorphine-induced rotation test. However, this conclusion does not necessarily apply to the amphetamine-induced rotation test because of the different mechanisms of these two rotation tests (see Appendix).

Our results suggest that persistent DBS effects in 6-OHDA-lesioned neuronal networks may be the result of the protection or regeneration of part of the physiological function of these networks in relation to locomotor activity in the absence of dopaminergic neurons. Alternatively, persistent effects of DBS could arise from DBS-induced effects that mimic a permanent lesion of the STN, for example, by space-consuming effects of the developing adventitia. Such mechanisms may explain our findings of persistent DBS effects on the initiation time of the contralateral forepaw in the stepping test (Figure 6) and, though with borderline significance, on sensorimotor neglect in the corridor test (Figure 10). A DBS-induced "mimicked" STN lesion would be in agreement with the lack of beneficial effects demonstrated in the open field behavior.

The different brain states and resulting behavioral effects are considered in Appendix. Figure 13 illustrates four different brain states in a single scheme of the lesioned hemisphere in the hemiparkinsonian rat: the healthy brain, the effects of a lesion, DBS after lesioning, and apomorphine administration after lesioning.

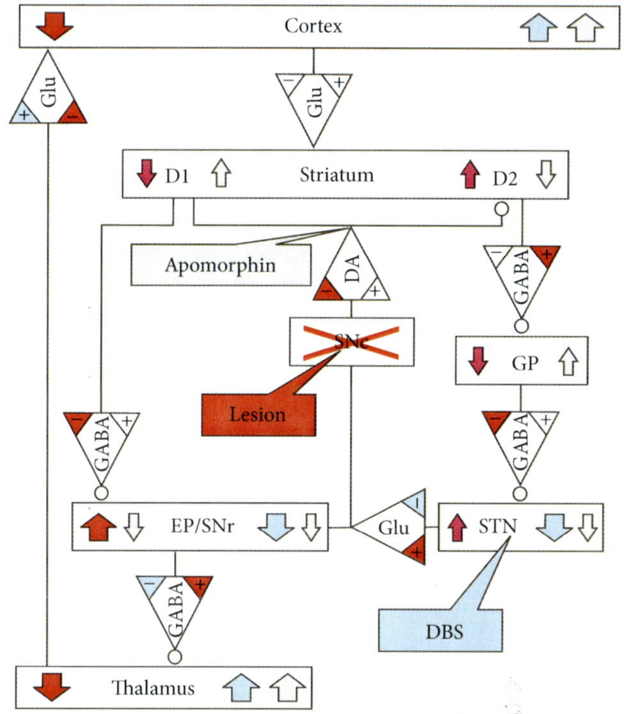

FIGURE 13: Simplified scheme of the lesioned hemisphere describing the effects of the lesion (red), DBS (blue), and apomorphine administration (light gray) on neurotransmitter release and on the activity (colored arrows) of different brain areas. Induced alterations in receptor numbers or sensitivities are not depicted; for explanation see Appendix. The brain areas are given in the boxes designated by SNc, GP, STN, and EP/SNr. The neurotransmitters glutamate (Glu), DA, and GABA are designated by triangular boxes pointing toward the affected brain areas that may be either excited (direct line input) or downregulated (input with circle). D1 and D2 stand for the dopaminergic receptors in the striatum, which are excited or inhibited by DA or apomorphine, respectively. Rectangular text balloons mark the input sites of lesioning, DBS, and apomorphine. The colored "+" and "−" signs in the neurotransmitter triangles designate the effects of lesioning (red) and DBS (blue) on transmitter release. Color-coding was not attempted for the effects of apomorphine on transmitter release.

4.3. Effects at the Molecular and Receptor Levels. Based on previous studies, apparently contradictory results have been obtained at both the molecular and receptor levels. The DBS-related decreases in the levels of extracellular DA and its metabolites in the dorsal part of the striatum described by Walker et al. [70] are in line with a decreased concentration of the DA metabolite DOPAC (3-4-dihydroxyphenylacetic acid) in the extracellular fluid of the striatum found by Yamamoto et al. [71]. In contrast, He et al. [72] described a DBS-induced increase in the extracellular striatal DA concentration. Recently, GABAergic activation by chronic DBS has been shown to be responsible for the compensation of motor asymmetries in hemiparkinsonian rats [73].

At the level of the receptors, missing neurotransmitter inputs are believed to induce a compensatory upregulation of receptor numbers or sensitivity. According to this view, a lesion-induced reduction in glutamate release to the cortex and the striatum resulting from alterations in activity along the striatum-D1 receptor-EP/SNr-thalamus pathway will result in an upregulation in glutamate receptors in the cortex and striatum. However, DBS after lesioning was found to reverse the increased striatal glutamate receptor numbers [57] and to increase the number of D1 receptors, which probably improves motor symptoms in PD patients [74]. At the same time, DBS decreases the number of D2/D3 receptors in the nucleus accumbens of rats, which may contribute to adverse DBS-induced neuropsychiatric side effects, such as apathy [74].

Most biochemical studies have been conducted under acute or subchronic (up to 7 days) STN-DBS. However, a deeper insight into the DBS-mechanisms and its long-term or persistent effects (≥6 weeks) require animal models that are suitable for combining biochemical, electrophysiological, optical microscopy, and other imaging methods, along with behavioral testing.

5. Conclusion and Outlook

To our knowledge, we present the first behavioral investigation in freely moving rats with chronic instrumentation for up to 6 weeks, which allowed the animals to adapt to the instrumentation and allowed us to conduct comparative behavioral tests at different times under acute DBS conditions and after the cessation of DBS. In our setup, we found unipolar stimulation to be more efficient for achieving several beneficial long-term DBS effects. In our tests of behavioral changes, the stepping and corridor tests were the most appropriate for the evaluation of DBS-induced locomotor and sensorimotor improvements. When DBS was stopped after 3 weeks, some effects persisted for at least 3 more weeks, such as the reduction of initiation time of the contralateral paw in the stepping test and the slight reduction of the contralateral bias in the corridor test. In contrast, performance in the apomorphine-induced rotation test showed no improvement after 6 weeks. Our findings may indicate a regeneration of neuronal circuits in the absence of dopaminergic neurons. This would make apomorphine-induced rotation a suitable test to determine the long-term success of 6-OHDA lesioning but not a very informative test for determining the beneficial effects of DBS. In interpreting anxiety-like behaviors, researchers must consider habituation effects in relation to the durations between test repetitions in both sham and experimental animals.

The determination of very fast reaction times was difficult. To improve the statistical power of these tests, a larger sample size should be combined with video detection of reaction times. Our model can be considered a versatile platform that allows for the independent testing of separate elements, such as electrodes and counter-electrodes. Relatively simple modifications to our model will allow for the testing of unexplored target regions in other neurodegenerative disorders.

In addition, various electrical parameters can be tested, such as stimulation frequency and signal shape. To our knowledge, no systematic investigations have been conducted on whether the frequencies applied to humans are suitable for use with much smaller animals. We believe that this topic needs further investigation, taking into account allometric effects for organisms with various brain sizes. Our results may help in developing a reduced set of test parameters to facilitate this research.

Major problem remains to be elucidated about the mechanism by which DBS acts. Although 6-OHDA lesioning induces PD-like symptoms, the long-term DBS effects in our model may be a result of the emergence of new or a strengthening of existing neuronal circuits that compensate for the absence of dopamine in the brains of young rats. This outcome may suggest that the DBS-related locomotor and sensorimotor improvements, with no detectable improvements in the results of the rotation test, indicate DBS effects in the activation of neuronal substitute circuits. If this hypothesis is supported by future research, investigations of the effects of stimulation may be helpful in other areas, such as stroke research.

Appendix

A Simplified Scheme of the Lesioned Hemisphere in the Hemiparkinsonian Rat

Figure 13 presents a simplified scheme of the lesioned hemisphere, illustrating different brain states, which are immediately induced by alterations in neurotransmitter release and in the activity of different brain areas. Long-term alterations in receptor numbers or sensitivities are not depicted. It should be noted that the scheme can attempt only a qualitative description of the separate effects. The interplay of the lesioned hemisphere with its nonlesioned counterpart must be considered to explain the overall effect, for example, the effect of amphetamine administration. The rotation effects may be explained by the assumption that the induced hyperactivation of the cortex of one hemisphere leads to a general pattern of muscle activation contralateral to the hyperactive side, which would result in a bending of the body toward this side and, subsequently, to rotation contralateral to the hyperactive hemisphere.

The depicted effects will, in principle, also apply when one of the successive treatments is omitted. Thus, the scheme allows for predicting multiple scenarios, such as the effects of DBS without a lesion or apomorphine administration without DBS. Nevertheless, the actual magnitudes of the combined effects on the activity of the various brain areas may vary significantly, leading to different individual responses. Short summaries of the different states illustrated by Figure 13 are given below.

Healthy Brain. No colors or arrows, which designate deviations from the normal brain activity, apply.

Lesion Effect. Obliteration of the SNc (red cross) stops DA input for D1 and D2 receptors in the striatum. Along the D1 pathway, the reduced GABAergic inhibition results in an increased activity of the entopeduncular nucleus/substantia nigra pars reticulata (EP/SNr). Along the D2 pathway, the effect on the globus pallidus (GP) is inverse. The increased GABAergic inhibition of the GP leads to a reduced inhibition of the STN, resulting in an increased activity of the EP/SNr in line with the effect on the D1 pathway (note that reduced arrow widths symbolize the parallel D1 and D2 signaling pathways to the EP/SNr). The simultaneous effects of the D1- and D2-signaling pathways result in an increase in EP/SNr activity, which leads to an increased inhibition of the thalamus and a subsequent reduction in the activity of the cortex of the lesioned hemisphere.

Apomorphine Effect (Induced Rotation) after Lesion. The missing DA input to the striatum after SNc obliteration leads to an oversensitization of the D1 and D2 receptors to apomorphine, a DA agonist, in the striatum of the lesioned side. After systemic administration of apomorphine, both the D1- and D2-mediated effects (gray arrows) lead to a downregulation of the EP/SNr and, consequently, a stronger output from the thalamus to the cortex of the ipsilateral hemisphere compared to the contralateral hemisphere, where D1 and D2 receptors retain normal sensitivity. Overactivity of the ipsilateral cortex increases muscle tension on the contralateral side of the body, resulting in a bending that leads to contralateral rotation.

DBS Effect. DBS reduces the hyperactivity of the STN, which results in a reduced activity of the EP/SNr. In an ideal case (as indicated by the width of the blue arrow in the STN box), this reduced activity may normalize the inhibition of the thalamus and consequently the cortex activity. This outcome requires that STN-DBS can overcompensate the effect of the lesion along the EP/SNr pathway. If so, unilateral DBS in nonlesioned animals should overactivate the thalamus and the cortex in the stimulated hemisphere. Indeed, like apomorphine in lesioned animals, DBS in nonlesioned rats has been shown to induce contralateral rotation [75]. In lesioned animals, DBS is unable to reverse the hypersensitivity of the D1 and D2 receptors and thus has no effect on apomorphine-induced rotation. The concordant DBS and apomorphine effects prevent the detection of therapeutic DBS effects in apomorphine-induced rotation tests.

Amphetamine Effect (Induced Rotation) after Lesion. Amphetamine induces an increased DA release and inhibits its reuptake. In 6-OHDA-lesioned rats, amphetamine effects can occur in only the contralateral hemisphere because the dopaminergic neurons are degenerated in the ipsilateral SNc. Systemic amphetamine administration hyperactivates the contralateral cortex, resulting in ipsilateral rotation. DBS should reduce the asymmetry in the cortex activities of the hemispheres by activating the cortex of the lesioned (ipsilateral) hemisphere. Indeed, a reduction or even reversion of the amphetamine-induced rotation by STN-DBS was found in 6-OHDA-lesioned rats [11].

These considerations suggest a higher relevance of amphetamine-induced rotation tests for assessing therapeutic DBS effects, although apomorphine-induced rotation tests are useful for determining the success and degree of lesion induction.

Disclosure

The present address for Immo Weber is Department of Neurology, University Hospital Giessen and Marburg, Marburg, Germany.

Acknowledgments

The authors wish to thank their keeper Gerda Brüsch for taking care of the animals and assistance with the behavioral tests. The authors are grateful to Professor Reiner Benecke for his encouraging support and for providing the facilities for the experiments and to Professor Andreas Wree and Karl Nowak who helped establish the surgical procedures and chronic instrumentation setup. The authors are indebted to Dr. Robert Arndt (Rückmann & Arndt, Berlin, Germany) and the Steinbeis-Zentrum STZ 1050 (Rostock, Germany) for a fruitful cooperation in the development of the stimulator systems. The authors are deeply indebted to Dr. Eilhard Mix for his help in designing the animal experiments. He was a source of constant guidance for Kathrin Badstuebner throughout the whole study. The authors regret that he refrained from a coauthorship for personal reasons after his retirement. The German Research Foundation (DFG, Research Training Group 1505/1,2 "welisa") financed a scholarship to Kathrin Badstuebner as well as small equipment and consumables for the experiments.

References

[1] P. Krack, M. I. Hariz, C. Baunez, J. Guridi, and J. A. Obeso, "Deep brain stimulation: From neurology to psychiatry?" *Trends in Neurosciences*, vol. 33, no. 10, pp. 474–484, 2010.

[2] S. A. Eisenstein, J. M. Koller, K. D. Black et al., "Functional anatomy of subthalamic nucleus stimulation in Parkinson disease," *Annals of Neurology*, vol. 76, no. 2, pp. 279–295, 2014.

[3] W. M. M. Schuepbach, J. Rau, K. Knudsen et al., "Neurostimulation for Parkinson's disease with early motor complications," *The New England Journal of Medicine*, vol. 368, no. 7, pp. 610–622, 2013.

[4] H. J. Kim, S. J. Beom, and S. H. Paek, "Nonmotor symptoms and subthalamic deep brain stimulation in parkinson's disease," *Journal of Movement Disorders*, vol. 8, no. 2, pp. 83–91, 2015.

[5] F. M. Weaver, K. Follett, M. Stern et al., "Bilateral deep brain stimulation vs best medical therapy for patients with advanced parkinson disease: a randomized controlled trial," *JAMA-Journal of the American Medical Association*, vol. 301, no. 1, pp. 63–73, 2009.

[6] E. Moro, A. M. Lozano, P. Pollak et al., "Long-term results of a multicenter study on subthalamic and pallidal stimulation in Parkinson's disease," *Movement Disorders*, vol. 25, no. 5, pp. 578–586, 2010.

[7] K. Nowak, E. Mix, J. Gimsa et al., "Optimizing a rodent model of parkinson's disease for exploring the effects and mechanisms of deep brain stimulation," *Parkinson's Disease*, vol. 2011, Article ID 414682, 19 pages, 2011.

[8] A. L. Benabid, P. Pollak, A. Louveau, S. Henry, and J. De Rougemont, "Combined (thalamotomy and stimulation) stereotactic surgery of the vim thalamic nucleus for bilateral parkinson disease," *Stereotactic and Functional Neurosurgery*, vol. 50, no. 1-6, pp. 344–346, 1987.

[9] W. M. M. Schüpbach, N. Chastan, M. L. Welter et al., "Stimulation of the subthalamic nucleus in Parkinson's disease: a 5 year follow up," *Journal of Neurology, Neurosurgery and Psychiatry*, vol. 76, no. 12, pp. 1640–1644, 2005.

[10] A. Castrioto, A. M. Lozano, Y.-Y. Poon, A. E. Lang, M. Fallis, and E. Moro, "Ten-year outcome of subthalamic stimulation in Parkinson disease: A blinded evaluation," *Archives of Neurology*, vol. 68, no. 12, pp. 1550–1556, 2011.

[11] S. Maesawa, Y. Kaneoke, Y. Kajita et al., "Long-term stimulation of the subthalamic nucleus in hemiparkinsonian rats: Neuroprotection of dopaminergic neurons," *Journal of Neurosurgery*, vol. 100, no. 4, pp. 679–687, 2004.

[12] D. Harnack, W. Meissner, J. A. Jira, C. Winter, R. Morgenstern, and A. Kupsch, "Placebo-controlled chronic high-frequency stimulation of the subthalamic nucleus preserves dopaminergic nigral neurons in a rat model of progressive Parkinsonism," *Experimental Neurology*, vol. 210, no. 1, pp. 257–260, 2008.

[13] A. L. Spieles-Engemann, K. Steece-Collier, M. M. Behbehani et al., "Subthalamic nucleus stimulation increases brain derived neurotrophic factor in the nigrostriatal system and primary motor cortex," *Journal of Parkinson's Disease*, vol. 1, no. 1, pp. 123–136, 2011.

[14] S. T. Wu, Y. Ma, K. Zhang, and J. G. Zhang, "Effect of deep brain stimulation on substantia nigra neurons in a rat model of Parkinson's disease," *Chinese Medical Journal*, vol. 125, pp. 4072–4075, 2012.

[15] A. Shinko, T. Agari, M. Kameda et al., "Spinal cord stimulation exerts neuroprotective effects against experimental Parkinson's disease," *PLoS ONE*, vol. 9, no. 7, Article ID e101468, 2014.

[16] H. Toda, C. Hamani, A. P. Fawcett, W. D. Hutchison, and A. M. Lozano, "The regulation of adult rodent hippocampal neurogenesis by deep brain stimulation: Laboratory investigation," *Journal of Neurosurgery*, vol. 108, no. 1, pp. 132–138, 2008.

[17] E. B. Montgomery Jr. and J. T. Gale, "Mechanisms of action of deep brain stimulation (DBS)," *Neuroscience and Biobehavioral Reviews*, vol. 32, no. 3, pp. 388–407, 2008.

[18] K. L. Collins, E. M. Lehmann, and P. G. Patil, "Deep brain stimulation for movement disorders," *Neurobiology of Disease*, vol. 38, no. 3, pp. 338–345, 2010.

[19] C. J. Wilson, B. Beverlin, and T. Netoff, "Chaotic desynchronization as the therapeutic mechanism of deep brain stimulation," *Frontiers in Systems Neuroscience*, vol. 5, no. 50, 2011.

[20] M. Delong and T. Wichmann, "Deep brain stimulation for movement and other neurologic disorders," *Annals of the New York Academy of Sciences*, vol. 1265, no. 1, pp. 1-8, 2012.

[21] G. Pizzolato and T. Mandat, "Deep brain stimulation for movement disorders," *Frontiers in Integrative Neuroscience*, vol. 6, no. 2, 2012.

[22] S. Santaniello, M. M. McCarthy, E. B. Montgomery, J. T. Gale, N. Kopell, and S. V. Sarma, "Therapeutic mechanisms of high-frequency stimulation in parkinson's disease and neural restoration via loop-based reinforcement," *Proceedings of the National Academy of Sciences of the United States of America*, vol. 112, no. 6, pp. E586–E595, 2015.

[23] P. Gubellini and P. Kachidian, "Animal models of Parkinson's disease: An updated overview," *Revue Neurologique*, vol. 171, no. 11, pp. 750–761, 2015.

[24] A. L. Spieles-Engemann, T. J. Collier, and C. E. Sortwell, "A functionally relevant and long-term model of deep brain stimulation of the rat subthalamic nucleus: Advantages and considerations," *European Journal of Neuroscience*, vol. 32, no. 7, pp. 1092–1099, 2010.

[25] Y. Temel, V. Visser-Vandewalle, S. Kaplan et al., "Protection of nigral cell death by bilateral subthalamic nucleus stimulation," *Brain Research*, vol. 1120, no. 1, pp. 100–105, 2006.

[26] Y. Liu, N. Postupna, J. Falkenberg, and M. E. Anderson, "High frequency deep brain stimulation: What are the therapeutic mechanisms?" *Neuroscience and Biobehavioral Reviews*, vol. 32, no. 3, pp. 343–351, 2008.

[27] R. Paulat, W. Meissner, R. Morgenstern, A. Kupsch, and D. Harnack, "Development of an implantable microstimulation system for chronic DBS in rodents," in *Proceedings of 2011 33rd Annual International Conference of the IEEE Engineering in Medicine and Biology Society*, pp. 660–662, Boston, MA, August 2011.

[28] C. Forni, O. Mainard, C. Melon, D. Goguenheim, L. Kerkerian-Le Goff, and P. Salin, "Portable microstimulator for chronic deep brain stimulation in freely moving rats," *Journal of Neuroscience Methods*, vol. 209, no. 1, pp. 50–57, 2012.

[29] R. de Haas, R. Struikmans, G. van der Plasse et al., "Wireless implantable micro-stimulation device for high frequency bilateral deep brain stimulation in freely moving mice," *Journal of Neuroscience Methods*, vol. 209, no. 1, pp. 113–119, 2012.

[30] S. G. Ewing, B. Porr, J. Riddell, C. Winter, and A. A. Grace, "SaBer DBS: A fully programmable, rechargeable, bilateral, charge-balanced preclinical microstimulator for long-term neural stimulation," *Journal of Neuroscience Methods*, vol. 213, no. 2, pp. 228–235, 2013.

[31] S. G. Ewing, W. J. Lipski, A. A. Grace, and C. Winter, "An inexpensive, charge-balanced rodent deep brain stimulation device: A step-by-step guide to its procurement and construction," *Journal of Neuroscience Methods*, vol. 219, no. 2, pp. 324–330, 2013.

[32] C. Chassain, C. Melon, P. Salin et al., "Metabolic, synaptic and behavioral impact of 5-week chronic deep brain stimulation in hemiparkinsonian rats," *Journal of Neurochemistry*, vol. 136, no. 5, pp. 1004–1016, 2016.

[33] K. Badstübner, T. Kröger, E. Mix, U. Gimsa, R. Benecke, and J. Gimsa, "Electrical impedance properties of deep brain stimulation electrodes during long-term in-vivo stimulation in the parkinson model of the rat," *Communications in Computer and Information Science*, vol. 357, pp. 287–297, 2013.

[34] P. Salin, C. Manrique, C. Forni, and L. Kerkerian-Le Goff, "High-frequency stimulation of the subthalamic nucleus selectively reverses dopamine denervation-induced cellular defects in the output structures of the basal ganglia in the rat," *Journal of Neuroscience*, vol. 22, no. 12, pp. 5137–5148, 2002.

[35] X. Fang, K. Sugiyama, S. Akamine, and H. Namba, "Improvements in motor behavioral tests during deep brain stimulation of the subthalamic nucleus in rats with different degrees of unilateral parkinsonism," *Brain Research*, vol. 1120, no. 1, pp. 202–210, 2006.

[36] D. Harnack, C. Winter, W. Meissner, T. Reum, A. Kupsch, and R. Morgenstern, "The effects of electrode material, charge density and stimulation duration on the safety of high-frequency stimulation of the subthalamic nucleus in rats," *Journal of Neuroscience Methods*, vol. 138, no. 1-2, pp. 207–216, 2004.

[37] J. Gimsa, B. Habel, U. Schreiber, U. V. Rienen, U. Strauss, and U. Gimsa, "Choosing electrodes for deep brain stimulation

experiments-electrochemical considerations," *Journal of Neuroscience Methods*, vol. 142, no. 2, pp. 251–265, 2005.

[38] U. Gimsa, U. Schreiber, B. Habel, J. Flehr, U. Van Rienen, and J. Gimsa, "Matching geometry and stimulation parameters of electrodes for deep brain stimulation experiments - Numerical considerations," *Journal of Neuroscience Methods*, vol. 150, no. 2, pp. 212–227, 2006.

[39] U. Ungerstedt, "6-hydroxy-dopamine induced degeneration of central monoamine neurons," *European Journal of Pharmacology*, vol. 5, no. 1, pp. 107–110, 1968.

[40] G. A. Metz, A. Tse, M. Ballermann, L. K. Smith, and K. Fouad, "The unilateral 6-OHDA rat model of Parkinson's disease revisited: An electromyographic and behavioural analysis," *European Journal of Neuroscience*, vol. 22, no. 3, pp. 735–744, 2005.

[41] K. E. Glajch, S. M. Fleming, D. J. Surmeier, and P. Osten, "Sensorimotor assessment of the unilateral 6-hydroxydopamine mouse model of Parkinson's disease," *Behavioural Brain Research*, vol. 230, no. 2, pp. 309–316, 2012.

[42] I. S. Pienaar, B. Lu, and T. Schallert, "Closing the gap between clinic and cage: Sensori-motor and cognitive behavioural testing regimens in neurotoxin-induced animal models of Parkinson's disease," *Neuroscience and Biobehavioral Reviews*, vol. 36, no. 10, pp. 2305–2324, 2012.

[43] U. Ungerstedt, L. L. Butcher, S. G. Butcher, N.-E. Andén, and K. Fuxe, "Direct chemical stimulation of dopaminergic mechanisms in the neostriatum of the rat," *Brain Research*, vol. 14, no. 2, pp. 461–471, 1969.

[44] U. Ungerstedt and G. W. Arbuthnott, "Quantitative recording of rotational behavior in rats after 6-hydroxy-dopamine lesions of the nigrostriatal dopamine system," *Brain Research*, vol. 24, no. 3, pp. 485–493, 1970.

[45] M. Olsson, G. Nikkhah, C. Bentlage, and A. Bjorklund, "Forelimb akinesia in the rat Parkinson model: differential effects of dopamine agonists and nigral transplants as assessed by a new stepping test," *Journal of Neuroscience*, vol. 15, no. 5, pp. 3863–3875, 1995.

[46] E. Dowd, C. Monville, E. M. Torres, and S. B. Dunnett, "The Corridor Task: A simple test of lateralised response selection sensitive to unilateral dopamine deafferentation and graft-derived dopamine replacement in the striatum," *Brain Research Bulletin*, vol. 68, no. 1-2, pp. 24–30, 2005.

[47] C. S. Hall and E. L. Ballechey, "A study of the rats behavior in a field: a contribution to a method in comparative psychology," *University of California Publications in Psychology*, vol. 6, pp. 1–12, 1932.

[48] G. Paxinos and C. Watson, *The Rat Brain in Stereotaxic Coordinates*, Academic Press, San Diego, USA, 6th edition, 2007.

[49] X. Fang, K. Sugiyama, S. Akamine, W. Sun, and H. Namba, "The different performance among motor tasks during the increasing current intensity of deep brain stimulation of the subthalamic nucleus in rats with different degrees of the unilateral striatal lesion," *Neuroscience Letters*, vol. 480, no. 1, pp. 64–68, 2010.

[50] W. Meissner, D. Harnack, G. Paul et al., "Deep brain stimulation of subthalamic neurons increases striatal dopamine metabolism and induces contralateral circling in freely moving 6-hydroxydopamine-lesioned rats," *Neuroscience Letters*, vol. 328, no. 2, pp. 105–108, 2002.

[51] R. Q. So, G. C. McConnell, A. T. August, and W. M. Grill, "Characterizing effects of subthalamic nucleus deep brain stimulation on methamphetamine-induced circling behavior in hemi-parkinsonian rats," *IEEE Transactions on Neural Systems and Rehabilitation Engineering*, vol. 20, no. 5, pp. 626–635, 2012.

[52] S. B. Ryu, E. K. Bae, J. Kim et al., "Neuronal responses in the globus pallidus during subthalamic nucleus electrical stimulation in normal and Parkinson's disease model rats," *Korean Journal of Physiology and Pharmacology*, vol. 17, no. 4, pp. 299–306, 2013.

[53] A. D. Dorval and W. M. Grill, "Deep brain stimulation of the subthalamic nucleus reestablishes neuronal information transmission in the 6-OHDA rat model of parkinsonism," *Journal of Neurophysiology*, vol. 111, no. 10, pp. 1949–1959, 2014.

[54] J. A. D. Dela Cruz, S. Hescham, B. Adriaanse et al., "Increased number of TH-immunoreactive cells in the ventral tegmental area after deep brain stimulation of the anterior nucleus of the thalamus," *Brain Structure and Function*, vol. 220, no. 5, pp. 3061–3066, 2014.

[55] L. K.-L. Goff, L. Jouve, C. Melon, and P. Salin, "Rationale for targeting the thalamic centre-median parafascicular complex in the surgical treatment of Parkinson's disease," *Parkinsonism and Related Disorders*, vol. 15, no. 3, pp. S167–S170, 2009.

[56] S. Lortet, E. Lacombe, N. Boulanger et al., "Striatal molecular signature of subchronic subthalamic nucleus high frequency stimulation in parkinsonian rat," *PLoS ONE*, vol. 8, no. 4, Article ID e60447, 2013.

[57] C. Melon, C. Chassain, G. Bielicki et al., "Progressive brain metabolic changes under deep brain stimulation of subthalamic nucleus in parkinsonian rats," *Journal of Neurochemistry*, vol. 132, no. 6, pp. 703–712, 2015.

[58] R. A. Ramdhani, A. Patel, D. Swope, and B. H. Kopell, "Early use of 60 Hz frequency subthalamic stimulation in parkinson's disease: a case series and review," *Neuromodulation*, vol. 18, no. 8, pp. 664–669, 2015.

[59] F. Hefti, E. Melamed, B. J. Sahakian, and R. J. Wurtman, "Circling behavior in rats with partial, unilateral nigro-striatal lesions: Effect of amphetamine, apomorphine, and DOPA," *Pharmacology, Biochemistry and Behavior*, vol. 12, no. 2, pp. 185–188, 1980.

[60] C. Da Cunha, E. C. Wietzikoski, M. M. Ferro et al., "Hemiparkinsonian rats rotate toward the side with the weaker dopaminergic neurotransmission," *Behavioural Brain Research*, vol. 189, no. 2, pp. 364–372, 2008.

[61] S. Grealish, B. Mattsson, P. Draxler, and A. Björklund, "Characterisation of behavioural and neurodegenerative changes induced by intranigral 6-hydroxydopamine lesions in a mouse model of Parkinson's disease," *European Journal of Neuroscience*, vol. 31, no. 12, pp. 2266–2278, 2010.

[62] G. A. Metz and I. Q. Whishaw, "Drug-induced rotation intensity in unilateral dopamine-depleted rats is not correlated with end point or qualitative measures of forelimb or hindlimb motor performance," *Neuroscience*, vol. 111, no. 2, pp. 325–336, 2002.

[63] J.-Y. Chang, L.-H. Shi, F. Luo, and D. J. Woodward, "High frequency stimulation of the subthalamic nucleus improves treadmill locomotion in unilateral 6-hydroxydopamine lesioned rats," *Brain Research*, vol. 983, no. 1-2, pp. 174–184, 2003.

[64] D. Kirik, C. Rosenblad, and A. Björklund, "Characterization of behavioral and neurodegenerative changes following partial lesions of the nigrostriatal dopamine system induced by intrastriatal 6-hydroxydopamine in the rat," *Experimental Neurology*, vol. 152, no. 2, pp. 259–277, 1998.

[65] G. Rozas, M. J. Guerra, and J. L. Labandeira-García, "An automated rotarod method for quantitative drug-free evaluation of overall motor deficits in rat models of parkinsonism," *Brain Research Protocols*, vol. 2, no. 1, pp. 75–84, 1997.

[66] J. Henning, U. Strauss, A. Wree et al., "Differential astroglial activation in 6-hydroxydopamine models of Parkinson's disease," *Neuroscience Research*, vol. 62, no. 4, pp. 246–253, 2008.

[67] J.-M. Reymann, F. Naudet, M. Pihan, S. Saïkali, B. Laviolle, and D. Bentué-Ferrer, "Subthalamic nucleus modulates social and anxogenic-like behaviors," *Behavioural Brain Research*, vol. 252, pp. 356–362, 2013.

[68] L. Jouve, P. Salin, C. Melon, and L. Kerkerian-Le Goff, "Deep brain stimulation of the center median-parafascicular complex of the thalamus has efficient anti-Parkinsonian action associated with widespread cellular responses in the basal ganglia network in a rat model of Parkinson's Disease," *Journal of Neuroscience*, vol. 30, no. 29, pp. 9919–9928, 2010.

[69] K. Badstuebner, M. Stubbe, T. Kroeger, E. Mix, and J. Gimsa, "Impedance detection of the electrical resistivity of the wound tissue around deep brain stimulation electrodes permits registration of the encapsulation process in a rat model," *Journal of Electrical Bioimpedance*, vol. 8, no. 1, pp. 11–24, 2017.

[70] R. H. Walker, R. J. Koch, C. Moore, and C. K. Meshul, "Subthalamic nucleus stimulation and lesioning have distinct state-dependent effects upon striatal dopamine metabolism," *Synapse*, vol. 63, no. 2, pp. 136–146, 2009.

[71] T. Yamamoto, T. Uchiyama, R. Sakakibara, J. Taniguchi, and S. Kuwabara, "The subthalamic activity and striatal monoamine are modulated by subthalamic stimulation," *Neuroscience*, vol. 259, pp. 43–52, 2014.

[72] Z. He, Y. Jiang, H. Xu et al., "High frequency stimulation of subthalamic nucleus results in behavioral recovery by increasing striatal dopamine release in 6-hydroxydopamine lesioned rat," *Behavioural Brain Research*, vol. 263, pp. 108–114, 2014.

[73] D. Petri, M. Pum, J. Vesper, J. P. Huston, and A. Schnitzler, "GABA A-receptor activation in the subthalamic nucleus compensates behavioral asymmetries in the hemiparkinsonian rat," *Behavioural Brain Research*, vol. 252, pp. 58–67, 2013.

[74] C. Carcenac, M. Favier, Y. Vachez et al., "Subthalamic deep brain stimulation differently alters striatal dopaminergic receptor levels in rats," *Movement Disorders*, vol. 30, no. 13, pp. 1739–1749, 2015.

[75] O. Bergmann, C. Winter, W. Meissner et al., "Subthalamic high frequency stimulation induced rotations are differentially mediated by D1 and D2 receptors," *Neuropharmacology*, vol. 46, no. 7, pp. 974–983, 2004.

8

Chaperone-Based Therapies for Disease Modification in Parkinson's Disease

Erik L. Friesen,[1,2] Mitch L. De Snoo,[1,2] Luckshi Rajendran,[3] Lorraine V. Kalia,[1,2,4,5] and Suneil K. Kalia[1,2,6]

[1] *Krembil Research Institute, Toronto Western Hospital, University Health Network, 60 Leonard Avenue, Toronto, ON, Canada*
[2] *Department of Laboratory Medicine and Pathobiology, University of Toronto, 1 King's College Circle, Toronto, ON, Canada*
[3] *Faculty of Medicine, University of British Columbia, 317-2194 Health Sciences Mall, Vancouver, BC, Canada*
[4] *Morton and Gloria Shulman Movement Disorders Clinic and The Edmond J. Safra Program in Parkinson's Disease, Division of Neurology, Department of Medicine, Toronto Western Hospital, University Health Network, 399 Bathurst Street, Toronto, ON, Canada*
[5] *Division of Neurology, Department of Medicine and Tanz Centre for Research in Neurodegenerative Diseases, University of Toronto, 190 Elizabeth Street, Toronto, ON, Canada*
[6] *Division of Neurosurgery, Department of Surgery, University of Toronto, 149 College Street, Toronto, ON, Canada*

Correspondence should be addressed to Suneil K. Kalia; suneil.kalia@utoronto.ca

Academic Editor: Cristine Alves da Costa

Parkinson's disease (PD) is the second most common neurodegenerative disorder and is characterized by the presence of pathological intracellular aggregates primarily composed of misfolded α-synuclein. This pathology implicates the molecular machinery responsible for maintaining protein homeostasis (proteostasis), including molecular chaperones, in the pathobiology of the disease. There is mounting evidence from preclinical and clinical studies that various molecular chaperones are downregulated, sequestered, depleted, or dysfunctional in PD. Current therapeutic interventions for PD are inadequate as they fail to modify disease progression by ameliorating the underlying pathology. Modulating the activity of molecular chaperones, cochaperones, and their associated pathways offers a new approach for disease modifying intervention. This review will summarize the potential of chaperone-based therapies that aim to enhance the neuroprotective activity of molecular chaperones or utilize small molecule chaperones to promote proteostasis.

1. Introduction

Parkinson's (PD) is the second most common neurodegenerative disorder affecting approximately 1% of the population over 60 [1]. People with PD typically present with cardinal motor symptoms including bradykinesia, muscular rigidity, rest tremor, or gait impairment but often also develop non-motor symptoms, such as cognitive impairment and psychiatric symptoms. Many but not all of the symptoms associated with PD result from loss of the dopaminergic neurons of the substantia nigra pars compacta (SN) [2]. Currently, PD is treated pharmacologically, by enhancing dopamine tone (e.g., dopamine replacement with L-dopa) and, surgically, by deep brain stimulation (DBS) [2]. As the disease progresses L-dopa treatment is associated with disabling complications including motor fluctuation and dyskinesia. DBS is restricted to a select group of patients presenting with L-dopa responsive motor symptoms and L-dopa-induced complications, but without significant cognitive impairment or psychiatric disturbance. Importantly, both interventions only provide symptomatic relief and do not slow the progression of PD. Consequently, there is a need for a treatment addressing the underlying causes of the disease.

Pathologically, PD is characterized by the presence of proteinaceous intracellular aggregates composed primarily of α-synuclein, termed Lewy pathology (Lewy bodies and Lewy neurites). Missense mutations and multiplications of the *SNCA* gene, which encodes for α-synuclein, cause heritable forms of PD and enhance the propensity of α-synuclein to self-aggregate thus implicating α-synuclein aggregation in the pathogenesis of the disease [3, 4]. While there is uncertainty regarding the specific form of aggregates ("species") that are neurotoxic, emerging evidence suggests that α-synuclein toxicity is conferred by soluble oligomeric species [5–8]. Given the central role of perturbed α-synuclein aggregation in PD, investigation into the nature and modification of the molecular pathways responsible for directing protein folding and misfolding, maintaining proper protein confirmation, and reducing abnormal protein aggregation, presents a promising avenue for identifying a disease modifying strategy.

2. Molecular Chaperones

Molecular chaperones are highly conserved proteins that function to maintain proteostasis by directing the folding of nascent polypeptide chains, refolding misfolded proteins, and targeting misfolded proteins for degradation. Molecular chaperones are also termed "heat shock proteins" (HSPs), as initial studies found them to be upregulated in response to high temperatures. In eukaryotes, HSPs are a large and heterogeneous group of proteins that have been classified into families based on their molecular weight: Hsp40, Hsp60, Hsp70, Hsp90, Hsp100, and the small HSPs [20]. The activity of HSP family members is modulated by another class of proteins termed "cochaperones" which can be subdivided based on the presence of a Bcl-2 Associated Athanogene (BAG) domain, a tetratricopeptide (TPR) domain, or a J domain. Each of the families of chaperones and cochaperones are composed of multiple proteins which, despite having similar functions and domain compositions, often vary significantly in terms of their expression pattern and subcellular localization. For a recent review of the complete set of chaperone and cochaperone proteins, see Kampinga and Bergink (2016) [20].

Due to the number and heterogeneity of chaperone and cochaperone proteins, the nomenclature has become complex, with some chaperones receiving multiple names. As such, a new nomenclature was developed where DNAJ, HSPD, HSPA, HSPC, HSPH, and HSPB are the preferred prefix terms for the Hsp40, Hsp60, Hsp70, Hsp90, Hsp100, and small Hsp family members, respectively [21]. For the purposes of this review, "Hsp" will be used when referring to an entire family of Hsp chaperones and the new nomenclature will be used when referring to specific members within a family.

The two main chaperone machines in eukaryotes are Hsp70 and Hsp90, which together account for at least half of the molecular chaperones present in eukaryotic cells [22]. The Hsp70 family members are the most studied molecular chaperones and have received significant attention in PD due to their abundance in Lewy bodies and their neuroprotective effect in preclinical models of the disease [23]. Only a subset of Hsp70 chaperones, namely, HSPA1A, HSPA1B, and HSPA6, show stress-induced expression patterns, whereas the other Hsp70 family members, such as HSPA8 (often referred to as Hsc70), are expressed constitutively at baseline conditions [20]. A signaling pathway involving the transcriptional activator, heat shock factor 1 (HSF-1), regulates the expression of inducible Hsp70 family members following stressful stimuli (Figure 1). At baseline conditions, HSF-1 is bound by Hsp90, maintaining HSF-1 in an inactive monomeric form [24]. Following proteotoxic stress, HSF-1 dissociates from Hsp90 and translocates to the nucleus where it upregulates transcription of its target genes [25]. Once proteostasis is reestablished, Hsp90 again sequesters HSF-1 into its inactive monomeric form, suppressing inducible Hsp70 expression. This crosstalk between chaperones and the presence of both constitutively active and stress-inducible chaperones on a negative feedback loop allows the cell to execute continuous "house-keeping" tasks in proteostasis, as well as respond to potentially devastating proteotoxic stress.

The primary role of Hsp70 is to ensure proper protein folding. Hsp70 accomplishes this by binding exposed hydrophobic domains on misfolded proteins ("clients") via its C-terminal substrate binding domain (SBD) and then undergoing multiple ATP hydrolysis cycles at the N-terminal ATPase domain [26, 27]. Hydrolysis of ATP to ADP stabilizes the Hsp70-client complex, which allows Hsp70 to hold the client protein and increases the likelihood of spontaneous refolding [22]. Subsequent ADP-ATP exchange reduces the stability of the Hsp70-client complex, allowing for client dissociation or subsequent ATP hydrolysis cycles. While there are multiple models of the mechanism by which Hsp70 mediates protein refolding, the cycling between ATP and ADP bound states is necessary for this function [28].

The ATP hydrolysis cycle on Hsp70 is modulated by Hsp40, HSPH2 (Hsp110), the TPR domain-containing Hsp70 interacting protein (Hip), and BAG family cochaperone proteins. Hsp40s are important for both client selection and facilitating ATP hydrolysis [29], and Hip stabilizes the ADP bound state of Hsp70 [30]. Both BAG family members and HSPH2 act as nucleotide exchange factors (NEFs), promoting the release of ADP from the ATPase domain [30–32]. As such, both Hsp40 and Hip promote Hsp70-client stability, whereas BAG family proteins and HSPH2 destabilize the interaction. Therefore, the relative abundance of cochaperone proteins may play an important role in the dynamics of Hsp70 refolding activity. A complex interplay between the nature of the client protein, the Hsp70 family member, and the cochaperone proteins present likely determines the efficacy and the mechanism by which a protein becomes refolded.

Outside of their primary function of protein refolding, molecular chaperones also play important roles in cellular processes such as guiding misfolded proteins for degradation through the ubiquitin-proteasome system (UPS) or autophagy-lysosome pathway (ALP), disaggregating protein aggregates, suppressing cell death pathways, and promoting mitochondrial health (Figure 1). Hsp70-mediated protein degradation via the UPS is largely regulated by cochaperone proteins, namely, the C-terminal Hsp70 interacting protein (CHIP), which is both an Hsp70 cochaperone and an E3 ubiquitin ligase, thus providing a mechanistic link between the chaperone system and the UPS [33, 34]. HSPA8 (Hsc70), in conjunction with lysosomal-associated membrane protein 2A (LAMP2A) and multiple cochaperones, can also facilitate

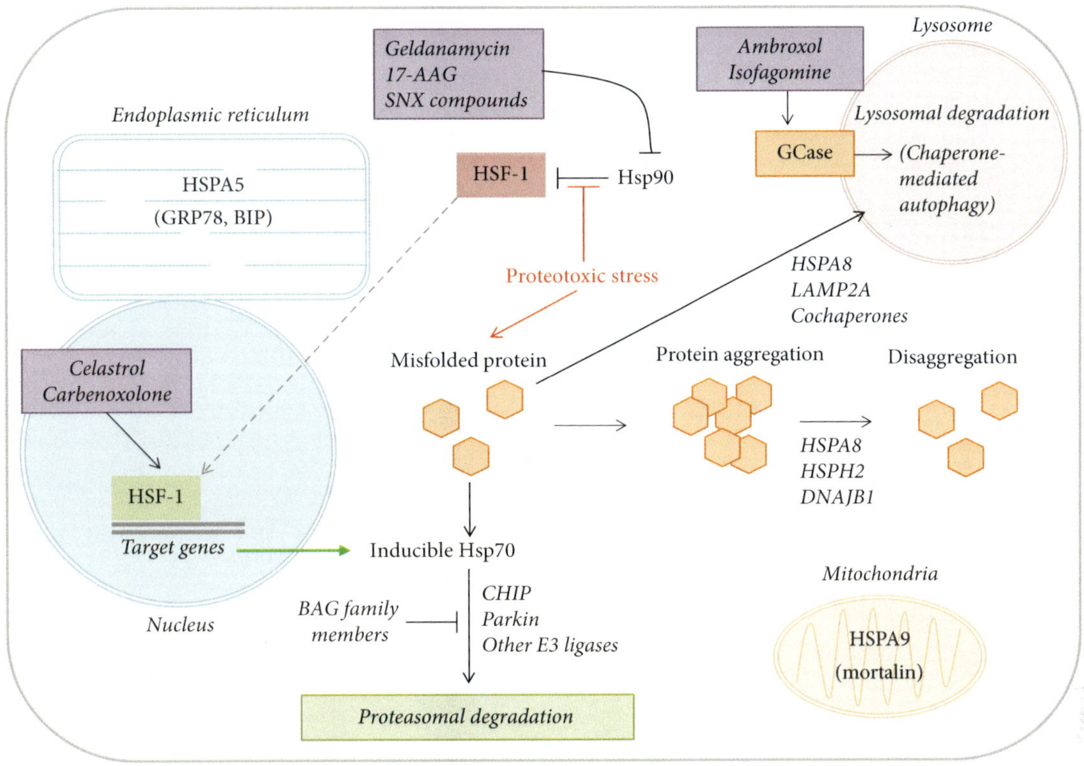

FIGURE 1: Proposed role of molecular and small molecule chaperones in proteostasis. At baseline, Hsp90 is bound to HSF-1, maintaining its inactive state. In the presence of proteotoxic stress, or the addition of Hsp90 inhibitors (i.e., geldanamycin, 17-AAG, and SNX compounds), active HSF-1 dissociates from Hsp90 and translocates into the nucleus where it induces Hsp70 expression. Inducible Hsp70 family members direct proteasomal degradation through a pathway mediated by CHIP, Parkin, and other E3 ligases. This process is inhibited by BAG family members and promoted by small molecule HSF-1 activators including celastrol and carbenoxolone. In response to proteotoxic stress, chaperones also direct misfolded proteins for degradation via the autophagy-lysosome system, through interactions with various cochaperones (chaperone-mediated autophagy). Chaperone/cochaperone complexes can also function to disaggregate already formed protein aggregates. The pharmacological chaperones, ambroxol, and isofagomine increase glucocerebrosidase (GCase) activity in the lysosome to further promote the process of chaperone-mediated autophagy. Chaperone functions within the endoplasmic reticulum and mitochondria are regulated by the specific members of the Hsp70 family, HSPA5 and HSPA9, respectively.

protein degradation via the ALP through a process termed chaperone-mediated autophagy (CMA) [35, 36] (Figure 1). Moreover, a chaperone machine composed of Hsp70, HSPH2 (Hsp110), and Hsp40 has a demonstrated "disaggregase" activity by which it can remove misfolded proteins from already formed aggregates [37, 38]. The close relationship between molecular chaperones and protein aggregation has led to their investigation in many neurodegenerative proteinopathies, including PD.

3. Molecular Chaperones in Parkinson's Disease

3.1. Molecular Chaperones Modulate α-Synuclein Aggregation and Toxicity. Early evidence implicating molecular chaperones in the pathobiology of PD stemmed from the observation by Auluck et al. (2002) that Hsp70 overexpression attenuated α-synuclein-mediated dopaminergic neurodegeneration in a *Drosophila* model [39]. This suggests that Hsp70 may play a neuroprotective role in PD. Subsequently, McLean et al. (2002) illustrated that multiple chaperone proteins colocalize with Lewy bodies and that the overexpression of several Hsp40 and Hsp70 family members antagonizes the formation of α-synuclein aggregates in vitro [40]. Molecular chaperones were further implicated in the pathobiology of PD by the observation that mutations within the promoter region upstream of both constitutively expressed and inducible Hsp70 family members increase the risk of PD in a patient population [41]. Furthermore, mutations in the mitochondrial Hsp70, HSPA9 (mortalin), were recently suggested to promote the development of PD [42–44]; however, other groups suggest mutations in HSPA9 are not a frequent cause of early-onset PD as they are also found in patient controls [45].

Since these initial studies, the capacity of Hsp70 overexpression to ameliorate α-synuclein aggregation and toxicity has been well characterized. Independent groups have shown that Hsp70 overexpression can attenuate α-synuclein-mediated cell death in yeast [46] and reduce high molecular weight aggregates and toxicity in rodent models of PD [47, 48]. Hsp70 overexpression was shown to be protective against cell death mediated by the mitochondrial complex I inhibitor,

1-methyl-4-phenyl-1,2,3,6-tetrahydropyridine (MPTP), both in vitro [49] and in vivo [50]. Although α-synuclein aggregation is not a feature of this toxin model, α-synuclein is required for MPTP-induced cell death as demonstrated by the resistance of α-synuclein null mice to MPTP [51]. Mitochondrial HSPA9, however, may play a role in the mitochondrial defects caused by the pathological A53T mutant α-synuclein as HSPA9 knockdown protects against the mitochondrial fragmentation and increased susceptibility to the complex I inhibitor, rotenone, induced by A53T overexpression [52].

In parallel with the Hsp70 overexpression results, recent studies have demonstrated that microRNA (miRNA) mediated translational repression of Hsp70 exacerbates α-synuclein aggregation and toxicity in vitro [53] and that miRNAs targeting Hsp70 are upregulated in brain regions with Lewy pathology [54]. Furthermore, the Hsp70 family members HSPA8 (Hsc70) and HSPA9 have lower expression in the SN (HSPA8/9) [55] and leukocytes (HSPA8) [56, 57] of PD patients relative to healthy controls, suggesting that chaperone levels and function may have a role in the pathogenesis of PD.

In contrast, the endoplasmic reticular Hsp70 family member, HSPA5 (GRP78/BiP), was found to be more abundant in the cingulate gyrus and parietal cortex of individuals with Dementia with Lewy Bodies (DLB) or PD with Dementia (PDD) relative to individuals with Alzheimer's disease (AD) and healthy controls [58]. The increase in HSPA5 in the cingulate gyrus was positively correlated with α-synuclein abundance, leading the authors to suggest that HSPA5 may be upregulated to mitigate α-synuclein toxicity [58]. This notion is supported by the observations that miRNA-mediated HSPA5 depletion enhances rotenone-induced cell death in vitro [59], and HSPA5 knockdown exacerbates the toxicity of AAV-delivered α-synuclein in rats [60]. Moreover, multiple studies have demonstrated that HSPA5 overexpression can suppress α-synuclein aggregation and toxicity in vitro and in vivo [61, 62].

The mechanism by which Hsp70 attenuates α-synuclein aggregation and toxicity seems to be dependent on both its refolding activity and its function in protein degradation via the UPS and ALP. Mutations that alter the ATPase function of Hsp70 (K71S) abolish its protective effect on α-synuclein toxicity, indicating that Hsp70 folding activity is necessary for its protective function [48]. Interestingly, this mutation has no effect on the capacity of Hsp70 to suppress α-synuclein aggregation [48], suggesting that Hsp70 uses distinct mechanisms to attenuate either the aggregation or the toxicity of α-synuclein. In addition to antagonizing the aggregation of α-synuclein, Hsp70 may also facilitate the disaggregation of already formed α-synuclein aggregates, similar to the Hsp70 "disaggregase" activity that has already been well characterized in other models of protein aggregation [38]. For example, Gao et al. (2015) recently demonstrated that an Hsp70 machine composed of HSPA8, DNAJB1, and HSPH2 could effectively disassemble preformed α-synuclein fibrils in vitro and in *C. elegans* [37] (Figure 1).

Hsp70/cochaperone complexes also mitigate α-synuclein-mediated toxicity by promoting the degradation of misfolded α-synuclein via either the UPS or ALP. Several studies have suggested that CMA may be playing an important role in mitigating α-synuclein toxicity and aggregation [35, 63, 64]. Enhanced α-synuclein expression in both transgenic and paraquat models of PD results in a concurrent enhancement of LAMP2A and HSPA8 expression and a greater movement of α-synuclein into the lysosomes [63]. Moreover, both LAMP2A and HSPA8 have lower expression in the SN of PD patients [55], and a recent study demonstrated a correlation between the loss of LAMP2A and α-synuclein aggregation in postmortem PD brains [65]. Interestingly, the observed decrease in LAMP2A and HSPA8 expression anatomically overlaps with an increase in miRNAs capable of translationally repressing both LAMP2A and HSPA8 [54], further implicating miRNAs in PD-associated chaperone dysregulation.

Outside of CMA, the Hsp70 cochaperone, CHIP, plays an important dual function in α-synuclein degradation, as it can target α-synuclein for degradation by either the proteasome or lysosome via its TPR domain or U-box domain, respectively [66]. CHIP may mediate this through ubiquitination of α-synuclein and suppression of oligomer formation [67]. However, not all Hsp70 cochaperones promote α-synuclein degradation. In contrast, overexpression of the BAG family member, BAG5, antagonizes CHIP-mediated α-synuclein ubiquitination, which prevents the ability of CHIP to suppress oligomer formation [67] and also enhances α-synuclein-mediated toxicity [68]. Therefore, the balance between multiple cochaperones may assist Hsp70 in triaging whether to refold or degrade a client substrate, and a disruption in the relative abundance or activity of cochaperones may compromise the chaperone system and subsequently proteostasis.

Taken together, the capacity of Hsp70 and its cochaperones to refold, disaggregate, and target for degradation potentially toxic α-synuclein species suggests that molecular chaperones may have a central and multifaceted role in the pathobiology of PD. Since multiple chaperones are downregulated, sequestered into protein aggregates, or face age-related loss-of-function in the brains of people with PD, it is possible that the depletion and dysfunction of molecular chaperones may further contribute to the progression of PD.

3.2. Molecular Chaperones and Other PD-Relevant Proteins. The potential role of chaperones in the pathobiology of PD is broadened by their capacity to regulate the stability and function of PD-relevant proteins other than α-synuclein, including LRRK2 *(PARK8)*, PINK1 *(PARK6)*, parkin *(PARK2)*, and DJ-1 *(PARK7)*. LRRK2 plays a regulatory role in vesicular trafficking, microtubule dynamics and mitochondrial health [69]. Mutations in LRRK2 are associated with autosomal dominant PD, and common genetic variants are associated with an increased risk of developing sporadic PD [70]. Pathological mutations in LRRK2 are associated with autophagy dysfunction (including CMA dysfunction), proteasome dysfunction, and mitochondrial stress. The pathogenic G2019S, R1441C, and Y1699C LRRK2 mutations were shown to enhance the clearance of the trans-Golgi network (TGN) via a protein complex including the chaperone proteins Hsp70 and BAG5 plus Rab7L1 and Cyclin G Associated Kinase (GAK), which are both located in risk loci for sporadic

PD [71]. TGN dynamics have a close relationship with the ALP suggesting that this chaperone-dependent clearance of the TGN by LRRK2 could explain how pathogenic LRRK2 mutations disrupt autophagy. CHIP and Hsp90 have been shown to play important and opposing roles in regulating LRRK2 stability, as CHIP mediates the ubiquitination and proteasomal degradation of LRRK2, whereas Hsp90 stabilizes it [72]. Ko et al. (2009) demonstrated that the toxicity of mutant LRRK2 could be enhanced by CHIP knockdown and attenuated by CHIP overexpression. Moreover, Hsp90 inhibition with the pharmacological agent 17-AAG (discussed below) was also protective against mutant LRRK2-mediated toxicity [72], presumably by promoting the degradation of the toxic gain-of-function mutant proteins. The G2385R LRRK2 variant is a risk factor for PD. G2385R LRRK2 demonstrates increased binding to Hsp90 and enhanced CHIP-dependent degradation resulting in lower steady state levels compared to wild-type LRRK2 [73]. Taken together, these results suggest that the interaction between chaperones and LRRK2 may regulate LRRK2 function, and these interactions may be compromised with PD-related mutations or variants of LRRK2.

Hsp70 and Hsp90 family members also regulate the stability of PINK1 and Parkin. PINK1 and Parkin function together in a pathway responsible for the selective autophagic clearance of damaged mitochondria, a process termed mitophagy [74]. The E3 ubiquitin ligase activity of Parkin also facilitates proteostasis via the UPS. Hsp90 regulates the processing and stability of PINK1, and the Hsp90 family member HSPC5, commonly known as TNF Receptor Associated Protein 1 (TRAP1), promotes mitochondrial health and compensates for the mitochondrial dysfunction caused by PD-associated PINK1 mutations [75]. Conversely, PINK1 and parkin mediated mitophagy protects cells against increased susceptibility to mitochondrial stress that results from the knockdown of mitochondrial HSPA9 [76, 77]. HSPA1L and the cochaperones, BAG2 and BAG4, have all been shown to modulate PINK1-Parkin mediated mitophagy [78, 79]. Outside of mitophagy, Hsp70 supports Parkin by preventing it from being sequestered [68] and acts in concert with CHIP to promote the E3 ubiquitin ligase activity of Parkin following proteotoxic stress [80]. In contrast, the cochaperone BAG5 inhibits Parkin E3 activity, which may provide a mechanistic explanation as to how BAG5 enhances dopaminergic neurodegeneration [68].

Molecular chaperones have also been shown to interact with DJ-1. Upregulation of DJ-1 results in a concurrent increase in Hsp70 expression [81], and PD-associated DJ-1 mutations enhance the association of DJ-1 with cytosolic Hsp70, HSPA9, and CHIP [82]. Furthermore, a recent study demonstrated that the cochaperone BAG5 interacts with DJ-1 and decreases its stability [83]. In turn, BAG5 suppresses the protective effect of DJ-1 on cell death caused by rotenone [83].

In summary, chaperones not only modulate α-synuclein but are implicated in multiple pathways that mediate the pathobiology of PD. Significant progress has been made in terms of understanding how chaperones and cochaperones can be manipulated to attenuate or reverse PD pathology. More recently, a mutation in J domain-containing cochaperone, DNAJC13, has been identified as a cause of autosomal dominant PD, further supporting a potentially important role for chaperone proteins in the pathogenesis of PD [84]. Considering their ability to protect against α-synuclein aggregation and neurodegeneration in preclinical models, as well as their effects on other PD-related proteins, the chaperone systems represent a suitable target for the design of novel therapeutics that have the potential to slow the progression of PD.

4. Potential Chaperone-Based Strategies for Treatment of PD

4.1. Small Molecule Chaperones. Small molecule chaperones are low molecular weight compounds that exhibit their own chaperone function by enhancing protein stabilization and folding processes and by antagonizing protein aggregation [10, 85]. These compounds are distinct from molecular chaperones in that they are neither proteins nor components of the cell's primary response mechanism to proteotoxic stress. Small molecule chaperones are subdivided into two groups: chemical chaperones and pharmacological chaperones [10]. Chemical chaperones are classified as either osmolytes or hydrophobic compounds and typically promote protein folding nonspecifically by creating a chemical environment that encourages proteins to acquire the proper conformation [10]. In contrast, pharmacological chaperones bind directly to their target protein(s) to modulate its conformation and stability [10, 85].

Osmolyte chemical chaperones include free amino acids and their derivatives, polyols, and methylamines. They are often enriched in conditions of environmental stress and denaturation to promote protein homeostasis and quality control processes [86]. Examples of relevant osmolytes include trehalose and mannitol. Oral 2% trehalose solution has demonstrated high effectiveness in a mouse model of Huntington's disease (HD) [87]. Similar to PD, HD is a neurodegenerative movement disorder associated with protein aggregation. Specifically, trehalose treatment resulted in decreased aggregation of the protein implicated in HD, huntingtin, and improved motor dysfunction [87]. More recently, it was shown that 2 and 5% oral trehalose solutions ameliorate the behavioural deficits and neurochemical pathology associated with a preclinical rat α-synuclein PD model [88]. Mannitol, which is currently widely used clinically as an FDA-approved osmotic diuretic [16] (Table 1), can reduce α-synuclein aggregation in vitro, in *Drosophila*, as well as in the hippocampus, basal ganglia, and SN of transgenic mouse models of PD [17, 89]. Moreover, mannitol-mediated reduction of α-synuclein aggregation correlates with significant neuroprotection and correction of behavioural deficits [17, 89]. The hydrophobic compound 4-phenylbutyrate (PBA) is another FDA-approved drug that serves as a chemical chaperone with beneficial in vitro and in vivo effects on α-synuclein aggregation and neurodegeneration [90]. This compound can be given via oral supplementation and is currently used for urea cycle disorders [17]. Though PBA can penetrate the blood brain barrier (BBB), work with HD mouse models has demonstrated that high doses are

TABLE 1: Examples of relevant therapeutics that either target endogenous molecular chaperones, exert their own chaperone function, or have promise for applying chaperone therapies in humans and their progress in preclinical research and clinical trials (CTs).

Chaperone therapies	Compounds	Current clinical trials (CTs)	Clinical utility
HSF-1 modulators			
Trigger HSF-1 activation induces downstream Hsp70 expression [9]	Celastrol	Short-term CTs for rheumatoid arthritis [10]	Limited: strong human toxicity [9]
	Carbenoxolone	Phase II CTs in UK for psoriasis [10]	Potential: trials in PD patients needed
Hsp90 inhibitors			
Inhibits the interaction between Hsp90 and HSF-1, leading to increased Hsp70 expression and activity [11, 12]	Geldanamycin		Limited: in vivo toxicity, poor solubility, and BBB penetration [13, 14]
	17-AAG	CTs for cancer treatment, discontinued	Limited: poor BBB penetration [13]
	17-DMAG	CTs for cancer treatment, discontinued	Limited: human toxicity [15]
	SNX-2112		Potential: trials in PD patients needed
Chemical chaperones			
Nonspecific compounds that benefit protein stabilization and folding and antagonize protein aggregation [10]	Osmolytes (i.e., 2% trehalose, mannitol)	Mannitol is FDA-approved osmotic diuretic [16]	Limited: high concentration dose likely needed for use in PD patients
	Hydrophobic compounds (i.e., 4-PBA)	4-Phenylbutyrate is FDA-approved, currently used for urea cycle disorders [17]	Limited: HD mouse model indicates needing high doses near max tolerability for human benefits [18]
Pharmacological Chaperones			
Specifically bind target protein for chaperone-mediated proteostasis [10]	Pharmacological chaperones (i.e., ambroxol, isofagomine)		Limited: high doses likely required for benefits in PD patients
Gene therapy			
Nonpharmacological modulation of chaperones	Adeno-associated virus vector of gene delivery	Several CTs for viral-mediated gene delivery in PD patients	Potential: safety of gene therapy has been established in PD patients [19]. It will require identification of appropriate chaperone targets

required to achieve benefits, which would likely translate to the maximum tolerability dosage for humans [18].

Pharmacological chaperones, such as ambroxol and isofagomine, can cross the BBB and have been demonstrated to increase the enzymatic activity of glucocerebrosidase (GCase) [91] (Figure 1). Mutations in the *GBA* gene, which encodes for GCase, are associated with an elevated risk of developing PD and decreased GCase activity in lysosomes. This reduction in GCase activity is associated with increased α-synuclein aggregation likely due to impairment of the ALP [92]. By enhancing GCase activity, pharmacological chaperones reduce α-synuclein accumulation in vitro and in the SN of mice [91, 93, 94]. Like chemical chaperones, pharmacological chaperones also require high doses to be beneficial which may limit their treatment efficacy.

4.2. HSF-1 Modulators. Endogenous molecular chaperone function can be modulated pharmacologically with compounds that augment endogenous chaperone levels. Several HSF-1 modulators including celastrol and carbenoxolone can trigger HSF-1 activation, leading to downstream induction of Hsp70 expression [9] (Figure 1). Celastrol has been demonstrated to be effective against protein aggregation and toxicity in various neurodegenerative disease models, including dopaminergic neuroprotection in a *Drosophila* model of PD [95]. However, this compound has been tested in short-term clinical trials for rheumatoid arthritis [10], and its clinical applicability may be restricted due to its toxicity [9]. Carbenoxolone has demonstrated the ability to attenuate α-synuclein and ubiquitin aggregation in vitro and in vivo [13, 96, 97]. Thus, it may have potential as a chaperone-mediated therapeutic option for PD. Carbenoxolone has reached phase II clinical trials in the UK for psoriasis treatment [10] so some safety and tolerability data should soon be available.

4.3. Hsp90 Inhibitors. The naturally occurring small molecule antibiotic, geldanamycin (GA), inhibits the interaction between Hsp90 and HSF-1, leading to increased Hsp70 expression [11] (Figure 1). In vitro cell studies have demonstrated the capability of this compound to decrease α-synuclein aggregation and reduce cell toxicity [98], and its neuroprotective effects have been shown in *Drosophila* and MPTP mouse models of PD [14, 99]. However, translation of this drug to the clinical setting is prevented by its in vivo toxicity, poor solubility, and limited penetration through the BBB [13, 14]. Other analogues of GA include 17-AAG and 17-DMAG, which similarly prevent α-synuclein aggregation and toxicity, but are more potent and less toxic than GA [12, 100]. However, 17-AAG and 17-DMAG were both tested in separate clinical trials relating to cancer treatment and were discontinued due to hepatotoxicity and limited efficacy [101]. Moreover, 17-AAG has poor permeability of the BBB, limiting its pharmacological usage for neurodegenerative diseases [13, 15] (Table 1). Consequently, compound library screening for small molecule Hsp90 inhibitors with improved pharmacokinetics, including BBB permeability, have led to the identification of SNX compounds [13]. These compounds are associated with an increase in Hsp70 activity in the brain and a reduction in α-synuclein oligomerization and toxicity in vitro [12]. An in vivo study using a rat model of PD has also demonstrated benefits of these compounds on rescuing striatal dopamine levels but not dopaminergic cell loss [102]. Although preclinical work suggests that there is therapeutic potential for the use of these compounds in PD, further drug development is required before translation to clinical trials.

4.4. Gene Therapy. Gene therapy represents a nonpharmacological approach to enhance chaperone function by exogenously elevating chaperone levels. Viral vectors (including adeno-associated virus (AAV) and lentivirus) have been demonstrated to be more efficient than nonviral vectors for gene delivery [103] and have been widely used to efficiently transduce postmitotic cells such as neurons, providing stable long-lasting expression [104]. AAV vectors are nonreplicating, rarely integrate, elicit minimal inflammation or toxicity in the brain, and do not induce disease, making it safe for clinical use [105–107]. Furthermore, intrinsic properties of the vector as well as the use of specific promoters can be engineered to regulate gene expression levels and cell-specificity [108].

Viral-mediated overexpression of chaperones has been demonstrated to increase survival of dopaminergic neurons in preclinical rodent models of PD [36, 39, 47, 50, 68, 109]. Another chaperone molecule with potential for gene therapy is the yeast, Hsp104, which has demonstrated disaggregase capacity [110]. Jackrel et al. (2014) engineered a highly active Hsp104 mutant that disassembles preformed protein aggregates from preexisting inclusions more rapidly and suppresses dopaminergic neurodegeneration in *C. elegans* more effectively than native Hsp104 [111]. Moreover, lentiviral delivery of yeast Hsp104 to the SN in a rat model attenuated α-synuclein toxicity [110], suggesting a similar approach could be taken in human patients. It should be noted, however, that although AAV vectors themselves elicit minimal immune response, foreign transgenic proteins may result in astrocyte and microglia activation with neuroinflammation and a potential neurotoxic response [112]. This can potentially limit the delivery of more specific or efficacious reengineered proteins, such as Hsp104.

Several clinical trials have demonstrated the safety of AAV- and lentivirus-mediated gene delivery in humans with PD [19] (Table 1). Although these trials mostly overexpress neurotrophic factors or deliver enzymes to enhance dopamine production, they provide proof-of-principle that chaperones could be modulated using viral vectors in humans. An alternative, less invasive approach for gene delivery involves the use of magnetic resonance imaging-guided focused ultrasound (MRIgFUS) to open the BBB. This method can be combined with the IV administration of a liposome-microbubble conjugated system containing genetic material, which allows for the targeted transfection of specific neuroanatomical regions [113]. MRIgFUS has been used in rodent models for gene delivery to the SN [113, 114]. Since the pathology of PD is not limited to the SN, viral delivery to multiple brain regions may be required for effective chaperone-based therapies. The minimally invasive nature of MRIgFUS may make it a more feasible delivery strategy than stereotactic injections.

5. Conclusions

Given the significant amount of evidence implicating molecular chaperones in the pathobiology of PD, this family of proteins may be a rational target in the design of novel therapeutics. While there is a high degree of complexity in molecular mechanisms of the Hsp70 and Hsp90 chaperone machines and the cochaperone proteins that regulate them, preclinical studies have clearly demonstrated that these proteins can be specifically and effectively targeted to slow or prevent disease progression. Currently, the major obstacle in applying these therapies to the patient population has been toxicity and reduced BBB penetrance. As such, gene therapy has emerged as a viable method by which to modulate chaperone activity within the brain. Preclinical and clinical trials have demonstrated the efficacy of intracranial gene delivery using viral vectors, indicating that this is a safe and effective method to specifically target molecular chaperones. Novel minimally invasive techniques, such as BBB permeabilization using MRIgFUS, represent a means by which pharmacological and genetic chaperone therapy delivery can be optimized, while minimizing the risk conferred to the patient. Significant work remains to be done in the preclinical domain to optimize methods to target chaperone proteins but the potential for the development of a novel therapeutic approach that slows neurodegeneration in PD remains high.

Authors' Contributions

Erik L. Friesen and Mitch L. De Snoo contributed equally to this paper.

Acknowledgments

The authors thank Megha Duggal and Alicia Triantafilou for proofreading the manuscript. Erik L. Friesen holds a Canadian Institutes of Health Research (CIHR) Canada Graduate Scholarship-Master's (CGS-M). Mitch L. De Snoo holds a Natural Sciences and Engineering Research Council of Canada (NSERC) CGS-M. Lorraine V. Kalia holds a CIHR Clinician-Scientist Award and received research support from NSERC, Michael J. Fox Foundation for Parkinson's Research, J. P. Bickell Foundation, University of Toronto Centre for Collaborative Drug Research, and Toronto General & Western Hospital Foundation and received research support from Parkinson's UK and educational support from Allergan. Suneil K. Kalia received research support from Michael J. Fox Foundation for Parkinson's Research, Parkinson Canada, and Toronto General & Western Hospital Foundation.

References

[1] L. M. de Lau and M. M. Breteler, "Epidemiology of Parkinson's disease," *The Lancet Neurology*, vol. 5, no. 6, pp. 525–535, 2006.

[2] L. V. Kalia and A. E. Lang, "Parkinson's disease," *The Lancet*, vol. 386, no. 9996, pp. 896–912, 2015.

[3] M. H. Polymeropoulos, C. Lavedan, E. Leroy et al., "Mutation in the α-synuclein gene identified in families with Parkinson's disease," *Science*, vol. 276, no. 5321, pp. 2045–2047, 1997.

[4] A. B. Singleton, M. Farrer, J. Johnson et al., "α-synuclein locus triplication causes Parkinson's disease," *Science*, vol. 302, no. 5646, article 841, 2003.

[5] K. A. Conway, J. D. Harper, and P. T. Lansbury, "Accelerated in vitro fibril formation by a mutant α-synuclein linked to early-onset Parkinson disease," *Nature Medicine*, vol. 4, no. 11, pp. 1318–1320, 1998.

[6] J. E. Tetzlaff, P. Putcha, T. F. Outeiro et al., "CHIP targets toxic α-synuclein oligomers for degradation," *Journal of Biological Chemistry*, vol. 283, no. 26, pp. 17962–17968, 2008.

[7] B. Winner, R. Jappelli, S. K. Maji et al., "In vivo demonstration that α-synuclein oligomers are toxic," *Proceedings of the National Academy of Sciences of the United States of America*, vol. 108, no. 10, pp. 4194–4199, 2011.

[8] L. V. Kalia, S. K. Kalia, P. J. McLean, A. M. Lozano, and A. E. Lang, "α-synuclein oligomers and clinical implications for parkinson disease," *Annals of Neurology*, vol. 73, no. 2, pp. 155–169, 2013.

[9] D. W. Neef, A. M. Jaeger, and D. J. Thiele, "Heat shock transcription factor 1 as a therapeutic target in neurodegenerative diseases," *Nature Reviews Drug Discovery*, vol. 10, no. 12, pp. 930–944, 2011.

[10] S. Bose and J. Cho, "Targeting chaperones, heat shock factor-1, and unfolded protein response: Promising therapeutic approaches for neurodegenerative disorders," *Ageing Research Reviews*, vol. 35, pp. 155–175, 2017.

[11] G. Chiosis and H. Tao, "Purine-scaffold Hsp90 inhibitors," *IDrugs: The Investigational Drugs Journal*, vol. 9, no. 11, pp. 778–782, 2006.

[12] P. Putcha, K. M. Danzer, L. R. Kranich et al., "Brain-permeable small-molecule inhibitors of Hsp90 prevent α-synuclein oligomer formation and rescue α-synuclein-induced toxicity," *Journal of Pharmacology and Experimental Therapeutics*, vol. 332, no. 3, pp. 849–857, 2010.

[13] D. Ebrahimi-Fakhari, L.-J. Saidi, and L. Wahlster, "Molecular chaperones and protein folding as therapeutic targets in Parkinson's disease and other synucleinopathies," *Acta neuropathologica communications*, vol. 1, no. 1, p. 79, 2013.

[14] P. K. Auluck and N. M. Bonini, "Pharmacological prevention of Parkinson disease in Drosophila [1]," *Nature Medicine*, vol. 8, no. 11, pp. 1185-1186, 2002.

[15] J. R. Porter, C. C. Fritz, and K. M. Depew, "Discovery and development of Hsp90 inhibitors: a promising pathway for cancer therapy," *Current Opinion in Chemical Biology*, vol. 14, no. 3, pp. 412–420, 2010.

[16] G.-Y. Pan, X.-D. Liu, and G.-Q. Liu, "Intracarotid infusion of hypertonic mannitol changes permeability of blood-brain barrier to methotrexate in rats," *Acta Pharmacologica Sinica*, vol. 21, no. 7, pp. 613–616, 2000.

[17] L. Cortez and V. Sim, "The therapeutic potential of chemical chaperones in protein folding diseases," *Prion*, vol. 8, no. 2, pp. 1–6, 2014.

[18] P. Hogarth, L. Lovrecic, and D. Krainc, "Sodium phenylbutyrate in Huntington's disease: a dose-finding study," *Movement Disorders*, vol. 22, no. 13, pp. 1962–1964, 2007.

[19] R. T. Bartus, M. S. Weinberg, and R. J. Samulski, "Parkinson's disease gene therapy: Success by design meets failure by efficacy," *Molecular Therapy*, vol. 22, no. 3, pp. 487–497, 2014.

[20] H. H. Kampinga and S. Bergink, "Heat shock proteins as potential targets for protective strategies in neurodegeneration," *The Lancet Neurology*, 2016.

[21] H. H. Kampinga, J. Hageman, M. J. Vos et al., "Guidelines for the nomenclature of the human heat shock proteins," *Cell Stress and Chaperones*, vol. 14, no. 1, pp. 105–111, 2009.

[22] A. Ciechanover and Y. T. Kwon, "Protein Quality Control by Molecular Chaperones in Neurodegeneration," *Frontiers in Neuroscience*, vol. 11, 2017.

[23] S. K. Kalia, L. V. Kalia, and P. J. McLean, "Molecular chaperones as rational drug targets for parkinson's disease therapeutics," *CNS & Neurological Disorders—Drug Targets*, vol. 9, no. 6, pp. 741–753, 2010.

[24] J. Zou, Y. Guo, T. Guettouche, D. F. Smith, and R. Voellmy, "Repression of heat shock transcription factor HSF1 activation by HSP90 (HSP90 complex) that forms a stress-sensitive complex with HSF1," *Cell*, vol. 94, no. 4, pp. 471–480, 1998.

[25] R. I. Morimoto, "Regulation of the heat shock transcriptional response: cross talk between a family of heat shock factors, molecular chaperones, and negative regulators," *Genes and Development*, vol. 12, no. 24, pp. 3788–3796, 1998.

[26] S. Rüdiger, L. Germeroth, J. Schneider-Mergener, and B. Bukau, "Substrate specificity of the DnaK chaperone determined by screening cellulose-bound peptide libraries," *EMBO Journal*, vol. 16, no. 7, pp. 1501–1507, 1997.

[27] B. Bukau and A. L. Horwich, "The Hsp70 and Hsp60 chaperone machines," *Cell*, vol. 92, no. 3, pp. 351–366, 1998.

[28] P. Goloubinoff and P. D. L. Rios, "The mechanism of Hsp70 chaperones: (entropic) pulling the models together," *Trends in Biochemical Sciences*, vol. 32, no. 8, pp. 372–380, 2007.

[29] W. L. Kelley, "Molecular chaperones: How J domains turn on Hsp70s," *Current Biology*, vol. 9, no. 8, pp. R305–R308, 1999.

[30] J. Höhfeld and S. Jentsch, "GrpE-like regulation of the Hsc70 chaperone by the anti-apoptotic protein BAG-1," *EMBO Journal*, vol. 16, no. 20, pp. 6209–6216, 1997.

[31] A. Arakawa, N. Handa, N. Ohsawa et al., "The C-terminal BAG domain of BAG5 induces conformational changes of the Hsp70 nucleotide- binding domain for ADP-ATP exchange," *Structure*, vol. 18, no. 3, pp. 309–319, 2010.

[32] H. Rampelt, J. Kirstein-Miles, N. B. Nillegoda et al., "Metazoan Hsp70 machines use Hsp110 to power protein disaggregation," *The EMBO Journal*, vol. 31, no. 21, pp. 4221–4235, 2012.

[33] G. C. Meacham, C. Patterson, W. Zhang, J. M. Younger, and D. M. Cyr, "The Hsc70 co-chaperone CHIP targets immature CFTR for proteasomal degradation," *Nature Cell Biology*, vol. 3, no. 1, pp. 100–105, 2001.

[34] S. Murata, Y. Minami, M. Minami, T. Chiba, and K. Tanaka, "CHIP is a chaperone-dependent E3 ligase that ubiquitylates unfolded protein," *The EMBO Reports*, vol. 2, no. 12, pp. 1133–1138, 2001.

[35] A. M. Cuervo, L. Stafanis, R. Fredenburg, P. T. Lansbury, and D. Sulzer, "Impaired degradation of mutant α-synuclein by chaperone-mediated autophagy," *Science*, vol. 305, no. 5688, pp. 1292–1295, 2004.

[36] M. Xilouri, O. R. Brekk, and L. Stefanis, "Autophagy and Alpha-Synuclein: Relevance to Parkinson's Disease and Related Synucleopathies," *Movement Disorders*, vol. 31, no. 2, pp. 178–192, 2016.

[37] X. Gao, M. Carroni, C. Nussbaum-Krammer et al., "Human Hsp70 Disaggregase Reverses Parkinson's-Linked α-Synuclein Amyloid Fibrils," *Molecular Cell*, vol. 59, no. 5, pp. 781–793, 2015.

[38] N. B. Nillegoda and B. Bukau, "Metazoan Hsp70-based protein disaggregases: emergence and mechanisms," *Frontiers in Molecular Biosciences*, vol. 2, 2015.

[39] P. K. Auluck, H. Y. E. Chan, J. Q. Trojanowski, V. M. Lee, and N. M. Bonini, "Chaperone suppression of α-synuclein toxicity in a Drosophila model for Parkinson's disease," *Science*, vol. 295, no. 5556, pp. 865–868, 2002.

[40] P. J. McLean, H. Kawamata, S. Shariff et al., "TorsinA and heat shock proteins act as molecular chaperones: Suppression of α-synuclein aggregation," *Journal of Neurochemistry*, vol. 83, no. 4, pp. 846–854, 2002.

[41] Y.-R. Wu, C.-K. Wang, C.-M. Chen et al., "Analysis of heat-shock protein 70 gene polymorphisms and the risk of Parkinson's disease," *Human Genetics*, vol. 114, no. 3, pp. 236–241, 2004.

[42] L. De Mena, E. Coto, E. Sánchez-Ferrero et al., "Mutational screening of the mortalin gene (HSPA9) in Parkinson's disease," *Journal of Neural Transmission*, vol. 116, no. 10, pp. 1289–1293, 2009.

[43] R. Wadhwa, J. Ryu, H. M. Ahn et al., "Functional significance of point mutations in stress chaperone mortalin and their relevance to parkinson disease," *Journal of Biological Chemistry*, vol. 290, no. 13, pp. 8447–8456, 2015.

[44] L. F. Burbulla, C. Schelling, H. Kato et al., "Dissecting the role of the mitochondrial chaperone mortalin in Parkinson's disease: Functional impact of disease-related variants on mitochondrial homeostasis," *Human Molecular Genetics*, vol. 19, no. 22, pp. 4437–4452, 2010.

[45] K. Freimann, K. Zschiedrich, N. Brüggemann et al., "Mortalin mutations are not a frequent cause of early-onset Parkinson disease.," *Neurobiology of aging*, vol. 34, no. 11, pp. 2694–e19, 2013.

[46] T. R. Flower, L. S. Chesnokova, C. A. Froelich, C. Dixon, and S. N. Witt, "Heat shock prevents alpha-synuclein-induced apoptosis in a yeast model of Parkinson's disease," *Journal of Molecular Biology*, vol. 351, no. 5, pp. 1081–1100, 2005.

[47] T. C. Moloney, R. Hyland, D. O'Toole et al., "Heat shock protein 70 reduces α-synuclein-induced predegenerative neuronal dystrophy in the α-synuclein viral gene transfer rat model of parkinson's disease," *CNS Neuroscience and Therapeutics*, vol. 20, no. 1, pp. 50–58, 2014.

[48] J. Klucken, Y. Shin, E. Masliah, B. T. Hyman, and P. J. McLean, "Hsp70 reduces α-synuclein aggregation and toxicity," *The Journal of Biological Chemistry*, vol. 279, no. 24, pp. 25497–25502, 2004.

[49] D. J. Quigney, A. M. Gorman, and A. Samali, "Heat shock protects PC12 cells against MPP+ toxicity," *Brain Research*, vol. 993, no. 1-2, pp. 133–139, 2003.

[50] Z. Dong, D. P. Wolfer, H.-P. Lipp, and H. Büeler, "Hsp70 gene transfer by adeno-associated virusi inhibits MPTP-induced nigrostriatal degeneration in the mouse model of Parkinson disease," *Molecular Therapy*, vol. 11, no. 1, pp. 80–88, 2005.

[51] W. Dauer, N. Kholodilov, M. Vila et al., "Resistance of α-synuclein null mice to the parkinsonian neurotoxin MPTP," *Proceedings of the National Academy of Sciences of the United States of America*, vol. 99, no. 22, pp. 14524–14529, 2002.

[52] F.-T. Liu, Y. Chen, Y.-J. Yang et al., "Involvement of mortalin/GRP75/mthsp70 in the mitochondrial impairments induced by A53T mutant α-synuclein," *Brain Research*, vol. 1604, pp. 52–61, 2015.

[53] Z. Zhang and Y. Cheng, "MiR-16-1 promotes the aberrant α -synuclein accumulation in parkinson disease via targeting heat shock protein 70," *Scientific World Journal*, vol. 2014, Article ID 938348, 2014.

[54] L. Alvarez-Erviti, Y. Seow, A. H. V. Schapira, M. C. Rodriguez-Oroz, J. A. Obeso, and J. M. Cooper, "Influence of microRNA deregulation on chaperone-mediated autophagy and α-synuclein pathology in parkinson's disease," *Cell Death and Disease*, vol. 4, no. 3, p. e545, 2013.

[55] L. Alvarez-Erviti, M. C. Rodriguez-Oroz, J. M. Cooper et al., "Chaperone-mediated autophagy markers in Parkinson disease brains," *Archives of Neurology*, vol. 67, no. 12, pp. 1464–1472, 2010.

[56] N. Papagiannakis, M. Xilouri, C. Koros et al., "Lysosomal alterations in peripheral blood mononuclear cells of Parkinson's disease patients," *Movement Disorders*, vol. 30, no. 13, pp. 1830–1834, 2015.

[57] G. Sala, G. Stefanoni, A. Arosio et al., "Reduced expression of the chaperone-mediated autophagy carrier hsc70 protein in lymphomonocytes of patients with Parkinson's disease," *Brain Research*, vol. 1546, pp. 46–52, 2014.

[58] J.-H. Baek, D. Whitfield, D. Howlett et al., "Unfolded protein response is activated in Lewy body dementias," *Neuropathology and Applied Neurobiology*, vol. 42, no. 4, pp. 352–365, 2016.

[59] M. Jiang, Q. Yun, F. Shi et al., "Downregulation of miR-384-5p attenuates rotenone-induced neurotoxicity in dopaminergic SH-SY5Y cells through inhibiting endoplasmic reticulum stress," *American Journal of Physiology - Cell Physiology*, vol. 310, no. 9, pp. C755–C763, 2016.

[60] M. Salganik, V. G. Sergeyev, V. Shinde et al., "The loss of glucose-regulated protein 78 (GRP78) during normal aging or from siRNA knockdown augments human alpha-synuclein (α-syn) toxicity to rat nigral neurons," *Neurobiology of Aging*, vol. 36, no. 6, pp. 2213–2223, 2015.

[61] P. Jiang, M. Gan, W.-L. Lin, and S.-H. C. Yen, "Nutrient deprivation induces α-synuclein aggregation through endoplasmic reticulum stress response and SREBP2 pathway," *Frontiers in Aging Neuroscience*, vol. 6, article no. 268, 2014.

[62] M. S. Gorbatyuk, A. Shabashvili, W. Chen et al., "Glucose regulated protein 78 diminishes α-synuclein neurotoxicity in a rat model of parkinson disease," *Molecular Therapy*, vol. 20, no. 7, pp. 1327–1337, 2012.

[63] S. K. Mak, A. L. McCormack, A. B. Manning-Bog, A. M. Cuervo, and D. A. Di Monte, "Lysosomal degradation of α-synuclein in vivo," *Journal of Biological Chemistry*, vol. 285, no. 18, pp. 13621–13629, 2010.

[64] M. Xilouri, O. R. Brekk, N. Landeck et al., "Boosting chaperone-mediated autophagy in vivo mitigates α-synuclein-induced neurodegeneration," *Brain*, vol. 136, no. 7, pp. 2130–2146, 2013.

[65] K. E. Murphy, A. M. Gysbers, S. K. Abbott et al., "Lysosomal-associated membrane protein 2 isoforms are differentially affected in early Parkinson's disease," *Movement Disorders*, vol. 30, no. 12, pp. 1639–1647, 2015.

[66] Y. Shin, J. Klucken, C. Patterson, B. T. Hyman, and P. J. McLean, "The Co-chaperone carboxyl terminus of Hsp70-interacting protein (CHIP) mediates α-synuclein degradation decisions between proteasomal and lysosomal pathways," *Journal of Biological Chemistry*, vol. 280, no. 25, pp. 23727–23734, 2005.

[67] L. V. Kalia, S. K. Kalia, H. Chau, A. M. Lozano, B. T. Hyman, and P. J. McLean, "Ubiquitinylation of α-synuclein by carboxyl terminus hsp70-interacting protein (chip) is regulated by bcl-2-associated athanogene 5 (bag5)," *PLoS ONE*, vol. 6, no. 2, Article ID e14695, 2011.

[68] S. K. Kalia, S. Lee, P. D. Smith et al., "BAG5 inhibits parkin and enhances dopaminergic neuron degeneration," *Neuron*, vol. 44, no. 6, pp. 931–945, 2004.

[69] A. R. Esteves, R. H. Swerdlow, and S. M. Cardoso, "LRRK2, a puzzling protein: insights into Parkinson's disease pathogenesis," *Experimental Neurology*, vol. 261, pp. 206–216, 2014.

[70] M. R. Cookson, "The role of leucine-rich repeat kinase 2 (*LRRK2*) in Parkinson's disease," *Nature Reviews Neuroscience*, vol. 11, no. 12, pp. 791–797, 2010.

[71] A. Beilina, I. N. Rudenko, A. Kaganovich et al., "Unbiased screen for interactors of leucine-rich repeat kinase 2 supports a common pathway for sporadic and familial Parkinson disease," *Proceedings of the National Academy of Sciences of the United States of America*, vol. 111, no. 7, pp. 2626–2631, 2014.

[72] H. S. Ko, R. Bailey, W. W. Smith et al., "CHIP regulates leucine-rich repeat kinase-2 ubiquitination, degradation, and toxicity," *Proceedings of the National Academy of Sciences of the United States of America*, vol. 106, no. 8, pp. 2897–2902, 2009.

[73] I. N. Rudenko, A. Kaganovich, R. G. Langston et al., "The G2385R risk factor for Parkinson's disease enhances CHIP-dependent intracellular degradation of LRRK2," *Biochemical Journal*, vol. 474, no. 9, pp. 1547–1558, 2017.

[74] A. M. Pickrell and R. J. Youle, "The roles of PINK1, Parkin, and mitochondrial fidelity in parkinson's disease," *Neuron*, vol. 85, no. 2, pp. 257–273, 2015.

[75] L. Zhang, P. Karsten, S. Hamm et al., "TRAP1 rescues PINK1 loss-of-function phenotypes," *Human Molecular Genetics*, vol. 22, no. 14, Article ID ddt132, pp. 2829–2841, 2013.

[76] L. F. Burbulla, J. C. Fitzgerald, K. Stegen et al., "Mitochondrial proteolytic stress induced by loss of mortalin function is rescued by Parkin and PINK1," *Cell Death and Disease*, vol. 5, no. 4, Article ID e1180, 2014.

[77] H. Yang, X. Zhou, X. Liu et al., "Mitochondrial dysfunction induced by knockdown of mortalin is rescued by Parkin," *Biochemical and Biophysical Research Communications*, vol. 410, no. 1, pp. 114–120, 2011.

[78] S. A. Hasson, L. A. Kane, K. Yamano et al., "High-content genome-wide RNAi screens identify regulators of parkin upstream of mitophagy," *Nature*, vol. 504, no. 7479, pp. 291–295, 2013.

[79] D. Qu, A. Hage, K. Don-Carolis et al., "BAG2 gene-mediated regulation of PINK1 protein is critical for mitochondrial translocation of PARKIN and neuronal survival," *Journal of Biological Chemistry*, vol. 290, no. 51, pp. 30441–30452, 2015.

[80] Y. Imai, M. Soda, S. Hatakeyama et al., "CHIP is associated with Parkin, a gene responsible for familial Parkinson's Disease, and enhances its ubiquitin ligase activity," *Molecular Cell*, vol. 10, no. 1, pp. 55–67, 2002.

[81] S. Batelli, D. Albani, R. Rametta et al., "DJ-1 modulates α-synuclein aggregation state in a cellular model of oxidative stress: Relevance for Parkinson's Disease and involvement of HSP70," *PLoS ONE*, vol. 3, no. 4, Article ID e1884, 2008.

[82] H. M. Li, T. Niki, T. Taira, S. M. M. Iguchi-Ariga, and H. Ariga, "Association of DJ-1 with chaperones and enhanced association and colocalization with mitochondrial Hsp70 by oxidative stress," *Free Radical Research*, vol. 39, no. 10, pp. 1091–1099, 2005.

[83] L. Qin, J. Tan, H. Zhang et al., "BAG5 Interacts with DJ-1 and Inhibits the Neuroprotective Effects of DJ-1 to Combat Mitochondrial Oxidative Damage," *Oxidative Medicine and Cellular Longevity*, vol. 2017, pp. 1–10, 2017.

[84] C. Vilariño-Güell, A. Rajput, A. J. Milnerwood et al., "DNAJC13 mutations in Parkinson disease," *Human Molecular Genetics*, vol. 23, no. 7, pp. 1794–1801, 2014.

[85] J. H. Zhao, H. L. Liu, H. Y. Lin et al., "Chemical chaperone and inhibitor discovery: potential treatments for protein conformational diseases," *Perspect Medicin Chem*, vol. 1, pp. 39–48, 2007.

[86] P. H. Yancey, M. E. Clark, S. C. Hand, R. D. Bowlus, and G. N. Somero, "Living with water stress: evolution of osmolyte systems," *Science*, vol. 217, no. 4566, pp. 1214–1222, 1982.

[87] M. Tanaka, Y. Machida, S. Niu et al., "Trehalose alleviates polyglutamine-mediated pathology in a mouse model of Huntington disease," *Nature Medicine*, vol. 10, no. 2, pp. 148–154, 2004.

[88] Q. He, J. B. Koprich, Y. Wang et al., "Treatment with Trehalose Prevents Behavioral and Neurochemical Deficits Produced in an AAV α-Synuclein Rat Model of Parkinson's Disease," *Molecular Neurobiology*, vol. 53, no. 4, pp. 2258–2268, 2016.

[89] R. Shaltiel-Karyo, M. Frenkel-Pinter, E. Rockenstein et al., "A Blood-Brain Barrier (BBB) disrupter is also a potent α-synuclein (α-syn) aggregation inhibitor: A novel dual mechanism of mannitol for the treatment of Parkinson Disease (PD)," *Journal of Biological Chemistry*, vol. 288, no. 24, pp. 17579–17588, 2013.

[90] M. Inden, Y. Kitamura, H. Takeuchi et al., "Neurodegeneration of mouse nigrostriatal dopaminergic system induced by repeated oral administration of rotenone is prevented by 4-phenylbutyrate, a chemical chaperone," *Journal of Neurochemistry*, vol. 101, no. 6, pp. 1491–1504, 2007.

[91] A. Migdalska-Richards, L. Daly, E. Bezard, and A. H. V. Schapira, "Ambroxol effects in glucocerebrosidase and α-synuclein transgenic mice," *Annals of Neurology*, vol. 80, no. 5, pp. 766–775, 2016.

[92] K. E. Murphy, A. M. Gysbers, S. K. Abbott et al., "Reduced glucocerebrosidase is associated with increased α-synuclein in

sporadic Parkinson's disease," *Brain*, vol. 137, no. 3, pp. 834–848, 2014.

[93] A. McNeill, J. Magalhaes, C. Shen et al., "Ambroxol improves lysosomal biochemistry in glucocerebrosidase mutation-linked Parkinson disease cells," *Brain*, vol. 137, no. 5, pp. 1481–1495, 2014.

[94] F. Richter, S. M. Fleming, M. Watson et al., "A GCase Chaperone Improves Motor Function in a Mouse Model of Synucleinopathy," *Neurotherapeutics*, vol. 11, no. 4, pp. 840–856, 2014.

[95] K. Faust, S. Gehrke, Y. Yang, L. Yang, M. F. Beal, and B. Lu, "Neuroprotective effects of compounds with antioxidant and anti-inflammatory properties in a Drosophila model of Parkinson's disease," *BMC Neuroscience*, vol. 10, article no. 1471, p. 109, 2009.

[96] P. Thakur and B. Nehru, "Long-term heat shock proteins (HSPs) induction by carbenoxolone improves hallmark features of Parkinson's disease in a rotenone-based model," *Neuropharmacology*, vol. 79, pp. 190–200, 2014.

[97] K. Kilpatrick, J. A. Novoa, T. Hancock et al., "Chemical induction of Hsp70 reduces α-synuclein aggregation in neuroglioma cells," *ACS Chemical Biology*, vol. 8, no. 7, pp. 1460–1468, 2013.

[98] P. J. McLean, J. Klucken, Y. Shin, and B. T. Hyman, "Geldanamycin induces Hsp70 and prevents α-synuclein aggregation and toxicity in vitro," *Biochemical and Biophysical Research Communications*, vol. 321, no. 3, pp. 665–669, 2004.

[99] H.-Y. Shen, J.-C. He, Y. Wang, Q.-Y. Huang, and J.-F. Chen, "Geldanamycin induces heat shock protein 70 and protects against MPTP-induced dopaminergic neurotoxicity in mice," *Journal of Biological Chemistry*, vol. 280, no. 48, pp. 39962–39969, 2005.

[100] N. Fujikake, Y. Nagai, H. A. Popiel, Y. Okamoto, M. Yamaguchi, and T. Toda, "Heat shock transcription factor 1-activating compounds suppress polyglutamine-induced neurodegeneration through induction of multiple molecular chaperones," *Journal of Biological Chemistry*, vol. 283, no. 38, pp. 26188–26197, 2008.

[101] K. Jhaveri and S. Modi, "Ganetespib: Research and clinical development," *OncoTargets and Therapy*, vol. 8, pp. 1849–1858, 2015.

[102] N. R. McFarland, H. Dimant, L. Kibuuka et al., "Chronic treatment with novel small molecule Hsp90 inhibitors rescues striatal dopamine levels but not α-synuclein-induced neuronal cell loss," *PLoS ONE*, vol. 9, no. 1, Article ID e86048, 2014.

[103] N. C. Rowland, S. K. Kalia, L. V. Kalia, P. S. Larson, D. A. Lim, and K. S. Bankiewicz, "Merging DBS with viral vector or stem cell implantation: "hybrid" stereotactic surgery as an evolution in the surgical treatment of Parkinson's disease," *Molecular Therapy—Methods and Clinical Development*, vol. 3, 2016.

[104] Z. Wu, A. Asokan, and R. J. Samulski, "Adeno-associated Virus Serotypes: Vector Toolkit for Human Gene Therapy," *Molecular Therapy*, vol. 14, no. 3, pp. 316–327, 2006.

[105] D. Pignataro, D. Sucunza, L. Vanrell et al., "Adeno-Associated Viral Vectors Serotype 8 for Cell-Specific Delivery of Therapeutic Genes in the Central Nervous System," *Frontiers in Neuroanatomy*, vol. 11, 2017.

[106] W. D. Lo, G. Qu, T. J. Sferra, R. Clark, R. Chen, and P. R. Johnson, "Adeno-associated virus-mediated gene transfer to the brain: Duration and modulation of expression," *Human Gene Therapy*, vol. 10, no. 2, pp. 201–213, 1999.

[107] M. G. Kaplitt, P. Leone, R. J. Samulski et al., "Long-term gene expression and phenotypic correction using adeno-associated virus vectors in the mammalian brain," *Nature Genetics*, vol. 8, no. 2, pp. 148–154, 1994.

[108] K. Albert, M. Voutilainen, A. Domanskyi, and M. Airavaara, "AAV Vector-Mediated Gene Delivery to Substantia Nigra Dopamine Neurons: Implications for Gene Therapy and Disease Models," *Genes*, vol. 8, no. 2, p. 63, 2017.

[109] P. Kermer, A. Köhn, M. Schnieder et al., "BAG1 is neuroprotective in in vivo and in vitro models of Parkinson's disease," *Journal of Molecular Neuroscience*, vol. 55, no. 3, pp. 587–595, 2015.

[110] C. Lo Bianco, J. Shorter, E. Régulier et al., "Hsp104 antagonizes α-synuclein aggregation and reduces dopaminergic degeneration in a rat model of Parkinson disease," *Journal of Clinical Investigation*, vol. 118, no. 9, pp. 3087–3097, 2008.

[111] M. E. Jackrel, M. E. Desantis, B. A. Martinez et al., "Potentiated Hsp104 variants antagonize diverse proteotoxic misfolding events," *Cell*, vol. 156, no. 1-2, pp. 170–182, 2014.

[112] L. Samaranch, W. S. Sebastian, A. P. Kells et al., "AAV9-mediated expression of a non-self protein in nonhuman primate central nervous system triggers widespread neuroinflammation driven by antigen-presenting cell transduction," *Molecular Therapy*, vol. 22, no. 2, pp. 329–337, 2014.

[113] C. Y. Lin, H. Y. Hsieh, C. M. Chen et al., "Non invasive, neuron-specific gene therapy by focused ultrasound-induced blood-brain barrier opening in Parkinson's disease mouse model," *Journal of Controlled Release*, vol. 235, pp. 72–81, 2016.

[114] L. Long, X. Cai, R. Guo et al., "Treatment of Parkinson's disease in rats by Nrf2 transfection using MRI-guided focused ultrasound delivery of nanomicrobubbles," *Biochemical and Biophysical Research Communications*, vol. 482, no. 1, pp. 75–80, 2017.

9

Classification and Characteristics of Pain Associated with Parkinson's Disease

Marcelo Rezende Young Blood,[1] Marcelo Machado Ferro,[2] Renato Puppi Munhoz,[3] Hélio Afonso Ghizoni Teive,[4] and Carlos Henrique Ferreira Camargo[1]

[1]*Neurology Service, Hospital Universitário, State University of Ponta Grossa, Ponta Grossa, PR, Brazil*
[2]*Neuropsychopharmacology Laboratory, State University of Ponta Grossa, Ponta Grossa, PR, Brazil*
[3]*Movement Disorders Centre, Toronto Western Hospital, University of Toronto, Toronto, ON, Canada*
[4]*Movement Disorders Unit, Neurology Service, Internal Medicine Department, Hospital de Clínicas, Federal University of Paraná, Curitiba, PR, Brazil*

Correspondence should be addressed to Carlos Henrique Ferreira Camargo; chcamargo@uol.com.br

Academic Editor: Ivan Bodis-Wollner

Neuropsychiatric symptoms and pain are among the most common nonmotor symptoms of Parkinson's disease (PD). The correlation between pain and PD has been recognized since its classic descriptions. Pain occurs in about 60% of PD patients, two to three times more frequent in this population than in age matched healthy individuals. It is an early and potentially disabling symptom that can precede motor symptoms by several years. The lower back and lower extremities are the most commonly affected areas. The most used classification for pain in PD defines musculoskeletal, dystonic, central, or neuropathic/radicular forms. Its different clinical characteristics, variable relationship with motor symptoms, and inconsistent response to dopaminergic drugs suggest that the mechanism underlying pain in PD is complex and multifaceted, involving the peripheral nervous system, generation and amplification of pain by motor symptoms, and neurodegeneration of areas related to pain modulation. Although pain in DP is common and a significant source of disability, its clinical characteristics, pathophysiology, classification, and management remain to be defined.

1. Introduction

Although the most commonly accepted criteria for the diagnosis of Parkinson's disease (PD) depend on motor symptoms, other signs and complaints related to the disease, such as a loss of sense of smell, constipation, depression, altered sleep patterns, and unexplained pain, may be detected years before the onset of any of the cardinal motor signs [1]. One landmark study showed that virtually all PD patients report at least one nonmotor symptom (NMS) when these manifestations are actively pursued using specific questionnaires, reaching an average of eight different symptoms per patient. In this same study, the most frequent NMS were neuropsychiatric, gastrointestinal, and pain related symptoms [2]. In the early stages of the disease, the most common NMS are hyposmia, pain, and sleep disturbances [3]. Additionally, pain, depression, and anxiety are associated with worse quality of life [3–5]. Although the correlation between pain and PD has been recognized since its first descriptions, including James Parkinson citation of "rheumatic pain extending from the arms to the fingers" [6], the issue of pain in PD has only recently received the deserved attention in both clinical and research settings.

Pain is present in around 60% of PD patients and occurs two to three times more frequently in this population than in age matched individuals without PD [7–9]. It is an early symptom and can precede motor symptoms by several years [1, 10, 11]. In individuals who have had the disease for less than six years, it can be the most disturbing NMS, particularly when it has musculoskeletal or visceral origin [12]. Although common in any disease stage [12], around 40% of patients may not report this complaint in routine visits to a physician [13].

Pain does not appear to be influenced by gender, age, or geographic/cultural variables [14]. Although some authors have reported a higher frequency in women [2, 7], this is not supported by most studies [8, 15–17]. Similarly, while some studies have reported a lower mean age for patients with pain [9, 15] and others have even suggested that onset of PD before the age of 65 is a risk factor for pain [9], most authors [8, 17–19] failed to find significant differences. An increase in the prevalence of pain should also be expected throughout the clinical and neurodegenerative progression of the disease; however, most studies showed no correlation between the presence or intensity of pain and clinical staging or disease duration [7, 19–21].

Pain usually occurs on the side on which motor symptoms first appear or are more severe [22]. While the main risk factors for developing spontaneous pain in PD are the presence of motor fluctuations and severity of motor symptoms [9, 16], this may not always be the case [23], as some patients with pain and motor complications present with pain on the side unaffected by the disease [16]. In a study of the influence of levodopa treatment and deep brain stimulation (DBS) on the "off" period in PD, both interventions improved somatic pain thresholds independently of any improvement in motor symptoms [24]. In terms of pain location, although it can be quite variable, the lower back and legs are the most commonly affected regions [14]. Shoulder pain, commonly reported by PD patients [2, 16], can be the first symptom of PD in 2–8% of patients and might even precede the onset of motor symptoms [25]. It is thought to stem from two different mechanisms: one, directly related to the neurological symptom, is pseudorheumatic and dopamine sensitive; the other is thought to be associated with degenerative lesions that may worsen with the progression of PD [18].

As depression and pain are prevalent NMS in PD and chronic pain is a known risk factor for depression [39], the association between the two symptoms is to be expected [40]. Indeed, individuals with pain and PD have higher scores on depression rating scales [41]. Although some studies failed to find any association [16, 17], current evidence suggests that the presence of depression is an important variable that should be taken into account in studies of pain in PD, particularly because of the frequency with which it is found and the fact that it can modify the perception of pain. Furthermore, it is potentially treatable [40].

Systemic diseases such as diabetes mellitus, osteoporosis, and rheumatic diseases are also associated with a greater prevalence of pain in PD [42]. Finally, there is also evidence of an association between genetic factors and musculoskeletal pain, a subtype of pain in PD. For example, mutations in the *SCN9A* (sodium channel Nav1.7) and *FAAH* (fatty acid amide hydrolase, a key cannabinoid metabolizing enzyme) genes have been associated with higher susceptibility to this symptom in PD [43, 44].

Table 1: Classification of pain related to Parkinson's disease.

Category	Characteristics
Musculoskeletal	Muscle and/or joint pain, inflammation, bone deformity, reduced joint mobility, and abnormal posture. Associated with muscle rigidity and can improve with levodopa therapy.
Dystonic	Associated with abnormal postures and can improve with levodopa therapy.
Neuropathic/radicular	Peripheral neuropathic pain: restricted to the territory of the affected nerve or nerve root.
Central or primary	Neuropathic pain that is not restricted to the affected nerve or nerve root. Varies with the medication cycle as a nonmotor fluctuation. Pain may have an autonomic character, with visceral sensations. Not associated with rigidity, dystonia, or musculoskeletal or structural lesions.
Akathisia	Subjective sensation of restlessness and an inability to remain still. Can vary with medication and improve with levodopa therapy.

2. Assessment and Classification of Pain in PD

The prevalence of pain in PD can vary from 34% [45] to 83% [7] depending on methodological assessments. Possible explanations for this large range include the tools and criteria used for the diagnosis and profile of the population studied. For instance, while some studies only considered this symptom to be present when it lasted more than three months [8, 9, 17, 46], others did not specify any time criterion [18, 19, 47]. Among the diagnostic tools for the assessment of pain in PD, the most widely used is the Brief Pain Inventory [5, 7, 9, 19–21]; however, because it only analyzes pain in the previous 24 hours, it can underestimate its prevalence. As pain is an unpleasant sensory and emotional experience [48], the use of a multidimensional scale to evaluate it is recommended [49]. The widely used McGill Pain Questionnaire [9, 18, 47, 50] is an example of this type of scale, evaluating sensory-discriminatory and affective-motivational domains [51].

Nonetheless, there is a lack of consensus regarding the assessment and classification of pain in PD patients. The first classification, published by Ford [52], is the most commonly used, but other proposals have been put forward as a result of the growing interest in the subject [9, 25, 53, 54].

2.1. The Ford Classification. The Ford classification [52] is based on studies by Goetz and Quinn [15, 55] and uses an approach that involves the etiology of pain and its association with motor symptoms (Table 1). It classifies PD related pain in five groups: musculoskeletal, dystonic, neuropathic/radicular, central or primary, and akathisia.

Musculoskeletal pain is the most common and easily identified type of pain [11]. It is associated with muscle rigidity and bradykinesia as well as a lack of mobility, postural abnormalities, and gait imbalance [56]. Lumbar pain is usually the most frequent complaint, but neck and leg pain are also common. Joint pain is most common in the shoulders, hips, knees, and ankles [56]. In cases of stiffness-related pain, adjustment of dopaminergic therapy together with physiotherapy and physical exercise is recommended to relieve symptoms. Nonsteroidal anti-inflammatory drugs and analgesics can help in orthopedic and rheumatologic conditions.

Dystonia is a movement disorder characterized by sustained or intermittent muscle contractions that result in abnormal, frequently repetitive movements and/or postures [57]. These contractions can cause the most intense pains PD patients experience and can be alleviated by intramuscular botulinum toxin injections as well as adjustment of dopaminergic therapy [58]. It is important to try to correlate the timing of dopaminergic therapy with the occurrence of pain as it can be observed as an early morning or as wearing off (WO) phenomenon, indicating dopaminergic deficiency [56]. Treatment with DBS of the subthalamic nucleus or internal globus pallidus may influence this symptom positively [59, 60].

Very localized pain with neuropathic characteristics (burning, electric-shock like, and paresthesia) limited to a nerve or nerve root territory was classified by Ford as neuropathic/radicular and can also be called peripheral neuropathic pain. It affects from 5% to 14% of PD patients with pain [9, 15, 19]. To our knowledge, there are no studies that have evaluated only peripheral neuropathic pain in PD; however, in most PD patients this type of pain is believed to be associated with focal compression associated with degenerative joint disease [56, 61] and assessments with electroneuromyography and neuroimaging may be necessary. The first-line drug treatments for neuropathic pain are amitriptyline, duloxetine, and pregabalin [62].

Central or primary pain presents with neuropathic characteristics and appears to be associated with impaired central modulation of pain caused by dopaminergic deficiency in the basal ganglia. It affects from 4% to 10% of PD patients with pain [7, 8]. It is typically not restricted to a nerve territory and has been described to affect atypical body areas such as face, head, pharynx, epigastrium, abdomen, pelvis, rectum, and genitalia [63]. This type of pain can be associated with autonomic manifestations, with visceral sensations, and can improve with administration of levodopa [52]. As it cannot be classified in any other group, it is considered a diagnosis of exclusion.

Akathisia is defined as a feeling of inner restlessness and an inability to remain still, presenting as a constant need to move or change position. Although it is sometimes described as a painful sensation, this is not normally the case and it should not be considered a sensory disturbance [7]. Javoy-Agid and Agid [64] suggest that akathisia is a result of a dopamine dysfunction in the dopaminergic mesocorticolimbic pathway, which originates in the ventral tegmental area and is impaired in PD. Restless legs syndrome is also caused by a similar dopamine dysfunction in this region, and both conditions respond to dopaminergic therapy [65].

2.2. Other Assessment Tools. The DoPaMiP study (*Douleur et maladie de Parkinson en Midi-Pyrénées*) suggests that an initial distinction can be made between pain related to PD (PRPD) and pain unrelated to PD (PUPD). This distinction was made by an expert group who based their conclusions on the relationship between pain and PD as reported by the patient, the clinical characteristics of the pain (such as location, duration, and frequency), aggravating factors and the association between pain and the disease symptoms, motor complications, and anti-Parkinsonian medication. PRPD can be further divided into (1) pain directly related to PD, when it cannot be attributed to any other health problem, and (2) pain indirectly related to PD, when it is caused by another disease (e.g., osteoarthritis) but is aggravated by PD because of rigidity and abnormal posture or movements. Hence, to be considered PRPD, the pain must be caused or aggravated by PD, while for it to be considered PUPD it should be related to other causes and not aggravated by PD [9].

The Marburg/São Paulo/Créteil Questionnaire uses a three-step approach. These consist of (1) establishing a temporal relation between pain and the symptoms of PD; (2) determining whether the pain is related to motor fluctuations; and (3) determining whether the pain is related to the anti-Parkinsonian treatment. If the answer in any of these three cases is affirmative, the pain is classified as PRPD; if not, it is classified as PUPD. In the former case, it can be further classified as musculoskeletal, neuropathic, or psychomotor/restlessness-related.

In some cases, the relation between pain and PD is difficult to determine. Despite obvious injury on imaging studies the cause and effect relationship can not be easily observed (e.g., disc herniation and low back pain). In DoPaMiP study, for example, patients with osteoarthritis were classified as either PRPD or PUPD. The authors agree that selection bias may have occurred in this approach [9]. There are two disadvantages to this approach: it does not define any subtype of pain and does not provide the individual response to dopaminergic therapy [66]. The perception of pain and other sensory modalities is clearly altered in individuals with PD [67], so it is not necessary to separate the pain related or unrelated to the disease.

"King's Parkinson's disease pain scale," which was proposed by a multicenter group that included King's College Hospital in London, is officially advocated by the "International Parkinson's and Movement Disorder Society Non-Motor PD Study Group" for evaluating pain in PD. It is a questionnaire with fourteen questions covering seven domains: (1) musculoskeletal pain; (2) chronic pain; (3) fluctuation-related pain; (4) nocturnal pain; (5) orofacial pain; (6) discoloration and edema/swelling; and (7) radicular pain. For each question, scores from 0 to 3 and 0 to 4 are assigned for the intensity and frequency of the symptom, respectively. The scores for severity and frequency are multiplied and the result is added to the result of the other items to obtain a score for each domain and, in the same way, the total score for the seven domains (0–168). The validation study found a strong correlation between this scale's scores and the Parkinson's disease-severity and quality of life scales scores. According to the authors, the score in each domain should be used to determine the type of pain the patient is presenting with, while the total score provides insight of the impact pain

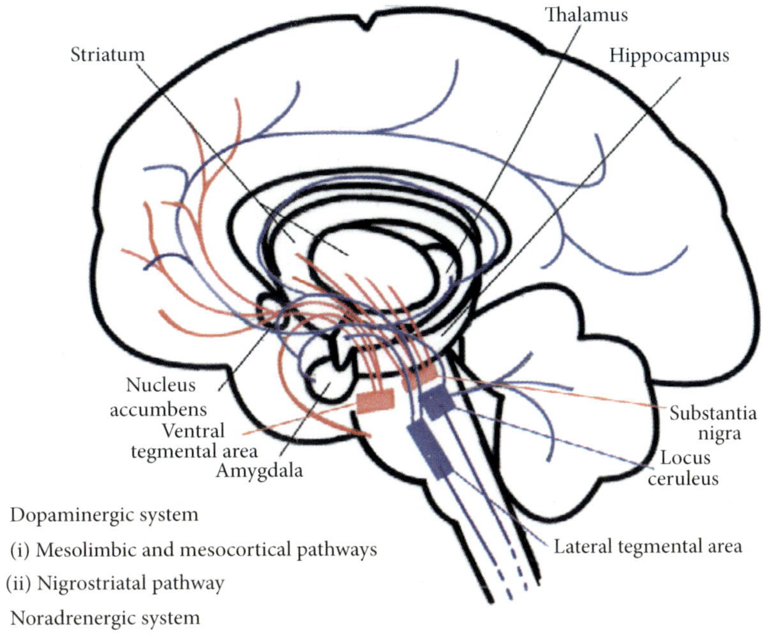

FIGURE 1: Dopaminergic and noradrenergic ascending pathways. This figure was drawn by the authors from information taken from texts and figures in literature [26–38].

has on the individual's life [53]. This is a new approach to pain in PD; although it may be too long to complete in routine clinical care, it will allow further in-depth testing in clinical trials for treatments of this specific aspect of PD.

3. The Pathophysiology of Pain in Parkinson's Disease

Motor symptoms in PD are mainly the result of degeneration of dopaminergic neurons in the substantia nigra pars compacta, affecting the nigrostriatal pathway and reducing stimulation of the motor cortex by the basal nuclei and thalamus (Figure 1). The pathological hallmark of the disease is the presence of Lewy bodies, which are spherical, eosinophilic, cytoplasmic inclusions in the degenerated neurons, containing mainly α-synuclein and ubiquitin. However, the changes are not restricted to this brain area and can be found in other nuclei of the brainstem and cortex and even peripheral neurons, such as those in the myenteric plexus [68]. Analysis of the distribution of these pathological markers in PD by Braak et al. [68] allowed the understanding of both motor and NMS of the disease through a logical six-stage ascending progression in a caudorostral direction. According to this hypothesis, the degenerative process starts in the caudal regions of the brainstem, such as the dorsal motor nuclei of the glossopharyngeal and vagus nerves and the anterior olfactory nucleus, passing through the locus coeruleus and Meynert's basal nucleus, the dorsal raphe nuclei, amygdalae, and hypothalamus and progressing through practically the whole cerebral cortex [68–70]. Motor symptoms are apparent in stage 3, after the mesencephalon has been affected. Prior to this stage, degeneration of the dorsal motor nucleus of the vagus (stage 1) can help to explain certain autonomic complaints such as obstipation and hypotension, while serotoninergic and noradrenergic dysfunction of the raphe nuclei and locus coeruleus, respectively (stage 2), can explain part of the pain related symptoms that occur in early PD [26, 27]. The exact mechanism by which cell degeneration occurs has yet to be elucidated but is thought to involve a cascade of events including interaction between genetic and environmental factors, impaired protein processing, oxidative stress, mitochondrial dysfunction, excitotoxicity, abnormal immune regulation, and inflammatory responses [28].

The basal nuclei play a central role in modulation of various pathways and function as components of a series of parallel circuits related to the motor, limbic, and associative systems (Figure 1). Striatal neurons can respond to different sensory stimuli applied to various body parts [29]. Of the four main dopaminergic pathways, two produce most of the dopamine in the brain: the nigrostriatal pathway, which is directly involved in PD, and the mesolimbic pathway, which is related to the reward system and central modulation of pain. The latter connects the ventral tegmental area of the mesencephalon to subcortical structures, such as the nucleus accumbens, thalamus, and the amygdala. A third pathway, the mesocortical pathway, is related to the affective and motivational dimensions of pain perception and allows the ventral tegmental area to communicate with the prefrontal cortex and the anterior cingulate cortex [30]. Lesions of the ventral tegmental area can increase sensitivity to pain, while electrical stimulation of the same area can have an analgesic effect [31]. A study using positron emission tomography found increased activation in the insula, prefrontal cortex, and anterior cingulate cortex during the "off" period [32]. All of these are areas of the limbic system associated with the affective-motivational dimension of pain [33]. Because the dopaminergic pathways and pain processing network overlap, hypofunction of the striatal dopaminergic system could result in amplification of sensory stimuli, leading to spontaneous pain sensation when dopamine levels are low [29].

Although the involvement of dopamine in central modulation of pain is well established, its role in the transmission of nociceptive stimuli from the periphery to the brain remains debatable [24]. Various studies have investigated the relationship between the threshold for pain triggered by thermal or electrical stimuli and treatment with levodopa or DBS [34–37]. Generally, the pain threshold is lower when levodopa levels are lower and tends to return to normal after administration of levodopa or after DBS even without an associated motor improvement. In other words, pain in these patients cannot be explained merely as a consequence of motor symptoms, such as rigidity, tremor, and dystonia [24].

Conte et al. [67] suggest two mechanisms in addition to striatal hypofunction to explain the different findings of their studies: degeneration of noradrenergic and serotoninergic neurons in the locus coeruleus and raphe nuclei, respectively, which can be even more pronounced than in the substantia nigra [38] and a loss of nerve fibers and Meissner corpuscles in the epidermis [71]. Together with the locus coeruleus, the gigantocellular nucleus, and the nuclei of the bulbar raphe, the periaqueductal gray matter and the parabrachial nuclei play an important role in the modulation of spinal nociceptive transmission, for example, on inhibition of nociceptive stimuli coming from the dorsal horn neuron. A disturbance in this pain-inhibiting region could cause an increase in the sensation of pain [72]. Degeneration of peripheral nociceptors also occurs in other chronic pain syndromes, such as fibromyalgia [73, 74].

Its different clinical characteristics, variable relationship with motor symptoms, and variable response to dopaminergic drugs suggest that pain in PD has a complex mechanism that involves the peripheral nervous system, the generation and amplification of pain by motor symptoms, and dopaminergic neuronal degeneration in areas responsible for central mechanisms.

4. The Relation between Levodopa Treatment and Pain in Parkinson's Disease

Levodopa is the most widely used and effective medication in the treatment of motor signs of PD. However, when used over a number of years, virtually all typical patients will present with complications related to pharmacokinetic and pharmacodynamic characteristics. The best-known of these include motor fluctuations such as WO, in which the therapeutic effects of levodopa do not last as long as they previously did, and dyskinesias [75]. Although only recently recognized, nonmotor fluctuations occur in a similar fashion in nearly all patients and can be main determinants of disability and worse quality of life [76]. NMS can be divided into three categories: neuropsychiatric, autonomic, and sensory. While most of these manifest during "off" periods and WO, some, such as agitation, psychosis, diaphoresis, and pain, can manifest when levodopa levels are at a peak. In this situation, pain appears to be more related to involuntary movements (dyskinesias or dystonia) than to dopamine levels per se. Fluctuation of sensory symptoms can be due to failure of primary somatosensory mechanisms [77].

Pain can be one of the main complaints reported during WO and occurs in around 50% of patients [78–80]. Chronic pain (i.e., pain lasting more than three months) is reported by more than 70% of patients with WO, suggesting that WO is a risk factor for development of chronic pain (unpublished personal data). Abdominal pain that does not respond to the use of analgesics and can only be alleviated with a new dose of levodopa can be considered a sign of WO [81, 82]. Pain that occurs only during WO can be considered of central origin, while if it is exacerbated during this period, it can be central, musculoskeletal, dystonic, or neuropathic/radicular [83].

The clinical characteristics of pain during WO and "off" periods are not well established. To our knowledge, only two studies in the literature analyzed pain during "off" periods and were only partial analyses [18, 50]. A recent study (unpublished personal data) using the McGill Pain Questionnaire found that patients with pain during WO had a higher score for the affective-motivational dimension. In the DoPaMiP study, the group with pain related to PD also had a higher score in this dimension than the pain unrelated to PD group [9]. This finding may be related to the hypothesis of dopaminergic dysfunction in the mesocorticolimbic pathway, which is associated with the affective/motivational dimension of pain [84]. In other words, degeneration of dopaminergic neurons in the ventral tegmental area may reduce pain thresholds and simultaneously activate structures in the limbic system associated with the unpleasant perception of pain.

5. Final Considerations

In recent years, NMS of PD have received increasing attention from physicians and researchers. Pain is present in the preclinical and initial stages of the disease and causes major impact on quality of life. Its clinical characteristics vary and can be associated with "off" periods or WO of levodopa. Although pain in PD is widespread and disabling, its clinical characteristics and pathophysiology and even the best way of classifying and treating it have yet to be defined. Further studies are required to clarify these points and elucidate the role of dopaminergic and nondopaminergic pathways in nociception, central modulation of pain, and the affective/motivational dimensions of pain perception.

References

[1] C. Pont-Sunyer, A. Hotter, C. Gaig et al., "The onset of nonmotor symptoms in parkinson's disease (the ONSET PD study)," *Movement Disorders*, vol. 30, no. 2, pp. 229–237, 2015.

[2] P. Barone, A. Antonini, C. Colosimo et al., "The PRIAMO study: a multicenter assessment of nonmotor symptoms and

their impact on quality of life in Parkinson's disease," *Movement Disorders*, vol. 24, no. 11, pp. 1641–1649, 2009.

[3] F. Baig, M. Lawton, M. Rolinski et al., "Delineating nonmotor symptoms in early Parkinson's disease and first-degree relatives," *Movement Disorders*, vol. 30, no. 13, pp. 1759–1766, 2015.

[4] A. Schrag, "Quality of life and depression in Parkinson's disease," *Journal of the Neurological Sciences*, vol. 248, no. 1-2, pp. 151–157, 2006.

[5] P. Valkovic, M. Minar, H. Singliarova et al., "Pain in Parkinson's disease: a cross-sectional study of its prevalence, types, and relationship to depression and quality of life," *PLoS ONE*, vol. 10, no. 8, Article ID e0136541, 2015.

[6] P. J. Garcia-Ruiz, K. R. Chaudhuri, and P. Martinez-Martin, "Non-motor symptoms of Parkinson's disease: a review...from the past," *Journal of the Neurological Sciences*, vol. 338, no. 1-2, pp. 30–33, 2014.

[7] A. G. Beiske, J. H. Loge, A. Rønningen, and E. Svensson, "Pain in Parkinson's disease: prevalence and characteristics," *Pain*, vol. 141, no. 1-2, pp. 173–177, 2009.

[8] G. Defazio, A. Berardelli, G. Fabbrini et al., "Pain as a nonmotor symptom of Parkinson disease: evidence from a case-control study," *Archives of Neurology*, vol. 65, no. 9, pp. 1191–1194, 2008.

[9] L. Nègre-Pagès, W. Regragui, D. Bouhassira, H. Grandjean, and O. Rascol, "Chronic pain in Parkinson's disease: the cross-sectional French DoPaMiP survey," *Movement Disorders*, vol. 23, no. 10, pp. 1361–1369, 2008.

[10] C.-H. Lin, R.-M. Wu, H.-Y. Chang, Y.-T. Chiang, and H.-H. Lin, "Preceding pain symptoms and Parkinson's disease: a nationwide population-based cohort study," *European Journal of Neurology*, vol. 20, no. 10, pp. 1398–1404, 2013.

[11] Y. E. Kim and B. S. Jeon, "Musculoskeletal problems in Parkinson's disease," *Journal of Neural Transmission*, vol. 120, no. 4, pp. 537–542, 2013.

[12] M. Politis, K. Wu, S. Molloy, P. G. Bain, K. R. Chaudhuri, and P. Piccini, "Parkinson's disease symptoms: the patient's perspective," *Movement Disorders*, vol. 25, no. 11, pp. 1646–1651, 2010.

[13] K. R. Chaudhuri, C. Prieto-Jurcynska, Y. Naidu et al., "The nondeclaration of nonmotor symptoms of Parkinson's disease to health care professionals: an international study using the nonmotor symptoms questionnaire," *Movement Disorders*, vol. 25, no. 6, pp. 704–709, 2010.

[14] A. Q. Rana, A. Kabir, M. Jesudasan, I. Siddiqui, and S. Khondker, "Pain in Parkinson's disease: analysis and literature review," *Clinical Neurology and Neurosurgery*, vol. 115, no. 11, pp. 2313–2317, 2013.

[15] C. G. Goetz, C. M. Tanner, M. Levy, R. S. Wilson, and D. C. Garron, "Pain in Parkinson's disease," *Movement Disorders*, vol. 1, no. 1, pp. 45–49, 1986.

[16] M. Tinazzi, C. Del Vesco, E. Fincati et al., "Pain and motor complications in Parkinson's disease," *Journal of Neurology, Neurosurgery and Psychiatry*, vol. 77, no. 7, pp. 822–825, 2006.

[17] H. A. Hanagasi, S. Akat, H. Gurvit, J. Yazici, and M. Emre, "Pain is common in Parkinson's disease," *Clinical Neurology and Neurosurgery*, vol. 113, no. 1, pp. 11–13, 2011.

[18] G. H. Letro, E. M. A. B. Quagliato, and M. A. Viana, *Pain in Parkinson's Disease*, vol. 67 of *Arquivos de Neuro-Psiquiatria*, 590, 585, 2009.

[19] M. A. Lee, R. W. Walker, T. J. Hildreth, and W. M. Prentice, "A survey of pain in idiopathic Parkinson's disease," *Journal of Pain and Symptom Management*, vol. 32, no. 5, pp. 462–469, 2006.

[20] A. Q. Rana, U. Saeed, M. S. Masroor, M. S. Yousuf, and I. Siddiqui, "A cross-sectional study investigating clinical predictors and physical experiences of pain in Parkinson's disease," *Functional Neurology*, vol. 28, no. 4, pp. 297–304, 2014.

[21] X.-J. Lin, N. Yu, X.-G. Lin et al., "A clinical survey of pain in Parkinson's disease in Eastern China," *International Psychogeriatrics*, vol. 28, no. 2, pp. 283–289, 2016.

[22] A. D. Ha and J. Jankovic, "Pain in Parkinson's disease," *Movement Disorders*, vol. 27, no. 4, pp. 485–491, 2012.

[23] N. E. Allen, C. M. Wong, C. G. Canning, and N. Moloney, "The Association between Parkinson's disease motor impairments and pain," *Pain Medicine*, 2015.

[24] R. G. Cury, R. Galhardoni, E. T. Fonoff et al., "Sensory abnormalities and pain in Parkinson disease and its modulation by treatment of motor symptoms," *European Journal of Pain*, vol. 20, no. 2, pp. 151–165, 2016.

[25] G. Wasner and G. Deuschl, "Pains in Parkinson disease—many syndromes under one umbrella," *Nature Reviews Neurology*, vol. 8, no. 5, pp. 284–294, 2012.

[26] H. Braak, K. Del Tredici, U. Rüb, R. A. I. de Vos, E. N. H. J. Steur, and E. Braak, "Staging of brain pathology related to sporadic Parkinson's disease," *Neurobiology of Aging*, vol. 24, no. 2, pp. 197–211, 2003.

[27] O.-B. Tysnes, B. Müller, and J. P. Larsen, "Are dysautonomic and sensory symptoms present in early Parkinson's disease?" *Acta Neurologica Scandinavica*, vol. 122, supplement 190, pp. 72–77, 2010.

[28] D. T. Dextera and P. Jenner, "Parkinson disease: from pathology to molecular disease mechanisms," *Free Radical Biology and Medicine*, vol. 62, pp. 132–144, 2013.

[29] C. Juri, M. Rodriguez-Oroz, and J. A. Obeso, "The pathophysiological basis of sensory disturbances in Parkinson's disease," *Journal of the Neurological Sciences*, vol. 289, no. 1-2, pp. 60–65, 2010.

[30] J. A. Obeso, C. Marin, C. Rodriguez-Oroz et al., "The basal ganglia in Parkinson's disease: current concepts and unexplained observations," *Annals of Neurology*, vol. 64, supplement 2, pp. S30–S46, 2008.

[31] F. Sotres-Bayón, E. Torres-López, A. López-Ávila, R. del Ángel, and F. Pellicer, "Lesion and electrical stimulation of the ventral tegmental area modify persistent nociceptive behavior in the rat," *Brain Research*, vol. 898, no. 2, pp. 342–349, 2001.

[32] C. Brefel-Courbon, P. Payoux, C. Thalamas et al., "Effects of levodopa on pain threshold in Parkinson's disease: a clinical and positron emission tomography study," *Movement Disorders*, vol. 20, no. 12, pp. 1557–1563, 2005.

[33] S. Potvin, S. Grignon, and S. Marchand, "Human evidence of a supra-spinal modulating role of dopamine on pain perception," *Synapse*, vol. 63, no. 5, pp. 390–402, 2009.

[34] R. Djaldetti, A. Shifrin, Z. Rogowski, E. Sprecher, E. Melamed, and D. Yarnitsky, "Quantitative measurement of pain sensation in patients with Parkinson disease," *Neurology*, vol. 62, no. 12, pp. 2171–2175, 2004.

[35] R. Nandhagopal, A. R. Troiano, E. Mak, M. Schulzer, M. C. Bushnell, and A. J. Stoessl, "Response to heat pain stimulation in idiopathic Parkinson's disease," *Pain Medicine*, vol. 11, no. 6, pp. 834–840, 2010.

[36] S.-Y. Lim, M. J. Farrell, S. J. Gibson, R. D. Helme, A. E. Lang, and A. H. Evans, "Do dyskinesia and pain share common pathophysiological mechanisms in Parkinson's disease?" *Movement Disorders*, vol. 23, no. 12, pp. 1689–1695, 2008.

[37] P. Schestatsky, H. Kumru, J. Valls-Solé et al., "Neurophysiologic study of central pain in patients with Parkinson disease," *Neurology*, vol. 69, no. 23, pp. 2162–2169, 2007.

[38] C. Zarow, S. A. Lyness, J. A. Mortimer, and H. C. Chui, "Neuronal loss is greater in the locus coeruleus than nucleus basalis and substantia nigra in Alzheimer and Parkinson diseases," *Archives of Neurology*, vol. 60, no. 3, pp. 337–341, 2003.

[39] A. L. J. Burke, J. L. Mathias, and L. A. Denson, "Psychological functioning of people living with chronic pain: a meta-analytic review," *British Journal of Clinical Psychology*, vol. 54, no. 3, pp. 345–360, 2015.

[40] A. Fil, R. Cano-de-la-Cuerda, E. Muñoz-Hellín, L. Vela, M. Ramiro-González, and C. Fernández-de-las-Peñas, "Pain in Parkinson disease: a review of the literature," *Parkinsonism and Related Disorders*, vol. 19, no. 3, pp. 285–294, 2013.

[41] U. Ehrt, J. P. Larsen, and D. Aarsland, "Pain and its relationship to depression in Parkinson disease," *The American Journal of Geriatric Psychiatry*, vol. 17, no. 4, pp. 269–275, 2009.

[42] G. Defazio, A. Gigante, P. Mancino, and M. Tinazzi, "The epidemiology of pain in Parkinson's disease," *Journal of Neural Transmission*, vol. 120, no. 4, pp. 583–586, 2013.

[43] L.-M. Zhang, Y.-Q. Chen, W.-J. Li, W. Sun, Y. Huang, and H.-Q. Zou, "Association between mutations of SCN9A gene and pain related to Parkinsonism," *Zhonghua Yi Xue Yi Chuan Xue Za Zhi*, vol. 30, no. 1, pp. 17–20, 2013.

[44] L. Greenbaum, I. Tegeder, Y. Barhum, E. Melamed, Y. Roditi, and R. Djaldetti, "Contribution of genetic variants to pain susceptibility in Parkinson disease," *European Journal of Pain*, vol. 16, no. 9, pp. 1243–1250, 2012.

[45] J. H. Roh, B.-J. Kim, J.-H. Jang et al., "The relationship of pain and health-related quality of life in Korean patients with Parkinson's disease," *Acta Neurologica Scandinavica*, vol. 119, no. 6, pp. 397–403, 2009.

[46] Ö. Skogar, P.-A. Fall, G. Hallgren et al., "Parkinson's disease patients' subjective descriptions of characteristics of chronic pain, sleeping patterns and health-related quality of life," *Neuropsychiatric Disease and Treatment*, vol. 8, pp. 435–442, 2012.

[47] M. D. G. W. de Sales Coriolano, J. M. de Siqueira Balbino, B. R. V. da Silva et al., "Pain characterization in patients with Parkinson's disease," *Revista Dor*, vol. 15, no. 2, pp. 78–82, 2014.

[48] IASP Task Force on Taxonomy, *Classification of Chronic Pain*, IASP Pain Terminology, IASP Press, Seattle, Wash, USA, 2nd edition, 2012, Edited by H. Merskey and N. Bogduk.

[49] R. Melzack, "The McGill pain questionnaire: major properties and scoring methods," *Pain*, vol. 1, no. 3, pp. 277–299, 1975.

[50] A. Nebe and G. Ebersbach, "Pain intensity on and off Levodopa in patients with Parkinson's disease," *Movement Disorders*, vol. 24, no. 8, pp. 1233–1237, 2009.

[51] C. A. Pimenta and M. J. Teixeira, "Questionário de dor McGill: proposta de adaptação para a língua Portuguesa," *Revista da Escola de Enfermagem da USP*, vol. 30, no. 3, pp. 473–483, 1996.

[52] B. Ford, "Pain in Parkinson's disease," *Clinical Neuroscience*, vol. 5, no. 2, pp. 63–72, 1998.

[53] K. R. Chaudhuri, A. Rizos, C. Trenkwalder et al., "King's Parkinson's disease pain scale, the first scale for pain in PD: an international validation," *Movement Disorders*, vol. 30, no. 12, pp. 1623–1631, 2015.

[54] V. Mylius, D. Ciampi de Andrade, R. G. Cury et al., "Pain in Parkinson's disease: current concepts and a new diagnostic algorithm," *Movement Disorders-Clinical Practice*, vol. 2, no. 4, pp. 357–364, 2015.

[55] N. P. Quinn, W. C. Koller, A. E. Lang, and C. D. Marsden, "Painful Parkinson's disease," *The Lancet*, vol. 1, no. 8494, pp. 1366–1369, 1986.

[56] B. Ford, "Pain in Parkinson's disease," *Movement Disorders*, vol. 25, supplement 1, pp. S98–S103, 2010.

[57] C. H. F. Camargo and H. A. G. Teive, "Evolução do conceito de distonia," *Arquivos de Neuro-Psiquiatria*, vol. 72, no. 7, pp. 559–561, 2014.

[58] C. Cordivari, V. P. Misra, S. Catania, and A. J. Less, "Treatment of dystonic clenched fist with botulinum toxin," *Movement Disorders*, vol. 16, no. 5, pp. 907–913, 2001.

[59] R. G. Cury, R. Galhardoni, E. T. Fonoff et al., "Effects of deep brain stimulation on pain and other nonmotor symptoms in Parkinson disease," *Neurology*, vol. 83, no. 16, pp. 1403–1409, 2014.

[60] A. Marques, O. Chassin, D. Morand et al., "Central pain modulation after subthalamic nucleus stimulation: a crossover randomized trial," *Neurology*, vol. 81, no. 7, pp. 633–640, 2013.

[61] G. Serratrice and B. Michel, "Pain in Parkinson's disease patients," *Revue du Rhumatisme English Edition*, vol. 66, no. 6, pp. 331–338, 1999.

[62] N. Attal, G. Cruccu, R. Baron et al., "EFNS guidelines on the pharmacological treatment of neuropathic pain: 2010 revision," *European Journal of Neurology*, vol. 17, no. 9, pp. 1113–1123, 2010.

[63] B. Ford, E. D. Louis, P. Greene, and S. Fahn, "Oral and genital pain syndromes in Parkinson's disease," *Movement Disorders*, vol. 11, no. 4, pp. 421–426, 1996.

[64] F. Javoy-Agid and Y. Agid, "Is the mesocortical dopaminergic system involved in parkinson disease?" *Neurology*, vol. 30, no. 12, pp. 1326–1330, 1980.

[65] A. Q. Rana, I. Siddiqui, A. Mosabbir et al., "Association of pain, Parkinson's disease, and restless legs syndrome," *Journal of the Neurological Sciences*, vol. 327, no. 1-2, pp. 32–34, 2013.

[66] G. Defazio, M. Tinazzi, and A. Berardelli, "How pain arises in Parkinson's disease?" *European Journal of Neurology*, vol. 20, no. 12, pp. 1517–1523, 2013.

[67] A. Conte, N. Khan, G. Defazio, J. C. Rothwell, and A. Berardelli, "Pathophysiology of somatosensory abnormalities in Parkinson disease," *Nature Reviews Neurology*, vol. 9, no. 12, pp. 687–697, 2013.

[68] H. Braak, K. Del Tredici, H. Bratzke, J. Hamm-Clement, D. Sandmann-Keil, and U. Rüb, "Staging of the intracerebral inclusion body pathology associated with idiopathic Parkinson's disease (preclinical and clinical stages)," *Journal of Neurology*, supplement 3, pp. III/1–III/5, 2002.

[69] L. V. Kalia and A. E. Lang, "Parkinson's disease," *The Lancet*, vol. 386, no. 9996, pp. 896–912, 2015.

[70] R. P. Munhoz, A. Moro, L. Silveira-Moriyama, and H. A. Teive, "Non-motor signs in Parkinson's disease: a review," *Arquivos de Neuro-Psiquiatria*, vol. 73, no. 5, pp. 454–462, 2015.

[71] M. Nolano, V. Provitera, A. Estraneo et al., "Sensory deficit in Parkinson's disease: evidence of a cutaneous denervation," *Brain*, vol. 131, no. 7, pp. 1903–1911, 2008.

[72] E. Scherder, E. Wolters, C. Polman, J. Sergeant, and D. Swaab, "Pain in Parkinson's disease and multiple sclerosis: its relation to the medial and lateral pain systems," *Neuroscience and Biobehavioral Reviews*, vol. 29, no. 7, pp. 1047–1056, 2005.

[73] A. L. Oaklander, Z. D. Herzog, H. M. Downs, and M. M. Klein, "Objective evidence that small-fiber polyneuropathy underlies some illnesses currently labeled as fibromyalgia," *Pain*, vol. 154, no. 11, pp. 2310–2316, 2013.

[74] N. Üçeyler, D. Zeller, A.-K. Kahn et al., "Small fibre pathology in patients with fibromyalgia syndrome," *Brain*, vol. 136, no. 6, pp. 1857–1867, 2013.

[75] F. Cardoso, "Fisiopatologia de flutuações e discinesias induzidas por levodopa em doença de Parkinson," in *Doença de Parkinson: Estratégias Atuais de Tratamento*, L. A. F. Andrade, E. R. Barbosa, F. Cardoso, and H. A. G. Teive, Eds., pp. 105–123, Omnifarma, São Paulo, Brazil, 4th edition, 2014.

[76] T. Witjas, E. Kaphan, J. P. Azulay et al., "Nonmotor fluctuations in Parkinson's disease: frequent and disabling," *Neurology*, vol. 59, no. 3, pp. 408–413, 2002.

[77] C. C. Aquino and S. H. Fox, "Clinical spectrum of levodopa-induced complications," *Movement Disorders*, vol. 30, no. 1, pp. 80–89, 2015.

[78] S.-M. Cheon, M. J. Park, W.-J. Kim, and J. W. Kim, "Non-motor off symptoms in Parkinson's disease," *Journal of Korean Medical Science*, vol. 24, no. 2, pp. 311–314, 2009.

[79] A. Rizos, P. Martinez-Martin, P. Odin et al., "Characterizing motor and non-motor aspects of early-morning off periods in Parkinson's disease: an international multicenter study," *Parkinsonism and Related Disorders*, vol. 20, no. 11, pp. 1231–1235, 2014.

[80] M. Seki, K. Takahashi, D. Uematsu et al., "Clinical features and varieties of non-motor fluctuations in Parkinson's disease: a Japanese multicenter study," *Parkinsonism and Related Disorders*, vol. 19, no. 1, pp. 104–108, 2013.

[81] A. Kulakowska, R. Pogorzelski, H. Borowik, and W. Drozdowski, "Wearing off phenomenon presenting with features of paroxysmal abdominal pain," *Neurologia i Neurochirurgia Polska*, vol. 37, supplement 5, pp. 197–202, 2003.

[82] A. Q. Rana and J. Depradine, "Abdominal pain: a symptom of levodopa end of dose wearing off in Parkinson's disease," *West Indian Medical Journal*, vol. 60, no. 2, pp. 223–224, 2011.

[83] A. Storch, C. B. Schneider, M. Wolz et al., "Nonmotor fluctuations in Parkinson disease: severity and correlation with motor complications," *Neurology*, vol. 80, no. 9, pp. 800–809, 2013.

[84] J. M. Jarcho, E. A. Mayer, Z. K. Jiang, N. A. Feier, and E. D. London, "Pain, affective symptoms, and cognitive deficits in patients with cerebral dopamine dysfunction," *Pain*, vol. 153, no. 4, pp. 744–754, 2012.

10

The Impact of Living with Parkinson's Disease: Balancing within a Web of Needs and Demands

Catharina Sjödahl Hammarlund,[1,2] Albert Westergren,[1,3] Ingrid Åström,[1] Anna-Karin Edberg,[3] and Peter Hagell[1]

[1]*The PRO-CARE Group, Faculty of Health Science, Kristianstad University, Kristianstad, Sweden*
[2]*Department of Health Sciences, Lund University, Lund, Sweden*
[3]*The Research Platform for Collaboration for Health, Faculty of Health Science, Kristianstad University, Kristianstad, Sweden*

Correspondence should be addressed to Catharina Sjödahl Hammarlund; catharina.sjodahl_hammarlund@med.lu.se

Academic Editor: Hélio Teive

This study explores the impact of living with Parkinson's disease (PD). Nineteen persons (11 women) aged 55–84 diagnosed with PD 3–27 years ago participated. Data were collected through semistructured interviews, which were recorded, transcribed verbatim, and analysed by qualitative content analysis. Four categories represented the impact of living with PD: "Changed prerequisites for managing day-to-day demands," "Loss of identity and dignity," "Compromised social participation," and "The use of practical and psychological strategies." There was a shift from an internal to an external locus of control in managing, control, competence, relatedness, and autonomy. According to self-determination theory, a shift towards extrinsically motivated behaviours may occur when these basic needs are thwarted, leading to compensatory strategies or needs substitutes with negative consequences on health and well-being. We suggest a needs-based approach as an important starting point to better understand the consequences of living with PD and to explore the means for people with PD to acquire an improved quality of life on their own terms. In conclusion, our findings suggest for a shift in focus, from a biomedical to a needs-based approach to understand the impact of living with PD and facilitate more person-centred care and person-centred outcome measurement.

1. Introduction

Parkinson's disease (PD) is a progressive, neurological disease involving motor (e.g., bradykinesia, tremor, rigidity, and postural impairment) and nonmotor (e.g., depression, anxiety, sleep disorders, fatigue, dysautonomia, and pain) symptoms [1, 2]. Its symptom profile and progression differ between individuals. The core pathology believed to cause the main motor symptoms is a striatal dopamine deficit due to progressive loss of nigrostriatal dopaminergic neurons [2]. Symptomatic dopaminergic therapy is initially successful, but a fluctuating drug response and dyskinesias often develop after some years. With the occurrence and progression of both motor and nonmotor symptoms, often in complex and fluctuating patterns [1, 3], the disease is typically perceived as unpredictable and difficult to control [4].

An increasing number of studies have considered the consequences of PD characterized symptomatic profiles, relationships among symptoms, and the impact of various features of the disease from the perspective of persons living with PD [5–7]. Previous studies have reported how persons with PD (PwPD) experience various disease aspects, such as loss of motor control, walking difficulties, environmental influences, cognitive and executive dysfunctions, emotional reactions, sleep disorders, difficulties in managing activities of daily living, neuropsychiatric reactions, social withdrawal and isolation, communication difficulties, and loss of physical and psychosocial competence [8–13]. Collectively, these and other studies have provided important insights into several aspects of PD. However, available studies have typically focused on relatively specific aspects of the disease (e.g., communication, fatigue, and walking) or subgroups of PwPD, such as women and middle-aged or older people

[14–17]. Few qualitative studies have attempted to capture the overall impact of PD on daily life, and available studies [18, 19] stem from the era before the introduction of, for example, modern dopamine agonists and enzyme inhibitors [20]. To the best of our knowledge, there are no studies that take a holistic approach when describing the consequences of living with PD. The aim of this study was therefore to explore the overall impact of living with PD.

2. Materials and Methods

2.1. Participants and Recruitment. Thirty consecutive Swedish-speaking people with clinically diagnosed PD from a Swedish movement disorder clinic were selected by purposeful sampling and invited to participate [21]. Specifically, we aimed to achieve variations regarding age, gender, disease duration, and PD severity. Exclusion criteria were ongoing psychiatric side effects from medication and clinically significant comorbidities that could compromise the ability to participate (e.g., dementia), as determined by a specialized PD nurse. Nineteen persons, 11 women and 8 men aged 55–84 (median: 66 years, q1–q3: 61–73 years), were able to participate and provided signed informed consent. They were diagnosed with PD since 3–27 years (median: 11 years, q1–q3: 7–14 years). Disease severity ranged from mild bilateral disease (Hoehn & Yahr stage II) to severe PD with inability to stand or walk unless aided (Hoehn & Yahr stage V) [22]. All participants were treated with levodopa, and additional antiparkinsonian therapy consisted of oral dopamine agonists (pramipexole and ropinirole), COMT inhibitors (entacapone and tolcapone), amantadine, subcutaneous apomorphine infusion, and deep brain stimulation. The study was conducted in accordance with the Declaration of Helsinki and was approved by the local research ethics committee.

2.2. Data Collection. Data were collected by means of face-to-face semistructured interviews, which were recorded and transcribed verbatim. The interviews lasted for 60 to 90 minutes and followed a preprepared interview guide. All interviews were conducted face to face in privacy, without the involvement of caregivers/family members. The interviewer started each interview with the phrase: "We are interested in learning more about how you have experienced the consequences of Parkinson's disease, now and in the past. Could you please tell me how you first noticed the disease?," followed by "Can you describe how the disease has influenced your daily life?." The interview guide consisted of a checklist of areas that might potentially add to the understanding of the consequences of PD. The areas were: at home, at work, in personal relationships and social life, cognitive ability, personal care, leisure activities, sleep, and rest. If not covered spontaneously by the respondent, these areas were explored by open-ended questions. When needed, prompts were used to encourage respondents to explore and expand statements in greater depth.

2.3. Data Analysis. Following verbatim interview transcription, data were analysed as described by Graneheim and Lundman [23] and Patton [21], according to the following steps: (1) All interviews were read separately several times in order to get an understanding of the essence of each interview and to identify primary patterns in the data. (2) Meaning units were identified and (3) coded with regard to the content. (4) Clusters of aspects that emerged in the coded data were organised in subcategories. (5) Subcategories were sorted by their conceptual representation, ending up in four main categories, representing a more abstract level of understanding. To assist and organise the analysis, the OpenCode 4.0 software for qualitative analysis was used. OpenCode 4.0 is a software for coding and categorising qualitative interview or observational data. The program was originally developed for grounded theory and qualitative content analysis, but can be used with most qualitative methods [24].

Table 1: The impact of living with Parkinson's disease.

Categories	Subcategories
Changed prerequisites for managing day-to-day demands	*Deteriorating physical functioning* *Fatigue* *Psychological changes and mood swings* *Cognitive impairments*
Loss of identity and dignity	*Altered family relationships* *A sense of lost identity* *A sense of being deprived of one's self-worth*
Compromised social participation	*Limited ability to meet with others* *Feeling socially isolated* *Social embarrassments* *Speech problems*
The use of practical and psychological strategies	*To be foreseeing and plan* *Various compensatory strategies were applied* *Trying to maintain a positive attitude* *Using downward comparisons* *Accepting healthcare support*

3. Results

The impact of living with PD can be understood as "Changed prerequisites for managing day-to-day demands," "Loss of identity and dignity," "Compromised social participation," and "The use of practical and psychological strategies" with internal variations seen as subcategories (Table 1).

3.1. Changed Prerequisites for Managing Day-to-Day Demands. The participants described how prerequisites for managing day-to-day demands had changed due to deteriorating physical, psychological, and cognitive functioning. This change affected most activities, which became difficult to manage, as some perceived their abilities to be severely affected or completely lost. The changed prerequisites concerned deteriorating physical functioning, fatigue, psychological changes, and mood swings as well as cognitive impairments.

Deteriorating physical functioning was evident in that the participants described that they had become slower no matter what they were doing and that everything took more time. Walking was more difficult because they felt stiff and it was increasingly hard to move the legs and feet. Walking pace had slowed down and keeping balance was more difficult. Fear of falling was common, and many had experienced several falls. They described that they sometimes suddenly could not move at all and felt like a statue, and there was nothing they could do about it.

> *I couldn't walk any further than maybe out of the house and into the garden . . . then I found myself in a world that was totally my own . . . . I became completely stiff . . . my wife shouted at me that "you have to move", but I was completely stuck* . . . . (Participant 8)

Other physical changes included painful cramps and pain in general. In combination with deteriorating fine motor abilities, daily activities (e.g., chores, shopping, getting dressed/undressed, and taking care of personal hygiene) became time-consuming, difficult to perform, and physically and psychologically challenging.

> *It takes time to do the buttons . . . . It's irritating sometimes. It takes a long time before you have finished dressing. . . .* (Participant 10)

The participants described *fatigue* as an overwhelming and general feeling of tiredness and loss of energy. A sense of feeling completely worn-out and unable to take action could appear suddenly and at any time. Most of the time nothing could be done to solve the situation except to go to bed. Fatigue was also described as being both physical and psychological.

> *I become so . . . utterly worn out. I can't hang my clothes. . . , put the dishes away. I can barely find the strength to go to the bathroom, or brush my teeth, because nothing works, you see. I just get slow, indifferent . . . . I don't care about anything but to go to bed . . . and just lie down. . . .* (Participant 1)

Psychological changes and mood swings were typically perceived as being related to physical deterioration and were described as difficult to control, for example, a sense of panic and powerlessness. Participants worried about the future and about what would happen when they could no longer care for themselves. Thoughts like these brought about anxiety and fear. Some felt depressed and downhearted most of the day, sad at being disabled, alone, and unable to do what they wanted to do. These thoughts could become destructive and murky, and some had feelings of wanting to die; what was the point of staying alive when life itself offered so little?

> *. . . maybe . . . . I need help to look back on my life . . . Well to . . . to be able to see the meaning of life . . . to shed some light over this darkness . . . . To go on living or not . . . there are . . . there are days when I feel that everything is really bad and . . . there is no point in anything . . . .* (Participant 15)

Participants described how *cognitive impairments* were manifested, for example, problems in remembering and concentrating. Those who used to read a lot found it difficult to remember what they just read and to understand the context. Communicating with others was difficult as names were often forgotten, and what to say and finding the right words became even worse when they were nervous. It became difficult to do things that they used to do, for example, cooking or carpentry as the ability to count and measure was compromised. They described problems organising and keeping papers and other things in order; it felt like the brain was in a state of chaos.

> *It's just like I . . . . I become indifferent . . . to some things. Very hard to keep things in order . . .* [laughs]. *I move things from one place to the other and I think that I have put everything right and then everything is . . . . There's some . . . there's some disorder . . . some chaos in the brain. . . .* (Participant 1)

3.2. Loss of Identity and Dignity. As the disease progressed, dependency on help with practical matters increased and family relationships changed. Participants expressed bitterness and shame of the person they had become and tried to conceal the disease. They noticed that the physical and mental changes affected their self-esteem, as well as how they were perceived by others. They felt humiliated and less confident when judged by others. Loss of identity and dignity altered family relationships, gave a sense of lost identity, and a sense of being worthless.

Altered family relationships involved affected the bond between husband and wife. Some described that their partner was afraid of future demands and responsibilities and was away more often. As the illness progressed, some families decided to redistribute household and family responsibilities. They found it difficult to ask for help as they wanted their families to treat them as they used to, without showing any special considerations. Participants became more dependent on practical help from their family members, for example, cooking and other chores, but also their personal hygiene and getting dressed, as well as concerns regarding their personal safety.

> *Well, I think that it feels very bad . . . needing to ask for help . . . to get dressed . . . and again when I want to go to bed . . . and at the same time one becomes really frightened . . . if I was alone in the house, what was I supposed to do . . . and imagining things like . . . . There is nobody here, what if I were to fall . . . .* (Participant 8)

A sense of lost identity was described by all participants. Although they felt that deep inside they were still the same person, they were also aware that they were physically changing. The posture became more stooped, their faces looked more tired, and they were not as fast and skilled as they once were. They could have held positions in management and family responsibilities, a person that others would seek advice from and see up to. Now, they had to give up doing things or taking responsibilities, both at home and at work. They found themselves being dependent on others. This made them feel belittled, insecure, and less confident, as if they no longer belonged to this world. They felt themselves to be a professional and a personal failure, something that deprived them of their self-image and identity.

> *...well, then you become sort of powerless...and indecisive.... You can't decide...you can't make up your mind....* (Participant 5)

A sense of being deprived of one's self-worth could appear when meeting with others. It made them feel uncomfortable and resented if they felt that someone pitied and felt sorry for them. They wanted to be treated as a valid citizen although they had PD, just like they had been treated before the diagnosis. Some also worried that they would be taken for an alcoholic due to physical symptoms such as balance problems and tremor. They noticed that people sometimes stared or looked at them in an odd way, and they also felt exposed to naive and hurtful comments.

> *Although I have Parkinson's disease, I want to be respected. I want to be able to do...take care of things like I always did in the past and I want to take an active part in society...hmmm...and I don't want to be looked down upon in any way...I want to be accepted even though I do have Parkinson's.* (Participant 15)

3.3. Compromised Social Participation. The prerequisites for taking part in social activities had changed and affected all aspects of their social life. They felt increasingly socially isolated, which in part was due to feeling embarrassed of their changed persona. In addition, some had speech problems, which made communicating difficult. Compromised social participation had to do with limited ability to meet with others, feeling socially isolated, social embarrassment, and speech problems.

Limited ability to meet with others and decreased activities in daily life were common. Not being able to drive was problematic as it made it more difficult to get around. Using public transportation required planning and was regarded as inconvenient. Other activities that were affected were holding cards whilst playing bridge, outings in the countryside, riding, playing football, or going out dancing. It was also difficult to manage stairs, to go in and out of shops, do the shopping, and other daily activities.

> *And when one needs to go into shops, which rarely happens, it's not easy when there is a flight of stairs that has to be managed.* (Participant 10)

Feeling socially isolated and being alone was hard. Even if it sometimes was preferable to be alone, there was also a feeling of being avoided, even by close friends. Participants often wished something would happen to break the silence of their secluded life, for example, a phone call or a letter. Even if there was only a bill it was read thoroughly as a strategy to feel connected to the outer world.

> *...well, from the moment I have the letter in my hand, I open it and it...it...just by doing that, it's something that makes you feel more alive...because it's a moment that feels exciting.... What's inside the envelope, what does the letter say...and then you start reading it...and if it's a bill I start to take an interest to it...you make as much of it as possible...in order to...live on....* (Participant 9)

The participants described *social embarrassments* as their facial expressions and nonverbal communication were reduced. Involuntary movements were a problem, for example, when having dinner with family and friends. Glasses and cups could suddenly be knocked over, tremors made it difficult to use cutlery and handling food or drink. Eating was time-consuming, and they felt embarrassed by keeping others waiting. They felt bitter at having the disease, which made them try to hide their symptoms.

> *It was like...when I had customers...and they sort of...why do you walk so funny? And then I ...oh, it's just because one of my toes is hurting...or something like that...hmm...that's how I kept it hidden for...well...at least...certainly for ten years....* (Participant 8)

Speech problems were frustrating to the point where some stopped talking altogether, and others found it difficult to articulate. Being nervous or stressed tended to make it worse. These problems could make it impossible to speak on the phone, and consequently people stopped calling.

> *...they told my children...to tell me that...that...we...we...we...don't understand what he's saying so there is no point calling.... And I understand that.... I find it equally...equally embarrassing....* (Participant 9)

3.4. The Use of Practical and Psychological Strategies. The participants used different strategies to adapt to various situations. Trying to find practical solutions were most common, for example, seeking information, planning, and using aids. Other examples of strategies used to promote psychological well-being were to have a positive attitude or to compare one's own situation to that of others. Practical and psychological strategies used were to be able to foresee and plan, to compensate for lost functioning, trying to maintain a positive attitude, using downward comparisons, and accepting support from health care.

To be foreseeing and plan was necessary when managing everyday life. Most things took more time, and those with cognitive difficulties needed detailed planning, taking notes, and doing things step-by-step. Medication required a great deal of planning and most participants followed a schedule. Even though all precautions were taken, it was still uncertain if they would manage to go through with their plans due to the unpredictability of the disease. They felt embarrassed when they had to cancel at the last minute.

... I don't always make plans just for myself. Sometimes there are others involved and it feels really bad to always be the one who cancels ... for example if we're going to the movies or something.... (Participant 5)

Various compensatory strategies were applied to compensate for lost functioning, for example, doing chores sitting down instead of standing up or to avoid reaching for things. Several situations were avoided altogether to minimise the risk of falling and being injured, for example, to shower instead of taking a bath. Some also chose to pay for the services that they were unable to do, for example, cooking and cleaning.

Well, I ... eh ... I ... eh ... do the dishes, when I've finished eating ... for other chores like cleaning up, I've help from others ... hired help ... and my children they cook ... when they cook for themselves, they also cook for me and then they freeze the food and bring it to me. I can take care of my personal hygiene. I take a shower every morning, but ... eh ... to take a bath, which I used to love doing ... it's not possible anymore. I can't get out of the bathtub. (Participant 9)

Trying to maintain a positive attitude was used to feel psychologically better, for example, trying to be optimistic, not to worry, enjoying the moment, making the best of the situation, trying to live life as normally as possible, and pushing all thoughts of the future aside. PD could progress in so many ways that they found it best to settle for what little they had and make the most of every moment. Some described the importance of fighting back and not giving up. For example, thinking of children and grandchildren was also helpful in finding enough strength to keep on living.

I have to start from how it is ... and make the best of the situation ... and so far, that's worked. It's not really a disaster to be ill.... Because you become sort of ... you look at life differently and become more grateful.... (Participant 14)

The participants were *using downward comparisons*, comparing themselves with those worse off, for example, while attending support group meetings. This strategy was helpful in realising that they still functioned relatively well, given the circumstances. However, others described the opposite reaction as it could make them worried and anxious that they might end up in a similar situation.

Well, of course you compare yourself with others.... You make certain comparisons with ... well, if you are sitting down ... having a conversation with someone, you tell yourself ... well, the things that he's doing aren't something that I do ... you sort of compare yourself with that person ... and then you choose to look at the best parts of the situation, and I tell myself that I'm much better off than he is.... (Participant 8)

The participants also used self-deception, that is, convincing themselves that things were not as bad as they might seem. Regardless of the individual's specific strategy, it was about finding a way that worked, to adapt and try to accept the situation.

Accepting healthcare support was important in managing the situation, even if accessibility was an issue. They wished that it would be possible to have one person to turn to for support and felt that the time between scheduled clinic visits was too long.

So she [the physician] *really helps me, you know ... and I feel that she's very supportive ... like ... she's always happy and kind when I call her and ... never ... never sort of stressed and she listens to what you have to say and ... so .... I think that ... that's very positive....* (Participant 1)

To use various kinds of aids was important, such as alarm devices to remind them when to take their medicines or a special chair to use in the shower. To be able to manoeuvre a wheelchair with a remote control improved independence. Some also found the use of a cane to be supportive, whereas others could consider walking aids as stigmatizing. However, using some of these aids, for example, a walker could be difficult in bad weather, such as snow or if there were stairs.

4. Discussion

This study explored the overall impact of living with PD from the perspective of PwPD. The results showed that living with PD incorporated a complex web of changed prerequisites for managing day-to-day demands and social participation, which in turn contributed to a perceived loss of identity and dignity. Living with PD also involved developing practical and psychological strategies to cope with the situation. These results may be thought of as a delicate balance within a web of needs and demands.

Psychological symptoms and mood swings were intertwined with cognitive and physical problems, adding to the struggle of managing the demands of everyday life. The participants felt depressed, low-spirited, and were worried about the future. Some held dark and destructive thoughts and considered intentionally ending their lives. In a previous study, suicidal and death ideation was present among one-third of persons with PD [25]. Depression is one of the most common nonmotor symptoms in PD [1] and has considerable impact on health-related quality of life [5, 6]. The physical changes also affected appearance. To look different provoked a sense of vulnerability due to feeling judged and evaluated by strangers. Those who suffered from tremor or balance impairments could be thought of as being intoxicated or worse. In agreement with earlier studies [17, 26, 27], this was found embarrassing and made participants feel deprived of their self-worth and shameful as they could no longer live up to social norms.

The results can be interpreted as a shift from an internal towards an external locus of control, in order to manage their sense of lost control and unpredictability, as the disease progressed (Figure 1). According to self-determination theory (SDT) [28, 29], this shift and the described distress and helplessness may be the result of thwarted basic needs. SDT

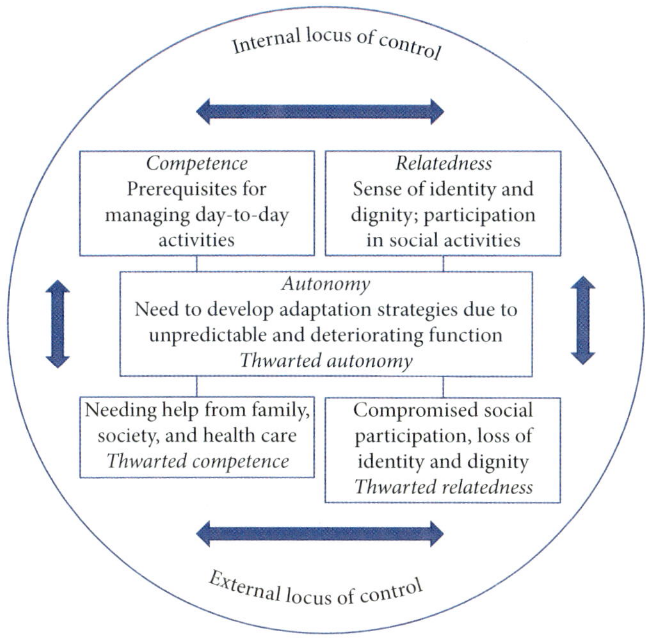

Figure 1: Balancing within a web of needs and demands. A model based on self-determination theory of how people with Parkinson's disease strive to manage the continuous shift between internal and external locus of control, in attempting to maintain competence, relatedness, and autonomy.

states that three basic psychological needs are necessary conditions for people's well-being and health: *competence* (a sense of confidence and feeling effective in interacting with the surrounding society), *relatedness* (belongingness, feeling connected to others) and *autonomy* (acting from interest and integrated values). When these needs become thwarted, a shift towards extrinsically motivated behaviours may occur. Such behaviours, for example, to no longer feel capable of changing one's situation (thwarted competence and autonomy) or feeling sad to be alone (thwarted relatedness), may lead to compensatory strategies or substitutes that will not benefit health and well-being. Interestingly, shifting locus of control and thwarted basic needs have been found to predict poor psychological well-being, depression, and ill health [28, 29]. SDT may thus help provide a deeper understanding of the complexity of the impact of living with PD, as the social conditions and other aspects that needed to be managed become more challenging as the disease progressed.

The vast range and complexity of PD-related symptoms and problems, and their impact on participants' needs and demands may seem overwhelming. Nevertheless, rather than a separable multidimensional array of disease manifestations, symptoms, and problems, these and other aspects are intermingled and appear to form a unity where all parts are facets of a single dimension of the impact of living with PD. This is similar to the findings in a previous study where PwPD and health care professionals (HCPs) conceptually mapped out the interrelationships among aspects deemed important to consider when evaluating interventional outcomes in PD [30]. While HCPs tended to group aspects into clinically distinct areas, PwPD mapped out a more intermingled pattern. This finding was strengthened in the present study, suggesting that the impact of PD from a patient perspective may be described as unidimensional but heterogeneous. Moreover, the impact as described here was largely expressed in terms of unmet needs that change over time, followed by different adaptation strategies. This has implications in terms of person-centred outcome measurement and supports a needs-based quality of life model [31–33]. This suggests that the impact of PD as well as needs-based outcomes may be interpreted in relation to SDT.

The changed ability to take part in various social activities restricted interactions with family, friends, and others. These aspects had consequences for the psychological and emotional aspects of reduced self-worth and the social identity. To facilitate meeting the needs and demands of everyday life, problem-focused and emotion-focused strategies were used to reduce stress and worry and to facilitate adaptation in various situations [34, 35]. However, for some, it was not always realistic to expect that everything would go according to plan. To be able to foresee possible problems and to plan ahead gave the participants a sense of control over the situation, but also reduced the possibility of acting spontaneously [16].

To maintain a positive attitude was one emotion-focused strategy that facilitated emotional balance and well-being. Some found new acquaintances in new contexts, for example, in a PD association, where they met others in similar situations. However, although some were comforted by being able to help those who were worse off, it could also be distressing for those who were afraid of ending up in a similar situation, which has been reported previously [36, 37].

The physical challenges and perceived distress in managing everyday activities and participating in society appear to be similar across different brain disorders [38]. It may thus well be that two persons with different disorders can have more in common than two persons with the same diagnosis, as their challenges not only relate to their health conditions. Therefore, the experienced impact of various disorders may be better represented by use of a needs-based rather than a function or symptom-based approach [31–33]. Arguably, the needs-based approach may also be beneficial from a clinical perspective, by being better positioned to facilitate a more person-centred care. The needs-based quality of life model postulates that life gains its quality from the ability and capacity of the individual to satisfy his/her needs [31–33]. This is in general agreement with the theory and empirical experiences of SDT [28, 29]. The results of our study point to the need for a shift from a biomedical to a more needs-based approach to better understand the impact of living with PD as well as interventional outcomes from the patient's perspective and to facilitate a more person-centred care.

Our findings illustrate the value of qualitative inquiry in order to gain a deeper knowledge and understanding of the impact of long-term illness from a patient perspective. Such information may also lay the foundations for novel and more person-centred outcome measures. It is well established that in addition to being conceptually and theoretically based, the content of any outcome measure intended to represent the patients' perspective should be derived directly from patients with experience from the target disorder [38, 39]. However, these two fundamental components do not appear to have been widely integrated in the development patient-reported outcome measures for PD [40–45].

5. Conclusion

We have found the impact of living with PD to be a complex unity of intermingled symptoms and problems that entail a balance within a web of needs and demands. Seen from this perspective, we suggest that a needs-based approach represents an important starting point to better understanding the consequences of living with PD and to explore the means for people with PD to acquire an improved quality of life on their own terms. This has important implications for understanding living with PD, as well as for designing improved and more person-centred interventions and outcome measures.

Acknowledgments

The authors wish to thank all participating patients for their cooperation, Dr. Klas-Göran Sahlén, Umeå University, Sweden, for valuable advice regarding the OpenCode program, and Mr. James Suckling for linguistic review of the manuscript. The study was supported by BAGADILICO (the Basal Ganglia Disorders Linnaeus Consortium) at Lund University, Sweden, the Faculty of Health Science, Kristianstad University, Kristianstad, Sweden, and the Faculty of Medicine, Lund University, Lund, Sweden.

References

[1] K. R. Chaudhuri and P. Odin, "The challenge of non-motor symptoms in Parkinson's disease," *Progress in Brain Research*' vol. 184, pp. 325–341, 2010.

[2] J. Jankovic, "Parkinson's disease: clinical features and diagnosis," *Journal of Neurology, Neurosurgery, and Psychiatry*' vol. 79, no. 4, pp. 368–376, 2008.

[3] D. Muslimovic, B. Post, J. D. Speelman et al., "Determinants of disability and quality of life in mild to moderate Parkinson disease," *Neurology*, vol. 70, no. 23, pp. 2241–2247, 2008.

[4] A. Haahr, M. Kirkevold, E. O. C. Hall, and K. Østergaard, "Living with advanced Parkinson's disease: a constant struggle with unpredictability," *Journal of Advanced Nursing*, vol. 67, no. 2, pp. 408–417, 2011.

[5] S. E. Soh, M. E. Morris, and J. L. McGinley, "Determinants of health-related quality of life in Parkinson's disease: a systematic review," *Parkinsonism and Related Disorders*, vol. 17, no. 1, pp. 1–9, 2011.

[6] J. M. van Uem, J. Marinus, C. Canning et al., "Health-related quality of life in patients with Parkinson's disease-a systematic review based on the ICF model," *Neuroscience and Biobehavioral Reviews*, vol. 61, pp. 26–34, 2016.

[7] M. Zhu, M. Li, D. Ye, W. Jiang, T. Lei, and K. Shu, "Sensory symptoms in Parkinson's disease: clinical features, pathophysiology, and treatment," *Journal of Neuroscience Research*, vol. 94, no. 8, pp. 685–692, 2016.

[8] M. Caap-Ahlgren and O. Dehlin, "Insomnia and depressive symptoms in patients with Parkinson's disease. Relationship to health-related quality of life. An interview study of patients living at home," *Archives of Gerontology and Geriatrics*, vol. 32, no. 1, pp. 23–33, 2001.

[9] R. M. Lamont, M. E. Morris, M. H. Woollacott, and S. G. Brauer, "Community walking in people with Parkinson's disease," *Parkinson's Disease*, vol. 2012, Article ID 856237, 8 pages, 2012.

[10] A. Lim, L. Leow, M. Huckabee, C. Frampton, and T. Anderson, "A pilot study of respiration and swallowing integration in Parkinson's disease: "on" and "off" levodopa," *Dysphagia*, vol. 23, no. 1, pp. 76–81, 2008.

[11] N. Miller, E. Noble, D. Jones, and D. Burn, "Hard to swallow: dysphagia in Parkinson's disease," *Age and Ageing*, vol. 35, no. 6, pp. 614–618, 2006.

[12] N. Miller, E. Noble, D. Jones, and D. Burn, "Life with communication changes in Parkinson's disease," *Age and Ageing*, vol. 35, no. 3, pp. 235–239, 2006.

[13] H. Sunvisson and S. L. Ekman, "Environmental influences on the experiences of people with Parkinson's disease," *Nursing Inquiry*, vol. 8, no. 1, pp. 41–50, 2001.

[14] M. Caap-Ahlgren and L. Lannerheim, "Older Swedish women's experiences of living with symptoms related to Parkinson's disease," *Journal of Advanced Nursing*, vol. 39, no. 1, pp. 87–95, 2002.

[15] D. Jones, L. Rochester, A. Birleson et al., "Everyday walking with Parkinson's disease: understanding personal challenges and strategies," *Disability and Rehabilitation*, vol. 30, no. 16, pp. 1213–1221, 2008.

[16] M. Olsson, L. Stafström, and S. Söderberg, "Meanings of fatigue for women with Parkinson's disease," *Qualitative Health Research*, vol. 23, no. 6, pp. 741–748, 2013.

[17] C. S. Hammarlund, K. Andersson, M. Andersson, M. H. Nilsson, and P. Hagell, "The significance of walking from the perspective of people with Parkinson's disease," *Journal of Parkinson's Disease*, vol. 4, no. 4, pp. 657–663, 2014.

[18] B. Habermann, "Day-to-day demands of Parkinson's disease," *Western Journal of Nursing Research*, vol. 18, no. 4, pp. 397–413, 1996.

[19] J. A. Marr, "The experience of living with Parkinson's disease," *Journal of Neuroscience Nursing*, vol. 23, no. 5, pp. 325–329, 1991.

[20] J. Jankovic and W. Poewe, "Therapies in Parkinson's disease," *Current Opinion in Neurology*, vol. 25, no. 4, pp. 433–447, 2012.

[21] M. Q. Patton, *Qualitative Evaluation and Research Methods*, Sage Publications Inc., Thousand Oaks, CA, USA, 2002.

[22] M. M. Hoehn and M. D. Yahr, "Parkinsonism: onset, progression and mortality," *Neurology*, vol. 17, no. 5, pp. 427–442, 1967.

[23] U. H. Graneheim and B. Lundman, "Qualitative content analysis in nursing research: concepts, procedures and measures to achieve trustworthiness," *Nurse Education Today*, vol. 24, no. 2, pp. 105–112, 2004.

[24] ICT Services and System, *Development and Division of Epidemiology and Global Health*, OpenCode 4.0, Umeå University, Umeå, Sweden, 2013, http://www.phmed.umu.se/enheter/epidemiologi/forskning/open-code/.

[25] S. Nazem, A. D. Siderowf, J. E. Duda et al., "Suicidal and death ideation in Parkinson's disease," *Movement Disorders*, vol. 23, no. 11, pp. 1573–1579, 2008.

[26] G. Nijhof, "Parkinson's disease as a problem of shame in

public appearance," *Sociology of Health and Illness*, vol. 17, no. 2, pp. 193–205, 1995.

[27] B. Thordardottir, M. H. Nilsson, S. Iwarsson, and M. Haak, ""You plan, but you never know"-participation among people with different levels of severity of Parkinson's disease," *Disability and Rehabilitation*, vol. 36, no. 26, pp. 2216–2224, 2014.

[28] E. L. Deci and R. M. Ryan, "The "what" and "why" of goal pursuits: human needs and the self-determination of behavior," *Psychological Inquiry*, vol. 11, no. 4, pp. 227–268, 2000.

[29] E. L. Deci and R. M. Ryan, "Self-determination theory: a macrotheory of human motivation, development, and health," *Canadian Psychology*, vol. 49, no. 3, pp. 182–185, 2008.

[30] C. Sjodahl Hammarlund, M. H. Nilsson, M. Idvall, S. R. Rosas, and P. Hagell, "Conceptualizing and prioritizing clinical trial outcomes from the perspectives of people with Parkinson's disease versus health care professionals: a concept mapping study," *Quality of Life Research*, vol. 23, no. 6, pp. 1687–1700, 2014.

[31] S. M. Hunt and S. P. McKenna, "The QLDS: a scale for the measurement of quality of life in depression," *Health Policy*, vol. 22, no. 3, pp. 307–319, 1992.

[32] S. P. McKenna, "Measuring patient-reported outcomes: moving beyond misplaced common sense to hard science," *BMC Medicine*, vol. 9, no. 1, 2011.

[33] S. P. McKenna and L. C. Doward, "The needs-based approach to quality of life assessment," *Value in Health*, vol. 7, no. 1, pp. S1–S3, 2004.

[34] S. Folkman and R. S. Lazarus, "If it changes it must be a process: study of emotion and coping during three stages of a college examination," *Journal of Personality and Social Psychology*, vol. 48, no. 1, pp. 150–170, 1985.

[35] R. S. Lazarus and S. Folkman, *Stress, Appraisal, and Coping*, Springer Publishing, New York, NY, USA, 1984.

[36] L. D. Frazier, "Coping with disease-related stressors in Parkinson's disease," *Gerontotogist*, vol. 40, no. 1, pp. 53–63, 2000.

[37] M. H. Nilsson, S. Iwarsson, B. Thordardottir, and M. Haak, "Barriers and facilitators for participation in people with Parkinson's disease," *Journal of Parkinson's Disease*, vol. 5, no. 4, pp. 983–992, 2015.

[38] L. C. Doward, D. M. Meads, and H. Thorsen, "Requirements for quality of life instruments in clinical research," *Value in Health*, vol. 7, no. 1, pp. S13–S16, 2004.

[39] D. L. Streiner and G. R. Norman, *Health Measurement Scales: A Practical Guide to Their Development and Use*, Oxford University Press, Oxford, UK, 2nd edition, 1995.

[40] L. Ambrosio, M. C. Portillo, C. Rodríguez-Blázquez, A. Carvajal, and P. Martínez-Martín, "Estudio piloto sobre la escala de convivencia con un proceso crónico en pacientes con enfermedad de Parkinson," *Revista de Neurologia*, vol. 61, no. 10, pp. 447–453, 2015.

[41] L. Ambrosio, M. C. Portillo, C. Rodríguez-Blázquez et al., "Living with chronic illness scale: international validation of a new self-report measure in Parkinson's disease," *NPJ Parkinson's Disease*, vol. 2, no. 1, p. 16022, 2016.

[42] S. Calne, M. Schulzer, E. Mak et al., "Validating a quality of life rating scale for idiopathic parkinsonism: Parkinson's Impact Scale (PIMS)," *Parkinsonism and Related Disorders*, vol. 2, no. 2, pp. 55–61, 1996.

[43] A. G. de Boer, W. Wijker, J. D. Speelman, and J. C. de Haes, "Quality of life in patients with Parkinson's disease: development of a questionnaire," *Journal of Neurology, Neurosurgery and Psychiatry*, vol. 61, no. 1, pp. 70–74, 1996.

[44] V. Peto, C. Jenkinson, R. Fitzpatrick, and R. Greenhall, "The development and validation of a short measure of functioning and well being for individuals with Parkinson's disease," *Quality of Life Research*, vol. 4, no. 3, pp. 241–248, 1995.

[45] M. Welsh, M. P. McDermott, R. G. Holloway, S. Plumb, R. Pfeiffer, and J. Hubble, "Development and testing of the Parkinson's disease quality of life scale," *Movement Disorders*, vol. 18, no. 6, pp. 637–645, 2003.

11

Absent Audiovisual Integration Elicited by Peripheral Stimuli in Parkinson's Disease

Yanna Ren,[1,2] Keisuke Suzuki,[3] Weiping Yang,[4] Yanling Ren,[5] Fengxia Wu,[2] Jiajia Yang,[2] Satoshi Takahashi,[2] Yoshimichi Ejima,[2] Jinglong Wu,[2,6,7] and Koichi Hirata[3]

[1]*Department of Psychology, Medical Humanities College, Guiyang University of Chinese Medicine, Guiyang 550025, China*
[2]*Cognitive Neuroscience Laboratory, Graduate School of Natural Science and Technology, Okayama University, Okayama 7008530, Japan*
[3]*Department of Neurology, Dokkyo Medical University, Tochigi 3210293, Japan*
[4]*Department of Psychology, Hubei University, Wuhan 430062, China*
[5]*Department of Light and Chemical Engineering, Guizhou Light Industry Technical College, Guiyang 550025, China*
[6]*Intelligent Robotics Institute, Beijing Institute of Technology, Beijing 100081, China*
[7]*Shenzhen Institute of Neuroscience, Shenzhen 518057, China*

Correspondence should be addressed to Jinglong Wu; wu@mech.okayama-u.ac.jp and Koichi Hirata; hirata@dokkyomed.ac.jp

Academic Editor: Hélio Teive

The basal ganglia, which have been shown to be a significant multisensory hub, are disordered in Parkinson's disease (PD). This study was to investigate the audiovisual integration of peripheral stimuli in PD patients with/without sleep disturbances. Thirty-six age-matched normal controls (NC) and 30 PD patients were recruited for an auditory/visual discrimination experiment. The mean response times for each participant were analyzed using repeated measures ANOVA and race model. The results showed that the response to all stimuli was significantly delayed for PD compared to NC (all $p < 0.01$). The response to audiovisual stimuli was significantly faster than that to unimodal stimuli in both NC and PD ($p < 0.001$). Additionally, audiovisual integration was absent in PD; however, it did occur in NC. Further analysis showed that there was no significant audiovisual integration in PD with/without cognitive impairment or in PD with/without sleep disturbances. Furthermore, audiovisual facilitation was not associated with Hoehn and Yahr stage, disease duration, or the presence of sleep disturbances (all $p > 0.05$). The current results showed that audiovisual multisensory integration for peripheral stimuli is absent in PD regardless of sleep disturbances and further suggested the abnormal audiovisual integration might be a potential early manifestation of PD.

1. Introduction

Parkinson's disease (PD) is traditionally recognized as a movement disorder and is characterized by bradykinesia, resting tremor, and rigidity. However, recent evidence suggests that patients with PD also have various nonmotor disturbances such as depression, cognitive impairment, sleep disorders, and olfactory disturbance [1, 2]. Moreover, nonmotor symptoms are sometimes evident prior to the onset of motor symptoms during the "premotor stage" and influence the patients' quality of life. Therefore, many studies have focused on the early detection and management of nonmotor symptoms associated with PD [1].

People obtain dynamic effective information from the complex environment through multiple senses. A number of studies have reported that people with PD present sensory and perceptual impairments [3], including delayed responses to auditory or visual stimuli compared with age-matched healthy controls [4–7]. However, a simple reaction time task includes many steps: identifying and evaluating the stimulus, selecting the appropriate response, and programming and executing the movement. Thus, delay at any one or all of these stages may lead to a delayed reaction time [5]. For PD patients, the observed increase in simple reaction time may result from slowness of movement compared with age-matched normal controls. To quantitatively assess sensory processing speed, it is necessary to remove the redundant time for executing the movement. Of note, individuals are often inundated with stimuli from various sensory modalities, and merging multisensory information is therefore often crucial in making a rapid and accurate response [8–12]. Therefore, the quantitative assessment of multisensory integration processing ability is very meaningful in the investigation of PD.

By comparing reaction times to multisensory stimuli and to individual component unisensory stimuli, quantitative assessment of multisensory integration can be performed while controlling for response time for executing movement in PD [13–15]. A substantial loss of dopaminergic neurons in the basal ganglia is observed in PD [16–18]. Using an extracellular single-cell recording technique, Nagy et al. confirmed that like the superior colliculus and related structures, the basal ganglia (e.g., the caudate nucleus and the substantia nigra) have the ability to integrate multisensory information [18]. The latest studies conducted by Noy et al. showed that individuals might optimally integrate audiovisual cues to synchronize steps during step-by-step walking [19], which indicated the importance of cross-modal integration of visual and auditory signals for PD patients. However, currently few studies have reported the audiovisual integration ability of PD patients. Fearon et al. [13] recently demonstrated that abnormal audiovisual processing occurs in PD patients compared with age-matched healthy controls; in their study, the visual stimuli were presented centrally. Previous studies have shown that the location of the presented stimuli may greatly affect detection and discrimination of the stimuli. The more peripherally a visual or auditory stimulus was located (from 0° to 60°), the slower both the response accuracy and the speed of the response were [20, 21]. Nidiffer et al. [21] found a similar response pattern to audiovisual stimuli. Furthermore, these authors also reported increasing performance facilitation as the stimuli were positioned at more peripheral locations, indicating that the location of the stimulus (central or peripheral) greatly influenced audiovisual integration [21]. However, it is still unknown whether the multisensory integration of peripheral stimuli is altered in the same way as the multisensory integration of centrally located stimuli.

Sleep disturbances that have a detrimental effect on health-related quality of life are a common disabling nonmotor symptom of PD. Such sleep disturbances can occur at any point during the course of PD and even at the initiative stage [22]. Sleep disturbances are estimated to occur in 60–98% of patients with PD [22–24]. Multiple factors contribute to the occurrence of sleep disturbances, including PD-related pathological changes, nocturnal motor/nonmotor symptoms, medication use, and comorbid primary sleep disorders [25]. However, because no investigation has focused on the audiovisual integration of PD patients with sleep disturbances, it is completely unknown whether or not sleep disturbances worsen the abnormal audiovisual integration that occurs in PD.

Using an auditory/visual stimulus discrimination task [26, 27], the present study aimed to quantitatively measure the ability of PD patients to integrate peripheral audiovisual stimuli and to evaluate the effect of sleep disturbances on PD-related peripheral audiovisual integration.

2. Methods

2.1. Subjects. A total of 36 age-matched healthy volunteers (62–78 years; mean age ± SD, 69.69 ± 4.41) and 30 PD patients (53–82 years; mean age ± SD, 67.53 ± 9.1) participated in this study and finished the experiment successfully. All of the age-matched healthy volunteers who made up the normal control group were randomly recruited from the Okayama Silver Human Resources Center, and all of the PD patients were recruited from outpatient clinics of the Department of Neurology, Dokkyo Medical University Hospital. All the recruited age-matched healthy volunteers agreed to participate in the experiment, and finished the experiment successfully. However, two of the PD patients in the outpatient clinics had no time to attend the experiment. A diagnosis of PD was made according to the established criteria by board-certified neurologists [28], and disease duration of the PD patients was recorded in Table 1. The participants were naïve to the device and to the task. All the participants provided written informed consent to the procedure, which was previously approved by the ethics committee of Okayama University (NC) or of Dokkyo Medical University Hospital (PD) specifically according to the location at which the examination was performed. Additionally, all of the participants in the NC group were in good physical condition and not taking any medications that might have central effects.

2.2. Stimuli. The visual stimulus was a black and white checkerboard image (52 × 52 mm), which was presented on a black background on a 21-inch computer monitor positioned 60 cm in front of the participant's eyes (Figure 1). All visual stimuli (V) were presented on the lower left or lower right quadrant of the screen for 150 ms (at a 12-degree visual angle to the left or right of the center and at a 5-degree angle below the central fixation point). The auditory stimulus was a 1000 Hz sinusoidal tone that was presented randomly to the left or right ear through earphones at approximately 60 dB SPL for 150 ms (10 ms of rise/fall cosine gate). The audiovisual stimuli (AV) were presented through a combination of the visual and auditory stimuli. Each subject participated in only one session consisting of 50 visual stimuli, 50 auditory stimuli, and 50 audiovisual stimuli.

2.3. Experimental Procedure. Each subject was instructed on how to complete the experiment, which consisted of two parts, a questionnaire assessment session and an auditory/visual stimuli discrimination session. All of the questionnaires were completed in the outpatient department or in a special quiet room with the assistance of professional staff. For the auditory/visual discrimination session, each subject was tested individually in a quiet room free from external noise and distraction, thereby minimizing the possible influence of any physiological effects.

TABLE 1: Demographics of Parkinson's disease patients with/without sleep disturbance according to PDSS-2, ESS, and PSQI scores.

	All PD patients	PD with sleep disturbances	PD without sleep disturbances
N	30	14	16
Age (y)	67.5 (1.6)	69.6 (2.3)	65.7 (0.2)
Gender (F : M)	17 : 13	7 : 7	10 : 6
H&Y stage	2.4 (0.1)	2.6 (0.2)	2.3 (0.2)
Disease duration (y)	4.5 (1.0)	5.8 (1.9)	3.4 (0.8)
Education (y)	12.4 (0.4)	12.1 (0.7)	12.6 (0.6)
PDSS-2***	15.2 (2.1)	24 (3.2)	7.6 (0.8)
ESS	7.8 (1.0)	8.5 (1.6)	7.2 (1.5)
PSQI	6.9 (1.2)	8.9 (2.2)	5.1 (1.1)
MOCA	24.2 (0.5)	24.3 (0.7)	24.1 (0.8)
LED (mg/day)	452 (67)	508 (90)	403 (100)

Data are presented as the mean ± standard error of the mean (SEM). F: female; M: male; H&Y stage: Hoehn & Yahr staging system (stages from 1 to 5; a higher score reflects more severe symptoms); PDSS-2: Parkinson's Disease Sleep Scale (score greater than the cutoff of 15 indicates a poor sleeper); ESS: Epworth Sleepiness Scale (score greater than the cutoff of 11 indicates excessive daytime sleepiness); PSQI: Pittsburgh Sleep Quality Index (score greater than the cutoff of 6 suggests possible insomnia); MOCA: Montreal Cognitive Assessment (score greater than the cutoff of 26 reflects normal cognition). ***$p < 0.001$ indicates a statistically significant difference between the PD group with sleep disturbances and the PD group without sleep disturbances.

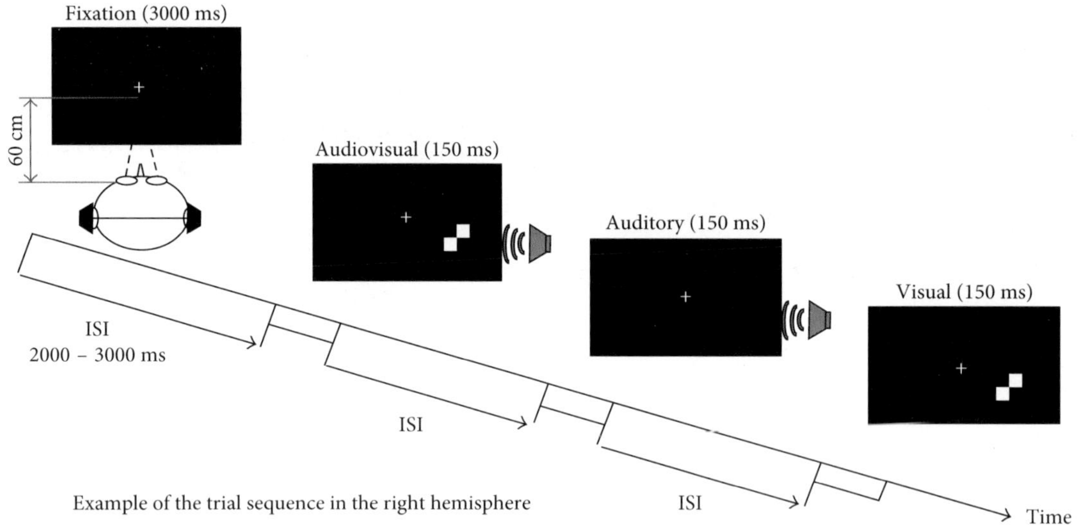

FIGURE 1: Schematic description of the experimental design. An example of a stimulus used to form a possible trial sequence is shown. After fixation for 3000 ms at the beginning of the session, all the auditory, visual, and audiovisual stimuli were presented randomly with a random interstimulus interval (ISI) of 2000–3000 ms. Following the presentation of each stimulus, the subject was instructed to identify which hemispace was presented by pressing the right or left button of a mouse as rapidly and accurately as possible.

2.3.1. Questionnaire Assessments. Each participant's overall cognitive function was estimated using the Montreal Cognitive Assessment (MOCA) [29]. The Japanese versions of the Parkinson's Disease Sleep Scale-2 (PDSS-2) [30], the Epworth Sleepiness Scale (ESS) [31, 32], and the Pittsburgh Sleep Quality Index (PSQI) [33] were used to evaluate sleep conditions. Additionally, for the PD patients, Hoehn and Yahr (HY) staging was used to rate disease severity [34], and the duration of the disease and Levodopa equivalent dose (LED) used were obtained from the attending physician after receiving the patient's permission. This session lasted approximately 40 mins.

2.3.2. Auditory/Visual Stimuli Discrimination Session. The subjects were instructed to perform an auditory/visual stimuli discrimination task in a quiet room (a laboratory room at Okayama University or at Dokkyo Medical University Hospital, Japan) with their eyes fixed on the fixation cross (Figure 1). All of the participants were naïve to the device and to the task. Stimulus presentation and response collection were conducted using Presentation software (Neurobehavioral Systems Inc., Albany, California, USA). At the beginning of the task, the subjects were presented with a fixation cross for 3000 ms. Following fixation, all stimuli were presented randomly, and the subjects were instructed to identify which hemispace the stimulus was presented in. They were instructed to press the appropriate button (the right button if the stimulus was presented in the right hemispace and the left button if the stimulus was presented in the left hemispace) as rapidly and accurately as possible. Each stimulus was followed by an interstimulus interval (ISI) that varied randomly in duration from 2000 to 3000 ms for subject response and rest. This session lasted approximately 6.3 mins.

TABLE 2: Comparisons of MOCA, PDSS-2, and ESS scores between NC and PD groups.

	Simple size, number	Female/male	Age (y)	Education (y)	MOCA***	PDSS-2*	ESS*	PSQI
NC	36	18/18	69.69 ± 0.74	12.86 ± 0.34	26.78 ± 0.33	10.03 ± 0.97	5.28 ± 0.65	6.33 ± 0.75
PD	30	16/14	67.53 ± 1.63	12.40 ± 0.44	24.17 ± 0.53	15.27 ± 2.10	7.80 ± 1.08	6.90 ± 1.20

Data are presented as the mean ± standard error of the mean (SEM). NC: age-matched normal controls; PD: Parkinson's disease patients. $^{*}p < 0.05$, $^{***}p < 0.001$; statistically significant difference between the NC group and the PD group.

2.4. Data Analysis

2.4.1. Questionnaire Assessments. The subject was defined as a poor sleeper if he or she had a global PDSS-2 score ≥15 [30]. The subject was recognized as having excessive daytime sleepiness if he or she had a total ESS score ≥11 [32] and was indicated as having insomnia if the overall PSQI score was ≥6 [35]. In the current study, we divided the PD patients into those with and those without sleep disturbances according to their PDSS-2 scores. The global score was computed separately for each subject in every assessment, and the resulting data were subjected to a one-sample t-test (two-tailed).

2.4.2. Mean Response Time and Hit Rates. In the auditory/visual discrimination session, the hit rates and mean response times were computed separately for each subject and in each condition. The hit rate is the percentage of correct responses (the response time falls within the average time period ± 2SD) relative to the total number of stimuli. The mean response time was determined as the average response time for all correct responses. Finally, the data were subjected to 2 groups (NC and PD) * 3 conditions (A, V, and AV) repeated measures ANOVA followed by post hoc tests to analyze the main effect and factors interaction.

2.4.3. Race Model. In the current study, audiovisual integration was evaluated using the redundant nature effect. To examine the redundant nature effect of multisensory integration for the bimodal stimuli condition, we reanalyzed the mean response times using cumulative distribution functions (CDFs). The bimodal AV data were compared with an independent race model, which is a statistical prediction model that uses the CDF of the summed probabilities of the visual and auditory responses [14, 15]. The model permits a direct comparison between the multisensory condition and the predicted probability of unimodal conditions, $[P(A) + P(V)] - [P(A) \times P(V)]$, by segmenting the subject-specific CDFs for each condition using 10 ms time bins. $P(A)$ is the probability of responding within a given time to a unimodal auditory trial, and $P(V)$ is the probability of responding within a given time to a unimodal visual trial. If the probability of a response to AV is significantly greater than that predicted by the summed probabilities of A and V, neural audiovisual integration of the two unimodal inputs is considered to be occurred [14, 15]. Then, the redundant nature effect of multisensory conditions was defined by subtracting a subject's race model from his or her audiovisual CDFs at each time bin to generate a difference curve for each subject. A one-sample t-test (two-tailed) was then performed for each time bin within each of the groups (the NC and PD groups) to identify significant deviations ($p < 0.05$) by comparing the value at each time bin with zero.

2.4.4. Correlation Analysis. For PD patients, there was no significant audiovisual integration; therefore, the bimodal response facilitation was assessed through the interactive index (ii) [36]. Correlation analysis was conducted to examine the relationship between the degree of response facilitation and H&Y stage or disease duration. The variables AV, V, and A represent the mean response times to each stimulus. All of the data were subjected to bivariate correlations analysis (*Pearson's correlation, two-tailed*):

$$\text{ii} = \frac{\max(A; V) - AV}{\max(A; V)} \times 100\%. \quad (1)$$

3. Results

3.1. Questionnaire Assessment. A one-sample t-test (two-tailed) was conducted between the NC and PD groups for Age, Education, MOCA score, PDSS-2 score, ESS score, and PSQI score, respectively. No significant difference was found between the two groups for Age ($p = 0.21$), Education ($p = 0.4$), or PSQI score ($p = 0.68$). However, there was a significant difference for MOCA score ($p < 0.001$), indicating the presence of cognitive impairment in PD. Furthermore, significant differences were also found for PDSS-2 score ($p = 0.02$) and ESS score ($p = 0.04$), showing that obvious sleep disturbances occurred in some PD patients (Table 2).

3.2. Mean Response Time and Hit Rates. The mean response times and hit rates for NC and PD patients are shown in detail in Table 3. Analysis using 3 (modality) * 2 (hemispace) repeated measures ANOVA showed main effects of modality in both the NC group $[F(2, 68) = 43.06, p < 0.001]$ and the PD patients $[F(2, 58) = 31.91, p < 0.001]$; however, no significant main effects of hemispace were found in either the NC group $[F(1, 34) = 5.46, p = 0.062]$ or the PD patients $[F(1, 29) = 1.63, p = 0.21]$. Therefore, the data from the left and right hemispaces were combined. The mean response times and hit rates for NC and PD are presented in Figure 2.

Analysis of the response times using 2 groups (NC and PD) * 3 modalities (A, V, AV) repeated measures ANOVA showed a significant main group effect $[F(1, 63) = 14.75, p < 0.001]$. The pairwise comparisons showed that for the NC group, the responses to bimodal AV stimuli were significantly faster than the responses to unimodal visual ($p < 0.001$) or auditory ($p < 0.001$) stimuli. However, there was no significant difference in the response of the NC group to unimodal visual and auditory stimuli ($p = 0.56$). For the PD group, the responses to bimodal AV stimuli were significantly faster than the responses to unimodal visual ($p < 0.001$) or auditory ($p < 0.001$) stimuli. However, there was no significant difference in the response

Table 3: The mean response times and hit rates for NC and PD patients.

	NC		PD	
	Right	Left	Right	Left
Response time (ms)				
Auditory	494.6 (8.8)	475.7 (10.9)	576.3 (18.7)	537.1 (17.9)
Visual	467.8 (9.1)	459.2 (8.4)	543.4 (18.8)	527.1 (21.4)
Audiovisual	431.2 (7.7)	425.7 (9.4)	482.0 (15.1)	481.7 (17.9)
Hit rates				
Auditory	0.95 (0.006)	0.95 (0.007)	0.91 (0.01)	0.91 (0.02)
Visual	0.95 (0.007)	0.95 (0.005)	0.91 (0.01)	0.91 (0.02)
Audiovisual	0.95 (0.005)	0.95 (0.007)	0.92 (0.02)	0.92 (0.01)

Data are presented as the mean ± standard error of the mean (SEM). A: auditory-only stimulus; V: visual-only stimulus; AV: audiovisual stimulus.

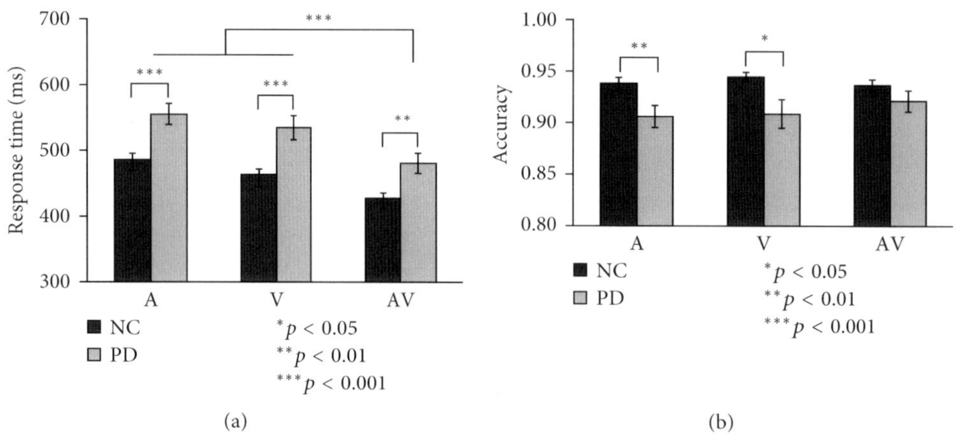

Figure 2: Average reaction times and hit rates by modality and group (error bars indicate the SEM) (A: auditory-only stimulus; V: visual-only stimulus; AV: audiovisual stimulus; $^{*}p < 0.05$).

to unimodal visual and auditory stimuli ($p = 0.13$). Additionally, there was a significant main effect of modality [$F(2, 126) = 72.78$, $p < 0.001$]. The pairwise comparisons between the NC and PD groups showed significantly faster responses for NC than those for PD to unimodal visual ($p < 0.001$), auditory ($p < 0.001$), and audiovisual stimuli ($p = 0.002$). However, there was no significant interaction between group and modality [$F(2, 126) = 1.62$, $p = 0.21$].

Analysis of the hit rates using 2 Group (NC and PD) * 3 Modality (A, V, AV) repeated measures ANOVA showed a significant main effect of group [$F(2, 63) = 8.68$, $p = 0.005$], with a higher accuracy for the NC group than for the PD group. The pairwise comparisons between the NC and PD groups showed significantly higher accuracy for NC than for PD to unimodal visual ($p = 0.012$) and auditory ($p = 0.008$) stimuli; however, no significant difference was found for the bimodal AV condition. However, there was no main effect of modality [$F(2, 126) = 0.52$, $p = 0.59$] and no interaction between group and modality [$F(2, 126) = 1.31$, $p = 0.27$].

3.3. Race Model Comparisons. A race model was used to analyze the RTs to evaluate the redundant nature effect of the multisensory stimuli under each of the experimental conditions (Figures 3(a) and 3(b)). The relationship was compared by subtracting the race model CDFs from the bimodal AV CDFs for each group (Figure 3(c)). Significant audiovisual interactions ($p < 0.05$, one-sample t-test) were found for the NC group (Figure 3(c), solid line); however, there were no significant differences between the responses to bimodal stimuli and the predicted race model for the PD patients (Figure 3(c), dotted line) ($p > 0.05$).

The foregoing results indicate that there was significant diversity in audiovisual interaction between the PD patients and the age-matched NC group. To further examine the possible cause of the significant cognitive functional difference between these two groups, we divided each group into two subgroups based on the individuals' MOCA scores (cutoff = 26). A similar race model analysis method was used for the further analyses. The results indicated that there was no significant difference between the NC subgroups ($p > 0.05$; Figure 4(a)) or between the PD subgroups ($p > 0.05$; Figure 4(b)). Additionally, we further divided PD patients into PD patients with sleep disturbance and PD patients without sleep disturbance based on their PDSS-2 scores (Table 1). The redundant nature analysis results showed no significant audiovisual integration for either the PD with sleep disturbance or the PD without sleep disturbance groups (Figure 5). Furthermore, the one-sample t-test (two-tailed) found that there was no significant difference between PD patients with sleep disturbance and PD patients without sleep disturbance ($p > 0.05$).

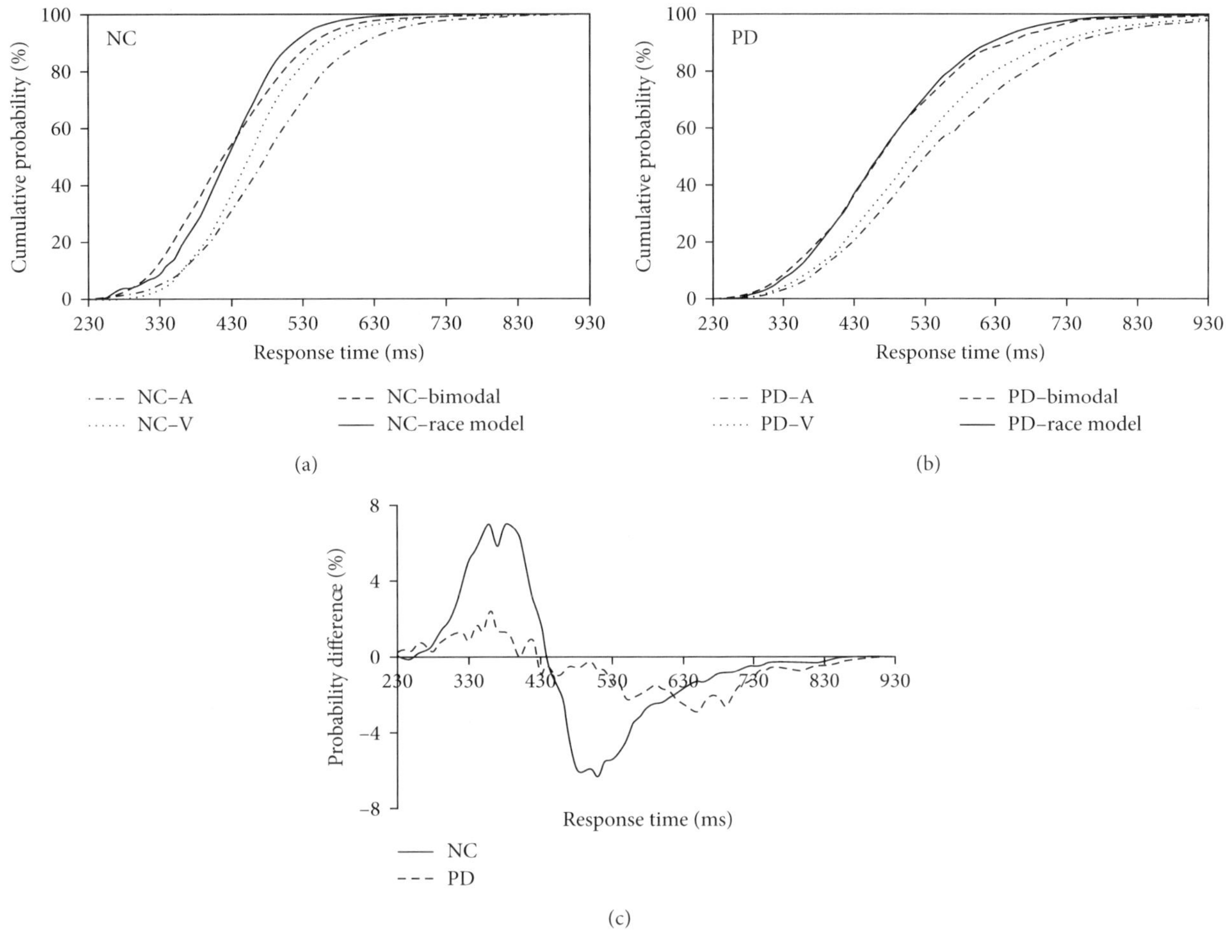

FIGURE 3: Distributions of response times. (a) Cumulative distribution functions (CDFs) for the discrimination response times to auditory, visual, and audiovisual stimuli and for the race model for NC. (b) CDFs for PD. (c) Significant audiovisual integration was found in NC (solid line), but not in PD patients (dotted line).

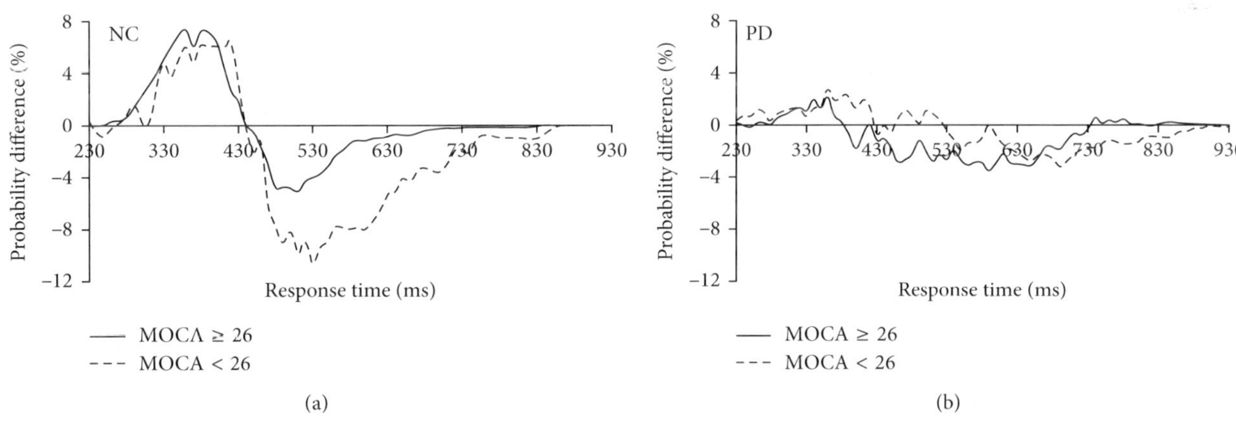

FIGURE 4: Direct comparison of audiovisual performance relative to the predicted race model. Significant audiovisual integration was found in both NC with (dotted line) and without (solid line) cognitive impairment (a). No significant audiovisual integration was occurred with (dotted line) or without (solid line) cognitive impairment (b).

3.4. Correlation Analysis. Figure 6 shows the results of the correlation analysis. The results indicate that there was no significant relationship between H&Y stage and response facilitation either for the PD with sleep disturbance group ($r = 0.437, p = 0.118$) or for the PD without sleep disturbance group ($r = -0.362, p = 0.169$), nor was there a significant relationship between disease duration and response facilitation for either the PD with sleep disturbance group ($r = 0.370, p = 0.193$) or the PD without sleep disturbance group ($r = -0.416, p = 0.109$).

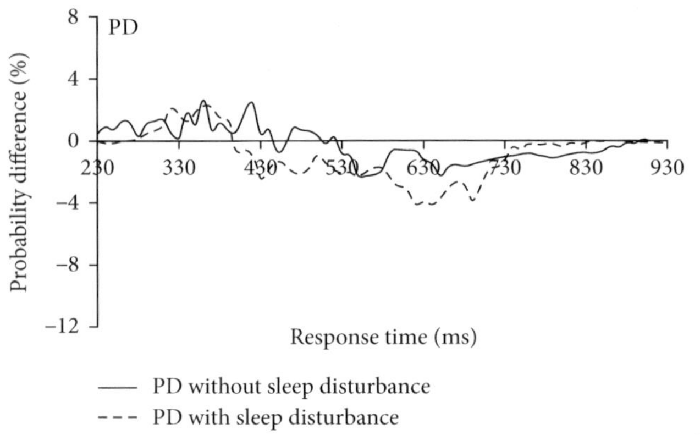

Figure 5: Direct comparison of audiovisual performance relative to the predicted race model. No significant audiovisual integration was found in both PD with sleep disturbance group (dotted line) and without sleep disturbance group (solid line).

4. Discussion

In this study, we examined the audiovisual multisensory integration elicited by peripheral stimuli in PD. The results showed that no significant audiovisual integration occurred in PD regardless of the presence of cognitive deficits or sleep disturbance; however, such integration did occur in age-matched normal controls. In addition, there were no significant correlations between audiovisual facilitation and H&Y stage or disease duration.

4.1. Absent Audiovisual Integration in PD. Regarding the investigation of multisensory integration in PD, this is the first study to quantitatively examine audiovisual multisensory integration to stimuli presented peripherally to PD patients and to report that no significant audiovisual integration was observed. Consistent with the results of a previous study, audiovisual processing in PD was found to be abnormal [13]. To some degree, the current results lead to a conclusion similar to that expressed by Fearon et al. They found that audiovisual processing in PD was attenuated but did exist and further reported that it was correlated with freezing of gait and disease duration [13]. Investigation of visual processing by fMRI showed that in PD patients, the neural response of the visual cortex to peripheral stimuli was weaker than the response to central stimuli [37]. Consistent with the inverse effectiveness principle of multisensory integration, audiovisual integration was greater when the stimuli were positioned at more peripheral locations (0° versus 30° and 60°) [21]. Therefore, the partial differences between our results and those of the previous study might be associated with the visual angle at which the stimuli were presented. To date, although there is no evidence of pathology in the visual cortex of PD patients, the present studies have implied the dysfunction of visual perception, and reduced activity in visual association cortices and primary visual cortex was found in PD [38, 39]. The regions traditionally considered to be sensory-specific (e.g., the primary visual cortex) have been proven an audiovisual integration effect as compensatory phenomena [40–43]. Therefore, it is reasonable for the abnormal audiovisual integration in PD patients.

Besides, recent studies have provided evidence that the subcortical basal ganglia have multisensory properties [17, 18]. Nagy et al. reported that the caudate nucleus and substantia nigra of anesthetized cats can respond to visual, auditory, or somatosensory stimulation alone as well to multisensory stimuli. In addition, the multisensory units of the caudate nucleus and substantia nigra showed significant cross-modal interaction, displaying additive or super-additive response facilitation to multisensory simulation. There is known to be a basal ganglia disorder in PD, as evidenced by cell death in the substantia nigra and the ventral (front) part of the pars compacta as well as substantial loss of dopaminergic neurons in the substantia nigra [24, 44, 45]. The higher audiovisual integration of peripheral stimuli might be susceptible to basal ganglia impairment; thus, it seems very possible that disorders of the basal ganglia may lead to the absence of audiovisual integration processing.

Additionally, attention can also greatly modulate audiovisual integration, and audiovisual integration has been shown to be greater in attended tasks than in unattended tasks [46–50]. Numerous behavioral and electroencephalographic studies have provided evidence for the existence of attentional deficits, for example, visual attention and auditory attention, in PD [49–54]. Therefore, the decrease in attention that occurs in PD might also contribute to the absence of audiovisual integration.

4.2. Absent Audiovisual Integration Independent of Cognitive Deficits and Sleep Disturbance in PD. In the present study, we examined 30 clinical PD patients who successfully completed the auditory/visual stimuli discrimination experiment independently without serious cognitive deficits or motor impairment. The demographic information showed lower MOCA scores for the PD patients than for their age-matched normal controls, and a further t-test (two-tailed) analysis revealed significant differences between the two groups. Our previous study showed decreased audiovisual integration both in divided attention and selective attention tasks for patients with mild cognitive impairment, and audiovisual integration further decreased significantly in Alzheimer's disease patients [55]. These results suggested that the cognitive deficits that occur in PD might lead to abnormal audiovisual integration. According to their MOCA scores, we divided the PD patients into two groups (cutoff = 26). The analysis revealed that there was no significant difference in audiovisual integration between the two sub-PD groups (MOCA scores of ≥26 and <26). According to the results, we propose that although cognitive deficits attenuate audiovisual integration, as found in our previous study, basal ganglia disorders might be the most critical factor associated with the lack of audiovisual integration in PD patients. In our study, we also divided the normal control group into two subgroups according to their MOCA scores. In that group, there were only three participants with MOCA scores below

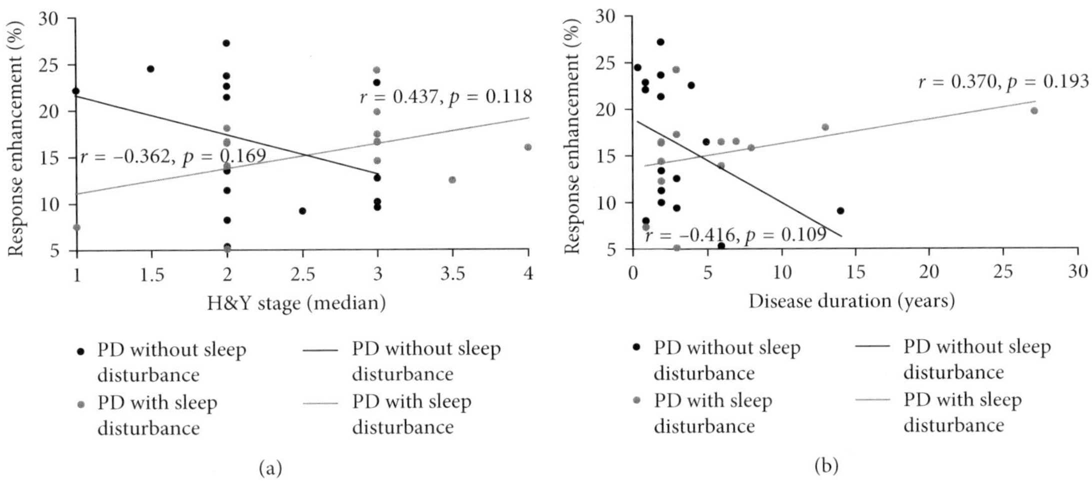

FIGURE 6: Correlation of H&Y stage and disease duration with response facilitation. (a) No significant relationship between H&Y stage and response facilitation. x-axis: H&Y stage; y-axis: response facilitation. (b) No significant relationship between disease duration and response facilitation. x-axis: disease duration; y-axis: response facilitation.

26 (two participants with scores of 25 and one with a score of 24), and these participants showed no significant cognitive impairment. Although the data for normal control participants with MOCA scores below 26 are insufficient for statistical analysis, the average probability difference curve of these participants is similar to that of the group with MOCA scores of 26 or greater. This result further suggests that audiovisual multisensory integration is much more sensitive to the basal ganglia disorder that occurs in PD than to slight alterations in cognitive function.

Additionally, in the present study, we examined the audiovisual integration of peripheral stimuli in PD patients with or without sleep disturbance. According to the PDSS-2 scores, 14 PD patients (47%) had sleep disturbances; based on these scores, we divided all the participants into two groups: those with and those without sleep disturbances. However, we found no significant difference in multisensory audiovisual integration in the two subgroups. These results further suggest that audiovisual integration of peripheral stimuli might be especially sensitive to basal ganglia disorders and that sleep disturbance was not the key factor determining the lack of audiovisual integration in these patients.

To further investigate whether the ability to integrate peripheral audiovisual stimuli is reserved in the early stage of PD and disappears with the progression of the disease in the current study, we evaluated the correlation of H&Y stage and disease duration with audiovisual multisensory integration through relative unisensory response time facilitation. No significant relationship was found between the bimodal response facilitation and H&Y stage or disease duration (all $p > 0.05$), regardless of the presence of sleep disturbance. The results confirm that the abnormal audiovisual multisensory processing occurred at an early PD stage. Together with the results of the previous study, these results further suggest that deficiencies in audiovisual multisensory processing might be a potential early manifestation of PD [13].

4.3. Limitations. The main limitation of the current study is the systemic alteration of audiovisual integration that occurred as a function of the change in the visual angle at which the stimuli are presented. The lack of objective assessments for the sleep status, such as polysomnography or actigraphy, and the limited battery (MOCA) used in this study could have influenced the results. The multiple comparisons employed in this study were not corrected because our study was exploratory in nature, which may have included some significant findings by chance. Additionally, as the sample was relatively small, we were unable to divide the PD patients according to motor symptoms and Levodopa equivalent dose in detail. Furthermore, EEG investigation is needed to evaluate the time course of audiovisual integration in PD to further verify whether the observed lack of audiovisual integration of peripheral stimuli occurs at the early stage of audiovisual integration.

5. Conclusions

The current study provides the first evidence that the audiovisual multisensory integration of peripheral stimuli is absent in PD patients regardless of the presence of sleep disturbances. The results of the study further suggest that abnormal audiovisual integration may be a potential early manifestation of PD.

Disclosure

Yanna Ren and Keisuke Suzuki contributed equally to this work and should be considered co-first authors.

Authors' Contributions

Yanna Ren and Weiping Yang conceived and designed the experiments. Yanna Ren, Fengxia Wu, and Keisuke Suzuki collected the data. Yanna Ren analyzed the data, wrote the draft manuscript, and received comments from Keisuke Suzuki, Yanling Ren, Jiajia Yang, Satoshi Takahashi, Yoshimichi Ejima, Jinglong Wu, and Koichi Hirata.

Acknowledgments

This study was supported by the Japan Society for the Promotion of Science (JSPS) KAKENHI Grant no. 16K18052; the National Natural Science Foundation of China (61473043; 61727807; 31600882; 31700973); the Beijing Municipal Science and Technology Commission (Z161100002616020); the Humanity and Social Science Youth Foundation of the Education Bureau of Hubei Province of China (16Q030, Weiping Yang); and the Humanity and Social Science Youth Foundation of the Ministry of Education of China (16YJC190025).

References

[1] K. R. Chaudhuri, D. G. Healy, and A. H. Schapira, "Non-motor symptoms of Parkinson's disease: diagnosis and management," *Lancet Neurology*, vol. 5, no. 3, pp. 235–245, 2006.

[2] K. R. Chaudhuri and A. H. Schapira, "Non-motor symptoms of Parkinson's disease: dopaminergic pathophysiology and treatment," *Lancet Neurology*, vol. 8, no. 5, pp. 464–474, 2009.

[3] K. A. E. Martens and Q. J. Almeida, "Dissociating between sensory and perceptual deficits in PD: more than simply a motor deficit," *Movement Disorders*, vol. 27, no. 3, pp. 387–392, 2012.

[4] J. Gauntlett-Gilbert and V. J. Brown, "Reaction time deficits and Parkinson's disease," *Neuroscience and Biobehavioral Reviews*, vol. 22, no. 6, pp. 865–881, 1998.

[5] K. A. Low, J. Miller, and E. Vierck, "Response slowing in Parkinson's disease," *Brain*, vol. 125, no. 9, pp. 1980–1994, 2002.

[6] A. Pascual-Leone, J. Valls-Sole, J. Brasil-Neto, L. Cohen, and M. Hallett, "Akinesia in Parkinson's disease. I. Shortening of simple reaction time with focal, single-pulse transcranial magnetic stimulation," *Neurology*, vol. 44, no. 5, p. 884, 1994.

[7] V. Paunikar, N. Shastri, and M. Baig, "Effect of Parkinson's disease on audiovisual reaction time in Indian population," *International Journal Of Biological and Medical Research*, vol. 3, no. 1, pp. 1392–1396, 2012.

[8] C. Spence, "Crossmodal correspondences: a tutorial review," *Attention, Perception, and Psychophysics*, vol. 73, no. 4, pp. 971–995, 2011.

[9] M. A. Meredith, J. W. Nemitz, and B. E. Stein, "Determinants of multisensory integration in superior colliculus neurons. I. Temporal factors," *Journal of Neuroscience*, vol. 7, no. 10, pp. 3215–3229, 1987.

[10] B. Stein and M. Meredith, *The Merging of the Sense*, Mit Press Cambridge, Cambridge, MA, USA, 1993.

[11] P. J. Laurienti, J. H. Burdette, J. A. Maldjian, and M. T. Wallace, "Enhanced multisensory integration in older adults," *Neurobiology of Aging*, vol. 27, no. 8, pp. 1155–1163, 2006.

[12] B. E. Stein, *The New Handbook of Multisensory Processing*, Mit Press Cambridge, Cambridge, MA, USA, 2012.

[13] C. Fearon, J. S. Butler, L. Newman, T. Lynch, and R. B. Reilly, "Audiovisual processing is abnormal in Parkinson's disease and correlates with freezing of gait and disease duration," *Journal of Parkinson's Disease*, vol. 5, no. 4, pp. 925–936, 2015.

[14] J. Miller, "Divided attention: evidence for coactivation with redundant signals," *Cognitive Psychology*, vol. 14, no. 2, pp. 247–279, 1982.

[15] J. Miller, "Timecourse of coactivation in bimodal divided attention," *Attention, Perception, and Psychophysics*, vol. 40, no. 5, pp. 331–343, 1986.

[16] M. Zhu, M. Li, D. Ye, W. Jiang, T. Lei, and K. Shu, "Sensory symptoms in Parkinson's disease: clinical features, pathophysiology, and treatment," *Journal of Neuroscience Research*, vol. 94, no. 8, pp. 685–692, 2016.

[17] A. Nagy, Z. Paróczy, M. Norita, and G. Benedek, "Multisensory responses and receptive field properties of neurons in the substantia nigra and in the caudate nucleus," *European Journal of Neuroscience*, vol. 22, no. 2, pp. 419–424, 2005.

[18] A. Nagy, G. Eördegh, Z. Paróczy, Z. Márkus, and G. Benedek, "Multisensory integration in the basal ganglia," *European Journal of Neuroscience*, vol. 24, no. 3, pp. 917–924, 2006.

[19] D. Noy, S. Mouta, J. Lamas, D. Basso, C. Silva, and J. A. Santos, "Audiovisual integration increases the intentional step synchronization of side-by-side walkers," *Human Movement Science*, vol. 56, pp. 71–87, 2017.

[20] R. A. Stevenson, J. K. Fister, Z. P. Barnett, A. R. Nidiffer, and M. T. Wallace, "Interactions between the spatial and temporal stimulus factors that influence multisensory integration in human performance," *Experimental Brain Research*, vol. 219, no. 1, pp. 121–137, 2012.

[21] A. R. Nidiffer, R. A. Stevenson, J. K. Fister, Z. P. Barnett, and M. T. Wallace, "Interactions between space and effectiveness in human multisensory performance," *Neuropsychologia*, vol. 88, pp. 83–91, 2016.

[22] T. J. Swick, "Parkinson's disease and sleep/wake disturbances," *Parkinson's Disease*, vol. 2012, Article ID 205471, 14 pages, 2012.

[23] M. J. Thorpy and C. H. Adler, "Parkinson's disease and sleep," *Neurologic Clinics*, vol. 23, no. 4, pp. 1187–1208, 2005.

[24] C. A. Davie, "A review of Parkinson's disease," *British Medical Bulletin*, vol. 86, no. 1, pp. 109–127, 2008.

[25] K. Suzuki, M. Miyamoto, T. Miyamoto, and K. Hirata, "Parkinson's disease and sleep/wake disturbances," *Current Neurology and Neuroscience Reports*, vol. 15, no. 3, pp. 1–11, 2015.

[26] Y. Ren, W. Yang, K. Nakahashi, S. takahashi, and J. Wu, "Audiovisual integration delayed by stimulus onset asynchrony between auditory and visual stimuli in older adults," *Perception*, vol. 46, no. 2, pp. 205–218, 2016.

[27] Y. Ren, *Study on Audiovisual Integration in Healthy Elderly and Parkinson Patients*, Okayama University, Okayama, Japan, 2017.

[28] A. J. Hughes, S. E. Daniel, L. Kilford, and A. J. Lees, "Accuracy of clinical diagnosis of idiopathic Parkinson's disease: a clinico-pathological study of 100 cases," *Journal of Neurology, Neurosurgery and Psychiatry*, vol. 55, no. 3, pp. 181–184, 1992.

[29] Y. Fujiwara, H. Suzuki, M. Yasunaga et al., "Brief screening tool for mild cognitive impairment in older Japanese: validation of the Japanese version of the montreal cognitive assessment," *Geriatrics and Gerontology International*, vol. 10, no. 3, pp. 225–232, 2010.

[30] K. Suzuki, M. Miyamoto, T. Miyamoto et al., "Nocturnal disturbances and restlessness in Parkinson's disease: using the Japanese version of the Parkinson's disease sleep scale-2,"

Journal of the Neurological Sciences, vol. 318, no. 1, pp. 76–81, 2012.

[31] M. Takegami, Y. Suzukamo, T. Wakita et al., "Development of a Japanese version of the Epworth Sleepiness Scale (JESS) based on item response theory," *Sleep Medicine*, vol. 10, no. 5, pp. 556–565, 2009.

[32] M. W. Johns, "A new method for measuring daytime sleepiness: the Epworth sleepiness scale," *Sleep*, vol. 14, no. 6, pp. 540–545, 1991.

[33] Y. Doi, M. Minowa, M. Uchiyama et al., "Psychometric assessment of subjective sleep quality using the Japanese version of the Pittsburgh Sleep Quality Index (PSQI-J) in psychiatric disordered and control subjects," *Psychiatry Research*, vol. 97, no. 2, pp. 165–172, 2000.

[34] M. M. Hoehn and M. D. Yahr, "Parkinsonism: onset, progression, and mortality," *Neurology*, vol. 50, no. 2, p. 318, 1998.

[35] D. J. Buysse, C. F. Reynolds, T. H. Monk, S. R. Berman, and D. J. Kupfer, "The Pittsburgh sleep quality index: a new instrument for psychiatric practice and research," *Psychiatry Research*, vol. 28, no. 2, pp. 193–213, 1989.

[36] R. A. Stevenson, D. Ghose, J. K. Fister et al., "Identifying and quantifying multisensory integration: a tutorial review," *Brain Topography*, vol. 27, no. 6, pp. 707–730, 2014.

[37] B. Wang, J. Guo, T. Yan et al., "Neural responses to central and peripheral objects in the lateral occipital cortex," *Frontiers in Human Neuroscience*, vol. 10, no. 54, pp. 1–11, 2016.

[38] A. M. Meppelink, B. M. de Jong, R. Renken, K. L. Leenders, F. W. Cornelissen, and T. van Laar, "Impaired visual processing preceding image recognition in Parkinson's disease patients with visual hallucinations," *Brain*, vol. 132, no. 11, pp. 2980–2993, 2009.

[39] D. Cheng, A. M. Jenner, G. Shui et al., "Lipid pathway alterations in parkinson's disease primary visual cortex," *PLoS One*, vol. 6, no. 2, Article ID e17299, 2011.

[40] E. Macaluso, "Multisensory processing in sensory-specific cortical areas," *Neuroscientist*, vol. 12, no. 4, pp. 327–338, 2006.

[41] Y. Wang, S. Celebrini, Y. Trotter, and P. Barone, "Visuo-auditory interactions in the primary visual cortex of the behaving monkey: electrophysiological evidence," *BMC Neuroscience*, vol. 9, no. 1, p. 79, 2008.

[42] G. A. Calvert, R. Campbell, and M. J. Brammer, "Evidence from functional magnetic resonance imaging of crossmodal binding in the human heteromodal cortex," *Current Biology*, vol. 10, no. 11, pp. 649–657, 2000.

[43] Y. Ren, Y. Ren, W. Yang et al., "Comparison for younger and older adults: stimulus temporal asynchrony modulates audiovisual integration," *International Journal of Psychophysiology*, vol. 124, pp. 1–11, 2018.

[44] A. H. V. Schapira, K. R. Chaudhuri, and P. Jenner, "Non-motor features of Parkinson disease," *Nature Reviews Neuroscience*, vol. 18, no. 7, pp. 435–450, 2017.

[45] J. A. Obeso, M. C. Rodríguez-Oroz, B. Benitez-Temino et al., "Functional organization of the basal ganglia: therapeutic implications for Parkinson's disease," *Movement Disorders*, vol. 23, no. S3, pp. S548–S559, 2008.

[46] D. Talsma, T. J. Doty, and M. G. Woldorff, "Selective attention and audiovisual integration: is attending to both modalities a prerequisite for early integration?," *Cerebral Cortex*, vol. 17, no. 3, pp. 679–690, 2007.

[47] D. Talsma, D. Senkowski, and M. G. Woldorff, "Intermodal attention affects the processing of the temporal alignment of audiovisual stimuli," *Experimental Brain Research*, vol. 198, no. 2-3, pp. 313–328, 2009.

[48] D. Talsma, D. Senkowski, S. Soto-Faraco, and M. G. Woldorff, "The multifaceted interplay between attention and multisensory integration," *Trends in Cognitive Sciences*, vol. 14, no. 9, pp. 400–410, 2010.

[49] S. Zhou, X. Chen, C. Wang, C. Yin, P. Hu, and K. Wang, "Selective attention deficits in early and moderate stage Parkinson's disease," *Neuroscience Letters*, vol. 509, no. 1, pp. 50–55, 2012.

[50] C. Pauletti, D. Mannarelli, M. C. De Lucia et al., "Selective attentional deficit in essential tremor: evidence from the attention network test," *Parkinsonism and Related Disorders*, vol. 21, no. 11, pp. 1306–1311, 2015.

[51] P. Vieregge, R. Verleger, E. Wascher, F. Stüven, and D. Kömpf, "Auditory selective attention is impaired in Parkinson's disease—event-related evidence from EEG potentials," *Cognitive Brain Research*, vol. 2, no. 2, pp. 117–129, 1994.

[52] M. Sharpe, "Auditory attention in early Parkinson's disease: an impairment in focused attention," *Neuropsychologia*, vol. 30, no. 1, pp. 101–106, 1992.

[53] K. Flowers and C. Robertson, "The effect of Parkinson's disease on the ability to maintain a mental set," *Journal of Neurology, Neurosurgery and Psychiatry*, vol. 48, no. 6, pp. 517–529, 1985.

[54] A. Hozumi, K. Hirata, H. Tanaka, and K. Yamazaki, "Perseveration for novel stimuli in Parkinson's disease: an evaluation based on event-related potentials topography," *Movement Disorders*, vol. 15, no. 5, pp. 835–842, 2000.

[55] J. Wu, J. Yang, Y. Yu et al., "Delayed audiovisual integration of patients with mild cognitive impairment and Alzheimer's disease compared with normal aged controls," *Journal of Alzheimer's Disease*, vol. 32, no. 2, p. 317, 2012.

12

Can a Smartphone Diagnose Parkinson Disease? A Deep Neural Network Method and Telediagnosis System Implementation

Y. N. Zhang[1,2]

[1]*School of Computer Science and Technology, Beijing Institute of Technology, Beijing 100081, China*
[2]*College of Computer Science and Information Engineering, Tianjin University of Science and Technology, Tianjin 300222, China*

Correspondence should be addressed to Y. N. Zhang; zh.y.n@163.com

Academic Editor: Hélio Teive

Parkinson's disease (PD) is primarily diagnosed by clinical examinations, such as walking test, handwriting test, and MRI diagnostic. In this paper, we propose a machine learning based PD telediagnosis method for smartphone. Classification of PD using speech records is a challenging task owing to the fact that the classification accuracy is still lower than doctor-level. Here we demonstrate automatic classification of PD using time frequency features, stacked autoencoders (SAE), and K nearest neighbor (KNN) classifier. KNN classifier can produce promising classification results from useful representations which were learned by SAE. Empirical results show that the proposed method achieves better performance with all tested cases across classification tasks, demonstrating machine learning capable of classifying PD with a level of competence comparable to doctor. It concludes that a smartphone can therefore potentially provide low-cost PD diagnostic care. This paper also gives an implementation on browser/server system and reports the running time cost. Both advantages and disadvantages of the proposed telediagnosis system are discussed.

1. Introduction

Parkinson's disease (PD) is a disorder of brain nervous system which can cause partial or full loss in movement, behavior, and mental processing, especially speech function [1]. Generally, PD can be observed in elderly people and causes disorders in speech [2]. At present, about 1% of the worldwide population over the age of fifty is suffering from PD [3]. Until now, many effective methods and medicines [4–6] are invented for relieving the symptoms of PD. Therefore, an early-diagnosis in time and available treatment can improve the prognosis of PD [7]. However, many patients diagnosed with PD are later found which resulted in delays in patient condition [8]. Moreover, many patients with Parkinson's disease in the community still remain undiagnosed and more patients get worse because of poor medical conditions in low income areas [9].

Even though many clinical examinations and diagnostic to PD have been proposed [10–14], it is important that we should exert more effort in automated diagnosis and telediagnosis [15] in real world. In the research of Esteva et al. [16], they deduced that billions of smartphones have the potential to provide medical care for skin cancer diagnosis. Inspired by this novel idea, a smartphone also has the potential to diagnose PD. Many clinical reports reveal that the dysphonic indicator is an important reference index in diagnosis [17]. Therefore, our method is based on the study of vocal impairment symptoms (dysphonia) (90% of people with PD have such symptom) [18].

The purpose of this research is to design a machine learning based telediagnosis PD system for patients by using a smartphone. We found that deep neural network [19] with K nearest neighbor (KNN) [20] method can achieve better performance on available speech datasets than other comparative methods. Not only is the proposed telediagnosis system compared with other researchers' methods, but also the running time cost is tested in browser/server system. To conclude, the contribution of this paper includes (1) achieving high performance and (2) proposing a feasible implementation with empirical test.

This paper is organized as follows: in Section 2, background and related works are presented. In Section 3, the proposed method and telediagnosis system are described.

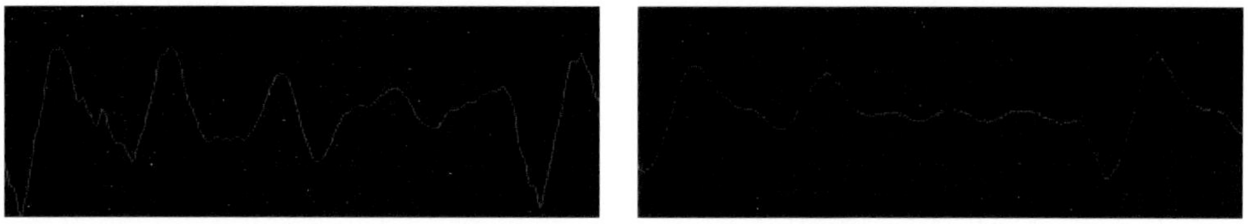

(a) Waveform of people with PD (b) Waveform of healthy people

FIGURE 1: Waveform of voice records from Istanbul University [21, 22] (x-axis: time duration, y-axis: amplitude of the signal).

Section 4 shows the experimental results. Conclusions are drawn in Section 5.

2. Background and Related Works

2.1. Parkinson's Disease and Speech Disorders. Many researchers have exerted much effort on PD in their researches. In 2006, Rao et al. [23] discussed diagnosis and treatment for PD. The author insisted that psychosis is usually drug induced; further it can be managed initially by reducing antiparkinsonian medications. Jankovic and Aguilar [24] reviewed approaches to the treatment of PD and the authors think that the new treatments are not necessarily better than the established conventional therapy and that the treatment options must be individualized and tailored to the needs of each individual patient. In 2010, Varanese et al. [25] showed treatment of advanced PD, and the research paper concluded that supportive care, including physical and rehabilitative interventions, speech therapy, occupational therapy, and nursing care, has a key role in the late stage of disease. Yitayeh and Teshome [26] reviewed the effectiveness of physiotherapy treatment on balance dysfunction and postural instability in persons with Parkinson's disease and the author also presented meta-analysis results, in 2016.

So far, it has been reported that of the 89% of PD patients with voice and speech disorders [27, 28], the reduced speech ability to communicate is considered to be one of the most important aspects of PD by many patients [29]. The common perceptual features of reduced loudness (hypophonia), reduced pitch variation (monotone), breathy and hoarse voice quality, and imprecise articulation [30], together with lessened facial expression (masked faces), contribute to limitations in communication in the majority of people with PD [31].

Figure 1 shows the comparison of waveforms between people with PD and healthy people. Intuitively, it can be observed that the waveform of healthy people is smooth and continuous, but the waveform of people with PD contains unexpected vibrations. The reason for this phenomenon is that the people with PD lose the ability of precise muscle control [32–34]. The vibrations can be detected by time frequency analysis; moreover machine learning based audio analysis methods are appropriate for diagnosing PD.

2.2. Machine Learning for Parkinson's Disease Diagnostic Care. Many researchers had proposed effective methods based on machine learning in automated diagnosis research. In 2014, Shahbakhi et al. [43] proposed a method using genetic algorithm and support vector machine for analysis of speech for diagnosis of PD. Little et al. [44] used support vector machine (SVM) with Gaussian radical basis kernel to diagnose PD. Shahbaba and Neal [35] showed a nonlinear model for the PD classification which is based on Dirichlet mixtures. Sakar and Kursun [45] applied mutual information measure to combine with SVM. Those methods achieve high classification accuracy but telediagnosis PD needs a better method with higher classification performance.

Recently, deep neural networks have shown potentials in speech recognition tasks; the classification and recognition accuracy is superior to conventional machine learning method. We proposed a method using deep neural network (stacked autoencoders, SAE) to reduce dimensions and K nearest neighbor classifier to diagnose PD. We also implemented a telediagnosis system based on the proposed method. Results of empirical test on smartphone are presented in Section 4.

3. Methodology

3.1. Structure of PD Telediagnosis Method and System Structure. The proposed structure of the PD telediagnosis method is as shown in Figure 2. A patient provides personal information and speech records by following instructions of smartphone. The personal information includes gender, age, and a brief health history. Patient is also asked to read a given text; then the speech records of the patient are parsed to be time frequency based features which are extracted from the voice samples. After the processing of SAE and KNN, patient can receive the diagnosis result.

Figure 3 shows the workflow of the proposed method in the view of machine learning, an appropriate set of time frequency features, SAE, and classifier dictated diagnostic accuracy. Therefore, the most important work is how to build a high accuracy diagnostic method.

Figure 4 briefly illustrates the architecture of the proposed method on B/S (browser/server) structure and details are shown in Section 4.4. The server should be installed on an operation system. In next step, an appropriate version of web service software should be deployed on this server. Usually a smartphone embedded Internet browser software (such as Google Chrome App). Therefore the smartphone can send/receive data (text and voice records) to server by Internet browser. The connection between smartphone and server can be 2/3/4G mobile network or WIFI. The server receives and processes audio files as Figures 1 and 2 present. Result of

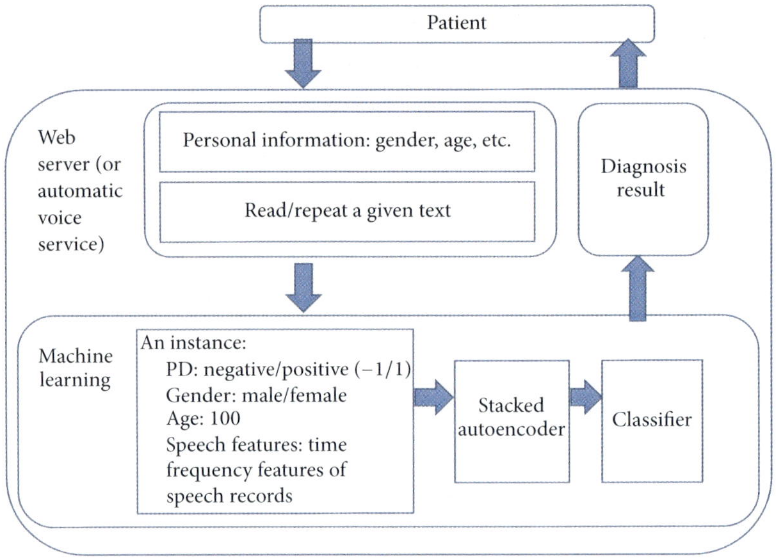

FIGURE 2: Acquisition and diagnosis of PD telediagnosis method.

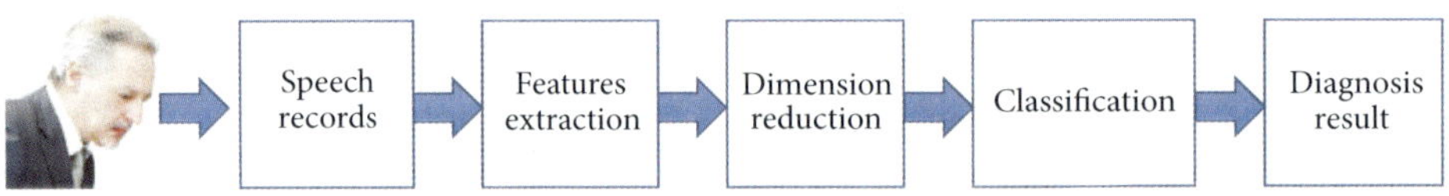

FIGURE 3: Workflow of the proposed method.

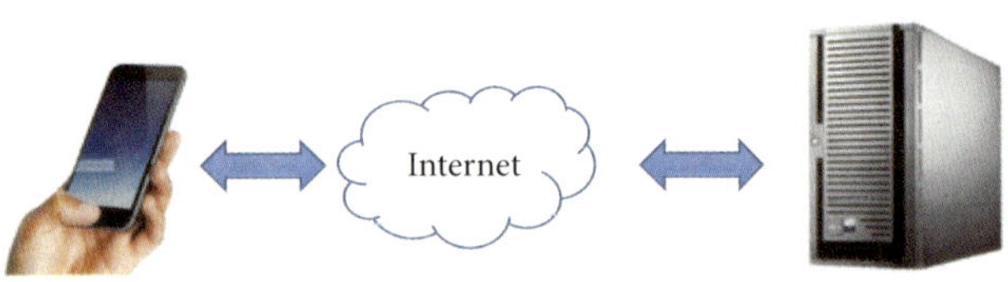

FIGURE 4: B/S (browser/server) structure.

PD diagnosis will be displayed on patient's smartphone. This B/S structure is not limited to smartphone, but it is suitable for other electronic devices too, such as iPad, notebook, and even a smart watch. Moreover, the automated voice service system (such as banks' telephone services) should fulfill the same task as B/S structure theoretically.

3.2. Speech Features. Dysphonia [17] is a typical speech problem of people with PD. Dysphonia is a human vocal problem which includes five major clinical features: loudness, decrease, breathiness, roughness, and exaggerated vocal tremor in voice. All those indications can be detected by analyzing time frequency in speech records. A set of 26 features is listed with the considering of the previous works held on this field of study [21, 46].

In Table 1, 6 types of parameters are listed; they are frequency parameters, pulse parameters, amplitude parameters, voicing parameters, pitch parameters, and harmonicity parameters. 26 features are also presented in Table 1.

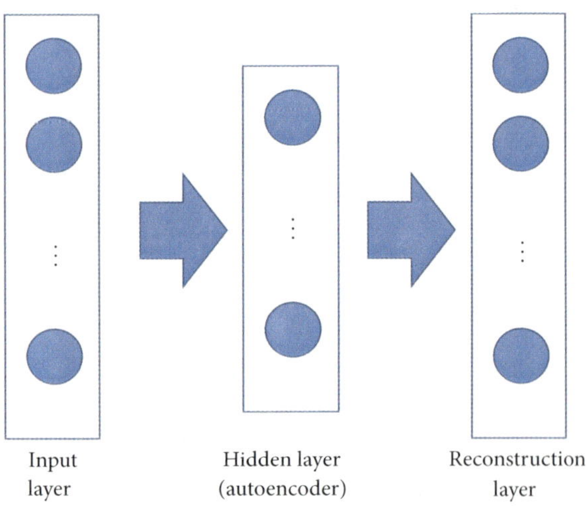

FIGURE 5: Autoencoder.

3.3. Stacked Autoencoders. Autoencoder [47] has been wildly used in unsupervised feature learning and speech recognition tasks. It can be built as a special three-layer neural network: the input layer, the hidden layer, and the reconstruction layer (as shown in Figure 5).

An autoencoder has two parts: (1) The encoder receives an input $x_0 \in R^{d0}$ to the hidden layer (latent representation feature) $x_1 \in R^{d1}$ via a mapping f_{encoder}:

$$x_1 = f_{\text{encoder}}(x_0) = s_{\text{encoder}}(W_1^T x_0 + b_1), \quad (1)$$

Table 1: Time frequency features.

Parameter type	Features
Frequency	Jitter (local)
Parameters	Jitter (rap)
(Number of features: 5)	Jitter (local, absolute)
	Jitter (ppq5)
	Jitter (ddp)
Harmonicity	Autocorrelation
Parameters	Noise-to-harmonic
(Number of features: 3)	Harmonic-to-noise
Pulse	Number of pulses
Parameters	Mean period
(Number of features: 4)	Number of periods
	Standard dev. of period
Amplitude	Shimmer (local)
Parameters	Shimmer (apq3)
	Shimmer (local, dB)
(Number of features: 6)	Shimmer (apq5)
	Shimmer (dda)
	Shimmer (apq11)
Pitch	Median pitch
Parameters	Mean pitch
	Minimum pitch
(Number of features: 5)	Maximum pitch
	Standard deviations
Voicing	Fraction of locally
Parameters	unvoiced frames
(Number of features: 4)	Number of voice breaks
	Degree of voice breaks
Types: 6	Total features: 26

where s_{encoder} is the activation function, whose input is called the activation of the hidden layer, and $\{W_1, b_1\}$ is the parameter set with a weight matrix $W_1 \in R^{d0*d1}$ and a bias value vector $b_1 \in R^{d1}$.

(2) The decoder maps the hidden representation x_1 back to reconstruction $x_2 \in R^{d0}$ via mapping function f_{decoder}:

$$x_2 = f_{\text{decoder}}(x_1) = s_{\text{decoder}}\left(W_2^T x_1 + b_2\right). \quad (2)$$

s_{decoder} is the activation function of the decoder with parameters $\{W_2, b_2\}$, $W_2 \in R^{d1*d0}$, $b_2 \in R^{d0}$. The input of s_{decoder} is defined as the activation of the reconstruction layer. Parameters are learned through backpropagation by minimizing the loss $L(x_0, x_2)$:

$$L(x_0, x_2) = L_r(x_0, x_2) + 0.5\varepsilon\left(\|W_1\|_2^2 + \|W_2\|_2^2\right) \quad (3)$$

In (3), $L(x_0, x_2)$ consists of the reconstruction error L_r and the L_2 regularization of W_1 and W_2. By minimizing the reconstruction error L_r, the hidden feature should be able to reconstruct the original input x_0 as much as possible.

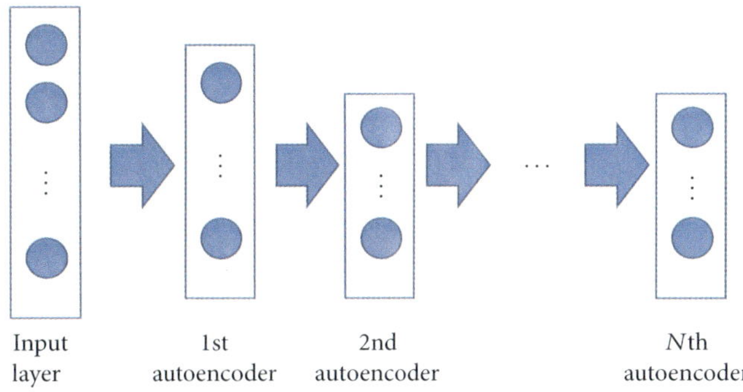

Figure 6: Stacked autoencoders.

The stacked autoencoders (SAE) [48] are multiple layers of autoencoders. They are a deep learning approach for dimensionality reduction and feature learning. As Figure 6 shows, there are n autoencoders which are trained one by one. The input vectors are fed to the first autoencoder. After finishing training the first autoencoder, the output hidden representation is propagated to the second auto layer. A typical activation function is sigmoid function which is used for activation functions s_{encoder} and s_{decoder}. After this pretraining stage, the whole SAE is fine-tuned [48] based on a predefined objective. The last hidden layer of the SAE encoder can further cooperate with other applications, such as SVM for classification task.

3.4. KNN Classifier. The KNN [49] classifier is quite simple: given a speech record of undiagnosed patient s, the system finds the K nearest neighbors to give diagnosis result. Formally, the decision rule can be written as

$$\text{score}(s, c_i) = \sum_{S_j \in \text{KNN}(S)} \text{Sum}\left(S, S_j\right)\delta\left(S_j, c_i\right). \quad (4)$$

Above, KNN(S) indicates the set of K nearest neighbors of speech records S. $\delta(S, c_i)$ is the classification for undiagnosed patient s with respect to class c_i, and

$$\delta(s, c_i) = \begin{cases} 1 & s \in c_i \\ -1 & s \notin c_i. \end{cases} \quad (5)$$

For undiagnosed patient, the patient could be given diagnosis result. K of KNN is 1 in this paper.

4. Experimental Results

4.1. Speech Datasets, Evaluation Criteria, and Classifiers. For comparison, we chose two research papers [21, 50] and the PD speech datasets they had used. We use Matlab as programming tool and all classification algorithms are determined by grid search method.

In the first paper, Sakar et al. [21] collected a speech dataset of diagnosis of PD and donated this speech dataset to UCI machine learning group for other researchers. This speech dataset contains a training set file, a testing set file, and a ZIP package of WMA files. Betul Erdogdu Sakar et al.

TABLE 2: Confusion matrix.

	Prediction as people with PD	Prediction as healthy people
Actual people with PD	True positive (TP)	False negative (FN)
Actual healthy people	False positive (FP)	True negative (TN)

designed a novel speech test; PD patients were asked to say only the sustained vowels "a" and "o" three times. Their work of speech dataset collection was finished at Istanbul University and we call the dataset "Istanbul Dataset" in the following experiments.

In the second paper, Ma et al. [50] proposed a kernel extreme learning machine with subtractive clustering features weighting approach. Their method compared with 15 researches' methods. Total 16 methods are compared in their research paper, and the method of Ma et al. gained top position. The dataset of their research was created by Little et al. [44] of the University of Oxford, in collaboration with the National Centre for Voice and Speech, Denver, Colorado, who recorded the speech signals. We call the dataset "Oxford Dataset" in the following experiments.

Accuracy, sensitivity, and other performance indexes are compared among those classifiers and these performance indexes are defined as follows:

$$\text{Accuracy} = \frac{\text{TP} + \text{TN}}{\text{TP} + \text{FP} + \text{TN} + \text{FN}}. \quad (6)$$

Sensitivity:

$$\text{Sensitivity} = \frac{\text{TP}}{\text{P}} = \frac{\text{TP}}{\text{TP} + \text{FN}}. \quad (7)$$

Specificity:

$$\text{specificity} = \frac{\text{TN}}{\text{N}} = \frac{\text{TN}}{\text{FP} + \text{TN}}. \quad (8)$$

F-score:

$$F\text{-score} = \frac{2\text{TP}}{2\text{TP} + \text{FP} + \text{FN}}. \quad (9)$$

MCC:

$$\text{MCC} = \frac{\text{TP} * \text{TN} - \text{FP} * \text{FN}}{\sqrt{(\text{TP} + \text{FP}) * (\text{TP} + \text{FN}) * (\text{TN} + \text{FP}) * (\text{TN} + \text{FN})}}, \quad (10)$$

where TP, FP, TN, and FN are the true and false positive and true and false negative classifications of a classifier and they are defined as shown in Table 2.

Involved classifiers are kernel extreme learning machine (KELM), Linear Support Vector Machine (LSVM), Multilayer perceptrons Support Vector Machine (MSVM), Radial basis function Support Vector Machine (RSVM), Classification and Regression Tree (CART), KNN, Linear Discriminant Analysis (LDA), and Naive Bayesian (NB) method.

TABLE 3: Results of comparative classifiers without SAE on Oxford Dataset.

Classifier	Classification accuracy (%)	Max	Mean	Min
KELM	ACC	83.23	71.32	68.49
LSVM	ACC	81.05	64.21	44.21
MSVM	ACC	84.21	61.98	43.16
RSVM	ACC	85.26	74.34	69.47
CART	ACC	89.47	73.95	58.95
KNN	ACC	**90.53**	**82.76**	**76.84**
LDA	ACC	87.37	69.61	53.68
NB	ACC	75.79	69.74	61.05

4.2. Experiment Results: Oxford Dataset and Algorithm Parameters. The Oxford Dataset [22, 46] consisted of voice measurements from 31 people and 23 of them were diagnosed with PD. There are total 195 samples comparing 147 PD and 48 healthy samples in the dataset. There are no missing values in the Oxford Dataset and each feature is real type value. The whole 22 features are contained in Table 1.

The SAE of the proposed method has two hidden layer: layer 1 and layer 2. The size of layer 1 is set as 10, 9, or 8 neurons and the size of layer 2 is set as 8, 7, or 6 neurons. The batch size of SAE is 20 in training and fine tuning step. All comparative classifiers are optimized by grid search method. We use 50-50% training-testing method as Polat [40] and Daliri [39] did. This experiment method tests comparative approaches with much less training data than 10-fold cross validation. Each classifier was tested 10 times and the results are presented in tables.

4.2.1. Classifiers without Deep Neural Network on Oxford Dataset. Table 3 summarized the detailed results of classification accuracy after 10 runs. From this table, it can be found that the classification performance of KNN is apparently differential. We can see that the KNN outperforms that with other 7 classifiers with a max, mean, and min accuracy of 90.53%, 82.76%, and 76.84%. All comparative classifiers give low classification results because the input samples are 22-dimensional data.

4.2.2. Classifiers with Deep Neural Network on Oxford Dataset. Tables 4 and 5 presented the comparison result of the classification accuracy and other performance indexes. Table 4 lists details of accuracy. For SAE, the influence of two layers in dimension reduction has been investigated. In this study, two hidden layers are tested as a subgrid search. As seen from Table 4, 1NN classifier gives more correct diagnosis results than other methods.

Comparing Tables 3 and 4, other 7 classifiers gave more correct classification result with the using of SAE (hidden layer 1 contains 9 neurons; hidden layer 2 contains 7 neutrons). KELM has obtained max classification accuracy as 98.81%; it is 16% higher than 82.23% in Table 3. LSVM gives 96.71% classification accuracy after dimensional reduction by SAE 8-7. In SAE 10-7 row, MSVM increased 11% in terms

Table 4: Results of comparative classifiers with SAE on Oxford Dataset.

Classification accuracy (%)		Classifiers							
		KELM	LSVM	MSVM	RSVM	CART	KNN	LDA	NB
SAE 10-8	Max	93.45	99.99	99.90	99.90	99.90	100.00	99.69	99.19
	Mean	77.74	95.89	94.47	96.32	96.04	**97.81**	95.17	94.29
	Min	66.67	93.66	89.23	93.43	93.81	93.23	92.85	93.73
SAE 10-7	Max	96.43	100.00	98.46	100.00	100.00	100.00	99.60	99.58
	Mean	80.18	96.20	95.76	96.58	96.82	**97.63**	96.16	95.22
	Min	63.69	94.13	93.46	93.52	94.53	94.52	93.01	93.61
SAE 10-6	Max	89.29	100.00	99.81	99.99	100.00	100.00	99.73	99.15
	Mean	71.73	96.26	94.74	96.51	96.43	**96.97**	94.59	95.18
	Min	45.83	93.74	89.13	93.51	94.64	93.22	91.37	93.62
SAE 9-8	Max	90.48	100.00	97.40	100.00	99.99	100.00	99.70	99.71
	Mean	78.27	95.87	95.04	96.87	96.87	**97.89**	96.08	95.12
	Min	56.55	92.36	89.04	93.99	94.24	92.70	92.71	93.54
SAE 9-7	Max	93.45	100.00	98.17	100.00	100.00	100.00	99.74	98.74
	Mean	80.77	96.23	93.88	**97.75**	96.82	97.13	97.01	95.82
	Min	65.48	94.22	89.04	93.59	94.49	93.14	93.28	93.93
SAE 9-6	Max	98.81	100.00	99.71	100.00	100.00	100.00	99.66	99.36
	Mean	84.59	96.22	95.63	96.46	96.01	**98.01**	94.03	95.51
	Min	70.83	93.31	90.58	94.16	94.30	93.26	93.55	93.94
SAE 8-8	Max	93.45	100.00	99.52	99.99	100.00	100.00	99.58	99.51
	Mean	76.61	96.02	95.39	95.64	96.22	**96.98**	95.45	94.32
	Min	55.95	94.19	92.21	93.37	94.36	92.75	93.75	92.25
SAE 8-7	Max	98.81	100.00	99.62	100.00	100.00	100.00	99.76	99.79
	Mean	84.23	96.71	95.48	96.82	96.23	96.63	95.69	**97.07**
	Min	70.83	94.40	92.21	93.92	94.57	94.10	92.99	94.14
SAE 8-6	Max	91.07	100.00	99.42	99.99	99.99	100.00	99.78	99.37
	Mean	78.22	96.01	94.52	96.21	95.91	**96.92**	95.57	95.98
	Min	57.74	93.37	90.87	93.59	92.53	93.42	93.44	92.49

of classification accuracy. RSVM gives 97.75% classification accuracy in the row of SAE 9-7. Similarly, CART produced average classification accuracy as 96% when applying SAE. LDA and NB also have got better performance than without using SAE; the classification accuracy of those 7 classifiers are improved by 10–15% with the using of SAE.

4.3. Experiment Results: Istanbul Dataset and Parameters Settings. The Istanbul University built a PD database. This database consists of training and test files. The training data belongs to 20 people with PD (6 females, 14 males) and 20 healthy individuals (10 females, 10 males) who participate in the PD database project at the Department of Neurology in Cerrahpasa Faculty of Medicine, Istanbul University. From all subjects, multiple types of sound recordings (26 voice samples including sustained vowels, numbers, words, and short sentences) are taken. A group of 26 linear and time frequency based features are extracted from each voice sample. Those features are presented in Section 3.2, as Table 2 shows.

28 PD patients are asked to say only the sustained vowels "a" and "o" three times, respectively, which makes a total of 168 recordings. The same 26 features are extracted from voice samples of this dataset. The researchers of the Istanbul University declared that [22] the PD dataset can be used as an independent test set to validate the results obtained on training set. The training file contains 1040 recordings and the testing file contains 168 files. Therefore, we used the training file and testing file to compare the proposed method with other methods.

The SAE of the proposed method has two hidden layer: layer 1 and layer 2. Layer 1 is set as 10, 9, or 8 neurons and layer 2 is set as 8, 7, or 6 neurons. The batch size of SAE is 20 in training and fine tuning step.

4.3.1. Classifiers without Deep Neural Network on Istanbul Dataset. Table 6 summarized the results of classification accuracy. According to the declaration of Istanbul University, fixed training set and testing set are given. Only one run will obtain final result. From this table, it can be found that the classification performance of RSVM is apparently differential. We can see that the RSVM outperforms that with other 7 classifiers with a classification accuracy of 76.41%. All comparative classifiers give low classification results because the input samples are 26-dimensional data. The Naive Bayesian method gives worst result among all classifiers.

TABLE 5: Performance indexes of comparative classifiers with SAE on Oxford Dataset *(average of 10 runs)*.

Performance indexes		Classifiers							
		KELM	LSVM	MSVM	RSVM	CART	KNN	LDA	NB
SAE 10-8	Specificity	0.2083	0.0889	0.0816	0.8148	0.7302	**0.9565**	0.4872	0.0286
	Sensitivity	0.0423	0.7	0.2174	0.3824	0.0625	**0.9306**	0.1429	0.2
	F-score	0.0645	0.5556	0.198	0.5253	0.0784	**0.9571**	0.1905	0.102
	MCC	−0.7719	−0.2635	−0.7095	0.1897	−0.245	**0.8425**	−0.3992	−0.8053
SAE 10-7	Specificity	0.3455	0.2794	0.3421	0.3256	0.7273	**0.9710**	0.6667	0.8571
	Sensitivity	0.775	0.7407	0.7193	0.7692	0.5616	**0.9231**	0.5581	0.7778
	F-score	0.5794	0.4167	0.6667	0.6612	0.6833	**0.9231**	0.7007	0.6512
	MCC	0.1304	0.0204	0.0653	0.1058	0.2438	**0.8941**	0.132	0.565
SAE 10-6	Specificity	0.5714	0.3387	0.7273	0.2581	**0.8621**	0.7432	0.0556	0.8806
	Sensitivity	0.5672	0.9091	0.7581	0.9375	0.3939	0.9048	0.0779	**0.9286**
	F-score	0.6496	0.5769	0.7966	0.8163	0.5417	0.6441	0.1200	**0.8387**
	MCC	0.1266	0.2715	0.4698	0.276	0.2536	0.5489	−0.7927	**0.7696**
SAE 9-8	Specificity	0.4462	0.2000	0.0274	0.1207	0.4615	**0.6066**	0.2500	0.6316
	Sensitivity	0.8333	**0.9091**	0.3182	0.3243	0.1829	0.8235	0.2069	0.7368
	F-score	0.5495	0.7299	0.1400	0.2400	0.2885	**0.6512**	0.3243	0.6437
	MCC	0.271	0.1567	−0.7202	−0.5726	−0.2897	**0.4142**	−0.3471	0.3612
SAE 9-7	Specificity	0.2597	0.125	0.0455	0.3667	0.4000	**0.9492**	0.4792	0.2917
	Sensitivity	0.0556	0.4366	0.2192	0.2857	0.6222	0.5000	0.2766	**0.7447**
	F-score	0.0263	0.5041	0.2909	0.2410	**0.7517**	0.6316	0.3059	0.6034
	MCC	−0.5503	−0.3827	−0.6362	−0.3354	0.0102	**0.5251**	−0.2493	0.0408
SAE 9-6	Specificity	0.8929	0.8462	0.0606	0.7857	0.3404	**0.9500**	0.0879	0.9241
	Sensitivity	0.7612	0.2558	0.0484	0.0256	0.7500	**0.8182**	0.2500	0.5000
	F-score	0.8430	0.3548	0.0625	0.0385	0.6261	**0.8824**	0.0227	0.5333
	MCC	0.6021	0.1269	−0.8850	−0.2700	0.0992	**0.7586**	−0.4156	0.4477
SAE 8-8	Specificity	0.1522	**1.0000**	0.9286	0.2683	0.8409	0.9889	0.6111	0.3542
	Sensitivity	0.1429	0.7647	0.5373	0.6111	0.5490	0.6000	**0.9870**	0.234
	F-score	0.1474	0.8667	0.6857	0.5641	0.6512	0.6667	**0.9500**	0.2472
	MCC	−0.705	**0.8529**	0.4336	−0.1264	0.4031	0.6548	0.7056	−0.4146
SAE 8-7	Specificity	0.7222	0.7500	0.3529	0.7500	0.1600	**0.9808**	0.2188	0.4118
	Sensitivity	**0.7805**	0.1205	0.0769	0.011	0.3143	0.7442	0.1290	0.4103
	F-score	0.7273	0.2083	0.1263	0.0215	0.3894	**0.8421**	0.0941	0.5333
	MCC	0.4980	−0.1252	−0.5701	−0.3344	−0.4651	**0.7579**	−0.6174	−0.1374
SAE 8-6	Specificity	0.8462	0.1333	0.375	0.125	0.2414	0.0308	**0.9231**	0.557
	Sensitivity	0.3415	0.6000	0.5057	0.7419	0.3333	0.1667	**0.7857**	0.6875
	F-score	0.5000	0.6809	0.6471	0.4182	0.4000	0.1020	**0.8544**	0.3548
	MCC	0.1387	−0.2028	−0.0663	−0.1667	−0.3928	−0.8271	**0.6974**	0.1831

TABLE 6: Results of comparative classifiers without SAE on Istanbul Dataset.

Classifier	Classification accuracy (%)	Value
KELM	ACC	57.83
L-SVM	ACC	39.88
M-SVM	ACC	75.60
R-SVM	ACC	**76.41**
CART	ACC	50.00
KNN	ACC	55.95
LDA	ACC	57.28
NB	ACC	30.95

4.3.2. Classifiers with Deep Neural Network on Istanbul Dataset. Tables 7 and 8 presented the comparison result of the classification accuracy and other 4 performance indexes. Table 7 lists details of classification accuracy. To SAE, two hidden layers are set as Oxford Dataset experiment. As seen from Table 6, KNN classifier gives more correct diagnosis results than other methods. The max, mean, and min classification accuracy of KNN classifier are not affected by network structure of SAE.

Comparing Tables 6 and 5, the other 7 classifiers gave more correct classification result with the using of SAE. And LSVM, RSVM, and CART show much more stability in classification accuracy. But KELM still did not obtain

TABLE 7: Results of comparative classifiers with SAE on Istanbul Dataset.

Classification accuracy (%)		Classifiers							
		KELM	LSVM	MSVM	RSVM	CART	KNN	LDA	NB
SAE 10-8	Max	93.45	100.00	99.90	100.00	100.00	100.00	100.00	100.00
	Mean	77.74	67.83	88.03	79.90	91.58	93.45	83.93	81.97
	Min	66.67	57.08	77.20	74.24	71.74	89.23	75.95	80.31
SAE 10-7	Max	96.43	100.00	98.46	100.00	100.00	100.00	100.00	100.00
	Mean	80.18	67.73	88.24	80.48	91.25	93.99	83.88	82.59
	Min	63.69	56.34	76.80	74.47	72.31	89.59	76.37	79.80
SAE 10-6	Max	89.29	100.00	99.81	100.00	100.00	100.00	100.00	99.90
	Mean	71.73	67.36	88.18	80.65	91.73	93.72	84.70	82.09
	Min	45.83	56.79	77.01	73.72	72.45	90.06	76.60	79.70
SAE 9-8	Max	90.48	100.00	97.40	100.00	100.00	100.00	99.81	100.00
	Mean	78.27	67.90	88.63	80.57	91.55	93.98	84.39	82.29
	Min	56.55	56.87	77.10	73.92	72.23	89.82	76.32	80.27
SAE 9-7	Max	93.45	100.00	98.17	100.00	100.00	100.00	99.90	99.71
	Mean	80.77	67.85	88.67	79.76	91.19	94.17	84.35	81.88
	Min	65.48	56.45	76.98	74.04	72.07	90.21	76.11	79.73
SAE 9-6	Max	98.81	100.00	99.71	100.00	100.00	100.00	100.00	100.00
	Mean	84.59	67.67	88.50	80.36	91.17	93.78	84.69	82.02
	Min	70.83	57.01	77.62	74.04	71.94	90.13	75.89	79.68
SAE 8-8	Max	93.45	100.00	99.52	100.00	100.00	100.00	99.81	100.00
	Mean	76.61	67.96	88.47	80.08	91.14	94.10	84.23	81.89
	Min	55.95	57.24	76.72	74.21	72.29	89.31	75.76	80.40
SAE 8-7	Max	98.81	100.00	99.62	100.00	100.00	100.00	100.00	100.00
	Mean	84.23	68.27	87.92	80.34	91.56	94.35	84.55	82.08
	Min	70.83	57.12	77.17	73.95	72.61	89.87	76.26	79.74
SAE 8-6	Max	91.07	100.00	99.42	100.00	100.00	100.00	100.00	100.00
	Mean	78.22	67.49	87.85	79.89	91.01	93.81	84.24	81.75
	Min	57.74	56.62	76.69	73.82	71.88	90.05	75.80	80.05

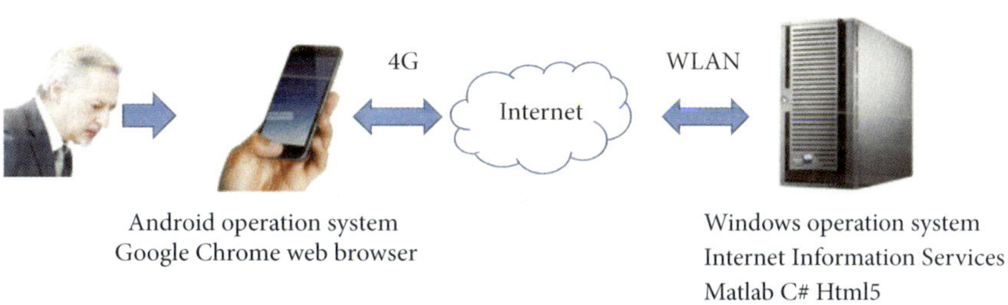

FIGURE 7: Implementation of the proposed system.

100.00% classification accuracy, Table 6. LSVM gives 92.00% classification accuracy after dimensional reduction by SAE 9-7. In SAE 10-7, SAE10-6, and SAE 9-6 row, LSVM did not give perfect performance. MSVM, LDA, and NB increased classification accuracy but still lack stability. In conclusion, every classifier has got better performance than without using SAE.

4.4. Implementation on B/S System. As Figure 7 shows, our smartphone is running Android system and it was installed from Google Chrome web browser. The server installed Windows operation system and Internet Information Services. We also installed Matlab 2016a and Visual Studio 2013 on this server. Programming techniques contain Matlab, C#, and HTML5.

We used Chrome to connect server via 4G mobile network in the street; we send 28 test speech records (WMA files) of Istanbul Dataset; a transmission of 12.1 MB data took less than 5 seconds to our laboratory. The server received speech records and ran the empirical experiments as Sections 4.2 and 4.3 present. No more than 2 minutes, results of all comparative classifiers were displayed on our smartphone. We also recorded our speech (as healthy samples) and send it to server for testing, but it should be noticed that a

TABLE 8: Performance indexes of comparative classifiers without SAE on Istanbul Dataset (average values of 10 runs).

Performance indexes		Classifiers							
		KELM	LSVM	MSVM	RSVM	CART	KNN	LDA	NB
SAE 10-8	Specificity	0.4474	0.7445	0.6667	0.8429	0.3684	0.8000	0.8904	0.8807
	Sensitivity	0.8692	0.3548	0.9149	0.5714	0.9799	0.9412	0.8000	0.6949
	F-score	0.8561	0.2857	0.9247	0.4848	0.9511	0.9600	0.8492	0.7257
	MCC	0.3297	0.0864	0.5577	0.369	0.4662	0.6391	0.6845	0.5884
SAE 10-7	Specificity	0.9551	0.9259	0.8046	0.5263	0.9231	0.9537	0.886	0.8193
	Sensitivity	0.6203	0.4368	0.963	0.8389	0.9052	0.9000	0.7222	0.8235
	F-score	0.7424	0.5802	0.8864	0.8834	0.9333	0.9076	0.7358	0.8235
	MCC	0.6179	0.4122	0.7737	0.2879	0.8021	0.8569	0.6144	0.6428
SAE 10-6	Specificity	0.7958	0.2545	0.9714	0.8397	0.9593	0.9275	0.8875	0.8293
	Sensitivity	0.2692	0.8761	0.7302	0.3333	0.800	0.9394	0.8068	0.7778
	F-score	0.2258	0.7826	0.8214	0.1951	0.8372	0.9442	0.8452	0.6931
	MCC	0.0573	0.1645	0.7473	0.1179	0.7829	0.8651	0.6943	0.5703
SAE 9-8	Specificity	0.9848	0.6842	0.9107	0.0909	0.9595	0.9375	0.9778	0.9067
	Sensitivity	0.0278	0.6712	0.8661	0.9110	0.5500	0.9318	0.7886	0.1111
	F-score	0.0513	0.6447	0.9065	0.8896	0.5946	0.9371	0.8778	0.1176
	MCC	0.0391	0.3530	0.7498	0.0022	0.5471	0.8689	0.6884	0.0187
SAE 9-7	Specificity	0.8874	0.5326	0.9063	0.8584	0.9478	0.9263	0.783	0.4706
	Sensitivity	0.0588	0.8421	0.8750	0.6545	0.7647	0.9589	0.9355	0.8543
	F-score	0.0571	0.6995	0.9225	0.6729	0.7761	0.9333	0.8112	0.8927
	MCC	−0.0524	0.3878	0.688	0.5207	0.7205	0.8807	0.6939	0.2558
SAE 9-6	Specificity	0.2778	0.7050	0.9764	0.7265	0.9833	0.9469	0.8257	1
	Sensitivity	0.9133	0.5172	0.5854	0.9804	0.8704	0.9091	0.8814	0.6517
	F-score	0.9133	0.3529	0.7059	0.7519	0.9261	0.9009	0.8000	0.7891
	MCC	0.1911	0.1782	0.657	0.6502	0.8252	0.8521	0.6832	0.6841
SAE 8-8	Specificity	0.7956	0.6964	0.8909	0.8500	0.65	0.9845	0.5714	0.7538
	Sensitivity	0.6129	0.6429	0.3333	0.7813	0.9459	0.7949	0.9098	0.8544
	F-score	0.4872	0.5714	0.0909	0.8547	0.9492	0.8611	0.8996	0.8502
	MCC	0.3530	0.3244	0.0938	0.5572	0.5836	0.8282	0.4977	0.6100
SAE 8-7	Specificity	0.7830	0.8455	0.7273	0.947	0.9292	0.9130	0.6792	0.9766
	Sensitivity	0.9355	0.2222	0.9111	0.2500	0.8727	0.9508	0.9217	0.3000
	F-score	0.8112	0.2703	0.9213	0.3462	0.8649	0.9587	0.8908	0.4364
	MCC	0.6939	0.0794	0.6181	0.2753	0.7983	0.8527	0.6307	0.4131
SAE 8-6	Specificity	0.9813	0.4468	0.9894	0.8165	0.9826	0.9048	0.8397	0.7300
	Sensitivity	0.4262	0.7603	0.7297	0.7627	0.7358	0.9841	0.8333	0.9412
	F-score	0.5843	0.7699	0.8372	0.7258	0.8298	0.9185	0.4255	0.8050
	MCC	0.5259	0.2034	0.7608	0.5677	0.7773	0.8696	0.4268	0.6612

quite environment is necessary. It is hard to achieve satisfied classification accuracy in a noisy circumstance.

4.5. Discussions and Future Work. Table 9 summarized the comparative results achieved from related researches. It can be seen that the proposed method achieves better results than other methods and our method shows a relatively fewer training samples. The reduced training dataset is meaningful when applying the proposed method in reality. The performance of SAE and KNN is robust to number of hidden neutrons of deep neural network.

We focus on classification accuracy, sensitivity, and other performance indexes to evaluate machine learning based PD diagnosis method; then we choose a B/S structure to test the proposed architecture. Advantages contain time saving, being convenient, and low cost. But we did not achieve 100% correct classification accuracy on smartphone. We deduced that there are still potential problems: (1) a good enough microphone should be taken into consideration. (2) Speech denoising may be fulfilled by multiple microphones. (3) An evolutionary system can overcome big testing data in real world. The future investigation will pay much attention on an evolutionary telediagnosis PD system and solve above issues. Moreover, we also noticed that two public datasets cannot guarantee that a machine learning based telediagnosis system can be trained very well and it is hard to satisfy hospitals,

Table 9: Comparative experiment results.

Related researches	Test method	Classification accuracy (%)	Training set
Shahbaba and Neal [35]	5-fold CV	87.70	80%
Psorakis et al. [36]	10-fold CV	89.47	90%
Guo et al. [37]	10-fold CV	93.10	90%
Ozcift and Gulten [38]	10-fold CV	87.10	90%
Daliri [39]	50-50% training-testing	91.20	**50%**
Polat [40]	50-50% training-testing	97.93	**50%**
Chen et al. [41]	10-fold CV	96.07	90%
Zuo et al. [42]	10-fold CV	97.47	90%
Rao et al. [23]	10-fold CV	99.49	90%
This study	50-50% training-testing	94.00–98.00	**50%**

clinics, and other medical institutions. And the stability and robustness of a telediagnosis system still need to be built urgently.

5. Conclusion

For building a convenient and feasible telediagnosis PD service via smartphone, we proposed a machine learning based method on browser/server architecture. In this paper, the proposed method contains stacked autoencoders and KNN classifier which is used to process speech records. The proposed method can remap time frequency features in low dimensional space. Results show that the proposed method with KNN classifier can give doctor-level classification results on public PD speech records. An experimental system is also built for testing; it is projected that telediagnosis of PD on a smartphone will be in the future.

References

[1] C. Marigliani, S. Gates, and D. Jacks, "Speech Pathology and Parkinson's Disease," in *Parkinson's Disease: A Team Approach*, M. S. Morris and R. N. Iansek, Eds., Melbourne, Australia, Buscombe Vicprint, 1997.

[2] N. Miller, E. Noble, D. Jones, and D. Burn, "Life with communication changes in Parkinson's disease," *Age and Ageing*, vol. 35, no. 3, pp. 235–239, 2006.

[3] G. F. Wooten, L. J. Currie, V. E. Bovbjerg, J. K. Lee, and J. Patrie, "Are men at greater risk for Parkinsons disease than women?" *Journal of Neurology, Neurosurgery & Psychiatry*, vol. 75, no. 4, pp. 637–639, 2004.

[4] J. M. Savitt, V. L. Dawson, and T. M. Dawson, "Diagnosis and treatment of Parkinson disease: molecules to medicine," *Journal of Clinical Investigation*, vol. 116, no. 7, pp. 1744–1754, 2006.

[5] Y. Wang, C.-L. Xie, L. Lu, D.-L. Fu, and G.-Q. Zheng, "Chinese herbal medicine paratherapy for Parkinson's disease: a meta-analysis of 19 randomized controlled trials," *Evidence-based Complementary and Alternative Medicine*, vol. 2012, Article ID 534861, 15 pages, 2012.

[6] W. Pan, S. Kwak, Y. Liu et al., "Traditional chinese medicine improves activities of daily living in parkinson's disease," *Parkinson's Disease*, vol. 2011, Article ID 789506, 7 pages, 2011.

[7] A. J. Lees, "Early diagnosis of Parkinson's disease," *British Journal of Hospital Medicine*, vol. 26, no. 5, pp. 511–518, 1981.

[8] D. P. Breen, J. R. Evans, K. Farrell, C. Brayne, and R. A. Barker, "Determinants of delayed diagnosis in Parkinson's disease," *Journal of Neurology*, vol. 260, no. 8, pp. 1978–1981, 2013.

[9] E. Cassani, M. Barichella, R. Cilia et al., "Simple and low-cost mucuna pruriens preparation for Parkinson's disease patients in low-income countries," *Journal of the Neurological Sciences*, vol. 357, 2015.

[10] G. Rizzo, M. Copetti, S. Arcuti, D. Martino, A. Fontana, and G. Logroscino, "Accuracy of clinical diagnosis of Parkinson disease," *Neurology*, vol. 86, no. 6, pp. 566–576, 2016.

[11] J. Jankovic, "Parkinson's disease: clinical features and diagnosis," *Journal of Neurology, Neurosurgery and Psychiatry*, vol. 79, no. 4, pp. 368–376, 2008.

[12] E. Tolosa, G. Wenning, and W. Poewe, "The diagnosis of Parkinson's disease," *Lancet Neurology*, vol. 5, no. 1, pp. 75–86, 2006.

[13] A. J. Hughes, Y. Ben-Shlomo, S. E. Daniel, and A. J. Lees, "What features improve the accuracy of clinical diagnosis in Parkinson's disease: a clinicopathologic study," *Neurology*, vol. 42, no. 6, pp. 1142–1146, 1992.

[14] M. Emre, D. Aarsland, R. Brown et al., "Clinical diagnostic criteria for dementia associated with Parkinson's disease," *Movement Disorders*, vol. 22, no. 12, pp. 1689–1707, 2007.

[15] H. Ozkan, "A comparison of classification methods for telediagnosis of Parkinson's disease," *Entropy*, vol. 18, no. 4, article 115, 2016.

[16] A. Esteva, B. Kuprel, R. A. Novoa et al., "Dermatologist-level classification of skin cancer with deep neural networks," *Nature*, vol. 542, no. 7639, pp. 115–118, 2017.

[17] G. K. Sewall, J. Jiang, and C. N. Ford, "Clinical evaluation of Parkinson's-related dysphonia," *Laryngoscope*, vol. 116, no. 10, pp. 1740–1744, 2006.

[18] W. S. Schley, E. Fenton, and S. Niimi, "Vocal symptoms in parkinson disease treated with levodopa: a case report," *Annals of Otology, Rhinology & Laryngology*, vol. 91, no. 1, pp. 119–121, 1982.

[19] A. De Brébisson and G. Montana, "Deep neural networks for anatomical brain segmentation," in *Proceedings of the IEEE Conference on Computer Vision and Pattern Recognition Workshops, CVPRW 2015*, pp. 20–28, June 2015.

[20] M.-L. Zhang and Z.-H. Zhou, "ML-KNN: a lazy learning approach to multi-label learning," *Pattern Recognition*, vol. 40, no. 7, pp. 2038–2048, 2007.

[21] B. E. Sakar, M. E. Isenkul, C. O. Sakar et al., "Collection and analysis of a Parkinson speech dataset with multiple types of sound recordings," *IEEE Journal of Biomedical and Health Informatics*, vol. 17, no. 4, pp. 828–834, 2013.

[22] http://archive.ics.uci.edu/ml/datasets/.

[23] S. S. Rao, L. A. Hofmann, A. Shakil et al., "Parkinson's disease: diagnosis and treatment," *American Family Physician*, vol. 74, no. 12, pp. 2046–2055, 2006.

[24] J. Jankovic and L. G. Aguilar, "Current approaches to the treatment of Parkinson's disease," *Neuropsychiatric Disease and Treatment*, vol. 4, no. 4, pp. 743–757, 2008.

[25] S. Varanese, Z. Birnbaum, R. Rossi, and A. Di Rocco, "Treatment of advanced Parkinson's disease," *Parkinson's Disease*, vol. 2010, Article ID 480260, 9 pages, 2010.

[26] A. Yitayeh and A. Teshome, "The effectiveness of physiotherapy treatment on balance dysfunction and postural instability in persons with Parkinson's disease: a systematic review and meta-analysis," *Sports Medicine, Arthroscopy, Rehabilitation, Therapy & Technology*, vol. 8, no. 1, 2016.

[27] L. Hartelins and P. Svensson, "Speech and swallowing symptoms associated with parkinson's disease and multiple sclerosis: a survey," *Folia Phoniatrica et Logopaedica*, vol. 46, no. 1, pp. 9–17, 1994.

[28] M. Oxtoby, *Parkinson's Disease People and Their Social Needs*, Parkinsons Disease Society, London, UK, 1982.

[29] R. A. Cools, D. V. Jh, W. M. Horstink et al., "Parkinson's disease: a reduced ability to shift to a new grouping if not prompted or guided," *Movement Disorders*, vol. 5, no. 2, 1990.

[30] J. Rusz, R. Cmejla, T. Tykalova et al., "Imprecise vowel articulation as a potential early marker of Parkinson's disease: effect of speaking task," *Journal of the Acoustical Society of America*, vol. 134, no. 3, pp. 2171–2181, 2013.

[31] B. Murdoch, T. Whitehill, M. De Letter, and H. Jones, "Communication impairments in parkinson's disease," *Parkinson's Disease*, vol. 2011, Article ID 234657, 2 pages, 2011.

[32] O. Blin, C. Desnuelle, O. Rascol et al., "Mitochondrial respiratory failure in skeletal muscle from patients with Parkinson's disease and multiple system atrophy," *Journal of the Neurological Sciences*, vol. 125, no. 1, pp. 95–101, 1994.

[33] S. Salenius, S. Avikainen, S. Kaakkola, R. Hari, and P. Brown, "Defective cortical drive to muscle in Parkinson's disease and its improvement with levodopa," *Brain*, vol. 125, no. 3, pp. 491–500, 2002.

[34] G. A. Fontana, T. Pantaleo, F. Lavorini, F. Benvenuti, and S. Gangemi, "Defective motor control of coughing in Parkinson's disease," *American Journal of Respiratory and Critical Care Medicine*, vol. 158, no. 2, pp. 458–464, 1998.

[35] B. Shahbaba and R. Neal, "Nonlinear models using Dirichlet process mixtures," *Journal of Machine Learning Research*, vol. 10, pp. 1829–1850, 2009.

[36] I. Psorakis, T. Damoulas, and M. A. Girolami, "Multiclass relevance vector machines: sparsity and accuracy," *IEEE Transactions on Neural Networks*, vol. 21, no. 10, pp. 1588–1598, 2010.

[37] P.-F. Guo, P. Bhattacharya, and N. Kharma, "Advances in detecting Parkinson's disease," in *Medical Biometrics*, vol. 6165 of *Lecture Notes in Computer Science*, pp. 306–314, Springer, Berlin, Germany, 2010.

[38] A. Ozcift and A. Gulten, "Classifier ensemble construction with rotation forest to improve medical diagnosis performance of machine learning algorithms," *Computer Methods and Programs in Biomedicine*, vol. 104, no. 3, pp. 443–451, 2011.

[39] M. R. Daliri, "Chi-square distance kernel of the gaits for the diagnosis of Parkinson's disease," *Biomedical Signal Processing and Control*, vol. 8, no. 1, pp. 66–70, 2013.

[40] K. Polat, "Classification of Parkinson's disease using feature weighting method on the basis of fuzzy C-means clustering," *International Journal of Systems Science*, vol. 43, no. 4, pp. 597–609, 2012.

[41] H.-L. Chen, C.-C. Huang, and X.-G. Yu, "An efficient diagnosis system for detection of Parkinson's disease using fuzzy *k*-nearest neighbor approach," *Expert Systems with Applications*, vol. 40, no. 1, pp. 263–271, 2013.

[42] W.-L. Zuo, Z.-Y. Wang, T. Liu, and H.-L. Chen, "Effective detection of Parkinson's disease using an adaptive fuzzy *k*-nearest neighbor approach," *Biomedical Signal Processing and Control*, vol. 8, no. 4, pp. 364–373, 2013.

[43] M. Shahbakhi, D. T. Far, and E. Tahami, "Speech analysis for diagnosis of parkinson's disease using genetic algorithm and support vector machine," *Journal of Biomedical Science and Engineering*, vol. 07, no. 04, pp. 147–156, 2014.

[44] M. A. Little, P. E. McSharry, E. J. Hunter, J. Spielman, and L. O. Ramig, "Suitability of dysphonia measurements for telemonitoring of Parkinson's disease," *IEEE Transactions on Biomedical Engineering*, vol. 56, no. 4, pp. 1015–1022, 2009.

[45] C. O. Sakar and O. Kursun, "Telediagnosis of parkinson's disease using measurements of dysphonia," *Journal of Medical Systems*, vol. 34, no. 4, pp. 591–599, 2010.

[46] M. A. Little, P. E. McSharry, S. J. Roberts, D. A. E. Costello, and I. M. Moroz, "Exploiting nonlinear recurrence and fractal scaling properties for voice disorder detection," *BioMedical Engineering Online*, vol. 6, article 23, 2007.

[47] Y. Wang, H. Yao, and S. Zhao, "Auto-encoder based dimensionality reduction," *Neurocomputing*, vol. 184, pp. 232–242, 2016.

[48] H.-I. Suk, S.-W. Lee, and D. Shen, "Latent feature representation with stacked auto-encoder for AD/MCI diagnosis," *Brain Structure and Function*, vol. 220, no. 2, pp. 841–859, 2015.

[49] Y. Huang and Y. Li, "Prediction of protein subcellular locations using fuzzy k-NN method," *Bioinformatics*, vol. 20, no. 1, pp. 21–28, 2004.

[50] C. Ma, J. Ouyang, H.-L. Chen, and X.-H. Zhao, "An efficient diagnosis system for Parkinson's disease using kernel-based extreme learning machine with subtractive clustering features weighting approach," *Computational and Mathematical Methods in Medicine*, vol. 2014, Article ID 985789, 14 pages, 2014.

13

CLOCK 3111T/C Variant Correlates with Motor Fluctuation and Sleep Disorders in Chinese Patients with Parkinson's Disease

Fan Lou,[1] Ming Li,[2] Xiaoguang Luo,[1] and Yan Ren[1]

[1]*Department of Neurology, First Affiliated Hospital of China Medical University, Shenyang, Liaoning, China*
[2]*Department of Neurology, The Fourth Affiliated Hospital of China Medical University, Shenyang, Liaoning, China*

Correspondence should be addressed to Yan Ren; renyan0411@163.com

Academic Editor: Joanne Trinh

Background. The clock genes controlling biological rhythm play an important role in the pathophysiology of aging. The purpose of this study was to determine whether there is an association between a variant of the circadian locomotor output cycles kaput (CLOCK) gene and circadian dysfunction of Parkinson's disease (PD). *Methods.* Six hundred and forty-six cases of Parkinson's disease from consecutive outpatients and inpatients ward from our hospital were included in this study. Kompetitive allele-specific PCR was used to determine the frequency distribution of genotypes and alleles. The examinations for the PD group were assessed in person in order to evaluate motor symptoms, cognitive function, sleep, and depression, including the Unified Parkinson's Disease Rating Scale (UPDRS), Mini-Mental State Examination (MMSE), Pittsburgh Sleep Quality Index (PSQI), and 17-item Hamilton Rating Scale for Depression (HAMD-17). *Results.* Motor fluctuation ($P < 0.001$) and sleep disorders ($P = 0.007$) were significantly different between the two groups. These correlations persisted after adjusting for confounding risk factors by further binary logistic regression analysis, suggesting that the CLOCK 3111T/C variant was associated with motor fluctuation (OR = 1.080, $P < 0.001$) and a subjective sleep disorder (OR = 1.130, $P = 0.037$). *Conclusion.* The CLOCK 3111T/C variant can be an independent risk factor for motor fluctuation and sleep disorder in Parkinson's disease.

1. Background

Parkinson's disease (PD) is a degenerative neurological disorder characterized by the loss of dopaminergic neurons in the substantia nigra. It is generally believed that the interaction between multiple genes and environmental factors contributes to an extremely complicated mechanism of PD [1]. Symptoms of circadian dysfunction are the typical symptoms of neurodegenerative diseases, such as Alzheimer's disease (AD) and PD [2–4]. Impaired circadian function in PD is implicated not only in impaired sleep and alertness but also in autonomic, behavior, mood, and fluctuating motor manifestations [5]. The daily life of patients with PD can be beset by circadian dysfunction, which may be more severe than motor symptoms alone and can become a heavy burden on the family.

The biological rhythm of the human body is regulated by the circadian system. Many physical activities are controlled by the circadian clock, such as the sleep-awake cycle, blood pressure, heart rate, respiration, temperature, visceral activity, immunity, neuroendocrine activity, cell division, and even DNA function. Recently, the clock genes that regulate the circadian rhythm in both the central and peripheral oscillators, located in the suprachiasmatic nucleus, including CLOCK (circadian locomotor output cycles kaput), BMAL1, Period (Per), and Cryptochrome (Cry) genes, have aroused the interest of many researchers [6]. Among those genes, CLOCK is the key gene that regulates the circadian rhythm in the brain and periphery, which can modulate the dopamine synthesis [7]. The 3111T/C is located in the 3′-untranslated region of the CLOCK gene, with a T→C transversion, which has previously been found to be associated with psychobehavioral control, hormone secretion, mood, and sleep [8, 9]. Recently, polymorphisms of some related clock genes have been reported to be associated with the circadian rhythm disturbances of PD [10, 11]. In a previous study, a significant association with CLOCK 3111T/C in the dominant model in PD was observed, when compared to that of the controls. This suggests that the circadian rhythm gene can be considered to promote the pathophysiology of PD [12]. However, current knowledge regarding the relationship between circadian dysfunction in PD and the CLOCK gene variant is scarce.

Studies on the relationship between a single-nucleotide polymorphism of clock genes and circadian dysfunctions of PD may provide more insight into the genetics of motor and nonmotor symptoms of PD. Therefore, in the present study, we examined the association between a polymorphism of the CLOCK gene with symptoms of circadian dysfunction in PD in a northeastern Chinese population using a retrospective case study.

2. Methods

2.1. Subjects. The present study included 646 patients with PD who were from an unrelated Chinese population in the northeastern provinces of China. The patients were recruited from the movement disorder clinic and inpatient ward of the Department of Neurology, the First Affiliated Hospital of China Medical University, Shenyang, China, from May 2010 to October 2015. The diagnosis of PD was made based on the UK PD Brain Bank Criteria by movement disorder neurologists [13]. Ages of the all participants ranged from 36 to 88 years. All patients underwent the Mini-Mental State Examination (MMSE). We excluded those whose score fell below 20 for individuals who received 6 years of schooling or less (primary school education) and below 24 for individuals who received more than 6 years of schooling (junior and above). Patients with Parkinsonism-plus and those who worked shift work were also excluded. All patients provided their written informed consent. The Ethics Committee of China Medical University approved the study. Demographic data were collected for all patients with PD.

2.2. Evaluation. We completed the following standard assessment measures when patients had not taken levodopa or other PD medications for at least 12 h (the "off state"):

(1) Hoehn and Yahr staging was used for determining the stage of the disease.

(2) Severity of Parkinsonism was evaluated using the Unified Parkinson's Disease Rating Scale (UPDRS) II + III, and the tremor, postural, and gait instability scores were further calculated according to the report from Kang et al. [14].

(3) Depression was determined by a score ≥8 on the 17-item Hamilton Rating Scale for Depression (HAMD-17).

(4) The motor fluctuation of the PD group was determined by a score of >1 on item 39 from the UPDRS IV [15].

(5) A subjective sleep disorder in the PD group was determined by a Pittsburgh Sleep Quality Index (PSQI) ≥ 7 [16].

(6) Orthostatic hypotension was determined by a decrease in the systolic blood pressure > 20 mmHg or a decrease in the diastolic pressure > 10 mmHg, accompanied by the symptoms of hypoperfusion, such as dizziness, within 3 minutes of moving into the upright position.

(7) Dyskinesia was determined using the total score of items 32 to 35 from the UPDRS IV.

2.3. DNA Extraction and Genotyping. Genomic DNA was extracted from leukocytes using the sodium dodecyl sulfate-proteinase K phenol-chloroform method. DNA purity was assessed by spectrophotometry, and DNA samples were stored at −20°C. Genotypes were determined using the Kompetitive allele-specific PCR (KASP) assay [17]. Each amplification reaction contained 50 ng/μl of template DNA, KASP 2x Master Mix standard ROX (LGC Genomics, UK), and KASP-by-Design assay mix (LGC Genomics, UK). For the allele-specific amplification of CLOCK gene 3111T/C, the primers (including forward primers marked by FAM and HEX) were 5′GAAGGTGACCAAGTTCATGCTAAAAC-ACTGTCAGAACTGGCTG3′ and 5′GAAGGTCGGAGT-CAACGGATTCCTAAAACACTGTCAGAACTGGCTA3′. During PCR, the thermocycling conditions of all the primers were 15 min at 94°C, followed by 10 cycles of 94°C for 20 s and 61°C for 1 min (dropping −0.6°C per cycle to achieve a 55°C annealing temperature), followed by 26 cycles of 94°C for 20 s and 55°C for 1 min. After amplification, PCR plates were read with a SpectraMax M5 FRET capable plate reader (LGC Genomics, UK) using the recommended excitation and emission values. Data were subsequently analyzed using KlusterCaller software (LGC Genomics, UK) to identify single-nucleotide polymorphism genotypes.

2.4. Statistical Analysis. The continuous variables are presented as mean ± SD and categorical variables as percentages. Differences of the continuous variables were evaluated by the Student's *t*-test, depending on the shape of the distribution curves. Categorical variables were compared using the χ^2 test. All genotype frequencies were checked using the Hardy-Weinberg analysis in two groups through the χ^2 test [18]. Differences in the distributions of the alleles and genotypes between the cases and controls were analyzed using the χ^2 test. The association between the CLOCK gene polymorphisms and circadian dysfunctions of PD was estimated by computing the odds ratios (ORs) and 95% confidence intervals (CIs) from a binary logistic regression analysis using the backward-stepwise method. The statistical analyses were performed using SPSS version 20.0 (IBM, USA) with the limit of significance set at $P < 0.05$ (two-tailed).

3. Results

We identified the CLOCK T3111C variant in 124 of 646 patients with PD, including the TC and CC genotypes, in a northeastern Chinese population, and we found a significant difference between patients with PD and the healthy controls in the dominant model [12]. Therefore, in order to further explore the clinical characteristics of the patients with variant, we divided the patients into the following two

TABLE 1: Demographic data and clinical profiles of carriers and noncarriers.

	CLOCK 3111T/C carriers (TC + CC) $n = 124$	CLOCK 3111T/C noncarriers (TT) $n = 522$	P value
Age (years)	62.35 ± 10.19	61.70 ± 10.13	0.515
Sex (%)	53 (42.7)	263 (50.4)	0.126
Onset age (years)	58.52 ± 10.33	58.02 ± 10.79	0.645
EOPD (%)	12 (9.7)	26 (5.0)	0.046^a
Disease duration (years)	3.90 ± 3.18	3.74 ± 3.04	0.550
Family history (%)	7 (5.6)	31 (5.9)	0.987
Formal education (years)	9.47 ± 3.38	9.63 ± 3.65	0.657
Hoehn-Yahr stage	1.84 ± 0.78	1.74 ± 0.73	0.165
UPDRS II + III	41.81 ± 19.73	40.26 ± 19.04	0.417
Mean tremor score	4.27 ± 4.19	4.00 ± 3.79	0.476
Mean PIGD score	7.71 ± 5.26	8.02 ± 5.25	0.691
Motor fluctuation	1.93 ± 1.88	0.83 ± 1.41	0.000^b
Dyskinesia	0.33 ± 0.94	0.25 ± 1.03	0.453
L-dopa therapy initial dosage (mg/day)	148.7 ± 38.86	154.6 ± 41.12	0.215
L-dopa therapy duration (year)	3.22 ± 2.57	2.95 ± 2.80	0.071
Good response to levodopa	107 (86.3)	474 (90.8)	0.133
MMSE	25.23 ± 3.51	25.37 ± 3.32	0.682
Sleep disorder (%)	48 (38.7)	138 (26.4)	0.007^a
Depression	10.26 ± 3.67	8.88 ± 3.73	0.183
Orthostatic hypotension (%)	16 (12.9)	69 (13.2)	0.926

The χ^2 square test was used to compare the categorical variables. Data are expressed as numbers with percentages in parentheses or as mean ± SE. UPDRS: Unified Parkinson's Disease Rating Scale; MMSE: Mini-Mental State Examination; EOPD: early-onset PD; PIGD: postural instability and gait difficulty. $^aP < 0.05$ and $^bP < 0.01$.

groups: T3111C variant carriers (TC and CC genotypes) and noncarriers (TT genotype). We compared the 124 carriers and 522 noncarrier patients using a complete set of clinical data. The demographic data and clinical profiles of the 3111T/C carriers and noncarriers are shown in Table 1. There were no significant differences in age, sex, course of diseases, years of education, Hoehn-Yahr stage, or severity of motor symptoms (UPDRS II + III) between the carriers and noncarriers ($P > 0.05$), indicating that the two groups were comparable.

As shown in Table 1, our study showed that the 3111T/C variant carriers scored significantly higher in motor fluctuation subitems than the noncarriers (1.93 ± 1.88 versus 0.83 ± 1.41, $P < 0.001$) did and also had more subjective sleep disorders (38.7% versus 26.4%, $P = 0.007$). We defined the onset age as the age at which the initial symptom appeared in confirmed patients. We defined early-onset PD (EOPD) as patients whose onset age was ≦50 years. The carriers had a significantly higher frequency of EOPD than the noncarriers (9.7% versus 5.0%, $P = 0.046$). However, no differences in dyskinesia, depression, or orthostatic hypotension were found between the carriers and the noncarriers ($P > 0.05$).

In order to further confirm the association between the gene variant and motor fluctuation and exclude other potential factors, binary logistic regression was used to examine the relationship. As shown in Table 2, after adjusting for age, disease duration, Hoehn–Yahr stage, impact of levodopa therapy, and EOPD, three variables, including the 3111T/C variant ($P < 0.001$), UPDRS II + III ($P < 0.001$), and Hoehn-Yahr stage ($P = 0.044$), were significantly associated with motor fluctuation in the logistic regression. These results showed that a polymorphism of CLOCK 3111T/C can be an independent risk factor for motor fluctuation (OR = 1.080, 95% CI = 1.057–1.104, $P < 0.001$). Similarly, as illustrated in Table 3, subjective sleep disorder was associated with a polymorphism of CLOCK 3111T/C ($P = 0.037$), UPDRS II + III ($P < 0.001$), and depression ($P < 0.001$). This showed that a polymorphism of CLOCK 3111T/C can be an independent risk factor for the sleep disorder in Parkinson's disease (OR = 1.130, 95% CI = 1.007–1.2689, $P = 0.037$).

4. Discussion

PD is multifactorial with many features exhibiting diurnal fluctuations, such as thermoregulation disorders, circadian variation of blood pressure and heart rate, emotional dysregulation, and even reactions to anti-PD pharmacotherapy that manifest as abnormalities in rhythm [3, 19–23]. Particularly, motor activity can vary throughout the day [24]. Recently, increasing studies show that these circadian rhythm dysfunctions of neurodegenerative disorders are associated with the abnormal regulation of clock genes [2, 4].

In the current study, we examined the association of a polymorphism of CLOCK gene with symptoms of circadian dysfunction in PD in a northeastern Chinese population using a retrospective case study. We found that 3111T/C variant carriers scored significantly higher than noncarriers in motor fluctuation, a subitem of UPDRS. Normal motor activity gradually increased during the

TABLE 2: Binary logistic regression of association between motor fluctuation and CLOCK 3111T/C variant.

Variable	OR	95% CI	P value
3111T/C variant	1.080	1.057–1.104	0.000[a]
Age (years)	0.645	0.202–2.067	0.461
Gender	0.962	0.649–1.424	0.845
Disease duration (years)	1.656	0.508–5.395	0.403
Hoehn-Yahr stage	0.940	0.885–0.998	0.044[b]
UPDRS II + III	4.698	2.868–7.695	0.000[a]
L-dopa therapy duration (year)	0.884	0.885–0.998	0.440
L-dopa therapy initial dosage (mg/day)	1.179	0.961–1.558	0.115
Response to levodopa	0.884	0.780–1.002	0.053
Mean PIGD score	1.002	0.945–1.062	0.957
EOPD	0.911	0.662–1.252	0.565

UPDRS: Unified Parkinson's Disease Rating Scale; MMSE: Mini-Mental State Examination; EOPD: early-onset PD. [a]$P < 0.01$ and [b]$P < 0.05$.

TABLE 3: Binary logistic regression of association between sleep disorders and CLOCK 3111T/C variant.

Variable	OR	95% CI	P value
3111T/C variant	1.130	1.007–1.268	0.037[a]
Age (years)	1.008	0.989–1.028	0.407
Gender	1.348	0.905–2.008	0.142
Disease duration (years)	1.039	0.971–1.111	0.266
Hoehn-Yahr stage	1.098	0.795–1.516	0.571
UPDRS II + III	1.044	1.022–1.066	0.000[b]
Mean PIGD score	0.976	0.917–1.038	0.443
Depression	3.872	2.455–6.135	0.000[b]
Response to levodopa	1.044	0.986–1.106	0.141

UPDRS: Unified Parkinson's Disease Rating Scale; MMSE: Mini-Mental State Examination. [a]$P < 0.05$ and [b]$P < 0.01$.

daytime and reached the lowest level at night. However, the rhythm is modified in patients with PD, and motor fluctuation is very common [25]. Motor fluctuation is considered to be associated with a longer disease progression and higher levodopa daily dose [26]. In our research, there were no differences in the initial dosage of levodopa and the levodopa therapy duration between the two groups ($P > 0.05$), which is consistent with the results from other studies [20, 27]. Therefore, we inferred that the main influencing factors of motor fluctuation could be attributed to the gene variant rather than the long-term effects of levodopa. In order to exclude the impact of related factors, we performed a logistical analysis. After adjusting for probable risk factors, such as age, sex, disease duration, severity of disease, and impact of levodopa therapy, motor fluctuation was still related to the 3111T/C variant and the risk of motor fluctuation of carriers was 1.077 times that of noncarriers, which shows that motor fluctuation may be associated with the variant of the CLOCK gene in the circadian system. Many studies found that fluctuations in motor activity may be caused by the circadian system. Boulamery found that rhythmic changes induced by lesions in unilateral 6-OHDA PD animal model, which has a loss of circadian rhythmicity, had reduced locomotor activity [28]. Other studies found that exposure to light or administration of the melatonin receptor antagonist facilitates recovery of motor function in chronic experimental models of PD [29, 30]. There is increasing evidence for the existence of interactions between the circadian rhythm and dopamine system and the modulation of dopamine synthesis by circadian genes. The CLOCK gene can regulate the transcription of tyrosine hydroxylase [31], which is the rate-limiting enzyme for dopamine synthesis. CLOCK can also affect the dopaminergic activity at the posttranscriptional level, which leads to the motor fluctuations [32]. Above all, our results indicate that patients with PD who are CLOCK 3111T/C variant carriers are more susceptible to the development of motor fluctuation than their wild-type counterparts.

Our study also found that since the 3111T/C variant carriers scored significantly higher than the noncarriers on the PQSI, carriers were associated with a higher risk of subjective sleep disorder when compared to that of the noncarriers. Numerous studies show that the polymorphism of CLOCK 3111T/C is associated with sleep disturbance in human beings, which could affect diurnal behavior pattern [33, 34]. Disturbed sleep-wake cycles are common nonmotor manifestations of PD, affecting up to 90% of the patients. It is suggested that the etiology of sleep disorders in PD depends on the adverse effects of antiparkinsonian medications and primary neurodegeneration of central sleep regulatory areas [35, 36]. We also found that patients with PD who have the CLOCK gene variant are more susceptible to the development of sleep disorders after adjusting for impact factors related to sleep, such as depression, severity of motor symptoms, age, sex, and disease duration. Therefore, we further confirmed that the polymorphism of CLOCK 3111T/C can be an independent risk factor for sleep disorders in PD. We also found that the proportion of patients with EOPD in the carrier group was significantly higher than that in the noncarrier group. This may reveal that the 3111T/C variant may play a role in lowering the onset age of PD and needs to be confirmed by further research.

In previous studies, different researchers have found that the polymorphism of CLOCK 3111T/C is associated with psychiatric disorders [37, 38]. Hua et al. [10] found that a polymorphism of Tef, which is a downstream regulatory gene of CLOCK, is associated with the depression of PD in Chinese population. Although in our study we found no statistical significant difference between the two groups in depression, a tendency could be found, which warrants further research. However, with regard to the other symptoms of circadian rhythm disorders, such as dyskinesia, orthostatic hypotension, and response to levodopa, no differences were found between the two groups. Different results may be attributed to the different loci of clock genes, sample size, different regions and nations, and different statistical methods.

Although the circadian timing controls the temporal patterning of molecular, cellular, and physiological processes throughout the body and the potential disruption of this timing system in PD would be expected to produce widespread symptoms [6], there is little known about the mechanism of the variant of clock genes leading to circadian dysfunctions in PD. However, pharmacotherapeutics and behavior pattern can intervene with pathological changes caused by circadian rhythm dysfunction [39]. Daily evening exposure to supplemental bright light improved sleep quality and mood, as well as bradykinesia and rigidity [40].

In conclusion, our results showed that the 3111T/C variant of CLOCK gene was closely related to the occurrence of motor fluctuation and sleep disorders in a northeastern Chinese population. It raises the possibility that circadian dysfunctions experienced by patients with PD may not merely be a subsidiary of the motor symptoms but an integral part of circadian system related to the disease itself. Our study confirmed a correlation between the symptoms of the circadian dysfunctions and Parkinson's disease from the view of the gene level. These findings suggest that circadian system may be a novel diagnostic and therapeutic target in motor fluctuation and sleep disorders with PD. However, multiple factors should be involved, such as genetic background, gene-environment interactions, and interaction of other clock genes. Therefore, more research is required to better understand the relationship between the polymorphism of clock genes and clinical profiles of PD.

5. Conclusion

CLOCK 3111T/C variant can be an independent risk factor for motor fluctuation and sleep disorder in Parkinson's disease in Chinese population.

References

[1] S. J. Chung, S. M. Armasu, K. J. Anderson et al., "Genetic susceptibility loci, environmental exposures, and Parkinson's disease: a case-control study of gene-environment interactions," *Parkinsonism & Related Disorders*, vol. 19, no. 6, pp. 595–599, 2013.

[2] L. D. Willison, T. Kudo, D. H. Loh, D. Kuljis, and C. S. Colwell, "Circadian dysfunction may be a key component of the non-motor symptoms of Parkinson's disease: insights from a transgenic mouse model," *Experimental Neurology*, vol. 243, pp. 57–66, 2013.

[3] A. Videnovic and D. Golombek, "Circadian and sleep disorders in Parkinson's disease," *Experimental Neurology*, vol. 243, pp. 45–56, 2013.

[4] E. S. Musiek, "Circadian clock disruption in neurodegenerative diseases: cause and effect?," *Frontiers in Pharmacology*, vol. 6, p. 29, 2015.

[5] A. Videnovic and G. L. Willis, "Circadian system-a novel diagnostic and therapeutic target in Parkinson's disease?," *Movement Disorders*, vol. 31, no. 3, pp. 260–269, 2016.

[6] J. Hirayama and P. Sassone-Corsi, "Structural and functional features of transcription factors controlling the circadian clock," *Current Opinion in Genetics & Development*, vol. 15, no. 5, pp. 548–556, 2005.

[7] D. B. Boivin, F. O. James, A. Wu, P. F. Cho-Park, H. Xiong, and Z. S. Sun, "Circadian clock genes oscillate in human peripheral blood mononuclear cells," *Blood*, vol. 102, no. 12, pp. 4143–4145, 2003.

[8] K. Mishima, T. Tozawa, K. Satoh, H. Saitoh, and Y. Mishima, "The 3111T/C polymorphism of hClock is associated with evening preference and delayed sleep timing in a Japanese population sample," *American Journal of Medical Genetics Part B: Neuropsychiatric Genetics*, vol. 133, pp. 101–104, 2005.

[9] A. R. Ozburn, K. Purohit, P. K. Parekh et al., "Functional implications of the CLOCK 3111T/C single-nucleotide polymorphism," *Frontiers in Psychiatry*, vol. 7, p. 67, 2016.

[10] P. Hua, W. Liu, S. H. Kuo et al., "Association of Tef polymorphism with depression in Parkinson disease," *Movement Disorders*, vol. 27, no. 13, pp. 1694–1697, 2012.

[11] P. Hua, W. Liu, Y. Zhao, H. Ding, L. Wang, and H. Xiao, "Tef polymorphism is associated with sleep disturbances in patients with Parkinson's disease," *Sleep Medicine*, vol. 13, no. 3, pp. 297–300, 2012.

[12] F. Lou, M. Li, Y. Ren, X. G. Luo, N. Liu, and X. Li, "CLOCK rs1801260 polymorphism is associated with susceptibility to Parkinson's disease in a Chinese population," *Neuroscience Bulletin*, vol. 33, no. 6, pp. 734–736, 2017.

[13] A. J. Hughes, S. E. Daniel, L. Kilford, and A. J. Lees, "Accuracy of clinical diagnosis of idiopathic Parkinson's disease: a clinico-pathological study of 100 cases," *Journal of Neurology, Neurosurgery, and Psychiatry*, vol. 55, no. 3, pp. 181–184, 1992.

[14] G. A. Kang, J. M. Bronstein, D. L. Masterman, M. Redelings, J. A. Crum, and B. Ritz, "Clinical characteristics in early Parkinson's disease in a central California population-based study," *Movement Disorders*, vol. 20, no. 9, pp. 1133–1142, 2005.

[15] C. Gao, H. Pang, X. G. Luo, Y. Ren, H. Shang, and Z. Y. He, "LRRK2 G2385R variant carriers of female Parkinson's disease are more susceptible to motor fluctuation," *Journal of Neurology*, vol. 260, no. 11, pp. 2884–2889, 2013.

[16] D. J. Buysse, C. F. Reynolds III, T. H. Monk, S. R. Berman, and D. J. Kupfer, "The Pittsburgh sleep quality index: a new instrument for psychiatric practice and research," *Psychiatry Research*, vol. 28, no. 2, pp. 193–213, 1989.

[17] C. He, J. Holme, and J. Anthony, "SNP genotyping: the KASP assay," *Methods in Molecular Biology*, vol. 1145, pp. 75–86, 2014.

[18] S. Rodriguez, T. R. Gaunt, and I. N. Day, "Hardy-Weinberg equilibrium testing of biological ascertainment for Mendelian randomization studies," *American Journal of Epidemiology*, vol. 169, no. 4, pp. 505–514, 2009.

[19] M. P. Bidikar, G. J. Jagtap, and R. T. Chakor, "Influence of deep breathing on heart rate variability in Parkinson's disease: co-relation with severity of disease and non-motor symptom scale score," *Journal of Clinical and Diagnostic Research (JCDR)*, vol. 8, no. 7, pp. BC01–BC03, 2014.

[20] U. Bonuccelli, P. Del Dotto, C. Lucetti et al., "Diurnal motor variations to repeated doses of levodopa in Parkinson's disease," *Clinical Neuropharmacology*, vol. 23, no. 1, pp. 28–33, 2000.

[21] B. Bruguerolle and N. Simon, "Biologic rhythms and Parkinson's disease: a chronopharmacologic approach to considering fluctuations in function," *Clinical Neuropharmacology*, vol. 25, no. 4, pp. 194–201, 2002.

[22] J. M. Senard, B. Chamontin, A. Rascol, and J. L. Montastruc, "Ambulatory blood pressure in patients with Parkinson's disease without and with orthostatic hypotension," *Clinical Autonomic Research*, vol. 2, no. 2, pp. 99–104, 1992.

[23] G. L. Willis, "Parkinson's disease as a neuroendocrine disorder of circadian function: dopamine-melatonin imbalance and the visual system in the genesis and progression of the degenerative process," *Reviews in the Neurosciences*, vol. 19, no. 4-5, pp. 245–316, 2008.

[24] J. J. van Hilten, G. Hoogland, E. A. van der Velde, H. A. Middelkoop, G. A. Kerkhof, and R. A. Roos, "Diurnal effects of motor activity and fatigue in Parkinson's disease," *Journal of Neurology, Neurosurgery, and Psychiatry*, vol. 56, no. 8, pp. 874–877, 1993.

[25] J. J. van Hilten, H. A. Middelkoop, G. A. Kerkhof, and R. A. Roos, "A new approach in the assessment of motor activity in Parkinson's disease," *Journal of Neurology, Neurosurgery, and Psychiatry*, vol. 54, no. 11, pp. 976–979, 1991.

[26] R. A. Hauser, M. P. McDermott, and S. Messing, "Factors associated with the development of motor fluctuations and dyskinesias in Parkinson disease," *Archives of Neurology*, vol. 63, no. 12, pp. 1756–1760, 2006.

[27] R. Cilia, A. Akpalu, F. S. Sarfo et al., "The modern pre-levodopa era of Parkinson's disease: insights into motor complications from sub-Saharan Africa," *Brain: A Journal of Neurology*, vol. 137, no. 10, pp. 2731–2742, 2014.

[28] A. Boulamery, N. Simon, J. Vidal, and B. Bruguerolle, "Effects of L-Dopa on circadian rhythms of 6-OHDA striatal lesioned rats: a radiotelemetric study," *Chronobiology International*, vol. 27, no. 2, pp. 251–264, 2010.

[29] L. E. Harrell and S. Balagura, "The effects of dark and light on the functional recovery following lateral hypothalamic lesions," *Life Sciences*, vol. 15, no. 12, pp. 2079–2087, 1974.

[30] G. L. Willis and A. D. Robertson, "Recovery of experimental Parkinson's disease with the melatonin analogues ML-23 and S-20928 in a chronic, bilateral 6-OHDA model: a new mechanism involving antagonism of the melatonin receptor," *Pharmacology, Biochemistry, and Behavior*, vol. 79, no. 3, pp. 413–429, 2004.

[31] T. Kawarai, H. Kawakami, Y. Yamamura, and S. Nakamura, "Structure and organization of the gene encoding human dopamine transporter," *Gene*, vol. 195, no. 1, pp. 11–18, 1997.

[32] S. Mukherjee, L. Coque, J. L. Cao et al., "Knockdown of Clock in the ventral tegmental area through RNA interference results in a mixed state of mania and depression-like behavior," *Biological Psychiatry*, vol. 68, no. 6, pp. 503–511, 2010.

[33] T. Iwase, N. Kajimura, M. Uchiyama et al., "Mutation screening of the human Clock gene in circadian rhythm sleep disorders," *Psychiatry Research*, vol. 109, no. 2, pp. 121–128, 2002.

[34] D. Katzenberg, T. Young, L. Finn et al., "A CLOCK polymorphism associated with human diurnal preference," *Sleep*, vol. 21, no. 6, pp. 569–576, 1998.

[35] E. L. Stack and A. M. Ashburn, "Impaired bed mobility and disordered sleep in Parkinson's disease," *Movement Disorders*, vol. 21, no. 9, pp. 1340–1342, 2006.

[36] D. B. Rye, "Sleepiness and unintended sleep in Parkinson's disease," *Current Treatment Options in Neurology*, vol. 5, no. 3, pp. 231–239, 2003.

[37] A. Serretti, F. Benedetti, L. Mandelli et al., "Genetic dissection of psychopathological symptoms: insomnia in mood disorders and CLOCK gene polymorphism," *American Journal of Medical Genetics Part B: Neuropsychiatric Genetics*, vol. 121, no. 1, pp. 35–38, 2003.

[38] F. Benedetti, S. Dallaspezia, M. C. Fulgosi et al., "Actimetric evidence that CLOCK 3111 T/C SNP influences sleep and activity patterns in patients affected by bipolar depression," *American Journal of Medical Genetics Part B: Neuropsychiatric Genetics*, vol. 144, no. 5, pp. 631–635, 2007.

[39] V. K. Datieva, A. V. Rosinskaia, and O. S. Levin, "The use of melatonin in the treatment of chronic fatigue syndrome and circadian rhythm disorders in Parkinson's disease," *Zhurnal Nevrologii I Psikhiatrii Imeni S.S. Korsakova*, vol. 113, pp. 77–81, 2013.

[40] G. L. Willis and E. J. Turner, "Primary and secondary features of Parkinson's disease improve with strategic exposure to bright light: a case series study," *Chronobiology International*, vol. 24, no. 3, pp. 521–537, 2007.

14

Apolipoprotein D Concentration in Human Plasma during Aging and in Parkinson's Disease: A Cross-Sectional Study

Andreas Waldner,[1] **Sarah Dassati**,[1,2] **Bernhard Redl**,[2] **Nicola Smania**,[3] **and Marialuisa Gandolfi**[3]

[1]*Department of Neurological Rehabilitation, Private Clinic Villa Melitta, Via Col di Lana 6, 39100 Bolzano, Italy*
[2]*Division of Molecular Biology, Biocenter, Innsbruck Medical University, Innrain 80-82, 6020 Innsbruck, Austria*
[3]*Neuromotor and Cognitive Neurorehabilitation Research Centre (CRRNC), Department of Neurosciences, Biomedicine and Movement Sciences, University of Verona UOC Neurorehabilitation—AOUI Verona, University Hospital, P.le L.A. Scuro 10, 37134 Verona, Italy*

Correspondence should be addressed to Andreas Waldner; andreas.waldner@villamelitta.it

Academic Editor: Ivan Bodis-Wollner

Apolipoprotein D (ApoD), a lipocalin transporter of small hydrophobic molecules, plays an important role in several neurodegenerative diseases. ApoD is expressed in and secreted from a variety of peripheral and brain tissues. Increments of ApoD have been reported in relation with oxidative stress conditions, aging, and degeneration in the nervous system. Preliminary findings support the role of ApoD in neuroprotection. However, its role in PD remains unclear. To date, no studies have been performed on the relationship between ApoD in the blood and PD, as neurodegenerative pathology related to oxidative damage. We investigated the concentration of ApoD in the blood of healthy control subjects and PD patients with mild-to-moderate neurological impairment. ApoD plasma levels were measured using sandwich enzyme-linked immunosorbent assays (ELISA) in 90 healthy subjects (aging-analysis cohort) and in 66 PD patients at different stages compared with 19 age-matched healthy subjects. Significant age-related increase of ApoD was detected in subjects older than 65 years of age ($p < 0.002$). In PD patients, a significant increase in ApoD plasma concentration was found compared with healthy subjects of the same age ($p < 0.05$). ApoD and PD stage are significantly correlated ($p < 0.05$). ApoD might be a valid marker for the progression of PD.

1. Introduction

Aging is the most significant risk factor for neurodegenerative disorders [1]. The progressive age-dependent increase in oxidative stress and inflammation ("inflamm-aging") represents a conserved and central mechanism of the functional decline occurring in old humans by impairing the dynamic organization of neuronal networks [2, 3]. It is involved in the pathogenesis of several of the major age-related diseases (i.e., cardiovascular disease, type 2 diabetes, and dementia) [4, 5]. The combined age-related induction of both proinflammatory cytokines, tumor necrosis factor α (TNF-α), and interleukine 6 (IL-6), in parallel with a decrease in antioxidant defence has been suggested to indicate morbidity and mortality in aged individuals [6]. The nervous system (NS) is the central regulator of aging [7]. Parkinson's disease (PD) is the second most common age-related neurodegenerative disorder beside Alzheimer's disease (AD) by affecting 1% of the population older than 65 years [8]. Parkinson's disease is a chronic progressive disease clinically manifested by bradykinesia, rigidity, postural instability, and tremor. Both idiopathic and the rare inherited PD reflect the pathological increase in the oxidative stress and inflammation-related events. The progressive loss of dopaminergic neurons of the substantia nigra (SN) and the presence of Lewy bodies within the same area are the main distinct and neuropathological hallmarks of PD [9]. The resulting dopamine (DA) depletion in their synaptic terminals leads to the cardinal motor symptoms of PD through the formation of dangerous hydroxyl radicals in the presence of ferrous ions [10–12].

The selective dopaminergic neuronal vulnerability is linked to the high iron levels characterizing the SN [11]. Increased levels of oxidized lipids, proteins, and DNA and decreased levels of the antioxidant reduced glutathione were detected in the SN of PD patient [13, 14]. Glutathione reduction is linked to an increased release of the arachidonic acid (AA) via phospholipase A2 followed by an accumulation of reactive oxygen species/reactive nitrogen species (ROS/RNS) and inflammatory mediators [15]. Thus, it has been suggested that limiting AA release and metabolism, a function performed by the atypical lipocalin apolipoprotein D (ApoD), will provide benefit in the early event in the pathogenesis of PD [16, 17].

Apolipoprotein D (ApoD) is a 29 kDa glycoprotein member of the lipocalin family [18]. It comprises an eight-stranded antiparallel β-barrel flanked by an α-helix. This structure forms a calyx consisting in a hydrophobic ligand pocket that binds AA and progesterone with higher affinity than other small ligands [18, 19]. In humans, ApoD is mainly produced in the plasma and in the brain, in which it is highly expressed in both the white frontal cortex and temporal cortex, in the SN and in the cerebellum. The lowest levels of this lipocalin were found in the hippocampus [20, 21]. In a healthy NS, ApoD is expressed by glia (astrocytes, oligoastrocytes, and Schwann cells) and other nonneuronal cells (e.g., pericytes), and it profoundly affects the function and survival of neurons [18]. In addition to its role in extracellular lipid transport, ApoD modulates AA metabolism in an antioxidant and anti-inflammatory manner [22]. ApoD stabilizes membranes-associated AA by attenuating its release from phospholipids [17]. It traps free AA via sequestration and prevents its consequent conversion into oxidants or into proinflammatory eicosanoids. In addition, ApoD was also demonstrated to reduce hydroperoxides of AA (i.e., eicosatetraenoic acid) to lipid hydroxides, thereby avoiding lipid peroxidation chain reactions and modulating inflammatory pathways [23]. According to its neuroprotective role, ApoD was found to be upregulated in brains affected by neurological (ischemic stroke), neurodegenerative (AD, PD, Niemann-Pick type C disease, transmissible spongiform encephalopathy), and psychiatric disorders (schizophrenia and bipolar disorder). These diseases are characterized by an altered brain AA metabolism and an increased excitotoxicity. Elevated levels of ApoD mRNA and protein were detected in brains after degeneration processes [15]. In contrast to the NS, the expression of ApoD in body fluids was not investigated in much detail during aging. Based on the emerging neuroprotective roles of ApoD the aim of this pilot study was to evaluate (1) ApoD levels in a cohort of healthy controls to verify the effect of aging on ApoD as well as the levels of TNF-α in order to get a better insight of the increase in ApoD during the "inflamm-aging" process [2, 24], (2) differences in ApoD levels between PD and age-matched healthy controls, and (3) differences in ApoD levels according to different levels of neurological impairment.

Thus, our pilot study was aimed to validate if ApoD may therefore be a reliable candidate as a marker for PD and/or in the progression of the disease.

2. Materials and Methods

2.1. Subjects. 66 patients with PD (mean age 72.84 ± 7.07 years) and 19 age-matched healthy controls (mean age 72.79 ± 1.55 years) were enrolled. They were white Americans, whose plasma was provided from the Harvard NeuroDiscovery Center Biomarker Study (HBS). They underwent neurological evaluation before enrollment. Inclusion criteria were a diagnosis of PD confirmed according to the United Kingdom Parkinson's Disease Society Brain Bank criteria (bradykinesia, muscular rigidity, rest tremor, and postural instability not caused by primary visual, vestibular, cerebellar, or proprioceptive dysfunction). PD patients were receiving pharmacological therapy (monoamine oxidase-B inhibitors) for PD because of ethical reasons.

Exclusion criteria were any other physiological/pathological factors that can exert an influence on the plasmatic ApoD concentration such as poststroke and/or traumatic brain injury, antipsychotic drugs treatment, obesity (body mass index > 27), idiopathic normal pressure hydrocephalus, Paget's disease, breast cancer, adenocarcinoma of the prostate, glucose- 6-phosphate deficiency, and insulin resistance-related disorders. Patients with PD were subdivided in the following two groups based on their stage of the disease (Hoehn and Yahr classification): 1.0–1.5 (group A, $n = 21$) and ≥ 2.0 (group B, $n = 45$).

90 healthy European Caucasian subjects were enrolled (mean age 52.05 ± 19.86 years) from Italy, Austria, and Eastern Europe. They were recruited from among persons who showed no sign of neurological disease and any physiological/pathological factors that can influence ApoD concentration. Healthy controls were subdivided in the following age groups: 20–40 years ($n = 30$), 41–65 years ($n = 30$), and >65 years ($n = 30$).

All participants provided written confirmed consent to participate in the study. The study protocol was approved by the local ethics committee of Gesundheitsbezirk Bozen/Comprensorio Sanitario di Bolzano (Prot 0107531-BZ and Prot 0002995-BZ).

2.2. Quantification of Plasma ApoD and TNF-α Level. Plasma ApoD and TNF-α levels were determined by commercially available enzyme-linked immunosorbent assay kits (USCN Life Science Inc., USA). In brief, human plasma was collected using ethylenediaminetetraacetic acid (EDTA) as an anticoagulant. Samples were centrifuged for 15 minutes at 1000 ×g. Plasma was removed and diluted 1 : 100 with Phosphate Buffered Saline (PBS) (pH = 7.0). Samples were tested in duplicates. 100 μl of each diluted standard, blank, and human samples were precoated with a monoclonal antibody specific to the related molecule (ApoD or TNF-α) and incubated for 2 hours. Subsequently, all the samples were incubated for 1 hour with 100 μl/well of a biotin-conjugated polyclonal antibody preparation, washed 3 times with a specific wash solution, and incubated for 30 min with 100 μl avidin conjugated horseradish peroxidase. Following the last 5 washes, 90 μl 3,3′,5,5′-tetramethylbenzidine (TMB) solution was added to each well. The enzyme-substrate reaction was terminated by addition of 50 μl sulphuric acid solution in each well and absorbance was measured spectrophotometrically at a wavelength of 450 nm. The sandwich ELISA used for detection of ApoD, and TNF-α had a sensitivity threshold of about 1.03 ng/ml and 0.1 pg/ml, respectively.

2.3. Statistical Analysis. Because the data of the 90 Healthy European Caucasian subjects were not normally distributed (Shapiro–Wilk test), nonparametric tests were used for inferential statistics. The Kruskal-Wallis H test ("one-way ANOVA on ranks") was used to determine if there were statistically significant differences between the three groups of an independent variable (APOD). Post hoc between-group comparisons were performed using the Mann–Whitney *U* test. Since the data of the white Americans (66 PD patients and 19 healthy subjects) were normally distributed (Shapiro–Wilk test), parametric tests were used for inferential statistics. The one-way analysis of variance (ANOVA) was used to determine any statistically significant differences between groups. Post hoc comparisons were performed using Tukey's multiple comparison test to evaluate whether there was any difference between groups after adjusting for multiple testing. Logistic regression was used to predict the probability that PD stage was influenced by ApoD levels. Age, gender, and PD medications were considered as covariates. Statistical analyses were carried out using the SPSS® Statistics version 20.0. $p < 0.05$ was set as a significant value for the first level of analysis.

Statistical analyses were carried out using the SPSS Statistics version 20.0. $p < 0.05$ was set as a significant value for the first level of analysis.

3. Results

3.1. Relationship between ApoD and Aging. Age-related ApoD levels in the plasma of healthy subjects are shown in Figure 1. The reported data were referred to subjects subdivided in different age groups: 20–40 years (group I, $n = 30$), 41–65 years (group II, $n = 30$), and >65 years (group III, $n = 30$). Increased ApoD levels were found only in older subjects aged >65 years, independently of gender. As shown in Figure 1, the increase in ApoD concentration was significant in subjects of group III (mean 34.61 ± 9.21 ng/ml) compared with subjects of group I (mean 28.28 ± 4.01 ng/ml) ($p < 0.001$) and group II (mean 27.73 ± 7.26 ng/ml) ($p < 0.002$). ApoD concentration did not significantly increase in subjects of group II (mean 27.73 ± 7.26 ng/ml) compared with younger subjects of group I (mean 28.28 ± 4.01 ng/ml) ($p > 0.5$). Thus, age-related ApoD concentration in human plasma increases significantly in older subjects >65 years. Table 1 shows the gender-unrelated and age-dependent ApoD increase in human plasma of healthy European Caucasian subjects.

3.2. Relationship between TNF-α and Aging. As shown in Figure 2, we found the following TNF-α concentrations: 0.188 ± 0.1 pg/ml in group I, 0.24 ± 0.05 pg/ml in group II,

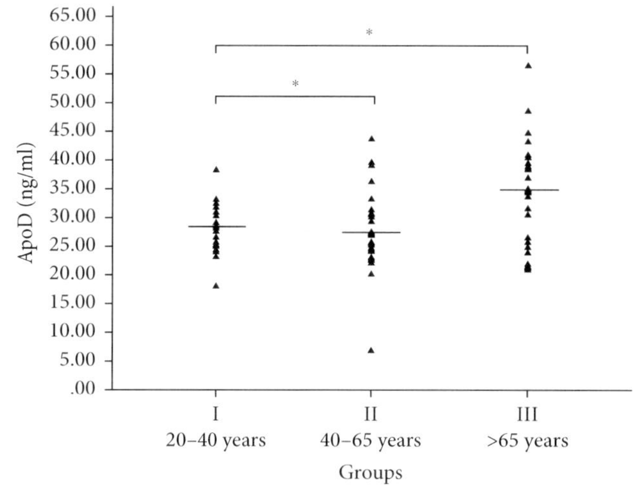

FIGURE 1: Age-dependent ApoD concentration in human plasma. Horizontal lines show the average distribution of age-related ApoD concentration in plasma in group I (mean 28.28 ± 4.01 ng/ml, $n = 30$, and 20–40 years), group II (mean 27.73 ± 7.26 ng/ml, $n = 30$, and 40–65 years), and group III (mean 34.61 ± 9.21 ng/ml, $n = 30$, and >65 years). The increase in ApoD concentration was significant in subjects of group III compared to subjects of group I ($p < 0.001$) and group II ($p < 0.002$).

and 0.61 ± 0.15 pg/ml in group III. Thus, the increase in TNF-α concentration in human plasma was significant between groups I and II ($p < 0.5$) and between groups II and III ($p < 0.0001$). In agreement with a previous study, TNF-α levels in human plasma of European Caucasian subjects during aging were found to be gender-unrelated in our study (Table 1) [6].

3.3. Relationship between ApoD and Disease Severity in Parkinson's Disease. ApoD levels were compared among control and PD subjects, who were in stages 1.0 to 5.0 in the scale of Hoehn and Yahr (H&Y). Plasmatic ApoD levels were higher in all PD patients (mean 104.15 ± 30.96 ng/ml) compared with age-matched healthy subjects (mean 79.35 ± 26.25 ng/ml) ($p < 0.005$) (Figure 3). PD subjects were subdivided in the following groups (Hoehn and Yahr classification): 1.0–1.5 (group A, $n = 21$) and ≥2.0 (group B, $n = 45$). Increased values of ApoD concentration were detected in PD patients of group B (mean 109.10 ± 32.31 ng/ml) ($p < 0.005$) compared with the healthy subjects. No difference was found between the 2 groups of patients. Stage and ApoD were significantly correlated ($p < 0.05$; Spearman's $r = 0.116$). Thus, ApoD is predictive of the stage (linear regression model) (Figure 4). ApoD levels in human plasma in PD were found to be gender-unrelated in human plasma of the white Americans group (Table 2).

4. Discussion

In the current study, we first investigated if and how "inflamm-aging" influences ApoD concentration in human plasma. The plasmatic increase in ApoD concentration

TABLE 1: Gender distribution of age-dependent ApoD and TNF-α levels in human plasma.

Group	Age (years)	ApoD concentration (ng/ml)			TNF-α concentration (pg/ml)		
		Females	Males	Total	Females	Males	Total
I	20–40	27.40 ± 4.17 (n = 14)	28.75 ± 2.85 (n = 16)	28.28 ± 4.01 (n = 30)	0.17 ± 0.02 (n = 14)	0.20 ± 0.13 (n = 16)	0.188 ± 0.1 (n = 30)
II	40–65	27.85 ± 5.77 (n = 14)	27.65 ± 8.55 (n = 16)	27.73 ± 7.26* (n = 30)	0.25 ± 0.05 (n = 13)	0.24 ± 0.05 (n = 15)	0.24 ± 0.05* (n = 28)
III	>65	31.37 ± 9.71 (n = 24)	34.65 ± 7.45 (n = 6)	34.61 ± 9.21* (n = 30)	0.65 ± 0.13 (n = 24)	0.62 ± 0.14 (n = 4)	0.61 ± 0.15* (n = 28)

*$p < 0.05$.

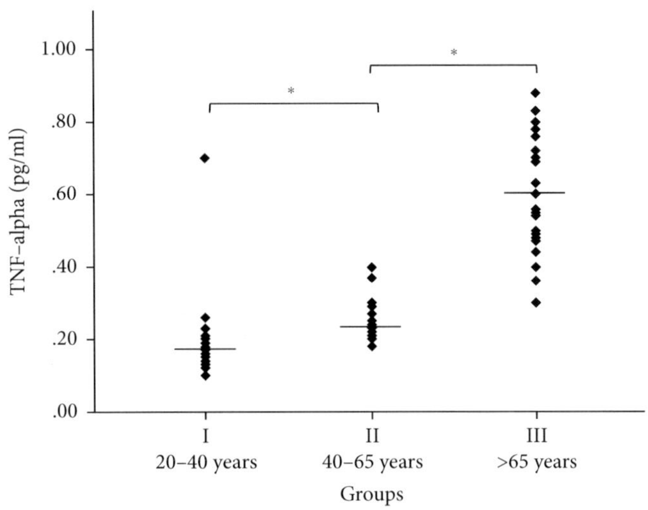

FIGURE 2: Age-dependent TNF-α concentration in human plasma. One-way analysis of variance (ANOVA) and Student's t-test with Tukey's post hoc were used. Horizontal lines show the average distribution of age-related ApoD concentration in human plasma in group I (mean 0.188 ± 0.1 pg/ml, n = 30, and 20–40 years), group II (mean 0.24 ± 0.05 pg/ml, n = 30, and 40–65 years), and group III (0.61 ± 0.15 pg/ml, n = 30, and >65 years). The increase in TNF-α concentration in human plasma was significant between groups I and II ($p < 0.05$) and between groups II and III ($p < 0.0001$).

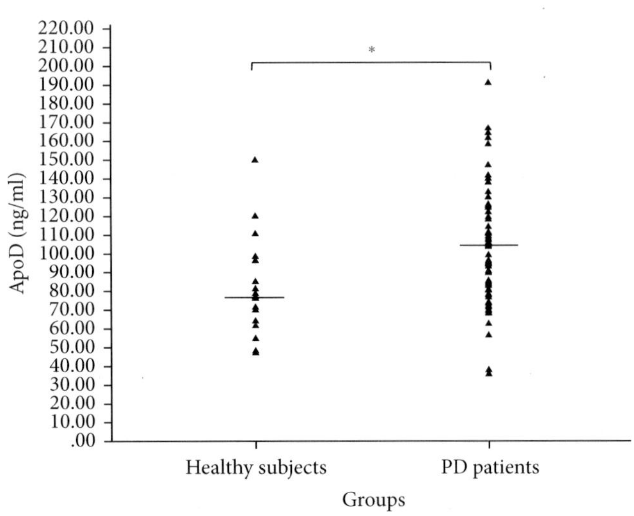

FIGURE 3: Plasma ApoD levels in healthy subjects and in PD.

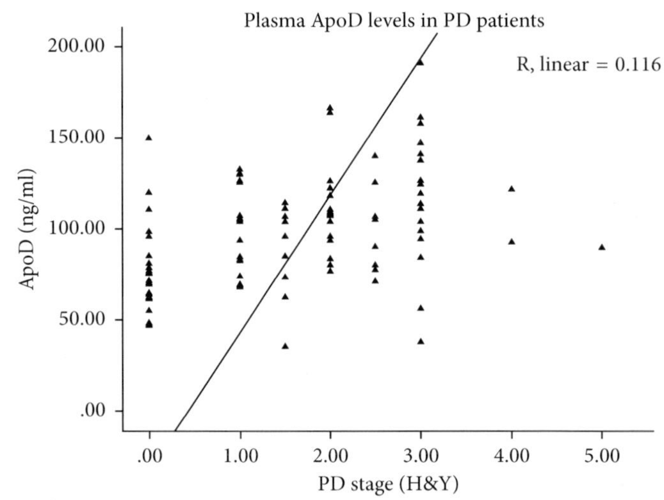

FIGURE 4: Plasma ApoD levels correlate with disease severity in PD. The linear regression analysis adjusted for age, gender, and PD medications reveal an increase in the plasmatic levels of ApoD, which is correlated with disease severity in PD ($p < 0.01$). Control data were included in the regression analysis as PD stage 0.

found in subjects older than >65 years supports our hypothesis. The detected velocity in ApoD increase between group II and III reflects the age-related overproduction of the ROS/RNS and inflammatory factors ($p < 0.002$). The plasmatic levels of ApoD start to increase at the age-related baseline upon which the entity of "inflamm-aging" slowly overwhelms the endogenous antioxidant and anti-inflammatory response. It would be hypothesized that "inflammatory tone" is observed to start rising before (in the group II age range) and that the increase in ApoD takes place later. This is highlighted by the significant increase in TNF-α concentration between the same groups ($p < 0.0001$). In addition, the incidence and prevalence of AD, which double every 5 years after an age of 65, contribute to the concept of the age-related baseline discussed above [24, 25]. Our findings are in agreement with the emerging role of ApoD as anti-stress protein in aging [15]. In a cross-species comparative analysis of transcription changes during brain aging, ApoD was identified as the most upregulated gene in the aged brain [3]. Overexpression of the human APOD gene increased survival under stress in the mouse and extended the mean lifespan in *Drosophila melanogaster* [26, 27].

Table 2: Gender distribution of ApoD levels in human plasma in PD.

Group	H&Y	Age (years)	ApoD (ng/ml)		
			Females	Males	Total
A	<2	71.57 ± 5.24	90.18 ± 25.70 ($n = 15$)	104.31 ± 17.90 ($n = 6$)	93.54 ± 24.47 ($n = 21$)
B	≥2	73.44 ± 8.99	107.67 ± 39.83 ($n = 21$)	111.81 ± 26.59 ($n = 24$)	109.10 ± 32.31 ($n = 45$)
All PD	1–5	72.84 ± 7.07	99.90 ± 34.63 ($n = 38$)	110.47 ± 25.25 ($n = 28$)	104.15 ± 30.96 ($n = 66$)
Healthy control group	72.79 ± 1.55	85.33 ± 24.32 ($n = 11$)	90.26 ± 14.29 ($n = 8$)	79.35 ± 26.25 ($n = 19$)	

$^{*}p < 0.05$.

The ApoD knockout (ApoD-KO) mouse model is characterized by prematurely aged, hyperkinesia and memory deficits. The loss of ApoD was found to affect the age-dependent transcriptome patterns of the cortex and hippocampus [28]. By contributing to the adaptability and plasticity occurring against the age-related morphological atrophic changes, ApoD protects the integrity of the NS by preserving organisms against the deleterious effects of aging [15, 27, 28]. In conclusion, the results of our pilot study provide the first evidence of an age-dependent increase of ApoD concentration in human blood plasma. In addition, they highlight the potential utility of ApoD as a promising candidate as a marker of the progressive inability to counterbalance the oxidative stress-inflammation-related insults by endogenous antioxidant defence.

Increasing evidences highlight the involvement of both oxidative stress and inflammation in the deregulation of plasma membrane lipid metabolism in PD and other neurodegenerative disorders [5, 14, 29, 30]. Specifically, an upregulation of the AA metabolic cascade was found in brain regions with a chronic SN lesion [31]. Consequently, a significant increase in ApoD expression was shown in glial cells in postmortem human brains of PD patients [32]. Thus, we investigated if and how ApoD concentration changes in human plasma of PD patients at different stages of their disease. We detected a higher increase of ApoD in PD patients compared to age-matched healthy subjects ($p < 0.005$). Increased values of ApoD concentration were found only in PD patients of the group B ($p < 0.005$). Stage and ApoD were significantly correlated ($p < 0.05$; Spearman's $r = 0.116$). Our findings are in agreement with the emerging role of ApoD in protecting cells against astrogliosis, whose increase contributes to the deterioration of motor symptoms of PD. By being required to compensate the loss of dopaminergic neurons as well as to control the spreading of consequent damages, reactive astrocytes can become dangerous once out of control. Thus, astrogliosis is a "double-edged sword." A role for ApoD in maintaining the glial response against the plethora of ROS/RNS and inflammatory mediators under fixed limits has been proposed [15, 33, 34]. The role of ApoD in modulating astrocyte reactivity has been well demonstrated both in mouse primary glial cultures and *in vivo* in controlling the on-off signals that tune the glial response to injury [33]. In addition, ApoD might be involved in removal of neurotoxic molecules released during cell dying [35]. ApoD has been also shown to contribute to an autocrine-protecting mechanism in astrocytes, avoiding accumulation of peroxidated lipids and altering the paraquat transcriptional response of genes involved in ROS managing and the inflammatory response to OS [30]. ApoD acts as a lipid transporter protein in neurite-promoting responses, in active myelination and in axonal outgrowth as well as a regeneration-promoting agent [33–37]. In addition, ApoD exerts its neuroprotective role by repairing the damaged lysosomal membranes. The pH recovery in PQ-treated lysosomes is mediated by ApoD [38]. Thus, all the emerging evidences supporting a central role of ApoD in PD-associated astrogliosis can explain our detected correlation of plasma ApoD levels with disease severity in PD. Given this perspective, new strategies aimed to augment ApoD neuroprotective properties together with therapeutic approaches targeting CNS-resident immune cells such as microglia and mast cells [15, 39]. All the patients enrolled in the study were receiving pharmacological therapy for PD because of ethical reasons. It has not been reported an influence of the different types of dopaminergic agents on the expression of ApoD, whereas an increase in AA and a decrease in docosahexaenoic acid (DHA) concentrations were found in postmortem brain in PD patients and parkinsonian monkeys treated with levodopa [40]. Consequently, a possible influence of levodopa on the detected ApoD levels cannot be excluded. In addition, a potential reduction in ApoD levels exerted from the antioxidant effects of monoamine oxidase (MAO) inhibitors has to be considered. These drugs reduced hyperactivity of MAO, which leads to an excessive production of hydrogen peroxide involved in neurotoxicity [41]. Interestingly, the combination of MAO inhibitors and levodopa was found to improve cognition, including probabilistic learning, working memory, and executive functions [42]. The potential contribution of ApoD as a lipid carrier in these drugs-related remodelling processes within the glial-neuronal networks has to be investigated. This is the first study of plasma ApoD in relation to PD and its progression. The strengths of the present study are the large patient sample for a preliminary study and the evaluation of effects within the brain by detecting changes in blood, a less intrusive procedure to collect from human subjects. Its limitation is the possibility that differences between TNF-α and ApoD concentration might also be the reflection of different tissue sources producing TNF-α (i.e., age). In conclusion, we found a significant increase in the plasmatic levels of ApoD in PD, which are correlated with disease severity ($p < 0.05$; Spearman's $r = 0.001$). Our study supports the idea that measuring the concentration of ApoD in human plasma may be used as a reliable marker for the progression of PD.

5. Conclusion

This study suggests a consistent age-related physiological increase of ApoD concentration in human plasma, especially in subjects over an age of 65 years. Although there is a general age-related increase in ApoD concentration during aging, we found that plasma levels of PD patients are significantly higher than age-matched healthy subjects. Parkinson's disease stage and ApoD are significantly correlated. The increase in the plasmatic levels of ApoD in PD is significant even in the presence of comorbidities, potentially compromising the lipid homeostasis as, for example, in hyperlipidemia. Considering the sample limitations and exploratory nature of this pilot study, further studies with larger sample size of healthy subjects and PD patients are recommended in order to verify the validity of ApoD that may therefore be a reliable candidate as a marker for disease progression.

Disclosure

Andreas Waldner and Sarah Dassati contributed equally to this work.

Conflicts of Interest

The authors declare that there are no conflicts of interest regarding the publication of this article.

Acknowledgments

The authors wish to gratefully acknowledge the support of Scherzer C. R., MD, Center for Neurologic Diseases, Harvard Medical School and Brigham and Women's Hospital, as well as his staff. Biospecimens were provided by the Harvard Biomarker Study. The Harvard Biomarker Study is supported by the Harvard NeuroDiscovery Center (HNDC), the Parkinson's Disease Biomarkers Program (PDBP) Grant U01 NS082157 of the NINDS, and the Massachusetts Alzheimer's Disease Research Center (ADRC) P50 AG005134 grant of the National Institute on Aging. The authors wish to gratefully acknowledge Frasnelli J. (Université du Québec à Trois-Rivières, Canada) and Yambire KF. (University Medical Center, Göttingen, Germany) for the statistical analysis. The authors thank Mutschlechner W. and Staudinger T. (Medical University of Innsbruck, Austria) as well as the entire staff of the Private Hospital Villa Melitta for technical support.

References

[1] B. A. Yankner, T. Lu, and P. Loerch, "The aging brain," *Annual Review of Pathology: Mechanisms of Disease*, vol. 3, no. 1, pp. 41–66, 2008.

[2] C. Franceschi, M. Bonafe, S. Valensin et al., "Inflamm-aging. An evolutionary perspective on immunosenescence," *Annals of the New York Academy of Sciences*, vol. 908, no. 1, pp. 244–254, 2000.

[3] N. A. Bishop, T. Lu, and B. A. Yankner, "Neural mechanisms of ageing and cognitive decline," *Nature*, vol. 464, no. 7288, pp. 529–535, 2010.

[4] A. Salminem, J. Ojala, K. Kaarniranta, and A. Kauppinen, "Mitochondrial dysfunction and oxidative stress activate inflammasomes: impact on the aging process and age-related diseases," *Cellular and Molecular Life Sciences*, vol. 69, no. 18, pp. 2999–3013, 2012.

[5] V. Calabrese, A. Santoro, D. Monti et al., "Aging and Parkinson's disease: inflammaging, neuroinflammation and biological remodeling as key factors in pathogenesis," *Free Radical Biology and Medicine*, vol. 115, pp. 80–91, 2018.

[6] D. De Gonzalo-Calvo, K. Neitzert, M. Fernández et al., "Differential inflammatory responses in aging and disease: TNF-alpha and IL-6 as possible biomarkers," *Free Radical Biology and Medicine*, vol. 49, no. 5, pp. 733–737, 2010.

[7] C. A. Wolkow, K. D. Kimura, M. S. Lee, and G. Ruvkun, "Regulation of *C. elegans* life-span by insulin like signaling in the nervous system," *Science*, vol. 290, no. 5489, pp. 147–150, 2000.

[8] M. J. Farrer, "Genetics of Parkinson disease: paradigm shifts and future prospects," *Nature Reviews Genetics*, vol. 7, no. 4, pp. 306–318, 2006.

[9] F. Blandini, "Neural and immune mechanisms in the pathogenesis of Parkinson's disease," *Journal of Neuroimmune Pharmacology*, vol. 8, no. 1, pp. 189–201, 2013.

[10] D. G. Graham, S. M. Tiffany, W. R. Bell Jr., and W. F. Gutknecht, "Autoxidation versus covalent binding of quinones as the mechanism of toxicity of dopamine, 6-hydroxydopamine and related compounds toward C1300 neuroblastoma cells in vitro," *Molecular pharmacology*, vol. 14, no. 4, pp. 644–653, 1978.

[11] E. Sofic, P. Rieder, H. Heinsen et al., "Increased iron (III) and total iron content in post mortem substantia nigra of parkinsonian brain," *Journal of Neural Transmission*, vol. 74, pp. 199–205, 1988.

[12] S. Fahn, "Description of Parkinson's disease as a clinical syndrom," *Annals of the New York Academy of Sciences*, vol. 991, no. 1, pp. 1–14, 2003.

[13] Y. Nakabeppu, D. Tsuchimoto, H. Yamaguchi, and K. Sakumi, "Oxidative damage in nucleic acids and Parkinson's disease," *Journal of Neuroscience Research*, vol. 85, no. 5, pp. 919–934, 2007.

[14] E. Sofic, K. W. Lange, K. Jellinger, and P. Riederer, "Reduced and oxidized glutathione in the substantia nigra of patients with Parkinson's disease," *Neuroscience Letters*, vol. 142, no. 2, pp. 128–130, 1992.

[15] S. Dassati, A. Waldner, and R. Schweigreiter, "Apolipoprotein D takeas center stage in the stress response of the aging and degenerative brain," *Neurobiology of Aging*, vol. 7, no. 7, pp. 1632–1642, 2014.

[16] A. A. Farooqui, W. Y. Ong, and L. A. Horrocks, "Inhibitors of brain phospholipase A2 activity: their neuropharmacological effects and therapeutic importance for the treatment of neurologic disorders," *Pharmacological Reviews*, vol. 58, no. 3, pp. 591–620, 2006.

[17] E. A. Thomas, R. C. George, and J. G. Sutcliffe, "Apolipoprotein D modulates arachidonic acid signaling in cultured cells: implications for psychiatric disorders," *Prostaglandins, Leukotrienes and Essential Fatty Acids*, vol. 69, no. 6, pp. 421–427, 2003b.

[18] E. Rassart, A. Bedirian, S. Do Carmo et al., "Apolipoprotein D," *Biochimica et Biophysica Acta*, vol. 1482, no. 1-2, pp. 185–198, 2000.

[19] A. Eichinger, A. Nasreen, H. J. Kim, and A. Skerra, "Structural insight into the dual ligand specificity and mode of high density lipoprotein association of apolipoprotein D," *Journal of Biological Chemistry*, vol. 282, no. 42, pp. 31068–31075, 2007.

[20] A. Navarro, J. Tolivia, A. Astudillo, and E. del Valle, "Pattern of apolipoprotein D immunoreactivity in human brain," *Neuroscience Letters*, vol. 254, no. 1, pp. 17–20, 1998.

[21] H. Li, K. Ruberu, T. Karl, and B. Garner, "Cerebral apolipoprotein-D is hypoglycosylated compared to peripheral tissues and is variably expressed in mouse and human brain regions," *PLoS One*, vol. 11, no. 2, article e0148238, 2016.

[22] P. R. Provost, L. Villeneuve, P. K. Weech, R. W. Milne, Y. L. Marcel, and E. Rassart, "Localization of the major sites of rabbit apolipoprotein D gene transcription by in situ hybridization," *Journal of Lipid Research*, vol. 32, no. 12, pp. 1959–1970, 1991.

[23] S. Bhatia, B. Knoch, J. Wong et al., "Selective reduction of hydroperoxyeicosatetraenoic acids to their hydroxy derivatives by apolipoprotein D: implications for lipid antioxidant activity and Alzheimer's disease," *Biochemical Journal*, vol. 442, no. 3, pp. 713–721, 2012.

[24] H. Brüünsgaard and B. K. Pedersen, "Age-related inflammatory cytokines and disease," *Immunology and Allergy Clinics of North America*, vol. 23, no. 1, pp. 15–39, 2003.

[25] C. Qiu, M. Kivipelto, and E. von Strauss, "Epidemiology of Alzheimer's disease: occurrence, determinants, and strategies toward intervention," *Dialogues in Clinical Neuroscience*, vol. 11, no. 2, pp. 111–128, 2009.

[26] D. Sanchez, B. Lopez-Arias, L. Torroja et al., "Loss of glial lazarillo, a homolog of apolipoprotein D. reduces lifespan and stress resistance in Drosophila," *Current Biology*, vol. 16, no. 7, pp. 680–686, 2006.

[27] P. M. Loerch, T. Lu, A. K. Dakin et al., "Evolution of the aging brain transcriptome and synaptic regulation," *PLoS One*, vol. 3, no. 10, article e3329, 2008.

[28] D. Sanchez, R. Bajo-Grañeras, M. Del Caño-Espinel et al., "Aging without Apolipoprotein D: molecular and cellular modifications in the hippocampus and cortex," *Experimental Gerontology*, vol. 67, pp. 19–47, 2015.

[29] E. del Valle, A. Navarro, A. Astudillo et al., "Apolipoprotein D expression in human brain reactive astrocytes," *Journal of Histochemistry & Cytochemistry*, vol. 51, no. 10, pp. 1285–1290, 2003.

[30] H. J. Lee, R. P. Bazinet, S. I. Rapoport, and A. K. Bhattacharjee, "Brain arachidonic acid cascade enzymes are upregulated in a rat model of unilateral Parkinson disease," *Neurochemical Research*, vol. 5, no. 4, pp. 613–619, 2010.

[31] C. Ordonez, A. Navarro, C. Perez, A. Astudillo, E. Martínez, and J. Tolivia, "Apolipoprotein D expression in substantia nigra of Parkinson disease," *Histology and Histopathology*, vol. 21, no. 4, pp. 361–366, 2006.

[32] R. Bajo-Grañeras, M. D. Ganfornina, E. Martín-Tejedor, E. Martín-Tejedor, and D. Sanchez, "Apolipoprotein D mediates autocrine protection of astrocytes and controls their reactivity level, contributing to the functional maintenance of paraquat-challenged dopaminergic systems," *Glia*, vol. 59, no. 10, pp. 1551–1566, 2011.

[33] M. D. Ganfornina, S. Do Carmo, J. M. Lora et al., "Apolipoprotein D is involved in the mechanisms regulating protection from oxidative stress," *Aging Cell*, vol. 7, no. 4, pp. 506–155, 2008.

[34] J. Kosacka, M. Gericke, M. Nowicki et al., "Apolipoproteins D and E3 exert neurotrophic and synaptogenic effects in dorsal root ganglion cell cultures," *Neuroscience*, vol. 162, no. 2, pp. 282–291, 2009.

[35] N. García-Mateo, M. D. Ganfornina, O. Montero et al., "Schwann cell-derived apolipoprotein D controls the dynamics of post-injury myelin recognition and degradation," *Frontiers in Cellular Neuroscience*, vol. 8, p. 374, 2014.

[36] W. Y. Ong, C. P. Lau, S. K. Leong, U. Kumar, S. Suresh, and S. C. Patel, "Apolipoprotein D gene expression in the rat brain and light and electron microscopic immunocytochemistry of apolipoprotein D expression in the cerebellum of neonatal, immature and adult rats," *Neuroscience*, vol. 90, no. 3, pp. 913–922, 1999.

[37] M. D. Ganfornina, S. Do Carmo, E. Martinez et al., "ApoD, a glia-derived apolipoprotein, is required for peripheral nerve functional integrity and a timely response to injury," *Glia*, vol. 11, pp. 1320–1334, 2010.

[38] R. Pascua-Maestro, S. Diez-Hermano, C. Lillo, M. D. Ganfornina, and D. Sanchez, "Protecting cells by protecting their vulnerable lysosomes: identification of a new mechanism for preserving lysosomal functional integrity upon oxidative stress," *PLoS Genetics*, vol. 13, no. 2, p. e1006603, 2017.

[39] S Brotini, C Schievano, and L Guidi, "Ultra-micronized palmitoylethanolamide: an efficacious adjuvant therapy for Parkinson's disease," *CNS & Neurological Disorders-Drug Targets*, vol. 16, no. 6, pp. 705–713, 2017.

[40] C. Julien, L. Berthiaume, A. Hadj-Tahar et al., "Postmortem brain fatty acid profile of levodopa-treated Parkinson disease patients and parkinsonian monkeys," *Neurochemistry International*, vol. 48, no. 5, pp. 404–414, 2006.

[41] S. G. Simonson, J. Zhang, A. T. Canada, Y.-F. Su, H. Benveniste, and C. A. Piantadosi, "Hydrogen peroxide production by monoamine oxidase during ischemia-reperfusion in the rat brain," *Journal of Cerebral Blood Flow & Metabolism*, vol. 13, no. 1, pp. 125–134, 1993.

[42] R. Krishna, M. Ali, and A. A. Moustafa, "Effects of combined MAO-B inhibitors and levodopa vs. monotherapy in Parkinson's disease," *Frontiers in Aging Neuroscience*, vol. 6, p. 180, 2014.

15

Clinimetrics of the 9- and 19-Item Wearing-Off Questionnaire

Carlos E. Mantese,[1,2] Artur Schumacher-Schuh,[1] and Carlos R. M. Rieder[1,3,4]

[1]*Postgraduate Program in Medical Sciences, Universidade Federal do Rio Grande do Sul, Porto Alegre, RS, Brazil*
[2]*Mãe de Deus Hospital, Porto Alegre, RS, Brazil*
[3]*Universidade Federal de Ciências da Saúde de Porto Alegre (UFCSPA), Porto Alegre, RS, Brazil*
[4]*Hospital de Clínicas de Porto Alegre (HCPA), Porto Alegre, RS, Brazil*

Correspondence should be addressed to Carlos R. M. Rieder; carlosrieder@gmail.com

Academic Editor: Peter Hagell

The treatment of Parkinson's disease (PD) with dopaminergic therapy improves functionality and quality of life. However, as the disease progresses, the wearing-off phenomenon develops, which necessitates complex posology adjustment or adjuvant therapy. This phenomenon may not be well recognized, especially if it is mild or involves nonmotor symptoms. Questionnaires were developed to improve the recognition of the wearing-off phenomenon. The questionnaires consist of a list of symptoms that patients must check if they have and if the symptoms improve with medication. A recent review by the Movement Disorder Society suggested the 19-item (WOQ-19) and 9-item (WOQ-9) questionnaires as screening tools for the wearing-off phenomenon. However, there has not been a systematic review to assess the questionnaires' clinimetric properties, such as sensitivity, specificity, test-retest reliability, and responsiveness. We conducted an extensive search for studies using these two tools. We identified 3 studies using WOQ-19 and 5 studies using WOQ-9. Both questionnaires seem to have good sensitivity (0.81–1). WOQ-19 has variable specificity (0.39–0.8), depending on the number of positive items, while WOQ-9 lacks specificity (0.1–0.69). Only one study using WOQ-19 reported test-retest, and only two studies reported responsiveness. Thus, this report describes the first independent systematic review to exam quantitatively the clinimetric properties of these two questionnaires.

1. Introduction

The treatment of Parkinson's disease (PD) with dopaminergic therapy improves functionality and quality of life. However, as the disease progresses, it causes motor and nonmotor fluctuations [1]. The well-described wearing-off (WO) phenomenon is the shortening effect of levodopa, which can be managed with dosage adjustment or adjuvant therapy, such as catechol-*O*-methyltransferase (COMT) inhibitors [2]. Clinical evaluation has been the gold standard for diagnosing this condition. However, the WO phenomenon may not be well recognized, mainly if it is mild or involves nonmotor symptoms. Several scholars argue that recognition of WO phenomenon could change the way that it is managed and improve patient's functionality [3].

To improve the recognition of WO phenomenon, a 32-item questionnaire (WOQ-32) was developed [3]. The questionnaire consists of a checklist of symptoms that patients must identify, and they must note if these symptoms improve with medication. For practical reasons, using the same research, this questionnaire was adapted to a 19-item questionnaire (WOQ-19), which had the same properties [4]. Later, a 9-item questionnaire (WOQ-9) was developed [5], containing the most valuable questions, and it was successfully tested [6]. The WOQ-9 has been used for a number of clinical studies, translated into several languages, and adapted with several different clinimetric properties [7]. A recent review by the Movement Disorder Society set both the WOQ-19 and WOQ-9 as recommended tools for screening for WO phenomenon [8]. However, this

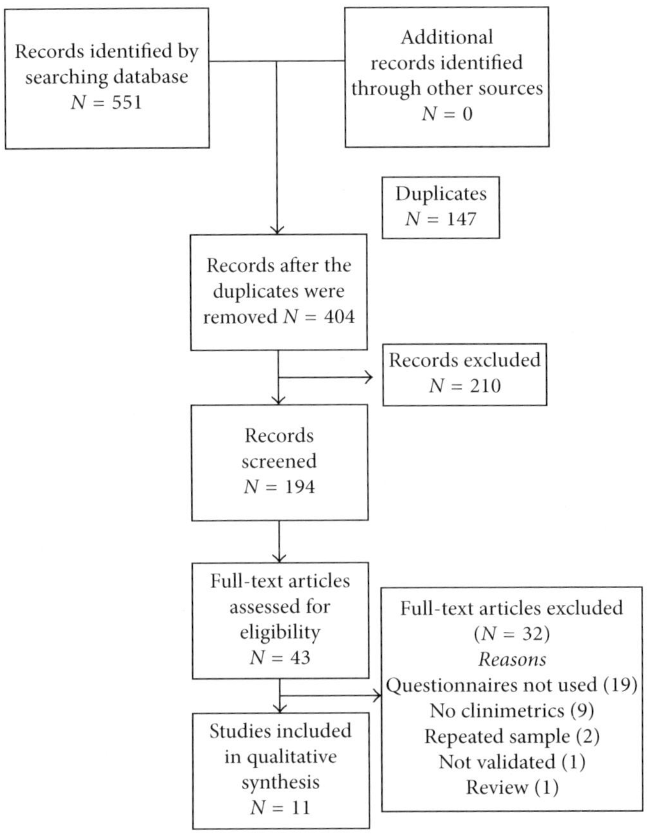

FIGURE 1: Flow diagram for data extraction.

review did not address quantitatively the clinimetric properties in Parkinson's disease patients compared to clinical evaluation.

Thus, we conducted a systematic review and analysis of the clinimetric properties of both the WOQ-19 and WOQ-9 questionnaires, such as sensitivity, specificity, predictive positive value (PPV), negative predictive value (NPV), and stability with test-retest and responsiveness.

2. Methods

We follow the PRISMA statement.

The inclusion criterion was studies using WOQ-9 or WOQ-19 in PD patients to diagnose WO compared to the gold-standard, clinical evaluation. The studies must examine sensitivity and specificity, or they must include data that we could calculate. Also, we include studies using one of the questionnaires if they employed data regarding test-retest or responsiveness. Formal validation was not required [9], but at least a translation and face validation for the given language was applied. Reviews, abstracts, and conference meetings were excluded. Responsiveness was calculated following Cohen's effect size [10].

The search was conducted in MEDLINE, Embase, and Web of Sciences between 01/06/2017 and 22/12/17. The terms were ((Parkinson's OR Parkinson's disease) AND (wearing off OR wearing-off OR motor fluctuation) AND (questionnaire)). There was also a bibliography review for the select articles and reviews already published. The articles were independently selected by title for abstract reading by two reviewers (Artur Schumacher-Schuh and Carlos E. Mantese). In case of disagreement, the articles were discussed by another author (Carlos R. M. Rieder). Later, a number of articles were selected for full reading based on abstract information.

3. Results

As shown in Figure 1, we observed 404 articles based on the title after excluding duplicates. We reviewed 194 abstracts and 43 full-text articles after excluding 4 abstracts. Ultimately, we selected 3 articles about WOQ-19 [11–13] and 5 articles about WOQ-9 [6, 14–17] for sensitivity and specificity, 1 for WOQ-19 test-retest [18], 2 for responsiveness, 1 for WOQ-9 [19], and 1 for WOQ-19 [20]. Of note, we did not include the original WOQ-19 description [4] because it was an adaptation of WOQ-32, as was WOQ-9 [5]. In addition to these articles, we exclude 17 more because they did not use the target questionnaires; among these 17, two more were from the same 32-item questionnaire [3, 21] and 15 from other means of assessment [22–36]. One article was not used because it lacked any type of language validation [37], and two articles presented post hoc analyses of the same populations outlined in other articles that we include [38, 39]. Nine articles did not present clinimetric properties [40–48], and among them, two provided data using which we could calculate only PPV [41, 43]. One was a review [7]. One paper [18] included for test-retest was not included for sensitivity and specificity because it used the same population as another article [13].

We did not identify any articles that were not included in the search from original libraries.

In WOQ-19, there are 3 trials selected (Table 1). One of them used 1-item cutoff [12], while the others [11, 13] used 2-item cutoff. The sensitivity ranged from 0.81 to 0.90, and the specificity was 0.39–0.80. PPV was 0.62–0.88, and NPV was 0.64–0.84. The wide range of specificity seems secondary to one study that used 1-item cutoff. This trial does not exhibit better aggregate sensitivity but has shown worse specificity.

In WOQ-9 (Table 2), all studies had 1-item cutoff. Sensibility was 0.87–1, specificity was 0.10–0.69, PPV was 0.48–0.86, and NPV was 0.71–1. All studies showed excellent sensitivity but lacked specificity.

Test-retest stability was assessed in one paper [18], two weeks apart from each test, which showed an intraclass correlation of number of positive items of 0.858. It was applied to stable patients; however, it did not mention the clinical stability or the type of intraclass correlation.

For responsiveness, two studies were analyzed [19, 20]. Both were clinical trials with COMT inhibitors. One of them [19] used WOQ-9 and reported improvement in most items in proportion of patients with improvements; however, it did not provide data to calculate the effect size. In the other trial [20], Cohen's effect size was 0.5.

4. Discussion

This report describes the first systematic review of quantitative clinimetric properties of WOQ-19 and WOQ-9.

Table 1: WOQ-19.

Author	Year	N	Cutoff	Sn	Sp	PPV	NPV
Martinez-Martin et al. [11]	2008	222	2	0.88	0.8	0.88	0.79
Seki et al. [12]	2013	464	1	0.81	0.39	0.62	0.64
Stocchi et al. [13]	2014	617	2	0.90	0.63	0.76	0.84

Sn: sensitivity; Sp: specificity; PPV: positive predictive value; NPV: negative predictive value.

Table 2: WOQ-9.

Author	Year	N	Cut-off	Sn	Sp	PPV	NPV
Stacy et al. [6]	2008	216	1	0.96	0.40	0.48	0.94
Chan et al. [14]	2011	101	1	0.87	0.69	0.86	0.71
Bares et al. [15]	2012	563	1	0.98	0.27	0.72	0.91
Santos et al. [16]	2014	60	1	1	0.10	0.54	1
Fukae et al. [17]	2015	180	1	0.94	0.39	0.66	0.83

Sn: sensitivity; Sp: specificity; PPV: positive predictive value; NPV: negative predictive value.

Systematic reviews are fundamental to summarize important data for research and clinical practices. Additionally, this report describes the first independent review of the clinimetric properties of these questionnaires.

The WOQ-19 seems to have good accuracy, which is an excellent tool in both research and clinical practice, when a 2-item cutoff is used. However, most of the trials used WOQ-9, which has excellent sensitivity but poor specificity. Thus, the WOQ-9 could be used as a screening tool to identify certain at-risk individuals, but it would need a clinical evaluation to confirm the diagnosis, as several trials have done [42, 46]. Stacy [7] has argued that office visits could fail to recognize WO, and its position as the gold standard of care may need reevaluation [6]. This hypothesis seems difficult to prove. Moreover, most clinical trials for Parkinson's disease treatment use wearing-off outcomes diaries or UPDRS (Unified Parkinson's Disease Rating Scale) wearing-off subitems. Raciti et al. [49] showed that UPDRS has 0.87 sensitivity and 0.43 specificity compared to clinical evaluation, which make it similar to WOQ-9 and considerably worse than WOQ-19.

The variability in WOQ-19 can be explained by several reasons. In WOQ-19, one clinical trial used the 1-item cutoff and therefore lost specificity. In a ROC curve plotted by Martinez-Martin et al. [11], the questionnaire showed better accuracy when the 2-item cutoff was used. As in WOQ-9, the 1-item cutoff seems to have the same lack of specificity. Fukae et al. [17] showed that when the 2-item cutoff is used, the WOQ-9's specificity improves (from 0.39 to 0.72) and loses a little sensitivity (from 0.94 to 0.87). Additionally, each study involved different languages, and the final result depended on, in part, the properties of each specific validation. Moreover, the gold standard could be different depending on the physician's expertise (i.e., if they are movement disorder specialists or in-training neurologists). Finally, while most clinical trials excluded patients who could not complete the questionnaires, certain differences in educational, cultural, and social backgrounds could explain a portion of the variability in the questionnaires.

Of note, we did not identify information regarding questionnaire reliability or validity other than criteria validity. Furthermore, only one article on WOQ-19 examined test-retest through intraclass correlation of number of positive items, and it did not mention the type, consistency, or agreement. The second is preferred [50]. For test-retest, even not mentioned clinical stability, two weeks apart from each test seems enough time in Parkinson's disease to avoid recall bias and ensure clinical stability. We have not found any paper with kappa agreement from individual question. Being a questionnaire with dichotomous responses, the use of kappa would seem appropriate. We did not identify any reports of test-retest for WOQ-9. Responsiveness was obtained from two clinical trials for WOQ-19 comparing add-on therapy with entacapone (a COMT inhibitor). This therapy is used to treat WO phenomenon, and both showed an improvement of questionnaire on the basis of number positive items. However, in one trial, we have no data to calculate the effect size [18]. The other one [19] showed effect size of 0.5, which means a moderate effect.

The lack of data regarding reliability and even validation by means other than criteria validation might be observed because the original study used WOQ-32, and later, the WOQ-19 and WOQ-9 were developed, and even those questionnaires were not tested for those properties by the developers. Additionally, we did not include conference meetings or abstracts, which can account for the loss of certain data (even so, we did not identify those data in the libraries we searched). This information is important to clinicians and researchers because it might influence how they use questionnaires. A questionnaire with poor test-retest performance is not reliable to use, and the results can change with no change in clinical status.

We excluded several important articles, such as Stacy et al.'s [3] description of the WOQ-32 questionnaire and its transformation into the WOQ-19 [4] and WOQ-9 [5]. However, this article involves data from a different questionnaire, which was later transformed into the WOQ-19 and WOQ-9 questionnaires. Several articles were post hoc analyses of primary data, which we had already included. One study did not have any type of validation and did not meet our inclusion criteria. Most of the excluded trials were with no comparator; therefore, we could not address clinimetric properties.

5. Conclusions

We conducted the first systematic review of WOQ-19 and WOQ-9, an important tool for screening and diagnosing

WO. The lack of certain data suggests caution when using the WOQ-9. However, the WOQ-19 exhibits reliability and was validated to use as a diagnostic tool. Moreover, we suggest that the authors report complete properties when they are publishing papers validating their methods.

Acknowledgments

Carlos R. M. Rieder was supported by the Brazilian government research grant agency CNPq (no. 311970/2014-1). The authors also thank the Fundo de Incentivo à Pesquisa e Eventos (FIPE), Hospital de Clínicas de Porto Alegre (HCPA), for article processing charges.

References

[1] C. C. Aquino and S. H. Fox, "Clinical spectrum of levodopa-induced complications," *Movement Disorders*, vol. 30, no. 1, pp. 80–89, 2015.

[2] R. Pahwa and K. E. Lyons, "Levodopa-related wearing-off in Parkinson's disease: identification and management," *Current Medical Research and Opinion*, vol. 25, no. 4, pp. 841–849, 2009.

[3] M. Stacy, A. Bowron, M. Guttman et al., "Identification of motor and nonmotor wearing-off in Parkinson's disease: comparison of a patient questionnaire versus a clinician assessment," *Movement Disorders*, vol. 20, no. 6, pp. 726–733, 2005.

[4] M. Stacy and R. Hauser, "Development of a patient questionnaire to facilitate recognition of motor and non-motor wearing-off in Parkinson's disease," *Journal of Neural Transmission*, vol. 114, no. 2, pp. 211–217, 2007.

[5] M. Stacy, R. Hauser, W. Oertel et al., "End-of-dose wearing off in Parkinson disease: a 9-question survey assessment," *Clinical Neuropharmacology*, vol. 29, no. 6, pp. 312–321, 2006.

[6] M. A. Stacy, J. M. Murphy, D. R. Greeley et al., "The sensitivity and specificity of the 9-item wearing-off questionnaire," *Parkinsonism and Related Disorders*, vol. 14, no. 3, pp. 205–212, 2008.

[7] M. Stacy, "The wearing-off phenomenon and the use of questionnaires to facilitate its recognition in Parkinson's disease," *Journal of Neural Transmission*, vol. 117, no. 7, pp. 837–846, 2010.

[8] A. Antonini, P. Martinez-Martin, R. K. Chaudhuri et al., "Wearing-off scales in Parkinson's disease: critique and recommendations," *Movement Disorders*, vol. 26, no. 12, pp. 2169–2175, 2011.

[9] D. E. Beaton, C. Bombardier, F. Guillemin, and M. B. Ferraz, "Guidelines for the process of cross-cultural adaptation of self-report measures," *SPINE*, vol. 25, no. 24, pp. 3186–3191, 2000.

[10] G. R. Norman, K. W. Wyrwich, and D. L. Patrick, "The mathematical relationship among different forms of responsiveness coefficients," *Quality of Life Research*, vol. 16, no. 5, pp. 815–822, 2007.

[11] P. Martinez-Martin, E. Tolosa, B. Hernandez, and X. Badia, "Validation of the "QUICK" questionnaire—a tool for diagnosis of "Wearing-Off" in patients with Parkinson's disease," *Movement Disorders*, vol. 23, no. 6, pp. 830–836, 2008.

[12] M. Seki, K. Takahashi, D. Uematsu et al., "Clinical features and varieties of non-motor fluctuations in Parkinson's disease: a Japanese multicenter study," *Parkinsonism and Related Disorders*, vol. 19, no. 1, pp. 104–108, 2013.

[13] F. Stocchi, A. Antonini, P. Barone et al., "Early detection of wearing off in Parkinson disease: the DEEP study," *Parkinsonism and Related Disorders*, vol. 20, no. 2, pp. 204–211, 2014.

[14] A. Chan, Y. F. Cheung, M. Au Yeung et al., "A validation study of the Chinese wearing off questionnaire 9-symptom for Parkinson's disease," *Clinical Neurology and Neurosurgery*, vol. 113, no. 7, pp. 538–540, 2011.

[15] M. Bareš, I. Rektorová, R. Jech et al., "Does WOQ-9 help to recognize symptoms of non-motor wearing-off in Parkinson's disease?," *Journal of Neural Transmission*, vol. 119, no. 3, pp. 373–380, 2012.

[16] J. G. Santos, H. F. Chien, and E. R. Barbosa, "Specificity and sensibility of 9-items wearing-off questionnaire in Brazilian Parkinson disease patient sample," *Arquivos de Neuro-Psiquiatria*, vol. 72, no. 11, pp. 867–873, 2014.

[17] J. Fukae, M. Higuchi, S. Yanamoto et al., "Utility of the Japanese version of the 9-item wearing-off questionnaire," *Clinical Neurology and Neurosurgery*, vol. 134, pp. 110–115, 2015.

[18] G. Abbruzzese, A. Antonini, P. Barone et al., "Linguistic, psychometric validation and diagnostic ability assessment of an Italian version of a 19-item wearing-off questionnaire for wearing-off detection in Parkinson's disease," *Neurological Sciences*, vol. 33, no. 6, pp. 1319–1327, 2012.

[19] K. Eggert, O. Skogar, K. Amar et al., "Direct switch from levodopa/benserazide or levodopa/carbidopa to levodopa/carbidopa/entacapone in Parkinson's disease patients with wearing-off: efficacy, safety and feasibility–an open-label, 6-week study," *Journal of Neural Transmission*, vol. 117, no. 3, pp. 333–342, 2010.

[20] E. Tolosa, B. Hernández, G. Linazasoro et al., "Efficacy of levodopa/carbidopa/entacapone versus levodopa/carbidopa in patients with early Parkinson's disease experiencing mild wearing-off: a randomised, double-blind trial," *Journal of Neural Transmission*, vol. 121, no. 4, pp. 357–366, 2014.

[21] J.-P. Azulay, F. Durif, R. Rogez et al., "Étude Précoce: évaluation d'un autoquestionnaire de déspistage et prise en charge précoces des fluctuations dans la maladie de Parkinson," *Revue Neurologique*, vol. 164, no. 4, pp. 354–362, 2008.

[22] N. Hattori, K. Fujimoto, and T. Kondo, "Patient perspectives on Parkinson's disease therapy in Japan and the United States: results of two patient surveys," *Patient Related Outcome Measure*, vol. 3, pp. 31–38, 2012.

[23] P. Santens and A. M. de Noordhout, "Detection of motor and non-motor symptoms of end-of dose wearing-off in Parkinson's disease using a dedicated questionnaire: a Belgian multicenter survey," *Acta Neurologica Belgica*, vol. 106, no. 3, pp. 137–141, 2006.

[24] P. Martinez-Martin and B. Hernandez, "Q10 study group. The Q10 questionnaire for detection of wearing-off phenomena in Parkinson's disease," *Parkinsonism Related Disorder*, vol. 18, no. 4, pp. 382–385, 2012.

[25] A. Schapira, S. Fox, R. Hauser et al., "Assessment of safety and efficacy of safinamide as a levodopa adjunct in patients with Parkinson disease and motor fluctuations: a randomized clinical trial," *JAMA Neurology*, vol. 74, no. 2, pp. 216–224, 2017.

[26] S. Cheon, M. Park, W. Kim et al., "Non-motor off symptoms in Parkinson's disease," *Journal of Korean Medical Science*, vol. 24, no. 2, pp. 311–314, 2009.

[27] R. Hauser, M. Panisset, G. Abbruzzese et al., "Double-blind trial of levodopa/carbidopa/entacapone versus levodopa/carbidopa in early Parkinson's disease," *Movement Disorders*, vol. 24, no. 4, pp. 541–550, 2009.

[28] A. Boiko, T. Batysheva, N. Minaeva et al., "Use of the new levodopa agent Stalevo (levodopa/carbidopa/entacapone) in

the treatment of Parkinson's disease in out-patient clinical practice (the START-M open trial)," *Neuroscience and Behavioral Physiology*, vol. 38, no. 9, pp. 933–936, 2008.

[29] M. Jog, M. Panisset, O. Suchowersky, B. Réhel, and R. Schecter, "Naturalistic evaluation of entacapone in patients with signs and symptoms of L-dopa wearing-off," *Current Medical Research and Opinion*, vol. 24, no. 11, pp. 3207–3215, 2008.

[30] W. Ondo, K. Sethi, and G. Kricorian, "Selegiline orally disintegrating tablets in patients with Parkinson disease and "wearing off" symptoms," *Clinical Neuropharmacology*, vol. 30, no. 5, pp. 295–300, 2007.

[31] G. Deuschl, A. Vaitkus, G. Fox et al., "Efficacy and tolerability of Entacapone versus cabergoline in parkinsonian patients suffering from wearing-off," *Movement Disorders*, vol. 22, no. 11, pp. 1550–1555, 2007.

[32] D. Brooks, Y. Agid, K. Eggert et al., "Treatment of end-of-dose wearing-off in Parkinson's disease: stalevo (levodopa/carbidopa/entacapone) and levodopa/DDCI given in combination with comtess/comtan (entacapone) provide equivalent improvements in symptom control superior to that of traditional levodopa/DDCI treatment," *European Neurology*, vol. 53, no. 4, pp. 197–202, 2005.

[33] T. Kondo and Y. Mizuno, "A long-term study of istradefylline safety and efficacy in patients with Parkinson disease," *Clinical Neuropharmacology*, vol. 38, no. 2, pp. 41–46, 2015.

[34] H. Hao, M. Shao, J. An et al., "Association of catechol-O-methyltransferase and monoamine oxidase B gene polymorphisms with motor complications in Parkinson's disease in a Chinese population," *Parkinson & Related disorders*, vol. 20, no. 10, pp. 1041–1045, 2014.

[35] W. F. Kum, J. Gao, S. S. Durairajan et al., "Risk factors in development of motor complications in Chinese patients with idiopathic Parkinson's disease," *Journal of Clinical Neuroscience*, vol. 16, no. 8, pp. 1034–1037, 2009.

[36] Q. Sun, T. Wang, T. F. Jiang et al., "Effect of a leucine-rich repeat kinase 2 variant on motor and non-motor symptoms in Chinese Parkinson's disease patients," *Aging and Disease*, vol. 7, no. 3, pp. 230–236, 2016.

[37] L. M. Melo, H. F. Chien, and E. R. Barbosa, "Identification of wearing-off manifestations (reduction of levodopa effect) in Parkinson's disease using specific questionnaire and comparison of the results with routine ambulatory evaluations," *Arquivos de Neuropsiquiatria*, vol. 68, no. 4, pp. 506–510, 2010.

[38] M. A. Stacy, H. Murck, and K. Kroenke, "Responsiveness of motor and nonmotor symptoms of Parkinson disease to dopaminergic therapy," *Progress in Neuro-Psychopharmacology & Biological Psychiatry*, vol. 34, no. 1, pp. 57–61, 2010.

[39] D. Colombo, G. Abbruzzese, A. Antonini et al., "The "gender factor" in wearing-off among patients with Parkinson's disease: a post hoc analysis of DEEP study," *Scientific World Journal*, vol. 2015, Article ID 787451, 10 pages, 2015.

[40] P. Martínez-Martín, E. Tolosa, B. Hernández, and X. Badia, "The patient card questionnaire to identify wearing-off in Parkinson disease," *Clinical Neuropharmacology*, vol. 30, no. 5, pp. 266–275, 2007.

[41] M. C. Altavista, E. Cassetta, L. Brusa et al., "Wearing-off detection in clinical practice: the wearing off real practice key (WORK-PD) study in Parkinson's disease," *Parkinsonism Related Disorders*, vol. 21, no. 2, pp. 95–100, 2015.

[42] P. A. Silburn, G. D. Mellick, B. I. Vieira et al., "Utility of a patient survey in identifying fluctuations in early stage Parkinson's disease," *Journal of Clinical Neuroscience*, vol. 15, no. 11, pp. 1235–1239, 2008.

[43] W. Chen, Q. Xiao, M. Shao et al., "Prevalence of wearing-off and dyskinesia among the patients with Parkinson's disease on levodopa therapy: a multi-center registry survey in mainland China," *Translational Neurodegeneration*, vol. 3, no. 1, pp. 1–8, 2014.

[44] H. Chen, J. Fang, F. Li, L. Gao, and T. Feng, "Risk factors and safe dosage of levodopa for wearing-off phenomenon in Chinese patients with Parkinson's disease," *Neurological Sciences*, vol. 36, no. 7, pp. 1217–1223, 2015.

[45] M. Picillo, R. Palladino, M. Moccia et al., "Gender and non motor fluctuations in Parkinson's disease: a prospective study," *Parkinsonism and Related Disorder*, vol. 27, pp. 89–92, 2016.

[46] M. Pistacchi, M. Gioulis, F. Sanson, and S. Marsala, "Wearing off: a complex phenomenon often poorly recognized in Parkinson's disease. A study with the WOQ-19 questionnaire," *Neurology India*, vol. 65, no. 6, pp. 1271–1279, 2017.

[47] H. Wu, F. Dong, Y. Wang et al., "Catechol-O-methyltransferase Val158Met polymorphism: modulation of wearing-off susceptibility in a Chinese cohort of Parkinson's disease," *Parkinsonism and Related Disorder*, vol. 20, no. 10, pp. 1094–1096, 2014.

[48] K. E. Rahne, C. Tagesson, and D. Nyholm, "Motor fluctuations and *Helicobacter pylori* in Parkinson's disease," *Journal of Neurology*, vol. 260, no. 12, pp. 2974–2980, 2013.

[49] L. Raciti, A. Nicoletti, G. Mostile et al., "Validation of the UPDRS section IV for detection of motor fluctuations in Parkinson's disease," *Parkinsonism and Related Disorder*, vol. 27, pp. 98–101, 2016.

[50] C. B. Terwee, S. D. Bot, M. R. de Boer et al., "Quality criteria were proposed for measurement properties of health status questionnaires," *Journal of Clinical Epidemiology*, vol. 60, no. 1, pp. 34–42, 2007.

16

Combination of Multifocal Electroretinogram and Spectral-Domain OCT Can Increase Diagnostic Efficacy of Parkinson's Disease

Jiang Huang ,[1] Yi Li,[2] Jianjiang Xiao,[2] Qin Zhang,[3] Guoxu Xu,[1] Guanhui Wu,[3] Tong Liu ,[4] and Weifeng Luo [3]

[1]*Department of Ophthalmology, Second Affiliated Hospital of Soochow University, Suzhou, China*
[2]*Department of Ophthalmology, Huashan Hospital North, Fudan University, Shanghai, China*
[3]*Department of Neurology, Second Affiliated Hospital of Soochow University, Suzhou, China*
[4]*Institute of Neuroscience, Soochow University, Suzhou, China*

Correspondence should be addressed to Weifeng Luo; luoweifengsz@sohu.com

Academic Editor: Hélio Teive

Background. The retinal changes have been identified in morphology and function in Parkinson's disease (PD). However, the controversial results suggest that it is incredible that only using a single method for testing retinal change to evaluate Parkinson's disease. The aim of this study was to assess retinal changes and increase the diagnostic efficacy of Parkinson's disease with a combination of multifocal electroretinogram (mf-ERG) and spectral domain optical coherence tomography (SD-OCT) examinations. *Method.* Fifty-three PD patients and forty-one healthy controls were enrolled. Subjects were assessed for retinal function using mf-ERG and retinal structure using SD-OCT. *Results.* The PD patients had a significantly decreased amplitude density of P1 and a delayed implicit time of P1 in some regions. The macular retinal thickness, macular volume, and average RNFL thickness were decreased in PD. The AUC of a single parameter of either retinal function or structure was low. Both of them were higher in diagnostic value to discriminate PD patients. *Conclusion.* The amplitude density of P1 combined with macular volume can get a high diagnostic efficacy to discriminate between participants with or without PD. It indicates that a combination of mf-ERG and SD-OCT provides a good clinical biomarker for diagnosis of PD.

1. Introduction

Parkinson's disease (PD) is the second most common neurodegenerative disorder affecting middle-aged and elderly people in the developed world [1, 2]. The clinical manifestations of Parkinson's disease are multisystem disorders with a wide variety of motor and nonmotor features [3, 4]. And the nonmotor aspects include mood disturbance, sleep disorder, cognitive decline dementia, autonomic failure, and vision dysfunction [5, 6]. Many PD patients have vision symptoms when examined [7], yet the vision-related problem of PD still remains under-recognized and less understood.

It is known that PD can cause neural impairment outside the central nervous system even before damage to the basal ganglia. Vision deficits of PD are common including visual acuity, contrast sensitivity, ocular movement, color perception, and other damages in the vision system [6, 7]. Lots of studies [8–10] have demonstrated that retina, especially the fovea, where dopaminergic amacrine cells have concentrated in, is the vulnerable site of vision function in PD.

Multifocal electroretinogram (mf-ERG) is a sensitive and specific method for monitoring the functional changes of the posterior retina, especially in the annular zone surrounding the fovea [11, 12]. Previous studies [13–15] have shown that the mf-ERG test can reflect the function of fovea in several retinal diseases, such as age-related macular degeneration, diabetic macular edema, Best's disease, and so on. Few studies [16, 17] have shown that mf-ERG values revealed decreased foveal electrical activity in PD patients.

Spectral-domain optical coherence tomography (SD-OCT) is a new, advanced, noninvasive technology, which can provide cross-sectional images of the retina and optic in a rapid, objective, reproducible manner for evaluation of the thickness of macular and retinal nerve fiber layer (RNFL) [18, 19]. Most studies [16, 20, 21] suggested the thinning of macular thickness and the loss of RNFL in patients with PD; however, some studies [22, 23] found neither a reduction in macular thickness nor the loss of RNFL.

These conclusions show that the retinal function and structure have changed in PD patients, and it may prove these retinal monitor techniques will be useful potential biomarkers for diagnosis or assessing disease progression in PD. However, studies with controversial results also suggest that it is incredible that only using a single method for testing retinal structure or function to evaluate PD.

To date, there are no studies of correlations of mf-ERG and SD-OCT in the macular function and structure in large participants. In this study, we combined mf-ERG with SD-OCT test in PD patients and healthy control subjects, and we analyzed the alterations in functional and structural changes in PD and the association between these changes in the diagnostic yield of PD.

2. Method

This was a cross-sectional study and was performed according to the principles outlined in the Declaration of Helsinki and was approved by the Institutional Review Board of the second affiliated Hospital of Soochow University. All participants gave written informed consent prior to study inclusion.

2.1. Participants. Patients with idiopathic PD and healthy controls (HC) participants were enrolled in the study. All patients were prospectively recruited from the local neurologic department and underwent a complete neurologic examination. The severity of the disease was described using Hoehn and Yahr scale and unified Parkinson disease rating scale III (UPDRS III). The Ophthalmic examination included best-corrected visual acuity (BCVA), intraocular pressure (IOP), visual field using Octopus instrument, slit-lamp examination, dilated ophthalmoscopy, fundus photography, SD-OCT, and mf-ERG examination. The diagnosis of idiopathic PD was confirmed by the treating neurologist based on the United Kingdom Brain Bank criteria for the clinical diagnosis of idiopathic PD [24].

The exclusion criteria included patients with diabetes mellitus, poor sitting stability, recognition disorder, and history of severe visual loss including cataract, glaucoma, age-related macular degeneration, hypermyopia (refractive diopter >−4.0D), and any ocular surgery.

2.2. mf-ERG Recording. Mf-ERG test was recorded according to the International Society for Clinical Electrophysiology of Vision guidelines [25] using a visually evoked test system (VETS V8.1; GOTEC, Chongqing). Pupils were dilated (≥7 mm) using 1.0% tropicamide and 2.5% phenylephrine. A Burian-Allen contact lens electrode was used, which was placed on the anesthetized (0.4% oxybuprocaine hydrochloride) cornea. A ground electrode was clipped to the right earlobe, and the electrode impedance was maintained below 5 kΩ. The patients were positioned at a distance of 33 cm from the stimulus monitor. The stimulus was presented on a 19-inch CRT. The mf-ERG system was used with a scaled 103-hexagon stimulus element displayed on a 19-inch CRT with a frame rate of 75 Hz. The hexagons were modulated between white (200 cd/m^2) and black (<2 cd/m^2) according to an m-sequence during the 8-minute recording sessions. The stimulus array was positioned on the retina at approximately 45° and centered on the fovea. Recordings were collected in sixteen segments of approximately 25 seconds. Fixation was controlled using an "x" target in the center of the stimulus. The contaminated segments were discarded and reevaluated.

2.3. SD-OCT Examination. Pupils were dilated (≥7 mm) using 1.0% tropicamide and 2.5% phenylephrine. SD-OCT was performed using Cirrus HD-OCT Model 4000 (Carl Zeiss Meditec Inc.). The macular zone including of the macular retinal thickness (MRT), central foveal thickness, and macular volume (MV) was assessed using a Macular Cube 512 × 128 scanning. The RNFL thickness was assessed using an Optic Disc Cube 200 × 200 scanning.

2.4. Data Analysis. Statistical analysis was performed using SPSS 20.0. Data were presented as mean ± SD as appropriate. Initial data analysis consisted of comparing the mean age between groups through a 2-tailed t-test. The parameters of mf-ERG and SD-OCT were evaluated using the Mann–Whitney U test. The Pearson chi-square test was employed for comparison of the frequencies. The correlation of the structural and functional changes in retina was evaluated using the Pearson correlation coefficient. A p value less than 0.05 was considered significant.

The mf-ERG test was analyzed to determine the amplitude density (AD) and implicit time (IT). The IT of P1 (first positive peak) and amplitudes (N1-P1) were analyzed for the specified areas in five rings including ring1, ring2, ring3, ring4, and ring5. The five rings represent the summed responses from five adjacent concentric ring-shaped areas.

The analysis of parameters of SD-OCT consisted of macular retinal thickness (MRT), central foveal thickness (CFT), macular volume (MV), and retinal nerve fiber layer (RNFL) thickness. The RNFL thickness was analyzed with the average RNFL and four quadrants including temporal quadrant thickness, superior quadrant thickness, nasal quadrant thickness, and inferior quadrant thickness.

3. Results

3.1. Basic Demographics Analysis. The participants' basic demographics are shown in Table 1. The two groups did not differ significantly in age, sex, intraocular pressure (IOP), or

TABLE 1: Demographics, disease characteristics, and visual field of all participants.

	HC	PD	p
Number of subjects	$n = 41$	$n = 53$	
Age (years)	62.29 ± 9.74	61.79 ± 9.89	0.807[a]
Male/female	24/17	35/18	0.456[b]
PD duration (months)	—	67.92 ± 45.52	—
BCVA	1.01 ± 0.03	0.99 ± 0.04	0.096[c]
MD of visual field (dB)	2.94 ± 3.25	7.00 ± 6.39	≤0.001[c]**
IOP (mmHg)	14.79 ± 2.93	14.19 ± 2.97	0.338[c]
Hoehn and Yahr scale	—	1.92 ± 0.54	—
UPDRS III	—	37.15 ± 16.61	—

Values are expressed as mean ± SD (unless otherwise stated). Statistical tests: [a]t-test; [b]Pearson's χ^2 test; [c]Mann-Whitney U test. $^{**}p < 0.01$. BCVA, best-corrected visual acuity; MD, mean deviation (dB); IOP, intraocular pressure (mmHg); UPDRS III, Unified Parkinson Disease Rating Scale III.

best-corrected visual acuity (BCVA). The PD group included male and female with a mean age of 61.79 ± 9.89 years (range: 32–81 years). The mean duration of PD was 67.92 ± 45.52 months (range: 10–204 months) with a median of 60 months since diagnosis.

There was a significant difference in the mean deviation (MD) of the visual field between the HC group and the PD group ($u = -4.060$, $p \le 0.001$). The basic demographics of parameters including age, sex, BCVA, and IOP had no difference between the two groups.

3.2. The mf-ERG Examination Results. The amplitude density (AD) of P1 differed significantly in ring1 and ring2 between the HC group and PD patients group ($p \le 0.001$). Compared with the HC group, the IT of P1 in ring1, ring2, and ring3 was significantly prolonged in the PD group ($p \le 0.001$). The AD and IT of N1 wave did not differ significantly among the rings (Table 2).

3.3. The SD-OCT Examination Results. The SD-OCT examinations results are summarized in Table 3. The macular retinal thickness (MRT) and macular volume (MV) were decreased in the PD group compared with healthy controls ($p = 0.027$, 0.001, resp.). The average of RNFL thickness and inferior quadrant thickness was obviously thinning in PD patients compared with the HC group ($p = 0.008$, 0.004, resp.). However, there was no significant difference in the other three quadrants of RNFL thickness between the two groups.

3.4. Correlation of Different Examination Results. The AD of P1 in ring1 was negatively correlated with the MD of the visual field ($p = 0.008$) and positively correlated with MV ($p = 0.005$). The AD of P1 in ring2 was negatively correlated with the MD of the visual field ($p = 0.003$) and positively correlated with MV ($p = 0.012$). The IT of P1 in ring3 was positively correlated with the MD of visual field ($p = 0.015$) and average RNFL thickness ($p = 0.027$) (Table 4).

TABLE 2: Retinal function analysis of PD patients and healthy subjects using mf-ERG.

	HC	PD	p
Number of eyes tested	$n = 82$	$n = 106$	
AD of P1 in ring1	139.43 ± 16.92	100.75 ± 21.13	≤0.001**
AD of P1 in ring2	36.93 ± 9.09	21.83 ± 7.49	≤0.001**
AD of P1 in ring3	15.79 ± 4.26	15.72 ± 4.00	0.692
AD of P1 in ring4	13.79 ± 3.23	13.30 ± 4.04	0.079
AD of P1 in ring5	10.08 ± 3.61	9.30 ± 1.74	0.062
IT of P1 in ring1	38.34 ± 4.85	42.72 ± 7.66	≤0.001**
IT of P1 in ring2	39.47 ± 6.21	42.72 ± 7.66	0.039*
IT of P1 in ring3	37.26 ± 4.42	41.09 ± 7.68	≤0.001**
IT of P1 in ring4	41.14 ± 4.53	41.67 ± 8.51	0.656
IT of P1 in ring5	43.24 ± 6.65	41.72 ± 8.14	0.159
AD of N1 in ring1	0.48 ± 0.22	0.43 ± 0.13	0.071
AD of N1 in ring2	0.27 ± 0.05	0.26 ± 0.07	0.121
AD of N1 in ring3	0.19 ± 0.13	0.16 ± 0.08	0.395
AD of N1 in ring4	0.20 ± 0.09	0.19 ± 0.07	0.872
AD of N1 in ring5	0.17 ± 0.10	0.16 ± 0.08	0.910
IT of N1 in ring1	19.76 ± 3.21	20.47 ± 4.67	0.149
IT of N1 in ring2	20.14 ± 5.41	21.94 ± 9.03	0.135
IT of N1 in ring3	23.06 ± 3.72	22.13 ± 6.58	0.230
IT of N1 in ring4	24.30 ± 7.06	23.03 ± 6.50	0.208
IT of N1 in ring5	21.61 ± 5.84	22.44 ± 6.58	0.675

Values are expressed as mean ± SD. Statistical tests: Mann-Whitney U test. AD = amplitude density (nV/deg^2); IT = implicit time (ms). $^{*}p < 0.05$; $^{**}p < 0.01$.

3.5. The ROC Curve Analyses of the Different Examinations Results. ROC (receiver operating characteristic) curves of single parameter were plotted in Figure 1. The AUC (area under curve) of the AD of P1 in ring1 and ring2 were 0.081 and 0.114, respectively. The IT of P1 in ring1, ring2, and ring3 to detect PD diagnosis was 0.674, 0.588, and 0.653, respectively. The MRT, MV, and RNFL revealed AUC of 0.406, 0.354, and 0.387, respectively. The MD of the visual field to detect PD diagnosis was 0.709.

ROC curves of the combinations of these parameters were plotted in Figure 2. The AUC (area under curve) of a combination of the AD of P1 in ring1, the MD and MV, to detect PD diagnosis, was 0.944. A combination of the AD of P1 in ring2, the MD and the MV, revealed AUC of 0.921. A combination of the AD of P1 in ring1 and the MV revealed AUC of 0.921. The AUC of the MD combined with the MV, the AD of P1 in ring1 combined with the MV, and the AD of P1 in ring2 combined with the MV were 0.746, 0.922, and 0.901, respectively. A combination of the IT of P1 in ring3, the MD, and the average RNFL thickness revealed AUC of 0.750 (Figure 2).

4. Discussion

Because of the relatively early stage of disease of recruited PD patients in our study, the visual acuity was normal and had no significant difference compared with the HC group.

Table 3: Macular thickness, macular volume, and RNFL thickness analysis using SD-OCT.

	HC	PD	p
Number of eyes	82	106	
Macular thickness			
Macular retinal thickness (microns ± SD)	269.93 ± 22.56	262.15 ± 25.80	0.027*
Central foveal thickness (microns ± SD)	239.68 ± 40.17	231.21 ± 49.28	0.100
Macular volume (mm^3)	9.87 ± 0.68	9.51 ± 0.85	0.001**
RNFL thickness (microns ± SD)			
Average	92.72 ± 11.50	88.93 ± 18.79	0.008**
Temporal quadrant thickness	68.23 ± 14.26	66.14 ± 18.26	0.117
Nasal quadrant thickness	65.96 ± 12.51	66.25 ± 20.53	0.347
Superior quadrant thickness	113.20 ± 22.53	111.27 ± 23.57	0.532
Inferior quadrant thickness	123.45 ± 25.93	113.08 ± 34.00	0.004**

Values are expressed as mean ± SD. Statistical tests: Mann–Whitney U test. RNFL = retinal nerve fiber layer. $^{*}p < 0.05$; $^{**}p < 0.01$.

Table 4: Correlation between visual functional parameters and structural parameters.

	MD	MRT	MV	Average RNFL
AD of P1 (R1)	(−0.191, 0.008)**	(0.193, 0.008)	(0.204, 0.005)**	(0.081, 0.267)
AD of P1 (R2)	(−0.214, 0.003)**	(0.139, 0.057)	(0.184, 0.012)*	(0.081, 0.267)
IT of P1 (R1)	(0.096, 0.190)	(−0.083, 0.255)	(−0.023, 0.749)	(−0.074, 0.311)
IT of P1 (R2)	(0.072, 0.328)	(−0.002, 0.973)	(−0.027, 0.716)	(−0.008, 0.918)
IT of P1 (R3)	(0.178, 0.015)*	(−0.102, 0.163)	(−0.010, 0.895)	(0.161, 0.027)*

Statistical tests: Pearson's correlation coefficient. AD = amplitude density (nV/deg^2); IT = implicit time (ms); MD = mean deviation; MRT = macular retinal thickness; MV = macular volume; RNFL = retinal nerve fiber layer $^{*}p < 0.05$; $^{**}p < 0.01$.

However, the abnormalities of the MD of the visual field were observed with the significant difference. Lots of studies [6, 23, 26] suggested that the MD of the visual field was a sensitive parameter of the visual function in patients with PD. The visual field test reflects the function of retinal ganglion cells, which have axons that project via the optic nerve to diverse targets in the brain.

Many previous studies [12, 18, 19] on the vision function of PD patients have used visual evoked potential (VEP). However, the VEP monitors the integrity of the entire visual pathway from the fovea to the visual cortex, so it can't be an accurate response to the fovea function. The mf-ERG test is specific and sensitive for reflecting the function of the fovea, where the density of the ganglion cell is much higher than other zones of the retina. To date, few studies [16, 17] have focused on PD with the mf-ERG test. In our study, we found that the amplitude of P1 was decreased and the IT of P1 was prolonged in ring1 and ring2 significantly compared with the HC group. The result was consistent with that of study of Kaur et al. [16], which showed that mf-ERG in central 2° revealed the reduced foveal activity in PD patients.

In recent years, since the application of SD-OCT instrument for measurement of the retinal thickness in patients with PD, lots of studies [16–23] focused on the structural changes in the retina of PD. However, the results had no agreement in conclusions. It may be because of the recruited patients with different disease stages or the difference of diversity of OCT apparatus.

The macular thickness analysis in our study revealed the thinning change in macular retinal thickness, macular volume, and average RNFL thickness of patients with PD compared with the HC group. Many studies [16, 20] confirmed this. However, some studies [23–29] had conflicting results. There are some possible reasons for it. First, in our study, the mean of Hoehn–Yahr scales is 1.92 ± 0.54 and UPDRS III scales is 37.15 ± 16.61, which suggested that the disease stage of recruited PD patients was early, but the motor manifestation was serious, so the change of thickness of RNFL may be obvious. Second, the age of recruited patients and the HC participants in our study was much younger than that of in previous studies [23, 29]. However, the RNFL is negatively correlated with age, making difficulties in detection of the subtle differences of RNFL in the older participants. So, when the patients are much older, it may be not easy to find the thinning changes caused by PD.

All of these reasons suggested that it was incredible to use a single method to evaluate the retinal change in patients with PD. Some studies confirmed that it was vital to combine functional and structural changes to evaluate the PD. Miri et al. [29] and Altintaş et al. [30] reported a near negative correlation between the total MV and P100 latency in PD and found that the pattern VEP combined with retinal foveal thickness had a high diagnostic yield for PD. Garcia-Martin et al. [21] reported that both of the AD of P-ERG and the thickness of macular and RNFL were decreased in PD patients.

These studies demonstrated that the retina of patients with PD had changed in both of morphology (retinal thickness) and retinal function including visual field, VEP test, and pattern ERG. We assumed that it could find more

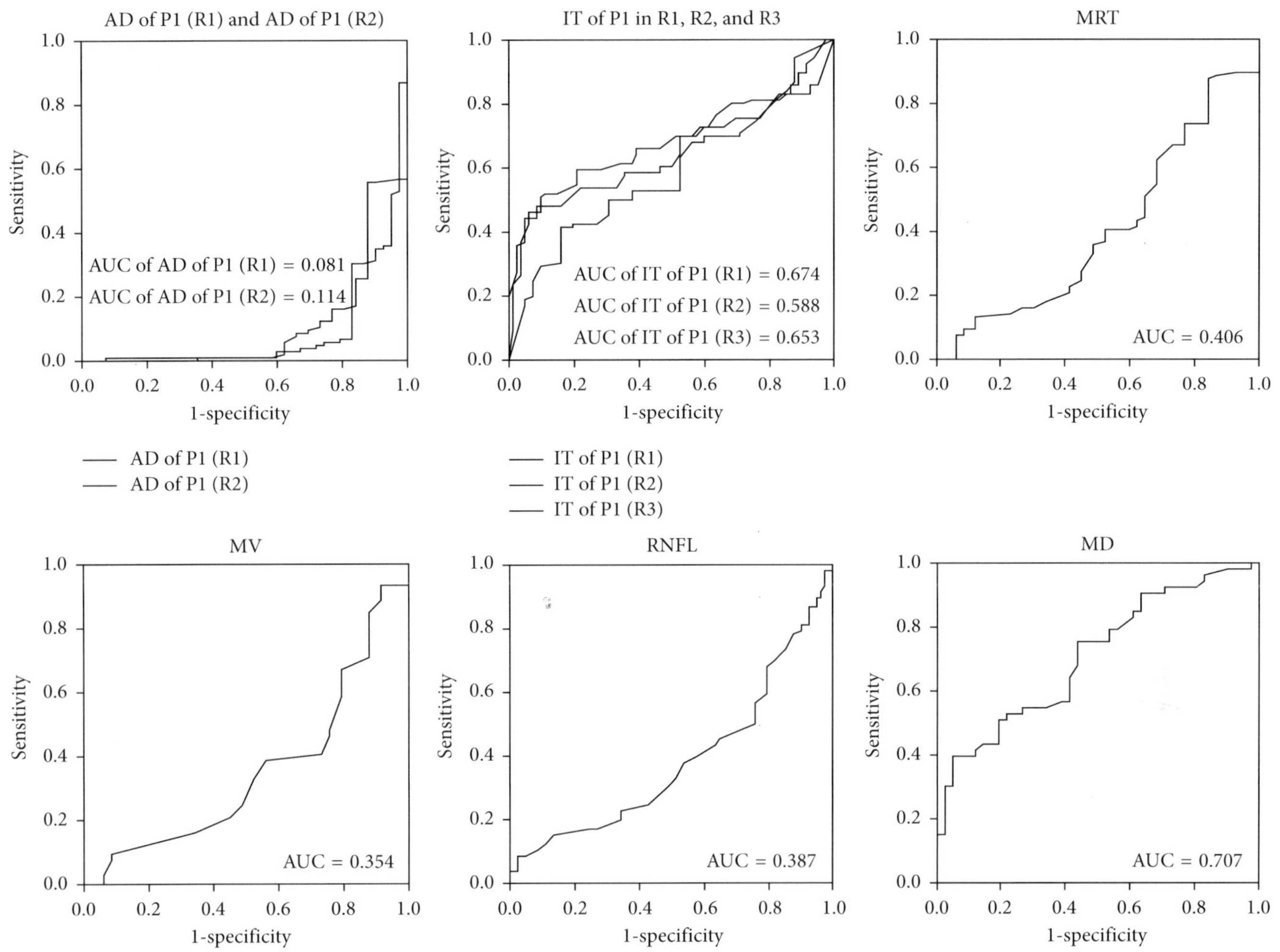

FIGURE 1: ROC curves of the single parameter of visual function or structure for discriminating Parkinson's disease. AD = amplitude density; IT = implicit time; R1 = ring1; R2 = ring2; R3 = ring3; MD = mean deviation of visual field; MRT = macular retinal thickness; MV = macular volume; RNFL = retinal nerve fiber layer.

clinical diagnostic values by integrating the test parameters. So, the main aim of our study was to evaluate retinal changes and increase the diagnostic yield of PD with a combination of mf-ERG and SD-OCT examinations.

We found an important correlation between macular morphology and function in patients with PD. The AD of P1 in some regions was negatively correlated with the MD of the visual field and positively correlated with MV. And the IT of P1 in some regions was positively correlated with the MD. That means there is a strong internal consistency between retinal structure and retinal function.

Further analysis of the ROC curve of multiparameter can lead to more information on clinical diagnostic value. This study indicates that the ROC curve for a combination of retinal structure and retinal function can much better discriminate between participants with PD and healthy controls than that for a single parameter. It demonstrated that the AD of P1 in ring1 combined with the MD and the MV had the highest diagnostic yield of PD. However, the less the parameters selected, the higher the diagnostic effectiveness. In our study, the AUC of the AD of P1 in ring2 combined with the MD of the visual field and the MV equaled that of the AD of P1 in ring1 combined with the MV. On the contrary, a combination of the IT of P1 in ring3 and the MD and the RNFL revealed a lower AUC. The AD of P1 in ring2 combined with the MV actually had a higher AUC, although there were only two parameters selected. It demonstrated that the AD of P1 combined with the MV could get a high diagnostic yield to discriminate between participants with or without PD.

By analysis of ROC curve, this study found that a single parameter of either function or structure revealed lower AUC significantly than that of the combined parameters. So, it indicates that a combination of mf-ERG and SD-OCT provides a good clinical biomarker for diagnosis of PD.

Acknowledgments

This work was supported by Suzhou "Rejuvenation of the Health through Science and Education" Youth Scientific

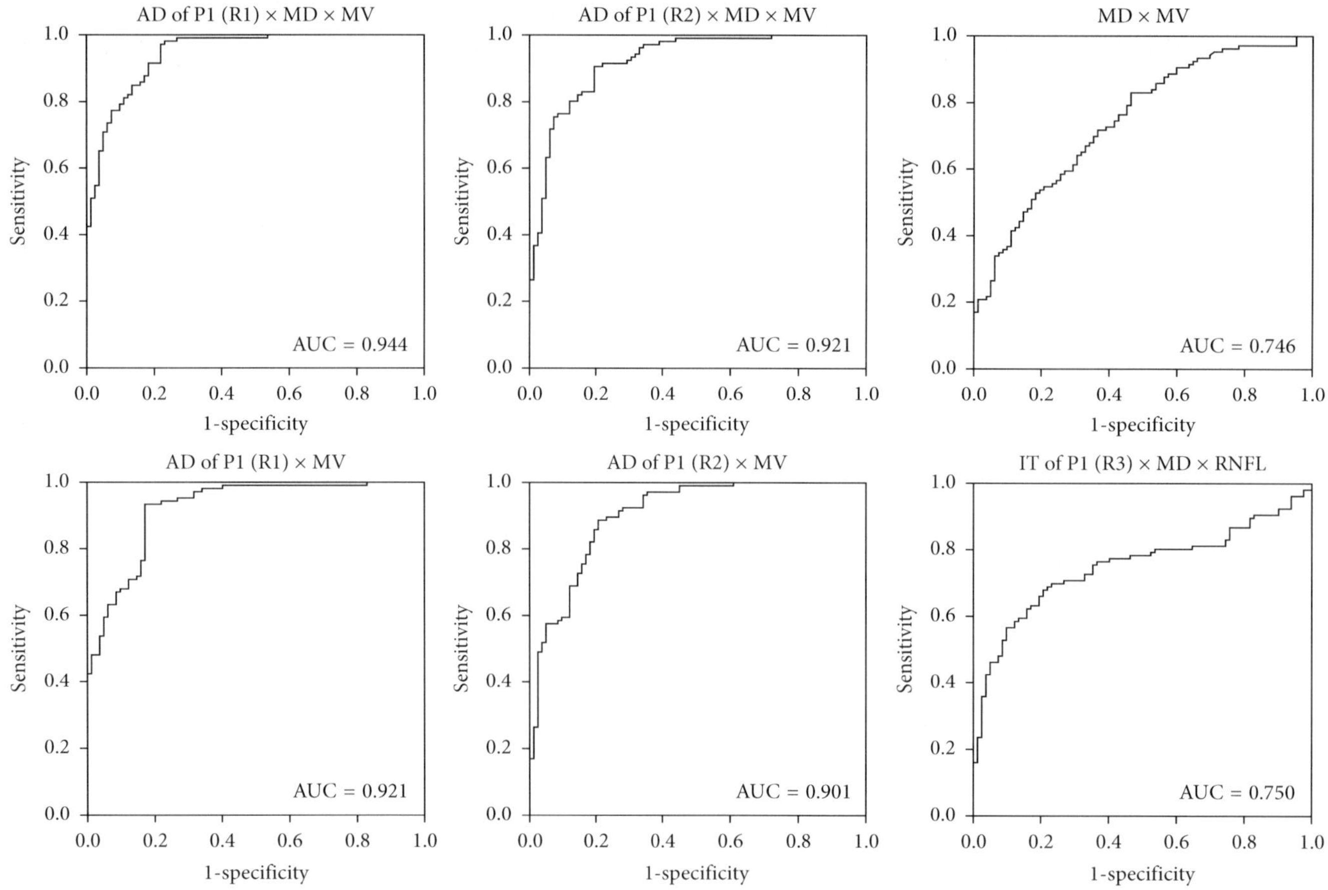

FIGURE 2: ROC curves of different combinations of visual function and structure parameters for discriminating Parkinson's disease. AD = amplitude density; IT = implicit time; R1 = ring1; R2 = ring2; R3 = ring3; MD = mean deviation of visual field, MRT = macular retinal thickness; MV = macular volume; RNFL = retinal nerve fiber layer.

Projects of China (KJXW2014014), Suzhou Science and Technology Development Project (SYSD2016091), and Project of Clinical Advantage Scientific Group of the Second Affiliated Hospital of Soochow University (XKQ2015002). The authors are especially grateful to the participants in this study.

References

[1] M. C. De Rijk, M. M. B. Breteler, G. A. Graveland et al., "Prevalence of Parkinson's disease in the elderly: the Rotterdam Study," *Neurology*, vol. 45, no. 12, pp. 2143–2146, 1995.

[2] L. M. L. De Lau and M. M. B. Breteler, "Epidemiology of Parkinson's disease," *The Lancet Neurology*, vol. 5, no. 6, pp. 525–535, 2006.

[3] L. M. Shulman, R. L. Taback, J. Bean, and W. J. Weiner, "Comorbidity of the nonmotor symptoms of Parkinson's disease," *Movement Disorders*, vol. 16, no. 3, pp. 507–510, 2001.

[4] P. Martinez-Martin, A. H. V. Schapira, F. Stocchi et al., "Prevalence of nonmotor symptoms in Parkinson's disease in an international setting; study using nonmotor symptoms questionnaire in 545 patients," *Movement Disorders*, vol. 22, no. 11, pp. 1623–1629, 2007.

[5] C. Lucetti, G. Gambaccini, P. Del Dotto et al., "Long-term clinical evaluation in patients with Parkinson's disease and early autonomic involvement," *Parkinsonism and Related Disorders*, vol. 12, no. 5, pp. 279–283, 2006.

[6] V. Biousse, B. C. Skibell, R. L. Watts, D. N. Loupe, C. Drews-Botsch, and N. J. Newman, "Ophthalmologic features of Parkinson's disease," *Neurology*, vol. 62, no. 2, pp. 177–180, 2004.

[7] I. Bodis-Wollner, "Foveal vision is impaired in Parkinson's disease," *Parkinsonism and Related Disorders*, vol. 19, no. 1, pp. 1–14, 2013.

[8] A. Sauerbier and K. R. Chaudhuri, "Parkinson's disease and vision," *Basal Ganglia*, vol. 3, no. 3, pp. 159–163, 2013.

[9] Z. Muresan and J. C. Besharse, "D2-like dopamine receptors in amphibian retina: Localization with fluorescent ligands," *Journal of Comparative Neurology*, vol. 331, no. 2, pp. 149–160, 1993.

[10] A. Akopian and P. Witkovsky, "D2 dopamine receptor-mediated inhibition of a hyperpolarization-activated current in rod photoreceptors," *Journal of Neurophysiology*, vol. 76, no. 3, pp. 1828–1835, 1996.

[11] D. C. Hood, J. G. Odel, C. S. Chen, and B. J. Winn, "The multifocal electroretinogram," *Journal of Neuro-Ophthalmology*, vol. 23, no. 3, pp. 225–235, 2003.

[12] M. Kondo, Y. Miyake, M. Horiguchi, S. Suzuki, and A. Tanikawa, "Clinical evaluation of multifocal electroretinogram," *Investigative Ophthalmology and Visual Science*, vol. 36, no. 10, pp. 2146–2150, 1995.

[13] V. Parisi, M. Tedeschi, G. Gallinaro, M. Varano, S. Saviano, and S. Piermarocchi, "Carotenoids and antioxidants in

age-related maculopathy Italian study: multifocal electroretinogram modifications after 1 year," *Ophthalmology*, vol. 115, no. 2, pp. 324.e2–333.e2, 2008.

[14] A. M. Palmowski, E. E. Sutter, M. A. Bearse, and W. Fung, "Mapping of retinal function in diabetic retinopathy using the multifocal electroretinogram," *Investigative Ophthalmology and Visual Science*, vol. 38, no. 12, pp. 2586–2596, 1997.

[15] I. V. Glybina and R. N. Frank, "Localization of multifocal electroretinogram abnormalities to the lesion site: findings in a family with Best disease," *Archives of Ophthalmology*, vol. 124, no. 11, pp. 1593–1600, 2006.

[16] M. Kaur, R. Saxena, D. Singh, M. Behari, P. Sharma, and V. Menon, "Correlation between structural and functional retinal changes in Parkinson disease," *Journal of Neuro-Ophthalmology*, vol. 35, no. 3, pp. 254–258, 2015.

[17] M. M. Moschos, G. Tagaris, I. Markopoulos et al., "Morphologic changes and functional retinal impairment in patients with Parkinson disease without visual loss," *European Journal of Ophthalmology*, vol. 21, no. 1, pp. 24–29, 2011.

[18] T. C. Chen, B. Cense, M. C. Pierce et al., "Spectral domain optical coherence tomography: ultra-high speed, ultra-high resolution ophthalmic imaging," *Archives of Ophthalmology*, vol. 123, no. 12, pp. 1715–1720, 2005.

[19] C. K. Leung, C. Y. Cheung, R. N. Weinreb et al., "Retinal nerve fiber layer imaging with spectral-domain optical coherence tomography: a variability and diagnostic performance study," *Ophthalmology*, vol. 116, no. 7, pp. 1257.e2–1263.e2, 2009.

[20] E. S. Sari, R. Koc, A. Yazici, G. Sahin, and S. S. Ermis, "Ganglion cell–inner plexiform layer thickness in patients with Parkinson disease and association with disease severity and duration," *Journal of Neuro-Ophthalmology*, vol. 35, no. 2, pp. 117–121, 2015.

[21] E. Garcia-Martin, D. Rodriguez-Mena, M. Satue et al., "Electrophysiology and optical coherence tomography to evaluate Parkinson disease severity," *Investigative Ophthalmology and Visual Science*, vol. 55, no. 2, pp. 696–705, 2014.

[22] J. Y. Lee, J. M. Kim, J. Ahn, H.-J. Kim, B. S. Jeon, and T. W. Kim, "Retinal nerve fiber layer thickness and visual hallucinations in Parkinson's disease," *Movement Disorders*, vol. 29, no. 1, pp. 61–67, 2014.

[23] E. E. Tsironi, A. Dastiridou, A. Katsanos et al., "Perimetric and retinal nerve fiber layer findings in patients with Parkinson's disease," *BMC Ophthalmology*, vol. 12, no. 1, p. 1, 2012.

[24] A. J. Hughes, S. E. Daniel, L. Kilford, and A. J. Lees, "Accuracy of clinical diagnosis of idiopathic Parkinson's disease: a clinico-pathological study of 100 cases," *Journal of Neurology, Neurosurgery and Psychiatry*, vol. 55, no. 3, pp. 181–184, 1992.

[25] D. C. Hood, M. Bach, M. Brigell et al., "ISCEV standard for clinical multifocal electroretinography (mf-ERG) (2011 edition)," *Documenta Ophthalmologica*, vol. 124, no. 1, pp. 1–13, 2012.

[26] H. R. Joo, B. B. Peterson, D. M. Dacey, S. Hattar, and S.-K. Chen, "Recurrent axon collaterals of intrinsically photosensitive retinal ganglion cells," *Visual Neuroscience*, vol. 30, no. 4, pp. 175–182, 2013.

[27] S. Miri, S. Glazman, L. Mylin, and I. Bodis-Wollner, "A combination of retinal morphology and visual electrophysiology testing increases diagnostic yield in Parkinson's disease," *Parkinsonism and Related Disorders*, vol. 22, pp. S134–S137, 2016.

[28] I. Gottlob, E. Schneider, W. Heider, and W. Skrandies, "Alteration of visual evoked potentials and electroretinograms in Parkinson's disease," *Electroencephalography and Clinical Neurophysiology*, vol. 66, no. 4, pp. 349–357, 1987.

[29] N. K. Archibald, M. P. Clarke, U. P. Mosimann, and D. J. Burn, "Retinal thickness in Parkinson's disease," *Parkinsonism and Related Disorders*, vol. 17, no. 6, pp. 431–436, 2011.

[30] Ö. Altintaş, P. Işeri, B. Özkan, and Y. Çağlar, "Correlation between retinal morphological and functional findings and clinical severity in Parkinson's disease," *Documenta Ophthalmologica*, vol. 116, no. 2, pp. 137–146, 2008.

17

Association of Gait Characteristics and Depression in Patients with Parkinson's Disease Assessed in Goal-Directed Locomotion Task

Péter Kincses,[1] Norbert Kovács,[2] Kázmér Karádi,[1] Ádám Feldmann,[1] Krisztina Dorn,[3] Zsuzsanna Aschermann,[2] Sámuel Komoly,[2] Tibor Szolcsányi,[1] Árpád Csathó,[1] and János Kállai[1]

[1] *Institute of Behavioral Sciences, University of Pécs, Pécs 7624, Hungary*
[2] *Clinical Center, Department of Neurology, University of Pécs, Pécs 7623, Hungary*
[3] *Pediatric Clinic, Clinical Center, University of Pécs, Pécs 7623, Hungary*

Correspondence should be addressed to János Kállai; janos.kallai@aok.pte.hu

Academic Editor: Ivan Bodis-Wollner

Introduction. In the genesis of Parkinson's disease (PD) clinical phenomenology the exact nature of the association between bradykinesia and affective variables is unclear. In the present study, we analyzed the gait characteristics and level of depression in PD and healthy volunteers. *Methods.* Patients with PD ($n = 48$) and healthy controls ($n = 52$) were recruited for the present study. Walking speed, stride length, and cadence were compared between groups while participants completed a goal-directed locomotion task under visually controlled (VC) and visually noncontrolled conditions (VnC). *Results.* Significantly higher depression scores were found in PD comparing to healthy control groups. In PD, depression was associated with gait components in the VC wherein the place of the target was visible. In contrast, in healthy subjects the depression was associated with gait components in VnC wherein the location and image of the target were memorized and recalled. In patients with PD and depression, the visually deprived multitask augments the rate of cadence and diminishes stride length, while velocity remains relatively unchanged. The depression associated with gait characteristics as a comorbid affective factor in PD, and that impairs the coherence of gait pattern. *Conclusion.* The relationship between depression and gait parameters appears to indicate that PD not only is a neurological disease but also incorporates affective disturbances that associate with the regulation of gait characteristics.

1. Introduction

Studies of gait characteristics in Parkinson's disease (PD) indicate that gait difficulties are commonly associated with affective disturbances [1–3]. In patients with PD, voxel-based morphometric and functional magnetic resonance imaging (fMRI) studies report a correlation between depression and gray matter impairment in the bilateral orbitofrontal cortex, right temporal region, and limbic system [4]. The neural networks involved in gait and balance control include the mesencephalic motor region and the primary and secondary motor cortex [5, 6]. In addition, the basal ganglia and supplementary motor area (SMA), which play a role in the affective organization of goal-directed locomotion, have been implicated in PD [7, 8]. The disruption of these regions induces deficits in action execution and preparation. The NPF's 2012 Parkinson's Outcomes Project [9] found that depression has the greatest impact on gait in patients with PD [7], but the association between depression and gait characteristic can be found in healthy elderly persons as well [10]. Previous studies have demonstrated that the treatment of depression can significantly alleviate motor symptoms. However, patients with PD who receive gait training and other forms of exercise therapy at an early stage demonstrate a significantly slower decline in quality of life than those who received intervention later [9].

In PD, the essential components of gait pattern include stride length, cadence, and velocity [11], wherein studies report decreased stride length and velocity and increased

Table 1: Demographic and clinical characteristics of Parkinson's disease patients and healthy control persons. MEMS = Mini-Exam of Mental Status; MADRS = Montgomery-Åsberg Depression Rating Scale; VC = visually controlled condition; VnC = visually noncontrolled condition; UPDRS = Unified Parkinson's Disease Rating Scale; LEDD = levodopa equivalent daily dose.

	Parkinson's disease ($N = 40$)	Healthy control ($N = 49$)	t; Z p value
Gender, males/females	24/16	24/25	1.0 ns.
Age, mean ± SD, Min–Max	68.0 ± 8.1; 57–80	65.6 ± 5.6; 56–79	1.6 ns.
MEMS (in %) mean ± SD	91.0 ± 16.6	89.4 ± 10.5	0.6 ns.
MADRS total, mean ± SD	18.1 ± 9.1	11.6 ± 8.2	3.5^{***}
Cadence VC (for 4 m)	9.9 ± 3.5	8.0 ± 2.2	3.1^{**}
Cadence VnC (for 4 m)	15.1 ± 6.9	9.8 ± 2.6	4.9^{***}
Step length VC (cm)	38.8 ± 11.1	45.9 ± 10.5	3.1^{**}
Step length VnC (cm)	28.1 ± 9.6	41.0 ± 10.8	5.9^{***}
Velocity VC (m/s)	0.6 ± 0.2	0.7 ± 2.3	1.2 ns.
Velocity VnC (m/s)	0.5 ± 0.2	0.6 ± 0.2	4.0^{***}
Disease duration, mean ± SD, Min–Max	6.7 ± 4.5; (1–16)	N/D	
UPDRS total mean ± SD, Min–Max	58.7 ± 25.5 (28–122)	N/D	
Mentation, mean ± SD	12.1 ± 6.2	N/D	
Daily activities mean ± SD	11.7 ± 7.5	N/D	
Motor examination mean ± SD	31.3 ± 13.7	N/D	
Complication mean ± SD	4.0 ± 3.4	N/D	
LEDD (mg) mean ± SD, Min–Max	712.2 ± 464.5 (154–1880)	N/D	

$p < 0.01^{**}$; $p < 0.001^{***}$.

cadence in patients with PD [12]. Many patients with PD experience dysfunctional coordination during walking, and falling is a frequent occurrence [13]. In particular, shorter stride length without surface cues is often detected, and as a compensatory mechanism, this plays an important role in the development of gait hypokinesia [12, 14].

The aim of this study was to examine associations between depression and gait characteristics in patients with PD and healthy elderly control. The present study explores between-group differences in gait pattern and investigates the association between depression and the components of goal-directed locomotion. The authors hypothesized that each examined gait component, velocity, cadence, and stride length, would significantly differ between patients with PD and age-matched healthy controls. In addition, the rate of gait disorder would demonstrate a strong association with depression and quality of life in patients.

2. Method

2.1. Participants. Patients with PD ($n = 48$) and healthy age and education in years fitted controls ($n = 52$) were recruited for the present study. Patient demographics and clinical characteristics are listed in Table 1. Healthy volunteer participants were recruited from a pensioners' club. Participants were able to walk unsupported and they had normal or corrected vision. All subjects had no history of psychiatric disease, previous treatment with depression, or significant cognitive impairment, were free of acute illness, and did not require nursing care. Patients were recruited from the Outpatients Clinics at the regional Department of Neurology UP Medical School. Considering the required free walk locomotion test condition, patients were only asked for participation who were classified as patients with PD in Hoehn and Yahr stages 3-4 and freezing was not detected [14, 15]. All patients were prescribed levodopa (L-dopa). Cognitive impairment was evaluated using the Mini Mental State Examination (MMSE) [16, 17]. Nondemented persons were only invited to participate in the experimental part of study. In addition, the Montgomery-Åsberg Depression Rating Scale (MADRS) was used to examine affective disturbances [18]. In addition, all subjects were right-handed, as assessed by the Edinburgh Handedness Inventory [19]. Handedness Laterality Quotients were 70% or higher for the right hand in all subjects.

The Unified Parkinson's Disease Rating Scale (UPDRS) [20] was applied to evaluate the PD symptoms (Table 1) and the total UPDRS scores have been used in the statistical analysis. Patients and healthy controls were excluded if they received an MMSE score of less than 23. Following MMSE examination, 40 patients with PD and 49 controls were recruited for experimental analysis. All participants provided written informed consent prior to experimentation. This study was performed in accordance with the Helsinki Declaration and approved by the Regional Research Ethics Committee of the Medical Center in the State University.

2.2. Procedure. Global motor function was assessed using the UPDRS by a movement disorder specialist (N.K), when medication was controlled during regular visits to the outpatient clinic. Patients' L-dopa equivalent dosage (LED) was calculated as described by Tomlinson et al. [21]. All patients took their medication in the morning approximately 2 h prior

TABLE 2: Pearson's correlation of gait characteristics and affective scales in the healthy control group in two conditions (VC = visually controlled condition; VnC = visually noncontrolled condition), MADRS (Montgomery-Åsberg Depression Rating Scale).

	(1)	(2)	(3)	(4)	(5)	(6)	(7)
(1) Velocity VC		$-.84^{***}$	$.87^{***}$	$.80^{***}$	$-.61^{***}$	$.71^{***}$	$-.21$
(2) Cadence VC			$-.94^{***}$	$-.64^{***}$	$.79^{***}$	$-.66^{***}$	$.27$
(3) Stride length VC				$.72^{***}$	$-.78^{***}$	$.75^{***}$	$-.21$
(4) Velocity VnC					$-.73^{***}$	$.78^{***}$	$-.32^{*}$
(5) Cadence VnC						$-.86^{***}$	$.39^{**}$
(6) Stride length VnC							$-.31^{**}$
(7) MADRS							

$p < 0.05^{*}$; $p < 0.01^{**}$; $p < 0.001^{***}$.

to examination. Participants were invited into a laboratory room and asked to perform two subsequent tasks that were originated from the clinical practice and modelled the everyday locomotion. To assess the gait characteristics, the patients and healthy controls were directed to approach a target in an examination room, where the main gait components of PD were evaluated using operationalized methods. At the beginning of the trial, participants were instructed to stand in front of a visible gray cross target (25 × 25 cm) placed 4 m away on a white wall. They were directed to lift their right arm and to point to a target with their right index finger. Next, while maintaining this arm and finger position, participants were instructed to approach the target and touch it. The goal-directed locomotion test contained two types of multiple task conditions: a simple visual control (VC) and complex nonvisual control (VnC). The first trial was conducted with VC and served as an introductory motor exercise to assess the gait characteristics of participants and to determine stability in circumstances with VC. Following the introductory VC task, three test trials were performed in the VnC condition. During this task, at the start line, after a visual fixation of the target, the participant's eyes were covered by nontransparent swimming glasses and asked to approach and touched the estimated place of the target. The participants were followed up by an assistant. The procedure was safe or falling or other complications did not happen. Under VC and VnC conditions, the participants' gait characteristics, including cadence, stride length, and velocity, were recorded and assessed on a large carpet using a visible scaled ruler. The measurement of gait components was initiated when patients took their first step toward the target and maintained throughout their route towards the goal. Offline video recordings of the route of locomotion were analyzed by two independent raters. Three main gait parameters were assessed, including velocity (m/s), cadence (number of steps from start to target), and stride length (distance in cm between successive heel contact points of the same foot).

2.3. Statistical Analysis. SPSS version 22.0 was used for statistical analysis (Chicago, IL, US). For group comparisons, patients with PD and healthy participants were compared. A two-tailed t-test for parametric and a Mann–Whitney U test for nonparametric data were used to assess between-group differences in age, sex, education level, MADRS, cadence, stride length, and velocity. Kolmogorov-Smirnov tests were used to assess the normality of variables. Logarithmic transformation was applied for cadence data in parametric comparisons. Moreover, Pearson's correlation analyses were used in the control group to assess within-group associations between movement parameters and MADRS data. In addition, in the patients' group, Pearson's correlation analyses were performed to evaluate the relationship between L-dopa dosage and MADRS, disease duration, cadence, stride length, and velocity variables. Gait data differences between groups were analyzed using multivariate test initially (MANCOVA, adjusted for age and gender), with follow-up univariate tests (ANOVA). For multiple comparisons between gait data and depression (following Feldmann et al.'s [4] method MADRS, cutoff = 13 was used) a 2 × 2 × 2 Analysis of Variance (ANOVA) was used with regard to the factors of velocity, cadence, stride length, and MADRS for all dependent variables (two conditions: locomotion with VC and locomotion with VnC) in healthy controls and patients with PD. Post hoc Scheffé-tests were applied to evaluate significant pairwise differences between variables. Reasonable results were listed in post hoc tables only. Levene's test was used to detect differences in the homogeneity of variance. Analyses were two-tailed and significance was set at 0.05.

3. Results

3.1. The Coherence of Gait Pattern and the Related Affective Associations in Visually Controlled and Visually Noncontrolled Conditions. Correlation analyses in the control group revealed a coherent pattern for velocity, stride length, and cadence. Under both VC and VnC conditions, the association of the three main gait components demonstrated the same coherent configuration (Table 2). During goal-directed locomotion, fast walkers typically exhibit a small cadence and long stride length while small cadence associated with long stride length. In the present task, the depression did not show a significant association with gait pattern under a simple VC conditions; however, in the multitask VnC condition, high depression scores correlated with low velocity, high cadence, and short stride length.

The correlation analysis of patients with PD demonstrated a coherent gait pattern (low velocity, high cadence, and long stride length) similar to that of healthy controls

Table 3: Persons' correlation of gait characteristics and depression scale in Parkinson's disease group in two conditions (VC = visually controlled condition; VnC = visually noncontrolled condition): MADRS (Montgomery-Åsberg Depression Rating Scale); UPDRS (Unified Parkinson's Disease Rating Scale); LED values; duration of disease.

	(1)	(2)	(3)	(4)	(5)	(6)	(7)	(8)	(9)	(10)
(1) Velocity VC		$-.86^{***}$	$.92^{***}$	$.75^{***}$	$-.74^{**}$	.21	$-.34^{*}$	$-.44^{**}$	$.34^{**}$	.21
(2) Cadence VC			$-.91^{***}$	$-.73^{**}$	$.82^{***}$	−.20	$.33^{*}$	$.37^{**}$	−.27	−.24
(3) Stride length VC				$-.75^{***}$	$-.79^{***}$	.16	$-.31^{*}$	$-.36^{*}$	$.34^{*}$	.22
(4) Velocity VnC					$-.85^{***}$	$.42^{**}$	−.25	$-.34^{*}$	.18	.16
(5) Cadence VnC						$-.34^{*}$	.25	$.38^{**}$	−.14	−.16
(6) Stride length VnC							−.13	−.15	.04	.08
(7) MADRS								$.47^{**}$	−.28	−.21
(8) UPDRS									−.03	.09
(9) LED values										$.63^{***}$
(10) Duration										

$p < 0.05^{*}$; $p < 0.01^{**}$; $p < 0.001^{***}$.

in both the VC and VnC conditions. However, contrary to healthy controls, the depression was linked to low velocity, high cadence, and short stride length in the VC condition. A similar association was not found in the multitask VnC condition between depression and gait parameters. This indicates that the depression associated gait pattern was reverted in the VC and VnC conditions for the control and PD groups. PD-specific UPDRS scores correlated with depression and all gait parameters excluding stride length in the VnC condition. LED values correlated with velocity and stride length only in the VC condition, and disease duration was found to associate with L-dopa dose (Table 3).

3.2. Multivariate Analyses and Multiple Comparisons. Comparison of the gait variables in the two groups (PD and healthy controls) showed the presence of significant differences concerning the mean gait scores [MANCOVA Wilks $\lambda = .569$; $F(6, 88) = 10.083$; $p < 0.001$], after controlling for age and gender. Analysis of covariance found significantly lower stride length and higher cadence in patients with PD compared with healthy controls in VC and VnC conditions. The velocity was significantly different in the two groups in the VnC condition only.

3.3. Pairwise Results by Scheffé-Test in Cadence. Comparisons of cadence between healthy controls and patients with PD indicated significant differences, wherein patients with PD demonstrated a significant increase in cadence (Table 4). Similar significant results were identified in comparisons of condition (VC × VnC) and with regard to affective disturbance (depression × nondepression). Higher cadence was identified in patients with PD, in the VnC condition, and in participants with a higher depression score. Healthy controls × the VnC condition demonstrated lower cadence compared to patients in the VnC condition. In addition, comparison of healthy controls with depression versus PD patients with depression revealed an increased cadence in PD patients who suffered from depression. Therefore, higher levels of depression and visuospatially deprived examination conditions (VnC) augmented the contrast in cadence between healthy controls and patients with PD, wherein cadence is increased in PD. Further analysis indicated that cadence was increased in the VC condition in patients with PD and depression, compared to the VnC condition. Therefore, patients with PD and higher depression scores demonstrated increased cadence in visuospatially deprived conditions.

3.4. Pairwise Results by Scheffé's Test in Stride Length. Differences in stride length between the VC and VnC conditions were significant, wherein stride length was reduced in the visually deprived condition. Patients demonstrated a significantly shorter stride length than healthy controls (Table 4). Participants with elevated depression scores exhibited shorter stride length than participants without indications of depression. In addition, significant differences were identified between nondepressed healthy subjects and nondepressed patients with regard to stride length, wherein the stride length of patients with PD was reduced. Next, stride length was found to decrease in the VnC condition in patients with PD, compared to the VC condition. Therefore, it is possible to suggest that, in patients with PD and depression, the VnC condition significantly decreases stride length.

3.5. Pairwise Results by Scheffé's-Test in Velocity. Higher velocity was detected in healthy controls compared to patients with PD. Moreover, lower velocity was identified in PD patients in the VnC condition compared to healthy participants (Table 4).

4. Discussion

The main result of this study is that when PD and control participants were tested during goal-directed locomotion high cadence was associated with reduced stride length, while slow walking velocity was associated with high cadence and short stride length in both groups but different in activity rate. When analyzing level of depression in controls, depression did not associate with velocity and other gait components in the common VC condition; however, high levels of depression showed an association with low velocity, high cadence,

Table 4: Multiple group comparison between patient x control, visually x nonvisually controlled conditions, and depression x nondepression groups with several gait parameters. He = healthy control condition, PD = Patient's condition, VC = visually controlled condition, VnC = visually noncontrolled condition, NoD = nondepressive condition, and DE = depressive condition.

Gait parameters	Mean (SD)						ANOVA intercept	Group comparisons	Scheffé post hoc p
	He	PD	VC	VnC	NoD	DE			
Cadence	8.9 (2.5)	12.5 (6.0)	8.86 (3.0)	12.7 (5.6)	9.07 (2.8)	11.08 (5.7)	$F = 904.14$ df = 1; $p < 0.001$	He versus PD	<0.001
								VC versus VnC	<0.001
								NoD versus DE	<0.001
								He × VnC versus PD × VnC	<0.001
								He × DE versus PD × DE	<0.004
								PD × VC × DE versus PD × VnC × DE	<0.006
Stride length (cm)	43,5 (10.8)	33.4 (11.6)	42,8 (11,2)	35,2 (12,1)	42.7 (11.3)	35.6 (12.1)	$F = 1813$ df = 1; $p < 0.001$	He versus PD	<0.001
								VC versus VnC	<0.001
								NoD versus DE	<0.001
								He × NoD versus PD × NoD	<0.005
								PD × VC × DE versus PD × VnC × DE	<0.047
Velocity (m/s)	0.65 (1.44)	0.54 (0.39)	0.65 (0.45)	0.53 (0.74)	0.59 (1.61)	0.40 (0.42)	$F = 185{,}48$ df = 1; $p < 0.001$	He versus PD	<0.001
								He × VnC versus PD × VnC	<0.048

and short stride length in the multitask VnC condition. In patients, the association of depression and gait components demonstrated a reverted pattern compared to controls. The depression was associated with velocity, stride length, and cadence in VC but not in VnC.

In addition, UPDRS scores were associated with all gait parameters excluding stride length in the VnC condition. The UPDRS, L-dopa equivalent doses, and illness duration showed the conventional syndrome specific associations but need to note that higher L-dopa equivalent doses associated with higher velocity and longer stride length but not with cadence and depression in patients with PD. With regard to intercorrelation analysis of the clinical components of gait, the gait pattern coherence remained intact while participants approached a target in both the VC and VnC conditions. The present results are consistent with the findings of previous studies, indicating that gait patterns are relatively coherent in the early stages of PD compared to healthy participants (low velocity, high cadence, and short stride length). However, in PD, velocity was reduced, cadence was increased, and stride length was shorter than in healthy controls [12]. The reduction in velocity relates to PD-specific visuospatial and proprioceptive impairments [11, 14], in the present case that was significant in complex multiple task in goal-directed locomotion without visual control condition. This indicates that, in patients with PD, depression linked to everyday activities, wherein walking (in a simple VC environment) is a difficult task for the majority of patients. Nevertheless, in the VnC (complex environment without visual guidance) condition, depression does not significantly associate with the goal-directed locomotion of patients with PD. To evaluate this data we need to note that depression-related gait pattern is linked to PD-specific visuospatial ability [22], which is associated with the hemispatial onset of PD symptoms [23], the applied L-dopa equivalent dose [24], disease duration, and current off/on effects [25]. In this study the off/on state had been controlled by the timing of examination, but the hemispatial onset of PD symptoms had not been the object of the present investigation.

It is necessary to establish that, in complex environmental conditions, when participants completed a VnC multitask, gait pattern remained relatively congruent, but patients with PD demonstrated a slower velocity, reduced stride length, and higher cadence compared to healthy controls. The reduction in velocity was significant in the visually deprived condition and in patients with elevated depression. Depression was associated with low velocity, reduced stride length, and elevated cadence in healthy controls in VnC conditions. However, in patients this effect was identified in the VC rather than the VnC condition.

The main results of this study arose from multiple comparisons of gait parameters and affective values between VC and VnC conditions in patients with PD and healthy controls. This analysis indicated that the visuospatially deprived multitask augments the rate of cadence and diminishes stride length in patients with PD and depression, while velocity remains unchanged. These results support previous findings that stride length and cadence are regulated by a bottom-up related reciprocal compensation mechanism [9, 12, 13, 26]. Our results indicate that this compensatory mechanism interacts with depression; however, the depression-related sensitivity of gait components differs. Multivariate analyses demonstrated that depression, first of all in visually noncontrolled multitask condition, produced a general reduction in stride length and increment in cadence in patients with PD to compare healthy controls. Velocity, first of all in visually noncontrolled multitask condition, was lower in patients with PD; however, the influence of depression on this condition has not been detected. It can be supposed that, in these patients, the reduction in the velocity of goal-directed locomotion was likely compensated by higher cadence and shorter stride length.

Lemke et al. [26] reported that depression, Parkinsonian posture, and gait demonstrate a number of similarities. The present evaluation of the relationship between depression and gait parameters appears to indicate that PD not only is a neurological disease but also incorporates a state of affective disturbance that influences the regulation of gait characteristics. In early stage of PD patients, first of all visually deprived multitask situation, depression specially modifies cadence and stride length but has no significant inhibition effect on the velocity of the gait. Consequently, the coherence of the gait pattern gets weaker. The correlation analyses indicated that in common visually controlled condition the depression and gate components showed a correlation pattern in PD (low velocity and stride length and high cadence); however, when multitask was applied in the visually noncontrolled condition the association between depression and gait features disappeared. Limitations to our study include consideration of depression as an aggregated score and its affective characteristic, apathy, quality of life, and the type of cognitive decline had not been detailed. Since the visuospatial disorder and the laterality of the first motor symptoms onset in PD are essential component in the gait control on these domains further research is needed.

5. Conclusion

The depression links to gait characteristics as a comorbid affective factor in PD. The findings reported above serve as a laboratory-based demonstration of gait specificity in PD and revealed depression-related dissimilarities in healthy and Parkinsonian gait patterns. Considering the associations between gait and depression these data might aid the development of exact clinical diagnoses, to conduct more efficient rehabilitation training for gait disturbances.

Authors' Contributions

P. Kincses, N. Kovács, S. Komoly, and J. Kállai contributed conception and design of the study. K. Karádi, Z. Aschermann, T. Szolcsányi, and K. Dorn were responsible for acquisition of data. Á. Feldmann and Á. Csathó performed analysis and interpretation of data. P. Kincses, S. Komoly, K. Dorn, and J. Kállai drafted the article. All authors made final approval of the version to be submitted.

Acknowledgments

The authors thank the patients and the healthy persons for their participation in the study. The study was supported by T-106176, OTKA Grant.

References

[1] J. L. Cummings, "Depression and parkinson's disease: a review," *American Journal of Psychiatry*, vol. 149, no. 4, pp. 443–454, 1992.

[2] D. Paleacu, A. Shutzman, N. Giladi, T. Herman, E. S. Simon, and J. M. Hausdorff, "Effects of pharmacological therapy on gait and cognitive function in depressed patients," *Clinical Neuropharmacology*, vol. 30, no. 2, pp. 63–71, 2007.

[3] K. R. Chaudhuri, P. Odin, A. Antonini, and P. Martinez-Martin, "Parkinson's disease: the non-motor issues," *Parkinsonism & Related Disorders*, vol. 17, no. 10, pp. 717–723, 2011.

[4] A. Feldmann, Z. Illes, P. Kosztolanyi et al., "Morphometric changes of gray matter in Parkinson's disease with depression: a voxel-based morphometry study," *Movement Disorders*, vol. 23, no. 1, pp. 42–46, 2008.

[5] T. Ziemssen and H. Reichmann, "Non-motor dysfunction in Parkinson's disease," *Parkinsonism and Related Disorders*, vol. 13, no. 6, pp. 323–332, 2007.

[6] D. Grabli, C. Karachi, M.-L. Welter et al., "Normal and pathological gait: what we learn from Parkinson's disease," *Journal of Neurology, Neurosurgery and Psychiatry*, vol. 83, no. 10, pp. 979–985, 2012.

[7] S. Lord, B. Galna, S. Coleman, D. Burn, and L. Rochester, "Mild depressive symptoms are associated with gait impairment in early Parkinson's disease," *Movement Disorders*, vol. 28, no. 5, pp. 634–639, 2013.

[8] P. A. Rocha, G. M. Porfírio, H. B. Ferraz, and V. F. M. Trevisani, "Effects of external cues on gait parameters of Parkinson's disease patients: a systematic review," *Clinical Neurology and Neurosurgery*, vol. 124, pp. 127–134, 2014.

[9] L. Almeida, M. S. Okun, D. Bowers et al., "Prevalence of depression in atypical Parkinsonian disorders versus Parkinson's Disease," *Movement Disorders*, vol. 30, pp. S634–S642, 2015.

[10] T. C. Brandler, C. Wang, M. Oh-Park, R. Holtzer, and J. Verghese, "Depressive symptoms and gait dysfunction in the elderly," *American Journal of Geriatric Psychiatry*, vol. 20, no. 5, pp. 425–432, 2012.

[11] A. J. Williams, D. S. Peterson, and G. M. Earhart, "Gait coordination in Parkinson disease: effects of step length and cadence manipulations," *Gait and Posture*, vol. 38, no. 2, pp. 340–344, 2013.

[12] M. E. Morris, R. Iansek, T. A. Matyas, and J. J. Summers, "Stride length regulation in Parkinson's disease: normalization strategies and underlying mechanisms," *Brain*, vol. 119, no. 2, pp. 551–568, 1996.

[13] A. Nieuwboer, R. Dom, W. De Weerdt, K. Desloovere, S. Fieuws, and E. Broens-Kaucsik, "Abnormalities of the spatiotemporal

characteristics of Gait at the onset of freezing in Parkinson's disease," *Movement Disorders*, vol. 16, no. 6, pp. 1066–1075, 2001.

[14] J.-P. Azulay, S. Mesure, and O. Blin, "Influence of visual cues on gait in Parkinson's disease: contribution to attention or sensory dependence?" *Journal of the Neurological Sciences*, vol. 248, no. 1-2, pp. 192–195, 2006.

[15] C. G. Goetz, W. Poewe, O. Rascol et al., "Movement Disorder Society Task Force report on the Hoehn and Yahr staging scale: status and recommendations," *Movement Disorders*, vol. 19, no. 9, pp. 1020–1028, 2004.

[16] M. F. Folstein, S. E. Folstein, and P. R. McHugh, "'Mini-mental state': a practical method for grading the cognitive state of patients for the clinician," *Journal of Psychiatric Research*, vol. 12, no. 3, pp. 189–198, 1975.

[17] E. P. Feher, R. K. Mahurin, R. S. Doody, N. Cooke, J. Sims, and F. J. Pirozzolo, "Establishing the Limits of the Mini-Mental State: examination of 'Subtests,'" *Archives of Neurology*, vol. 49, no. 1, pp. 87–92, 1992.

[18] S. A. Montgomery and M. Asberg, "A new depression scale designed to be sensitive to change," *British Journal of Psychiatry*, vol. 134, no. 4, pp. 382–389, 1979.

[19] R. C. Oldfield, "The assessment and analysis of handedness: the Edinburgh inventory," *Neuropsychologia*, vol. 9, no. 1, pp. 97–113, 1971.

[20] S. Fahn, R. Elton, and UPDRS Program Members, "Unified Parkinson's disease rating scale," in *Recent Developments in Parkinson's Disease*, S. Fahn, C. Marsden, M. Goldstein, and D. Calne, Eds., vol. 2, pp. 153–163, Macmillan Healthcare Information, Florham Park, NJ, USA, 1987.

[21] C. L. Tomlinson, R. Stowe, S. Patel, C. Rick, R. Gray, and C. E. Clarke, "Systematic review of levodopa dose equivalency reporting in Parkinson's disease," *Movement Disorders*, vol. 25, no. 15, pp. 2649–2653, 2010.

[22] S. Stuart, S. Lord, E. Hill, and L. Rochester, "Gait in Parkinson's disease: a visuo-cognitive challenge," *Neuroscience and Biobehavioral Reviews*, vol. 62, pp. 76–88, 2016.

[23] K. Karádi, T. Lucza, Z. Aschermann et al., "Visuospatial impairment in Parkinson's disease: the role of laterality," *Laterality*, vol. 20, no. 1, pp. 112–127, 2015.

[24] V. Fleury, E. Cousin, V. Czernecki et al., "Dopaminergic modulation of emotional conflict in Parkinson's disease," *Frontiers in Aging Neuroscience*, vol. 6, article 164, 2014.

[25] S. T. Moore, H. G. MacDougall, J.-M. Gracies, H. S. Cohen, and W. G. Ondo, "Long-term monitoring of gait in Parkinson's disease," *Gait and Posture*, vol. 26, no. 2, pp. 200–207, 2007.

[26] M. R. Lemke, T. Wendorff, B. Mieth, K. Buhl, and M. Linnemann, "Spatiotemporal gait patterns during over ground locomotion in major depression compared with healthy controls," *Journal of Psychiatric Research*, vol. 34, no. 4-5, pp. 277–283, 2000.

18

LSVT-BIG Improves UPDRS III Scores at 4 Weeks in Parkinson's Disease Patients with Wearing Off: A Prospective, Open-Label Study

Tatsuya Ueno,[1] Megumi Sasaki,[2] Haruo Nishijima,[1] Yukihisa Funamizu,[1] Tomoya Kon,[1] Rie Haga,[1] Akira Arai,[1] Chieko Suzuki,[1] Jin-ichi Nunomura,[1] Masayuki Baba,[1] and Masahiko Tomiyama[1]

[1]*Department of Neurology, Aomori Prefectural Central Hospital, Aomori, Japan*
[2]*Department of Rehabilitation, Aomori Prefectural Central Hospital, Aomori, Japan*

Correspondence should be addressed to Tatsuya Ueno; lacote19thg@gmail.com

Academic Editor: Eng King Tan

The efficacy of LSVT-BIG for advanced Parkinson's disease (PD) patients with wearing off remains to be determined. Therefore, we evaluated whether LSVT-BIG improves motor disability in eight PD patients with wearing off. Unified Parkinson's Disease Rating Scale (UPDRS) scores, daily off time, and mobility assessments were evaluated during the "on" time before and after the LSVT-BIG course. LSVT-BIG significantly improved UPDRS III scores at 4 weeks and UPDRS II scores in the "off" state at 12 weeks, with no changes in the other measures. The findings suggest that LSVT-BIG may be an effective therapy for advanced PD patients with wearing off.

1. Introduction

Wearing off is a gradual decrease in the duration of effect of each dose of medication for Parkinson's disease (PD) [1], which leads to a reduced quality of life in patients with PD [2]. Dopamine replacement therapy alone cannot satisfactorily treat patients with advanced PD with motor fluctuations, such as those resulting from wearing off [3, 4]. Deep brain stimulation is considered for severe wearing off and troublesome dyskinesia; however, it has been reported that axial symptoms affecting speech, gait, and postural instability progressively worsened 5 years after surgery [5]. Therefore, an alternative procedure, such as exercise, is needed for the treatment of advanced PD with wearing off.

Exercise is an established adjunctive therapy in PD. Lee Silverman Voice Treatment- (LSVT-) BIG is an exercise course that focuses on intensive high-amplitude movements to restore normal movement amplitude by recalibrating the patient's perception of movement [6] and improves motor performance measured by the Unified Parkinson's Disease Rating Scale (UPDRS) III in patients with PD [7–10]. However, previous studies demonstrating the efficacy of LSVT-BIG did not address the effect on "off" time [7–10]. Therefore, the efficacy of LSVT-BIG for PD patients with wearing off remains to be determined. To our knowledge, this is the first study to evaluate whether LSVT-BIG improves motor disability and reduces daily off time in PD patients presenting with wearing off motor fluctuations. We hypothesized that LSVT-BIG treatment would improve UPDRS II and III scores, reduce daily off time, and improve performance on the 10-meter walk test and Time Up and Go (TUG) test.

2. Participants and Methods

Eight Japanese patients with idiopathic PD referred from our outpatient clinic were enrolled between May 2013 and March 2014. Participants were required to fulfill diagnostic criteria for idiopathic PD [11] and had a daily off time of more than 2 hours per day. Other inclusion criteria comprised Hoehn and Yahr (H-Y) Stages II–III, outpatient treatment, and stable

TABLE 1: Clinical characteristics of patients with Parkinson's disease.

Patients	Age (years)	Sex	Hoehn and Yahr	Disease duration (years)	Daily off time (hours)	UPDRS-III	Medication (daily dose)
1	61	F	3	11	3.2	14	L/C 400 mg, ROP 12 mg, AMA 150 mg
2	66	F	3	13	5	13	L/C 650 mg, PRA 1.5 mg, AMA 300 mg, SEL 2.5 mg
3	58	F	2.5	8	3.2	20	L/C 300 mg, CAB 3 mg, AMA 150 mg
4	72	M	2	11	5.2	0	L/B 700 mg, ENT 600 mg, PRA-CR 4.5 mg, PER 750 μg, SEL 5 mg, ZON 25 mg, IST 20 mg
5	53	M	2	13	5.2	8	L/C 600 mg, CAB 2 mg, AMA 150 mg, ZON 25 mg, IST 40 mg, TRI 6 mg
6	71	F	2	8	6	12	L/C 600 mg, PRA 1.5 mg, AMA 150 mg, IST 20 mg
7	69	M	3	24	4.8	9	L/C 350 mg, PER 1500 μg, ENT 300 mg, AMA 100 mg, ZON 25 mg, IST 40 mg
8	56	F	3	14	4.9	26	L/C 1000 mg, PRA-CR 4.5 mg, AMA 300 mg, ZON 50 mg, TRI 3 mg

L/C, levodopa/carbidopa; L/B, levodopa/benserazide; PRA, pramipexole; PRA-CR, pramipexole continuous release; ROP, ropinirole; CAB, cabergoline; AMA, amantadine; SEL, selegiline; ENT, entacapone; ZON, zonisamide; IST, istradefylline; TRI, trihexyphenidyl; UPDRS-III, Unified Parkinson's Disease Rating Scale part III.

medication 4 weeks prior to beginning the study. Exclusion criteria were as follows: patients without informed consent; unavailable self-report on/off diary (for 3 consecutive days); patients with untreated cancer, dementia (MMSE < 24), severe depression, anemia, or hypotension; abnormal liver, renal, cardiopulmonary function; or a comorbidity affecting mobility or ability to exercise. This study was conducted in accordance with the Declaration of Helsinki and was approved by the ethics committee of Aomori Prefectural Central Hospital, Japan. All participants provided informed consent.

One physiotherapist (MS) certified as an LSVT-BIG instructor delivered all BIG sessions and also provided instructions for patients. LSVT-BIG is delivered face-to-face at a treatment dosage of 4 days/week for 4 weeks (1-hour sessions). Training has previously been described in detail [6]. After the 4-week course of LSVT-BIG, participants were encouraged to exercise for 15 to 20 minutes (some parts of LSVT-BIG) regularly at home in addition to the LSVT-BIG session. They had been on a stable regimen of drugs for at least 4 weeks before the entry and during the evaluation period.

All participants reported their on/off state using the self-report on/off diary for 3 consecutive days before assessment. UPDRS III was scored by an experienced neurologist (MT) [12]. The evaluating neurologist was not blinded to the subject's participation in this study. We made an effort to pay attention to the nonspecific effect of increased attention from hospital staff. We analyzed the following measures for changes from baseline to post-LSVT-BIG (4, 8, and 12 weeks): daily off time, UPDRS parts II and III [12], 10 m walk test, and TUG test [13] during "on" periods. UPDRS III, 10 m walk test, and TUG at 4 weeks were evaluated before the final LSVT-BIG session.

Statistical analyses were performed with the freely available EZR software version 1.32 (Saitama Medical Center, Jichi Medical University, Saitama, Japan) [14]. A probability level of 5% ($P < 0.05$) was considered statistically significant. Variables are presented as median [interquartile range]. The quantitative data were evaluated to determine whether they followed a normal distribution using the Shapiro-Wilk test. UPDRS II "off" score and III "on" score were normally distributed in the Shapiro-Wilk test, and we performed a one-way ANOVA with repeated measures followed by the paired t-test, with Bonferroni correction for multiple comparisons. UPDRS II score (on), TUG, 10 m walk test, and daily off time were not normally distributed in the Shapiro-Wilk test ($P < 0.05$), so we performed the Friedman test followed by the Wilcoxon test, with Bonferroni correction for multiple comparisons.

3. Results

Clinical characteristics of the patients are listed in Table 1. All eight patients completed the LSVT-BIG program and received all evaluations. Male/female ratio was 3/5. Their mean age (SD) was 63.2 (7.2), disease duration was 12.8 (5.1) years, and levodopa equivalent daily dosage (not including trihexyphenidyl, istradefylline, and zonisamide) was 1040 (395) mg [15].

LSVT-BIG significantly improved UPDRS III "on" scores at 4 weeks compared with baseline scores (baseline median UPDRS III "on" scores [interquartile range]: 12.5 [8.8–15.5]; 4 weeks: 8.5 [6.5–11.5]; 8 weeks: 8.0 [6.0–11.0]; 12 weeks: 9.5 [7.8–13.3]) (Table 2). However, the UPDRS III "on" score increased again at 12 weeks.

The UPDRS II score during the "off" state was significantly ameliorated at 12 weeks (baseline median UPDRS II "off" scores [interquartile range]: 14.5 [10.8–18.2]; 4 weeks: 13.0 [9.0–15.3]; 8 weeks: 14.0 [7.0–15.8]; 12 weeks: 12.5 [8.3–16.0]) (Table 2).

Daily off time, UPDRS II during the "on" state, and gait performance of the 10 m walk test and TUG were not significantly different from baseline measures at 4, 8, or 12 weeks (Table 2).

TABLE 2: Outcome measures from baseline to 12 weeks.

	Baseline	4 weeks	8 weeks	12 weeks
UPDRS II (off)	14.5 [10.8–18.2]	13.0 [9.0–15.3]	14.0 [7.0–15.8]	12.5 [8.3–16.0]*
UPDRS II (on)	0.5 [0–2.5]	0 [0–1.3]	0 [0–1.5]	0.5 [0–2.3]
UPDRS III (on)	12.5 [8.8–15.5]	8.5 [6.5–11.5]†	8.0 [6.0–11.0]	9.5 [7.8–13.3]
Daily off time (hours)	5.0 [4.4–5.2]	3.2 [1.8–3.6]	3.7 [2.8–4.3]	3.8 [3.5–4.6]
TUG (sec)	7.8 [7.3–8.1]	6.7 [5.9–7.4]	7.5 [6.4–8.9]	7.0 [6.6–8.2]
Timed 10 m (sec)	8.7 [7.4–9.7]	8.3 [7.3–9.1]	8.0 [7.0–8.5]	8.2 [8.0–8.4]

Data are median [interquartile range]. *Baseline versus 12 weeks: $P < 0.05$; †baseline versus 4 weeks: $P < 0.05$.
UPDRS- III, Unified Parkinson's Disease Rating Scale part III; TUG, Timed Up and Go.

4. Discussion

This prospective open-label study revealed two important outcomes of LSVT-BIG in PD patients with wearing off. First, LSVT-BIG improved UPDRS III scores during the "on" state throughout the training course. However, this efficacy did not last long, because the scores increased at the end of the study. Second, LSVT-BIG ameliorated the UPDRS II score during the "off" state at the end of this study.

Several studies showed that this training led to improved motor performance in PD patients [7–10]. The ameliorating effect of LSVT-BIG was higher in H-Y stage I than in H-Y stage III [7]. We showed that LSVT-BIG improved UPDRS III scores in patients with wearing off, which may provide a therapeutic option for the management of advanced PD patients. However, this efficacy did not continue for more than 4 weeks after the final LSVT-BIG session. Our results suggest that motor skill learning is maintained in advanced PD patients with wearing off, but the progressive degeneration of nigrostriatal dopaminergic neurons may result in an unsustained motor learning system. This problem may also contribute to a lack of effects of self-exercise at home [16, 17]. LSVT-BIG is delivered one-to-one with intensive motivation and feedback [6], an approach considered to be more effective than self-exercise [8]. Therefore, it appears to be well-advised to continue active intervention after the 4-week training course to maintain the improvements.

LSVT-BIG also ameliorated UPDRS part II score during the "off" state at the end of this study. There were a tendency for a decrease of UPDRS II scores at 4 weeks and 8 weeks, but statistical analysis showed no significant differences. The UPDRS II score reflects activity of daily living [12]. Indices of quality of life, such as Parkinson's Disease Questionnaire-39, were used in previous studies, but the studies did not evaluate UPDRS II scores [7–10]. Amelioration of motor performance in PD patients with wearing off may impact their activity of daily living [18]. Therefore, these results may be associated with improvement of motor performance in PD patients with wearing off.

Our findings showed that LSVT-BIG did not decrease the daily off time but improved motor performance for levodopa. Wearing off is caused by a progressive loss of nigrostriatal dopaminergic neurons and altered postsynaptic responses to dopamine [1]. Thus, we speculate that LSVT-BIG may directly or indirectly alter the postsynaptic response to dopamine in the basal ganglia by relearning normal movement.

Generalization of our findings is limited by the open-label study design and sample size. Daily off time did not significantly decrease in this study, but there was a tendency for a decrease of 1.8 hours from baseline to 4 weeks. Investigation of a larger sample size may have a different outcome. Additionally, we did not investigate the UPDRS part III score in the "off" state. This study was performed in patients attending outpatient visits, but who were not hospitalized. In PD patients with wearing off, the "on" state is required to visit hospital, so we evaluated the UPDRS part III score during the "on" state. This study showed that LSVT-BIG improved motor performance in the "on" state. More research is needed to determine if LSVT-BIG would be useful to raise the level of motor performance in "off" state patients. Finally, this study did not have a matched comparison group. An open-label noncontrolled study may show positive results due to the nonspecific effect of more intensive treatment staff contact and interaction.

In conclusion, our findings suggest that LSVT-BIG may provide a therapeutic option for the management of PD patients with wearing off. However, satisfactory amelioration may last only a short time. Accordingly, it is necessary to continue active interventions to maintain the improvements even after the LSVT-BIG course has been completed. Further studies addressing these matters are needed to confirm whether LSVT-BIG is useful for advanced PD patients with wearing off motor fluctuations.

References

[1] P. Jenner, "Wearing off, dyskinesia, and the use of continuous drug delivery in parkinson's disease," *Neurologic Clinics*, vol. 31, no. 3, pp. S17–S35, 2013.

[2] J. Sławek, M. Derejko, and P. Lass, "Factors affecting the quality of life of patients with idiopathic Parkinson's disease—a cross-sectional study in an outpatient clinic attendees," *Parkinsonism & Related Disorders*, vol. 11, no. 7, pp. 465–468, 2005.

[3] C. W. Olanow, "The scientific basis for the current treatment of Parkinson's disease," *Annual Review of Medicine*, vol. 55, pp. 41–60, 2004.

[4] C. W. Olanow, J. A. Obeso, and F. Stocchi, "Continuous dopamine-receptor treatment of Parkinson's disease: scientific rationale and clinical implications," *Lancet Neurology*, vol. 5, no. 8, pp. 677–687, 2006.

[5] L. M. Romito and A. Albanese, "Dopaminergic therapy and subthalamic stimulation in Parkinson's disease: a review of 5-year reports," *Journal of Neurology*, vol. 257, supplement 2, pp. S298–S304, 2010.

[6] B. G. Farley, C. M. Fox, L. O. Ramig, and D. H. McFarland, "Intensive amplitude-specific therapeutic approaches for Parkinson's disease: toward a neuroplasticity-principled rehabilitation model," *Topics in Geriatric Rehabilitation*, vol. 24, no. 2, pp. 99–114, 2008.

[7] B. G. Farley and G. F. Koshland, "Training BIG to move faster: the application of the speed-amplitude relation as a rehabilitation strategy for people with Parkinson's disease," *Experimental Brain Research*, vol. 167, no. 3, pp. 462–467, 2005.

[8] G. Ebersbach, A. Ebersbach, D. Edler et al., "Comparing exercise in Parkinson's disease—the Berlin LSVT®BIG study," *Movement Disorders*, vol. 25, no. 12, pp. 1902–1908, 2010.

[9] J. Janssens, K. Malfroid, T. Nyffeler, S. Bohlhalter, and T. Vanbellingen, "Application of LSVT BIG intervention to address gait, balance, bed mobility, and dexterity in people with Parkinson disease: a case series," *Physical Therapy*, vol. 94, no. 7, pp. 1014–1023, 2014.

[10] G. Ebersbach, U. Grust, A. Ebersbach, B. Wegner, F. Gandor, and A. A. Kühn, "Amplitude-oriented exercise in Parkinson's disease: a randomized study comparing LSVT-BIG and a short training protocol," *Journal of Neural Transmission*, vol. 122, no. 2, pp. 253–256, 2015.

[11] A. J. Hughes, S. E. Daniel, L. Kilford, and A. J. Lees, "Accuracy of clinical diagnosis of idiopathic Parkinson's disease: a clinico-pathological study of 100 cases," *Journal of Neurology Neurosurgery and Psychiatry*, vol. 55, no. 3, pp. 181–184, 1992.

[12] C. C. Goetz, "The Unified Parkinson's Disease Rating Scale (UPDRS): status and recommendations," *Movement Disorders*, vol. 18, no. 7, pp. 738–750, 2003.

[13] S. Morris, M. E. Morris, and R. Iansek, "Reliability of measurements obtained with the Timed "Up, & Go" test in people with Parkinson disease," *Physical Therapy*, vol. 81, no. 2, pp. 810–818, 2001.

[14] Y. Kanda, "Investigation of the freely available easy-to-use software 'EZR' for medical statistics," *Bone Marrow Transplantation*, vol. 48, no. 3, pp. 452–458, 2013.

[15] C. L. Tomlinson, R. Stowe, S. Patel, C. Rick, R. Gray, and C. E. Clarke, "Systematic review of levodopa dose equivalency reporting in Parkinson's disease," *Movement Disorders*, vol. 25, no. 15, pp. 2649–2653, 2010.

[16] H. Nakae and H. Tsushima, "Problems with daily living and performing home exercise in Japanese home-care patients with Parkinson's disease," *Hirosaki Medical Journal*, vol. 65, no. 1, pp. 55–64, 2014.

[17] L. A. King, J. Wilhelm, Y. Chen et al., "Effects of group, individual, and home exercise in persons with Parkinson disease: a randomized clinical trial," *Journal of Neurologic Physical Therapy*, vol. 39, no. 4, pp. 204–212, 2015.

[18] H. Reichmann, J. Boas, D. Macmahon, V. Myllyla, A. Hakala, and K. Reinikainen, "Efficacy of combining levodopa with entacapone on quality of life and activities of daily living in patients experiencing wearing-off type fluctuations," *Acta Neurologica Scandinavica*, vol. 111, no. 1, pp. 21–28, 2005.

19

Stigma Experienced by Parkinson's Disease Patients: A Descriptive Review of Qualitative Studies

Marina Maffoni,[1] Anna Giardini,[1] Antonia Pierobon,[1] Davide Ferrazzoli,[2] and Giuseppe Frazzitta[2]

[1]*Psychology Unit, Istituti Clinici Scientifici Maugeri, IRCCS Montescano (PV), Pavia, Italy*
[2]*Parkinson's Disease and Brain Injury Rehabilitation Department, Moriggia-Pelascini Hospital, Gravedona ed Uniti, Italy*

Correspondence should be addressed to Anna Giardini; anna.giardini@icsmaugeri.it

Academic Editor: Shey-Lin Wu

Parkinson's disease (PD) is a neurodegenerative disease characterized by motor and nonmotor symptoms. Both of them imply a negative impact on Health-Related Quality of Life. A significant one is the stigma experienced by the parkinsonian patients and their caregivers. Moreover, stigma may affect everyday life and patient's subjective and relational perception and it may lead to frustration and isolation. Aim of the present work is to qualitatively describe the stigma of PD patients stemming from literature review, in order to catch the subjective experience and the meaning of the stigma construct. Literature review was performed on PubMed database and Google Scholar (keywords: Parkinson Disease, qualitative, stigma, social problem, isolation, discrimination) and was restricted to qualitative data: 14 articles were identified to be suitable to the aim of the present overview. Results are divided into four core constructs: stigma arising from symptoms, stigma linked to relational and communication problems, social stigma arising from sharing perceptions, and caregiver's stigma. The principal relations to these constructs are deeply analyzed and described subjectively through patients' and caregiver's point of view. The qualitative research may allow a better understanding of a subjective symptom such as stigma in parkinsonian patients from an intercultural and a social point of view.

1. Introduction

At first blush, Parkinson's disease (PD) is characterized by motor symptoms. Indeed, the four cardinal features of this pathology are identified in the tremor at rest, rigidity, akinesia (or bradykinesia,) and postural instability [1]. Nevertheless, nonmotor symptoms are as much as relevant, even if invisible or not immediately detectable, and they often imply a negative impact on Health-Related Quality of Life (HRQoL) [2, 3]. A significant one is the stigma experienced by the parkinsonian patients and their caregivers. In fact, this phenomenon has not a secondary importance: stigma appears to provide a determinant contribution to HRQoL in patients with PD [4]. Moreover, stigma may characterize everyday life with a gloomy filter, marked by disability and isolation [5].

The general meaning of the word *stigma* is linked to a complex experience concerning a devaluating, discriminant, and discomfort feeling. According to one of the first contemporary conceptualizations of this construct, stigma is an attribute implying a discredit of the subject who is considered "bad, or dangerous, or weak. She/he is thus reduced in our minds from a whole and usual person to a tainted, discounted one" [6, p. 3]. A stigmatized person, that is a person with stigma, is someone who appears changed and different from what is considered normal and accepted. As a consequence, the subject could be isolated and the social identity may be deeply threatened and mined, too [7].

When stigma is present in PD, it originates from the interface of the patient with the outside world [4]. That is, it is not only an individual construct but rather a social one. Indeed, it is a sort of mark underlining the deviant nature of the stigmatized subject from the perspective of those who are the stigmatizers [8]. Indeed, despite different theories, approaches, and models developed over the years [9–11], there is always a social component to consider when speaking about stigma. Therefore, stigma is a complex phenomenon due to the interaction between a context and a subject who receives a devaluating mark [7].

Scales and tools have been developed in order to better describe and quantify stigma in chronic illnesses, such as PD ([12, 13]; for a review, [14]). Nevertheless, being a personal experience, stigma is difficult to be objectively described. The core meaning of this construct could be better defined by collecting the subjective point of view of PD patients [15].

Aim of the present work is to qualitatively describe the stigma of PD patients stemming from literature review, focusing on qualitative international research.

2. Method

The authors applied a research strategy to sum up a descriptive overview of the complex and motley experience of stigma in PD linked both to disabling physical conditions and to social, relational, and communicative obstacles. The review was restricted to qualitative published articles in order to catch the subjective experience and meaning of the stigma construct.

Literature review was performed on PubMed database and Google Scholar (keywords: Parkinson Disease, qualitative, stigma, social problem, isolation, discrimination) and was not limited to any country neither to any period of time. 26 papers were identified. The authors read all materials in order to identify where the experience of a devaluating and discriminant feeling linked to the PD effectively emerged and/or was exhaustively discussed. The authors excluded papers in which stigma was an introductive or very marginal, not informative theme. Duplicates were also deleted. Another exclusion criterion adopted was the focus on quantitative reports. Consensus was reached by a vis-à-vis discussion and followed by email discussions. An article was included in the study only when a general consensus was provided.

After that procedure, 6 articles were selected. Subsequently, other 8 additional qualitative studies were selected from references to chosen articles, according to the same methodology previously adopted. At the end of the process, 14 articles were identified to be suitable to the aim of the present overview.

In order to understand and identify the stigma experience, two authors (MM, AG) read the selected 14 articles and took notes of each aspect linked to the construct, discussing online and trying to reach an agreement. In order to reach a consensus among all authors, an iterative process of continuous analysis of data was applied. First, an initial or open coding procedure was carried on, afterwards MM and AG extrapolated the meaningful issues, and AP, DF, and GF read the articles verifying the coherence among the extrapolated key words and reported themes. All emerging issues were considered in the review, considering that even the less quoted experience could contribute to better understanding of the complex stigma phenomenon. All authors contributed to conceptualize stigma experience, critically organizing the emerging themes into major categories. Memos, diagrams, and maps were used as tools enabling data sharing and to reach a consensus.

Results are presented in a descriptive/narrative way, describing the thematic issues linked to stigma experience; in order to simplify comprehension, the results and the identified categories are also presented in a table and graphically summed up.

3. Results

As for other chronic and progressive disabling diseases, PD drove patients to experience stigma day after day. From patients' point of view, stigma appears as a complex construct with multiple undesirable facets. This emerged from the plethora of expressions linked to stigma used by patients addressing PD: shame, disgrace, embarrassment, feeling dishonorable, and feeling awkward, terrible, or horrible, and so on [5, 16, 17, 23, 24, 28].

In Table 1, the 14 articles included in our descriptive review are described. In order to organize data that emerged from literature review, results were divided into paragraphs according to identified key words; results are quantitatively described in Table 2 and represented as a whole in Figure 1.

3.1. Stigma Arising from Symptoms. Elements and conditions determining stigma are different. One of the main causes identified by patients of this phenomenon are motor, physical, and visible symptoms [5, 16, 18–20]. It is not casual that ancient Greeks coined the term stigma referring to "*bodily signs* designed to expose something unusual and bad" [6, p. 1]. Indeed, symptoms are impossible to hide and become a clear and concrete statement of the subjective perception of a capricious disease that speaks by means of the body [17, 21]. In the selected article, the perception of stigma emerges directly linked to PD symptoms and their manifestation in public [18]. In this regard, Israeli women describe their visible body as a traitor, since it unscrupulously reveals PD to the public [16]. That is, body becomes a servant of PD acting by means of its visible symptoms. In this regard, Hermanns's ethnographic approach reveals that the observable traits of disturbances such as drooling, balance difficulties, shaking problems, and other similar symptoms are additional challenges for the patient [5]. PD disrupts the experience of an autonomous and integrated human being due to the exterior signs of the illness condition [22]. Moreover, the deteriorated body image provokes feelings of shame and embarrassment leading to isolation [19, 20].

Nevertheless, stigma is not only linked to the changing exterior image of PD patient but also to the progressive loss of functionality. The contribution of PD to the stigma experience is double: an undesirable self-image and a loss of autonomy and self-efficacy. Indeed, when asking to freely tell their life history with PD thorough in-depth interviews, subjects describe their symptoms as a matter of shame because of the physical dependence and the need for help to do even the simplest tasks [16, 23, 25]. Stigma may arise from the consciousness of the awkwardness and inability to perform not only usual work activities but also simple motor actions [24]. An impoverishment of physical functionality conducts to a reduction of activity and social engagement linked to stigma perception [18].

Table 1: Study characteristics of the 14 articles included in the qualitative review.

Study	Location of patients' recruitment	Number of participants	Qualitative methods	Study aim
Nijhof, 1995	Amsterdam, The Netherlands	23 PD pts (10 F; 13 M)	In-depth interviews with qualitative analysis of content	To explore PD subjective interpretations
Posen et al., 2000	Tel Aviv, Israel	15 PD pts (F)	Sessions of psychoeducational work-group (MacKenzie and Livesley, 1983)	To describe the PD experience in a female work-group
Sunvisson and Ekman, 2001	Sweden	11 PD pts (no gender details)	Interviews during a period of 2 years and phenomenological data analysis	To elucidate environmental influences on lived PD experiences
Van Der Bruggen and Widdershoven, 2004	/	4 novels	Existential-phenomenological analysis of narrative materials of PD patients	To catch the meaning of being a PD patient
Bramley and Eatough, 2005	Nottingham, UK	1 PD pts (F) (single case study)	Semi-structured interviews analyzed using interpretative phenomenological analysis (IPA)	To catch the subjective PD daily experience
Miller et al., 2006 (a)	Sunderland, UK	37 PD pts (14 F; 23 M)	In-depth interviews with qualitative analysis of content	To study changes in communication impact on daily PD patients' lives
Miller et al., 2006 (b)	Sunderland, UK	37 PD pts (14 F; 23 M)	In-depth interviews with qualitative analysis of content	To establish if and how changes in swallowing impact on daily PD patients' lives
Mshana et al., 2011	Mwanza, Tanzania	28 PD pts, 28 caregivers, 4 health workers, 2 traditional healers (no gender details)	In-depth interviews and focus groups	To detect how PD is perceived and treated in a rural African population
Chiong-Rivero et al., 2011	USA	48 PD pts (26 F; 22 M) 15 caregivers (13 F; 2 M)	Focus groups and one-on-one interviews	To collect Health-Related Quality of Life consequences of Parkinson's disease from the patient's and caregivers' perspective
Hermanns, 2013	Texas, USA	14 PD pts (7 F; 7 M)	Ethnographic approach using interview data, participant observations, and fieldwork (2-year exposure)	To discuss the visible and invisible stigma
Soleimani et al., 2014	Iran	10 PD pts (3 F; 7 M)	Semistructured, face-to-face interviews and content analysis approach	To explore the effects of PD on people's social interactions
Soundy et al., 2014	/	37 qualitative articles (review)	Metaethnography	To summarize and to synthesize qualitative studies concerning the PD experience and perception
Giardini et al., 2016	Montescano (PV), Italy	27 PD pts (14 F; 13 M)	Semi-structured interviews with PD patients analyzed using the Grounded Theory methodology	To qualitatively describe the rehabilitation experience of PD inpatients
Soleimani et al., 2016	Iran	17 PD pts (7 F; 10 M)	Semistructured, face-to-face interviews and content analysis approach	To explore the primary concerns and perceptions of daily PD patients' lives

Legend: PD = Parkinson's disease; Pts = patients; F = female; M = male.

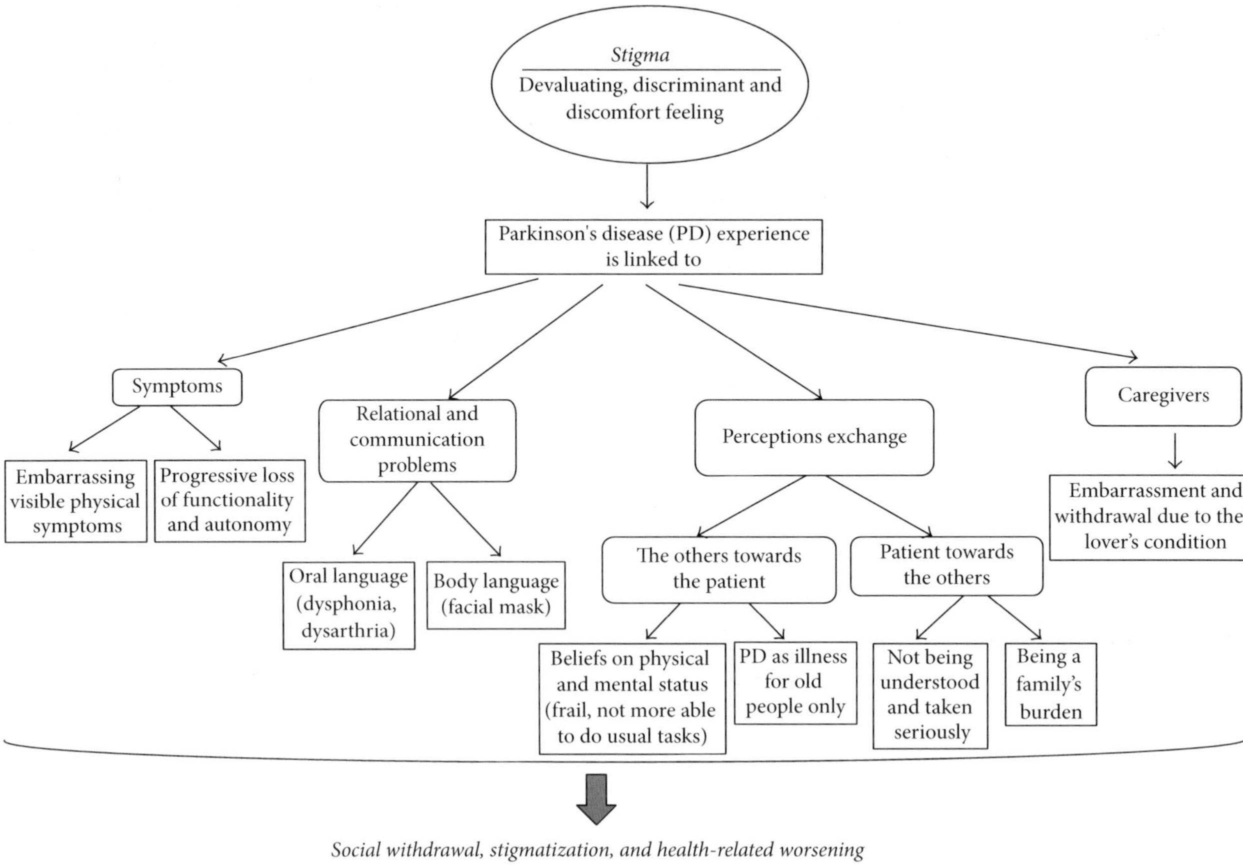

Figure 1: Stigma's core constructs in Parkinson's disease.

Table 2: Thematic issues related to stigma experience identified in the reviewed articles.

Thematic issues	Reference number of each reviewed article
Symptoms	
Embarrassing visible physical symptoms	[5, 16–22]
Progressive loss of functionality and autonomy	[5, 16, 18, 23–25]
Relational and communication problems	
Oral language (dysphonia, dysarthria)	[5, 19, 26, 27]
Body language (facial mask)	[5, 24]
Perceptions exchange	
The others towards the patient	
Beliefs on physical and mental status	[5, 16, 21, 23, 24, 26]
PD as an illness for old people only	[5, 16, 28]
Patient towards the others	
Not being understood and taken seriously	[5, 26, 27],
Being a family burden	[5, 16, 18, 24–26]
Caregivers	
Embarrassment and withdrawal due to their lover's condition	[24, 25, 28]

3.2. Stigma Linked to Relational and Communication Problems. Stigma experience arises also from the hindrances to communication and relational life imposed progressively by PD. Indeed, the relationship with the others becomes complex and contradictory since the PD patient has to find the right balance between contact and distance [21].

First of all, relations and communications are a matter of complaint; patients state to be frequently mislabelled, for example, as drunkard [5]. Moreover, the delayed thinking process and the difficulty to convey beliefs easily may cause a subjective experience of frustration and isolation, since the others take their own decisions without waiting for the patient's feedback [26]. Communication changes may have an impact on the patients' and their caregivers' life; subjects attribute to voice and articulation changes many disabling impacts: formulation problems and attention difficulties and subjective feelings of frustration and neglecting linked to withdrawal [27]. Indeed, all these issues conduct the PD patient to remain confined at home, where she/he feels normal and more comfortable since they can bypass the comparison with the outside society [5, 19].

However, communication is not only a matter of speaking. Human beings communicate by means of gesture and body language too. In this regard, face is a sensitive topic to PD patients. Indeed, one of the most visible and undesirable features is the typical rigid and unexpressive face of PD patients, the facial mask. Patients describe other people's difficulty to decipher their mute expression and this condition inexorably causes isolation of the stigmatized person, who perceives a progressive sense of alienation and disconnection from the others [5, 24].

3.3. Social Stigma Arising from Perceptions Exchanges. Stigma is a complex matter of feeling and perceptions; the interface between inside and outside is determinant. This means that the contribution of patients and caregivers is equally important and the starting point of a stigmatizing perception is usually shared without clear boundaries.

3.3.1. The Others' Perceptions towards the PD Patient. Taking into account the others' point of view, Hermanns highlights that a PD patient notices to be seen as frail by the others [5]. Moreover, subjects describe a perceived sense of unease and uncomfortable feelings of individuals that are in front of their physical problems and that cannot escape from their sight [24]. Indeed, it is the response of the others that is a matter of shame [23]. When the disease proceeds and disability increases, the patient has to struggle with the experience of marginalization and isolation due to the forced abandonment of work and responsibilities [21].

As to symptoms (i.e., hallucinations), patients may avoid telling their family members, since they worry they could perceive them as cognitively impaired or not being reliable anymore [26]. Indeed, a group of women highlights the difference when speaking of functional aspects that are more socially accepted than of mental and degenerative issues: PD is linked to a diffused and stigmatizing belief of being a disease characterized by a cognitive impairment transforming patient into an insane [16].

Another main reason of social stigmatization is linked to common belief that PD is a disease only for old people; this prejudice may be strong in society, including family members [5, 16]. Interestingly, from a qualitative research conducted within a rural zone of Tanzania, PD is called "old age illness" in Swahili language due to the common prejudice of the age range in which PD may appear [28].

3.3.2. The PD Patient' Perceptions towards the Others. From the patient's perspective, stigma may be linked to patient's metaperceptions of the other people's beliefs towards PD [18]. Patients frequently complain to be misunderstood or even not to be understood and be taken seriously from the outside normal society [5]. A reason of misunderstanding may stem from the fluctuating nature of PD symptoms that leads family members and formal caregivers to believe she/he is pretending [26]. Moreover, some interviewed PD patients complain not to receive the right time to express themselves by the others who replace them in discussions or decisions, without fully understanding their communication difficulties [27].

Stigma arises also from the patient's perception to be a burden for caregivers, also due to the uncertain progression of the disease [5, 16, 18, 24, 26]. Subjects may report feelings of guilt and selfishness towards their caregivers due to the increasingly demanding request of special attention in the daily chores [25]. Moreover, PD patients experience a stigma feeling due to the change or loss of their social roles: they are not the providers of their families and they are often forced to leave their workplace [24].

3.4. Caregiver's Stigma. Stigma not only is an experience of the patients but rather may be also a feeling characterizing the family caregivers. PD is something unwanted that marks all the family, leading to difficulties also in public settings and to undesirable feeling of shame and pity [24]. In this regard, Mshana et al. show that, in rural communities of Tanzania, there is a trend to stigmatize the entire PD patient's family because of the dishonorable condition experienced [28]. Indeed, the PD patient's family members may be totally absorbed by taking care of the ill family member, since they are not able any more to take part in social and working life of their community. Equally, also in a European context, the patient's families have been frequently led to a forced withdrawal, in particular during meal time when it becomes difficult to invite guests [25] or at least dealing with the embarrassing and visible symptoms of their ill family member [24].

4. Clinical Implications

Being in contact with the patient and discovering her/his experience and inner psychological needs may guide health care professionals and caregivers to take care of the ill person in a more fitted and tailored manner. In fact, by understanding a disease as a whole, from a holistic point of view, one could provide clues to be more effective in patient's management. The capricious and unpredictable nature of this progressive neurological disorder makes the comprehension of a patient's experience and psychosocial correlates even more fundamental. Stereotypes, misunderstandings, shame, isolation, discriminations, and stigmatization are a silent, partly visible, and partly invisible phenomenon, which is necessary to be considered [5]. Indeed, stigma has an important negative effect on the illness progress and management: it may contribute to avoiding or interrupting treatment, as well as to manifesting depressive symptoms [29, 30]. Although dedicated to mental illness and presenting still controversial results, specific psychotherapeutic approaches to stigma seem to be effective, enhancing skills to deal with self-stigma through self-esteem, empowerment, and help-seeking behavior enhancement [31, 32]. Further studies on patients with chronic diseases intended to implement a focused intervention on stigma, may be deserved, adapting protocols and outcome measures on this specific population.

Moreover, stigma has an intrinsic complexity that deserves to be better understood [30]; there is an important need to reach and educate who is foreign to being chronically ill and as an outsider nurtures the stigma phenomenon. By disseminating information and by educating the others, starting from the informal caregivers, we could treat properly this source of sufferance, in line with the WHO ICF model, where disability stems from the interaction of a health condition with personal and environmental factors [33].

Finally, the choice of a holistic and multidisciplinary treatment of all symptoms of PD appears of great importance to guarantee a satisfying health management of the patient [17, 34]. The need to focus on nonmotor symptoms in PD, which stigma belongs to, moves a step forward to a tailored patient-centered medicine, enabling the health professionals to see the patient as a person, living in an everyday life.

5. Conclusions

The social consideration and attitude towards a disease are important, since they contribute in determining the environment in which the patient has to live and interact in [5, 35]. Indeed, disability stems from the interaction between the individual and the environment [36]. Stigma is a complex phenomenon well attested and in need of comprehension in the context of chronic diseases and PD is not an exception [37]. Even if stigma could be a silent and invisible phenomenon [5], it may have direct relevant impact on HRQoL [4].

Our focus on qualitative approaches could contribute to sustain a subjective insight into patient's experience [15]. In fact, patients are the most trustworthy witnesses of their lives. They are the main protagonists of their changing illness experience: day after day, they live on with their body and continuously come to terms with the PD [5, 17].

Stemming from our review stigma could be considered as a nonmotor symptom as relevant as the other ones. In fact, stigma is not only a feeling of shame and embarrassment arising from a self-perception of inadequacy due to loss of autonomy and visible symptoms but also an experience related to the attitudes and beliefs of the social context towards the PD patient who is stigmatized and forced to withdrawal. That is, it is the negative or positive response of the outside world that may do the difference. Indeed, according to the recent ICF conceptualization, disability is not only a state linked to personal limitations and impairments but also a condition interconnected with the environment and the interface with it [36, 38].

To date, what PD patients and their caregivers seem to experience is a mark [8], a shameful sign of different needs and impaired behaviors. Indeed, PD manifestations break social rules and all what is normally attended by a healthy social community [23]. Further qualitative studies on this topic are needed in order to better understand a subjective symptom as stigma in parkinsonian patients from an intercultural and a social point of view.

References

[1] J. Jankovic, "Parkinson's disease: clinical features and diagnosis," *Journal of Neurology, Neurosurgery & Psychiatry*, vol. 79, no. 4, pp. 368–376, 2008.

[2] D. Santos-García and R. De La Fuente-Fernández, "Impact of non-motor symptoms on health-related and perceived quality of life in Parkinson's disease," *Journal of the Neurological Sciences*, vol. 332, no. 1-2, pp. 136–140, 2013.

[3] L. Kadastik-Eerme, M. Rosenthal, T. Paju, M. Muldmaa, and P. Taba, "Health-related quality of life in Parkinson's disease: a cross-sectional study focusing on non-motor symptoms," *Health and Quality of Life Outcomes*, vol. 13, no. 1, article 83, 2015.

[4] H. I. Ma, M. Saint-Hilaire, C. A. Thomas, and L. Tickle-Degnen, "Stigma as a key determinant of health-related quality of life in Parkinson's disease," *Quality of Life Research*, vol. 25, no. 12, pp. 3037–3045, 2016.

[5] M. Hermanns, "The invisible and visible stigmatization of Parkinson's disease," *Journal of the American Association of Nurse Practitioners*, vol. 25, no. 10, pp. 563–566, 2013.

[6] E. Goffman, *Stigma: Notes on the Management of Spoiled Identity*, Prentice-Hall, New York, NY, USA, 1963.

[7] B. Major and L. T. O'Brien, "The social psychology of stigma," *Annual Review of Psychology*, vol. 56, pp. 393–421, 2005.

[8] E. E. Jones, A. Farina, A. H. Hastorf, H. Markus, D. T. Miller, and R. A. Scott, *Social Stigma: The Psychology of Marked Relationships*, Freeman, New York, NY, USA, 1984.

[9] L. H. Yang, A. Kleinman, B. G. Link, J. C. Phelan, S. Lee, and B. Good, "Culture and stigma: adding moral experience to stigma theory," *Social Science and Medicine*, vol. 64, no. 7, pp. 1524–1535, 2007.

[10] B. A. Pescosolido, J. K. Martin, A. Lang, and S. Olafsdottir, "Rethinking theoretical approaches to stigma: a Framework Integrating Normative Influences on Stigma (FINIS)," *Social Science & Medicine*, vol. 67, no. 3, pp. 431–440, 2008.

[11] J. E. Pachankis, "The psychological implications of concealing a stigma: a cognitive-affective-behavioral model," *Psychological Bulletin*, vol. 133, no. 2, pp. 328–345, 2007.

[12] S. C. Burgener and B. Berger, "Measuring perceived stigma in persons with progressive neurological disease: Alzheimer's dementia and Parkinson's disease," *Dementia*, vol. 7, no. 1, pp. 31–53, 2008.

[13] D. Rao, S. W. Choi, D. Victorson et al., "Measuring stigma across neurological conditions: the development of the stigma scale for chronic illness (SSCI)," *Quality of Life Research*, vol. 18, no. 5, pp. 585–595, 2009.

[14] S. A. M. Stevelink, I. C. Wu, C. G. Voorend, and W. H. van Brakel, "The psychometric assessment of internalized stigma instruments: a systematic review," *Stigma Research and Action*, vol. 2, no. 2, 2012.

[15] J. M. Corbin and A. L. Strauss, *Basics of Qualitative Research: Techniques and Procedures for Developing Grounded Theory*, Sage, Thousand Oaks, Calif, USA, 2008.

[16] J. Posen, O. Moore, D. Sadeh Tassa, K. Ginzburg, M. Drory, and N. Giladi, "Young women with PD: a group work experience," *Social Work in Health Care*, vol. 32, no. 1, pp. 77–91, 2000.

[17] A. Giardini, A. Pierobon, S. Callegari, G. Bertotti, M. Maffoni, and G. Frazzitta, "Towards proactive active living: patients with Parkinson's disease experience of a multidisciplinary intensive rehabilitation treatment," *European Journal of Physical and Rehabilitation Medicine*, In press.

[18] A. Soundy, B. Stubbs, and C. Roskell, "The experience of Parkinson's disease: a systematic review and meta-ethnography," *The Scientific World Journal*, vol. 2014, Article ID 613592, 19 pages, 2014.

[19] M. A. Soleimani, R. Negarandeh, F. Bastani, and R. Greysen, "Disrupted social connectedness in people with Parkinson's disease," *British Journal of Community Nursing*, vol. 19, no. 3, pp. 136–141, 2014.

[20] M. A. Soleimani, F. Bastani, R. Negarandeh, and R. Greysen, "Perceptions of people living with Parkinson's disease: a qualitative study in Iran," *British Journal of Community Nursing*, vol. 21, no. 4, pp. 188–195, 2016.

[21] H. Van Der Bruggen and G. Widdershoven, "Being a Parkinson's patient: immobile and unpredictably whimsical literature and existential analysis," *Medicine, Health Care, and Philosophy*, vol. 7, no. 3, pp. 289–301, 2004.

[22] N. Bramley and V. Eatough, "The experience of living with Parkinson's disease: an interpretative phenomenological analysis case study," *Psychology & Health*, vol. 20, no. 2, pp. 223–235, 2005.

[23] G. Nijhof, "Parkinson's disease as a problem of shame in public appearance," *Sociology of Health & Illness*, vol. 17, no. 2, pp. 193–205, 1995.

[24] H. Chiong-Rivero, G. W. Ryan, C. Flippen et al., "Patients' and caregivers' experiences of the impact of Parkinson's disease on health status," *Patient Related Outcome Measures*, vol. 2011, no. 2, pp. 57–70, 2011.

[25] N. Miller, E. Noble, D. Jones, and D. Burn, "Hard to swallow: dysphagia in Parkinson's disease," *Age and Ageing*, vol. 35, no. 6, pp. 614–618, 2006.

[26] H. Sunvisson and S.-L. Ekman, "Environmental influences on the experiences of people with Parkinson's disease," *Nursing Inquiry*, vol. 8, no. 1, pp. 41–50, 2001.

[27] N. Miller, E. Noble, D. Jones, and D. Burn, "Life with communication changes in Parkinson's disease," *Age and Ageing*, vol. 35, no. 3, pp. 235–239, 2006.

[28] G. Mshana, C. L. Dotchin, and R. W. Walker, "'We call it the shaking illness': perceptions and experiences of Parkinson's disease in rural northern Tanzania," *BMC Public Health*, vol. 11, article 219, 2011.

[29] K. Oehlberg, F. K. Barg, G. K. Brown, D. Taraborelli, M. B. Stern, and D. Weintraub, "Attitudes regarding the etiology and treatment of depression in Parkinson's disease: a qualitative study," *Journal of Geriatric Psychiatry and Neurology*, vol. 21, no. 2, pp. 123–132, 2008.

[30] E. J. Henshaw, "Too sick, not sick enough? Effects of treatment type and timing on depression stigma," *Journal of Nervous and Mental Disease*, vol. 202, no. 4, pp. 292–299, 2014.

[31] D. Mittal, G. Sullivan, L. Chekuri, E. Allee, and P. W. Corrigan, "Empirical studies of self-stigma reduction strategies: a critical review of the literature," *Psychiatric Services*, vol. 63, no. 10, pp. 974–981, 2012.

[32] P. T. Yanos, A. Lucksted, A. L. Drapalski, D. Roe, and P. Lysaker, "Interventions targeting mental health self-stigma: a review and comparison," *Psychiatric Rehabilitation Journal*, vol. 38, no. 2, pp. 171–178, 2015.

[33] J. M. T. van Uem, J. Marinus, C. Canning et al., "Health-Related Quality of Life in patients with Parkinson's disease—a systematic review based on the ICF model," *Neuroscience and Biobehavioral Reviews*, vol. 61, pp. 26–34, 2016.

[34] G. Frazzitta, G. Bertotti, D. Uccellini et al., "Short- and long-term efficacy of intensive rehabilitation treatment on balance and gait in parkinsonian patients: a preliminary study with a 1-year followup," *Parkinson's Disease*, vol. 2013, Article ID 583278, 5 pages, 2013.

[35] S. Moore and S. Knowles, "Beliefs and knowledge about Parkinson's disease," *Sensoria—A Journal of Mind, Brain, and Culture*, vol. 2, no. 1, pp. 15–21, 2006.

[36] World Health Organization (WHO), *International Classification of Functioning, Disability, and Health: ICF*, World Health Organization, Geneva, Switzerland, 2001.

[37] J. Engebretson, "Understanding stigma in chronic health conditions: implications for nursing," *Journal of the American Association of Nurse Practitioners*, vol. 25, no. 10, pp. 545–550, 2013.

[38] A. Giardini, P. Ferrari, E. M. Negri, G. Majani, C. Magnani, and P. Preti, "The positive role of caregivers in terminal cancer patients' abilities: usefulness of the ICF framework," *European Journal of Physical and Rehabilitation Medicine*, vol. 52, no. 2, pp. 214–222, 2016.

20

Benefit from the Chin-Down Maneuver in the Swallowing Performance and Self-Perception of Parkinson's Disease Patients

Annelise Ayres,[1] Geraldo Pereira Jotz,[1] Carlos R. M. Rieder,[2,3] and Maira Rozenfeld Olchik[4]

[1]*Postgraduate Program in Health Sciences, Universidade Federal de Ciências da Saúde de Porto Alegre, Porto Alegre, RS, Brazil*
[2]*Postgraduate Program in Medical Sciences, Universidade Federal do Rio Grande do Sul, Porto Alegre, RS, Brazil*
[3]*Department of Neurology and Postgraduate Program in Rehabilitation, Universidade Federal de Ciências da Saúde de Porto Alegre (UFCSPA), Porto Alegre, RS, Brazil*
[4]*Department of Surgery and Orthopaedics, Universidade Federal do Rio Grande do Sul, Porto Alegre, RS, Brazil*

Correspondence should be addressed to Maira Rozenfeld Olchik; mairarozenfeld@hotmail.com

Academic Editor: Ivan Bodis-Wollner

Aims. To verify the effectiveness of the maneuver application in swallowing therapy with PD. *Materials and Method.* We performed an open-label trial, with three groups compounds by PD individuals: the experimental group, control group, and orientation group. The study included PD patients with dysphagia. A cognitive screening, through a questionnaire about depression and quality of life, was conducted. Swallowing assessment was performed through (1) fiberoptic endoscopic evaluation of swallowing (FEES); (2) clinical evaluation and Functional Oral Intake Scale (FOIS); and (3) assessment of the quality life related to swallowing (SWALQOL). A therapeutic program, which consisted of chin-down postural maneuver and orientations on feeding, was applied. Both groups (EG and OG) received on-month therapeutic program. *Results.* A significant improvement in swallowing, evaluated by clinical assessment, was observed in solid ($p < 0.001$) and liquid ($p = 0.022$) consistencies in EG when compared to OG and CG. Patients in EG presented improvement in QoL, with the significant difference in comparison with the other groups, about domain frequency of symptoms ($p = 0.029$) in SWALQOL questionnaire. *Conclusion.* The postural maneuver chin-down improved swallowing performance and self-perception, but not the laryngeal signs. This trial is registered with registration number NCT02973698.

1. Introduction

Dysphagia is a highly prevalent symptom in Parkinson's disease (PD) [1]. In the early stages of the disease, it may be present in up to 80% of patients and, in advanced stages, the incidence may increase to 95% [1–3]. Signs and symptoms of dysphagia in PD may occur in oral, pharyngeal, and esophageal swallowing phases. Laryngeal penetration and pulmonary aspiration are the most aggravating symptoms [4–6]. Such signs and symptoms may result in complications, such as malnutrition, dehydration and lung problems. Respiratory infection by aspiration is the leading direct cause of death in patients with PD, and it is highly associated with immobility and dysphagia [7]. There is prevalence from 30% to 45% of pneumonia among the death causes in patients with PD [8–11].

Although dysphagia is a complicated PD symptom, the number of studies about the effects of swallowing therapy in this disease is still limited. There are studies on the use of biofeedback for the therapeutic intervention [12–14], about the use of expiratory muscle strength training for swallowing [15], about the effects of surface electrical stimulation [16], and on myofunctional exercises for swallowing [17, 18]. However, these pieces of evidence are far from conclusive. The only studies on rehabilitation and management of oropharyngeal dysphagia in patients with PD still do not have conclusive results [4, 19].

In a literature review on swallowing therapy for PD, we found only nine studies on this subject [4]. From these, only two [20, 21] reported the effect of chin-down posture maneuver. Logemann et al. [20] conducted, so far, the largest study on compensatory approaches for oropharyngeal dysphagia in PD. The authors compared chin-down posture maneuver with changes in food consistency in the treatment of oropharyngeal dysphagia. The results showed that the postural maneuver was the less effective strategy in the prevention of liquids aspiration than changes in food consistency. The same was found in a study by Robbins et al. [21]. This study demonstrated profound differences of interventions to prevent pneumonia. However, the authors suggest that swallowing becomes safer as the food consistency changes (thickened liquids). Other articles show improvements in some swallowing parameters, after the investigated treatment strategies (change of food texture, tactile and thermal oral stimulation, myofunctional exercises, Lee Silverman Voice, exercises with biofeedback, and expiratory muscle training), but no significant improvements in swallowing global function.

As was previously described, up to this moment, studies which investigate the effectiveness of the chin-down postural maneuver in the rehabilitation of dysphagia PD patients have applied it only in an isolated moment, during the performance of a swallowing objective examination. It does not enable a therapeutic process to learn the maneuver correctly. They have tested it only in one food consistency (liquid consistency), or they have applied it to other therapeutic strategies, with no opportunity to verify its isolated effectiveness. So, this study has the purpose of verifying the efficiency of the maneuver application, in isolation, in a therapeutic program, as well as testing its effectiveness with different food consistencies.

2. Materials and Methods

This study is an open-label trial performed in PD patients with oropharyngeal dysphagia, from March 2014 to May 2015. Clinical trial is registered with ClinicalTrails.gov number NCT02973698.

2.1. Participants. Participants were PD patients recruited from a Parkinson's disease and Movement Disorders Clinic from Hospital de Clínicas de Porto Alegre (HCPA), a reference hospital, in Rio Grande do Sul, Brazil. The written free and informed consent to participate in the research was obtained from participants. This study was approved by the hospital central research ethics committee.

2.2. Inclusion and Exclusion Criteria. The included subjects were patients with the diagnosis of Parkinson's disease, according to the criteria from the United Kingdom Parkinson's Disease Society Brain Bank criteria for idiopathic PD [22] that have the diagnosis of oropharyngeal dysphagia. The diagnosis of oropharyngeal dysphagia was made by fiberoptic endoscopic evaluation of swallowing (FEES), according to the criteria from Santoro et al. [23]. PD staging was based on the Hoehn and Yahr Staging Scale (H&Y, Degree of Disability Scale) (Hoehn & Yahr, 1967), used to assess the severity of PD. As exclusion criteria, there were the following aspects: presenting language and hearing disorders, which could complicate the understanding of an intervention program, diagnosis of dementia, or other neurological illnesses.

2.3. Patient Evaluation. Cognitive screening which consists of Mini-Mental State Examination (MMSE) and Montreal Cognitive Assessment (MoCA) in all patients was performed before the intervention. The instruments Parkinson Disease Questionnaire-39 (PDQ-39), translated to Portuguese, and the Beck Depression Inventory (BDI) were also applied. These tests were used to verify the influence of cognitive aspects, depression, and quality of life in the therapeutic process.

To evaluate the intervention's effectiveness, an evaluation of swallowing was conducted in two moments (before and after intervention). Three kinds of assessments were performed: (1) fiberoptic endoscopic evaluation of swallowing (FEES); (2) clinical evaluation; and (3) assessment of the quality of life related to swallowing (SWALQOL).

(i) Fiberoptic Endoscopic Evaluation of Swallowing (FEES). This objective examination of swallowing was performed according to the following protocol: First, the prior state of secretion in the nasopharyngeal structures, oropharynx, and laryngopharynx was tested. Next, the individual received liquid consistency offered through a syringe, 3 and 5 mL of water with edible blue food coloring. For the sticky consistency, 3 and 5 mL of thickened water were provided through a needle with edible blue food coloring. A half a glass of water and salt biscuits with real blue food coloring were offered to assess the solid consistency. No anesthetic was used for the examination. The images were later analyzed by an otolaryngologist physician, experienced in the dysphagia area. The presence of thickening on the posterior laryngeal wall, tremor in structures (base of tongue and vallecula), early escape (characterized by the presence of food in the hypopharynx or larynx before the swallowing reflex was triggered), vallecular stasis in glossoepiglottic folds and pyriform sinus (characterized by accumulation of food after the third swallowing on the mentioned structures), penetration (characterized by the presence of food in the laryngeal vestibule), tracheal aspiration (characterized by food intake in the region located below the vocal folds, in the subglottic region and in the trachea, at any time of swallowing), and cough reflex was observed. The alterations were classified as present or absent. The equipment used was the flexible nasopharyngoscope Maschida ENT-III, 3.2 mm, with Xerônio Storz light source.

(ii) Clinical Evaluation and Functional Oral Intake Scale (FOIS). Clinical evaluation of swallowing was performed by a certified speech therapist, previously trained to apply the protocols. All the assessments were conducted by the same professional. This assessment had the purpose of checking signs and symptoms of oropharyngeal dysphagia. Solid food consistency (half portion of bread) and liquid (100 mL of water) evaluated by free demand were used. The analyzed signs and symptoms were based on the area literature [24], which are history of aspiration pneumonia; alert state; interaction attention/ability; awareness of the swallowing problem; awareness of secretion; ability to manipulate flows; postural control; fatigability; anatomy and oral, pharyngeal, and laryngeal physiology; orofacial tonus; oral apraxia; orofacial sensitivity; gag pharyngeal contraction;

saliva swallowing; cough and hawk; swallowing apraxia; oral residue; delayed swallowing reflex; reduction in laryngeal elevation; wet voice; and multiple swallowing. A total of 21 signs and symptoms were evaluated as present or absent. At the end of the objective and clinical evaluation, the intake of food was scored according to Functional Oral Intake Scale (FOIS). This scale scores the level of oral food intake of patients at specific levels, from 0 (restricted to alternative food pathway) to 7 (total oral intake with no restrictions), with the aim of monitoring the patients' evolution during the therapeutic process. The valid and reliable instrument has a coefficient of interrater reliability from 0.98 to 0.99, with Kappa coefficient average values between 0.86 and 0.91, with appropriate consensual validity (Kendall 0,90 agreement) and criterion validity (based on the Mann Assessment test of Swallowing Ability) [25]. A translated and validated version for Brazilian Portuguese was used [26].

(iii) The Quality of Life in Swallowing Disorders. The questionnaire Quality of Life in Swallowing Disorders (SWAL-QOL) was applied, to verify the symptoms presented by the patients, as well as their influence on the quality of life. This instrument has Alpha Cronbach coefficient higher than 0.80, except in one domain. Thus, it presents excellent internal consistency and short-term reproducibility. It is a sensitive scale to differentiate oropharyngeal dysphagia degrees of severity. The version translated and validated for Brazilian Portuguese was used [27]. All questionnaires were applied in a waiting room. The questions and possible answers were read by the researcher for all patients. The questionnaires application was performed individually, for each patient.

2.4. Intervention. Individuals who agreed to participate in this study were allocated to one of the three interventions groups: (1) experimental group (patients performed the chin-down posture maneuver), (2) control group (PD individuals without any intervention), and (3) orientation group (PD participants that received swallowing orientations).

(1) The Experimental Group (EG) (Chin-Down Posture Maneuver Group). Patients received an intervention program consisting of four weekly individual sessions of 30 minutes. In these sessions, the training of chin-down postural maneuver with saliva and water was performed. The participants were trained to perform the maneuver twice a day, swallowing saliva, and during meals, throughout the week, at home. The participants received a form, so they recorded the number of times they performed the maneuver at home. It allowed the control of adherence, the importance of adherence to treatment being reinforced at each session. Besides, the subjects received instructions regarding feeding as follows.

Swallowing Orientations

Environment during Feeding Time

(i) Do the meals in a quiet location.

(ii) Keep off television, radio or any other device that can distract you.

(iii) Keep your attention on the food.

(iv) Do not talk during feeding.

(v) Avoid making meals at times when you are sleepy or tired.

(vi) Try to make meals when in the ON period of medication.

Posture during Feeding

(i) Sit next to the table.

(ii) Keep your torso upright and your head up.

(iii) Avoid lying down right after the end of the meal.

(iv) Put small portions of food in the mouth.

(v) Try to chew the food well and many times before swallowing.

(vi) Swallow more than once, until you are sure there is no residue in the mouth.

(vii) If you have the sensation of food "stuck in the throat" swallow more your saliva.

Meal Time

(i) Maximum time of the main meal (breakfast, lunch, and dinner) is 30 minutes.

(ii) Do not eat in a hurry.

Oral Hygiene

(i) Do not forget to brush your tooth after meals.

(ii) Remember to brush your tongue.

(iii) If you use the dental prosthesis, it should be removed and cleaned with tooth brushing after every meal, and the tongue should be brushed.

(iv) In patients that do not have teeth, washing the mouth should be done with a brushing of the tongue and the remaining with gauze soaked with water and mouthwash.

All the instructions, as well as the explanation about the maneuver, were submitted to the patients through a written document.

(2) The Control Group (CG) (PD Individuals without Any Intervention). The participants of this group underwent evaluation of swallowing, and the same assessment was repeated after four weeks, without any intervention during that period.

(3) Orientations Group (OG). The individuals participated in an intervention program which consisted of four individual sessions a week, with 30 minutes. In these sessions, the instructions about feeding were performed. The people received all the instructions on a written document (see Swallowing Orientations). In the sessions, doubts about the guidelines and treatment adherence were verified. In this group, the chin-down postural maneuver was not applied.

The chin-down postural maneuver is performed by requesting the patient to swallow lowering the head with the

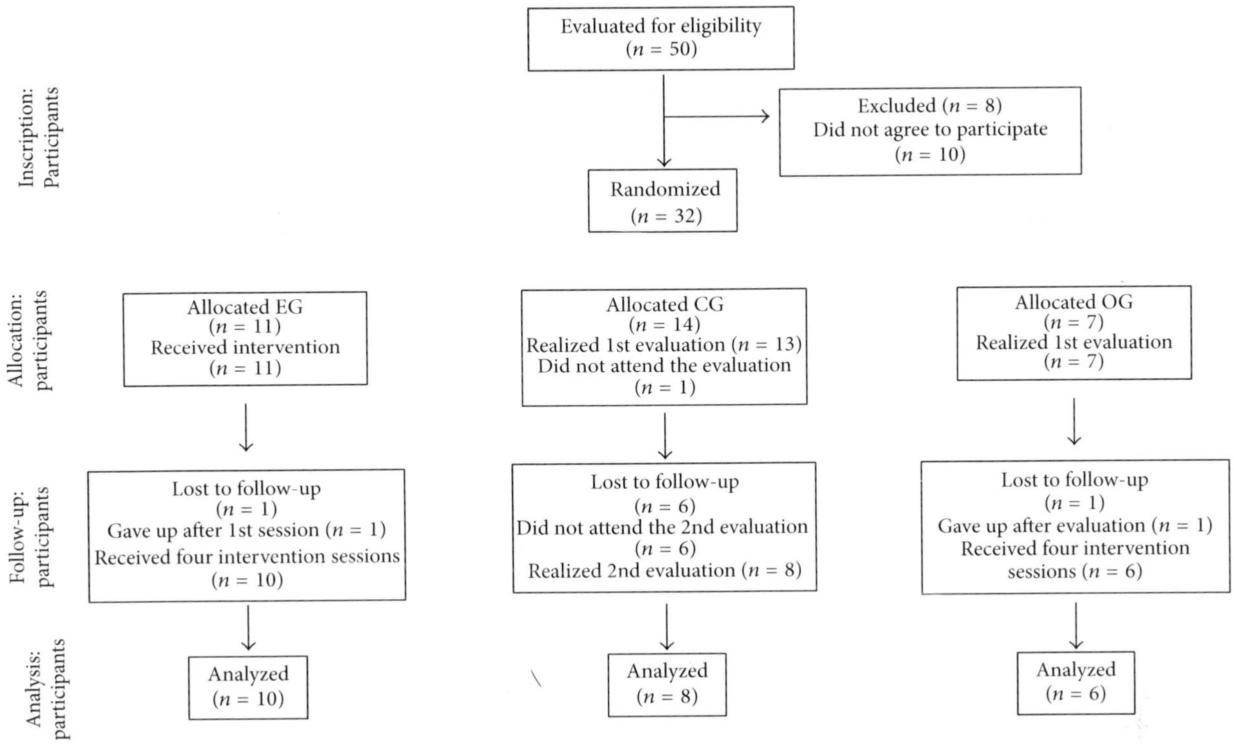

FIGURE 1: Steps of study.

intention of touching the chin in the neck. This maneuver promotes the major protection of the airways by posteriorization of the base of the tongue, with an enlargement of the vallecular space and displacement of the epiglottis to a more protective position.

The EG and OG interventions were used by the same researcher, previously trained. After the end of the research, the same swallowing therapy performed to the GE was offered to the CG and OG individuals.

2.5. Statistical Analysis. Statistical analysis was performed through the Statistical Package for Social Sciences (SPSS), version 20.0. For the primary outcome analysis, the Shapiro-Wilk normality test, the Student's t-test (clinical evaluation of swallowing variable), and the Generalized Estimating Equations (GEE) (SWALQOL variable) were used. Data from the FEES variable did not allow inferential statistical analysis. The Spearman correlation test was used, with separate groups, to check the relationship between the demographic and clinical variables of the three groups and the clinical evaluation of the swallowing variable. The regression test and the Pearson correlation test were applied to check the influence of the BDI and the PDQ variables in the swallowing clinical evaluation. To verify the group's similarities in the preintervention assessment, the Shapiro-Wilk normality test was performed. Next, to the standard variables (age, MOCA, PDQ, and BDI), the ANOVA was applied. For the nonnormal variables (disease duration, education, and H&Y stages), the Kruskal-Wallis test for independent samples was used. For all tests, 5% of error was provided.

3. Results

The selection process of the participants consisted of 4 steps as it is shown in Figure 1. The sociodemographic and clinical profile of this study's participants are described in Table 1.

Patients that received the program of chin-down posture maneuver presented significant improvements in signals and symptoms of dysphagia by clinical evaluation when compared with the other two groups (control and orientation group) regarding solid ($p < 0.001$) and liquid ($p = 0.022$) consistencies (Table 2).

The analysis by fiberoptic endoscopic evaluation of swallowing (FEES) did not show differences between patients that received and did not receive the intervention.

Regarding quality of life, patients that received the intervention of chin-down maneuver (EG) presented a significant improvement in scores of domains frequency of symptoms and mental health on the SWAL-QOL when compared with the groups that did not receive this intervention (Table 3).

In the analysis of the correlation between the groups and cognitive variables with an evaluation of swallowing no correlations were found. Thus, no influence of the cognitive aspects of the therapeutic process was evidenced, in this population.

4. Discussion

Our results showed that patients that received the intervention of chin-down postural maneuver have improvement in clinical evaluation of dysphagia and quality of life evaluated by SWAL-QOL. These findings suggest that a simple and

Table 1: Sociodemographic and clinical data.

Groups	Experimental (EG) $n = 10$	Control (CG) $n = 8$	Orientation (OG) $n = 6$	p value
Male gender	80%	75%	66.70%	—
Age*	62.0 (±11.5)	62.8 (±6.2)	64.5 (±5.6)	0.694[a]
Schooling*	5.9 (±4.1)	10.3 (±8.4)	12.0 (±9.1)	0.142[b]
Time of disease*	10.7 (±4.7)	11.8 (±8.0)	8.8 (±6.0)	0.524[b]
H&Y*	2.8 (±0.8)	2.5 (±0.7)	2.5 (±0.8)	0.363[b]
MEEM*	26.6 (±3.8)	25.6 (±3.7)	25.3 (±4.1)	0.702[b]
MOCA*	21.9 (±4.9)	20.5 (±7.7)	21.2 (±8.4)	0.834[a]
PDQ-39*	41.4 (±13.8)	38.7 (±16.7)	36.5 (±17.1)	0.704[a]
BDI*	13.8 (±7.7)	17.1 (±9.2)	14.7 (±9.3)	0.523[a]
FOIS*	5.9 (±1.3)	6.8 (±0.5)	6.8 (±0.4)	—

[a]ANOVA; [b] Kruskal-Wallis test; *Representation of the data as mean and standard deviation; H&Y: Hoehn & Yahr Scale; MMSE: Mini-Mental State Examination; MOCA: Montreal Cognitive Assessment; PDQ-39: Parkinson's Disease Questionnaire-39; BDI: Beck Depression Inventory; FOIS: Functional Oral Intake Scale. — indicates that statistical testing was not applied to this variable (FOIS).

Table 2: Correlation between the periods before and after clinical evaluation of swallowing.

Groups	Solid Pre Mean (PD)	Solid Post Mean (PD)	p	Liquid Pre Mean (PD)	Liquid Post Mean (PD)	p
Experimental (EG)	4.56 (±0.631)	2.40 (±0.290)	0.002*	3.33 (±0.609)	1.56 (±0.388)	0.01*
Control (CG)	4.88 (±1.007)	3.00 (±0.354)	0.083	2.13 (±0.874)	1.13 (±0.482)	0.26
Orientation (OG)	2.67 (±0.304)	3.17 (±0.495)	0.33	0.50 (±0.312)	0.83 (±0.281)	0.39

Student's t-test; PD: standard deviation; p: p value; *$p < 0.005$.

inexpensive dysphagia therapy as the chin-down postural maneuver is effective to improve dysphagia in PD patients. This intervention demonstrated benefits, even in a short period. Cognitive ability, depression, and quality of life did not influence this process.

In literature, there is heterogeneity studies about swallowing therapy in PD patients. At this moment, only eight studies about this topic in this population were found. These five studies [12, 14, 16–18] led to improvements in some participants' swallowing parameters, but with no global function changes. Three studies [13, 15, 28] found improvements in swallowing after therapy. These changes have been demonstrated through better scores in FOIS scale and Penetration-Aspiration Scale. Although our study had much less time of intervention, the results are similar to the literature [12, 14, 16–18]. Regarding SWALQOL, we observed that these results corroborated with other studies that found that swallowing-related QoL improved after an SLP intervention. This finding demonstrates the importance of dysphagia therapy in this population, as a way of reducing swallowing-related complaints and improving QoL [29].

In addition to the motor symptoms of PD, there is a high prevalence of nonmotor symptoms, such as cognitive decline, loss of facial expression, micrograph, and sleep disorders [30]. Therefore, clinical studies on swallowing therapy in PD need to control the influence of these symptoms in the therapeutic process. Among these symptoms, the cognitive decline is highlighted, which has a prevalence from 25% to 38.2% in early stages of PD [31, 32], and it may result in significant rehabilitation impacts. The lack of cognitive data associated with therapeutic improvements is critical to the right study evaluation, described in the literature [13, 15, 28].

Swallowing treatment in a neurodegenerative disease seeks functionality of safe swallowing and maintenance of nutritional status and respiratory conditions. According to the literature [20, 21], the choice of introducing a therapeutic strategy must follow the order: first, postural techniques; then, oral sensitivity improvements techniques; next, swallowing maneuvers; and, finally, change of food consistency. This law is based on the easiest way patients learn, and it aims at delaying the food texture change, which, in many cases, will not be reversed. Thus, the chin-down postural maneuver was chosen based on previous studies which have shown that it is among the two most recommended maneuvers in the therapeutic process for individuals with PD and based on its effectiveness to prevent aspiration pneumonia in patients with PD, when combined with liquid thickening [18, 20, 21, 28].

Also, this strategy aims to improve the protection of the airways, reducing the possibility of penetration in the larynx or aspiration, being frequently recommended for thin liquids swallowing, to reduce early escape and possible entry into the air pathway [18, 28]. Added to these aspects, according to a larger study [20] patients who received swallowing therapy in PD suggest that the chin-down posture is easier and more pleasant, compared to other used therapeutic strategies.

The therapeutic process involves changing habits and new learning. The postural maneuver performance involves

TABLE 3: SWALQOLL analysis before and after intervention.

Domain		Experimental (EG)		Control (CG)		Orientation (OG)		p value
		Mean (standard deviation)						
(1) Swallowing as a burden	Pre	71.5	9.4	98.2	6.8	89.3	8.0	0.279
	Post	60.4	13.8	85.7	9.9	95.6	8.4	
(2) Desire to eat	Pre	68.2	7.0	91.2	7.6	82.3	7.9	0.306
	Post	71.5	7.9	81.8	7.7	92.0	9.3	
(3) Eating duration	Pre	66.4	11.2	26.5	9	24.7	10.6	0.812
	Post	72.6	10.6	25	10.2	24.7	15.4	
(4) Frequency of symptoms	Pre	63.5	3.6	72.4	3.7	72.2	4.1	0.029*
	Post	73.3	4.3	71.6	4	75.7	5.6	
(5) Food selection	Pre	74.2	7.8	87.6	3.9	85.5	5.1	0.539
	Post	86.8	8.7	89.1	4.5	81.3	5	
(6) Communication	Pre	47.3	4.4	45.6	6.2	45.3	5.5	0.713
	Post	57.9	7	50.3	6.1	57.8	6.9	
(7) Fear to eat	Pre	72.5	5.3	71.6	4.6	73.2	5.4	0.662
	Post	80.9	6.6	73.9	5	74.3	5.9	
(8) Mental health	Pre	74	6.7	87.8	7.6	92.1	6.2	0.004*
	Post	70.9	9.6	90.3	5.7	82.9	12.3	
(9) Social function	Pre	76.1	5.7	86.7	5.1	88.8	4.7	0.425
	Post	83.4	7.1	88.6	4.6	80.5	8.6	
(10) Sleep	Pre	50.9	11.4	15.5	11	25.1	10.2	0.093
	Post	65.9	11.4	26.4	10.2	18.9	11.2	
(11) Fatigue	Pre	65.7	7.5	51.4	7.7	60.4	4.8	0.298
	Post	81.4	5	58.7	4.2	56.2	10	
Total	Pre	63.9	3.5	67.5	4.1	68.9	3.1	0.288
	Post	72.2	4.7	69.3	3.2	69.6	4.3	

Statistical test: GEE; $^{*}p < 0.005$; SWAL QOL: Quality of Life in Swallowing Disorders Questionnaire.

learning the proper movement for its implementation, as well as inhibition of an automatic behavior for the implementation of a new way of swallowing. Thus, the individuals go through a learning process, which causes changes in structures and functioning of their neural cells and connections [33]. The consolidation of a new learning process depends on the plasticity of the central nervous system, which occurs in three stages: development, learning, and after lesional processes, translated into the nervous system attempting to form new connections and recovery of lost connections [33]. Thus, the lack of changes in the swallowing pattern, in an objective examination of the EG participants, may be a result of the short therapy time, which did not allow the complete knowledge consolidation.

The findings generalization is limited because the changes occur only from the clinical judgment. Although significant changes in the objective evaluation of swallowing have been observed, the results expressed impacts on participants' swallowing performance and self-perception, as evidenced by improvements in quality of life (SWALQOL) in the experimental group.

Also, the absence of changes in the FEES evaluated parameters must be analyzed with caution. It raises the hypothesis that this is a short intervention period for improvements in these parameters, and the FEES evaluates a unique feeding moment, with small food quantities and in an unusual manner to the patient. On the other hand, the clinical evaluation performed according to the demand allows a swallowing evaluation in an environmental situation. Besides, a high number of patients felt uncomfortable when they performed the FEES, which may negatively influence the findings.

Furthermore, the small sample is a limiting aspect of the findings, and it may have affected the results. However, these results may support larger and randomized studies to ensure the effectiveness of the chin-down postural maneuver for swallowing dynamics, quality of life, and swallowing difficulties in PD.

5. Conclusions

In conclusion, the present study shows that the chin-down posture maneuver, a free and easy procedure, improves the swallowing performance and self-perception of PD patients.

References

[1] J. G. Kalf, B. J. M. de Swart, B. R. Bloem, and M. Munneke, "Prevalence of oropharyngeal dysphagia in Parkinson's disease: a meta-analysis," *Parkinsonism & Related Disorders*, vol. 18, no. 4, pp. 311–315, 2012.

[2] A. R. Wintzen, U. A. Badrising, R. A. C. Roos, J. Vielvoye, L. Liauw, and E. K. J. Pauwels, "Dysphagia in ambulant patients with Parkinson's disease: common, not dangerous," *The Canadian Journal of Neurological Sciences*, vol. 21, no. 1, pp. 53–56, 1994.

[3] M. Nagaya, T. Kachi, T. Yamada, and A. Igata, "Videofluorographic study of swallowing in Parkinson's disease," *Dysphagia*, vol. 13, no. 2, pp. 95–100, 1998.

[4] S. K. Smith, H. Roddam, and H. Sheldrick, "Rehabilitation or compensation: time for a fresh perspective on speech and language therapy for dysphagia and Parkinson's disease?" *International Journal of Language & Communication Disorders*, vol. 47, no. 4, pp. 351–364, 2012.

[5] N. Argolo, M. Sampaio, P. Pinho, A. Melo, and A. C. Nóbrega, "Swallowing disorders in Parkinson's disease: impact of lingual pumping," *International Journal of Language and Communication Disorders*, vol. 50, no. 5, pp. 659–664, 2015.

[6] Y. H. Kim, B.-M. Oh, I.-Y. Jung, J. C. Lee, G. J. Lee, and T. R. Han, "Spatiotemporal characteristics of swallowing in Parkinson's disease," *Laryngoscope*, vol. 125, no. 2, pp. 389–395, 2015.

[7] G. C. Fernandes, M. P. Socal, A. F. S. Schuh, and C. R. M. Rieder, "Clinical and epidemiological factors associated with mortality in Parkinson's disease in a Brazilian cohort," *Parkinson's Disease*, vol. 2015, Article ID 959304, 6 pages, 2015.

[8] M. D'Amelio, P. Ragonese, L. Morgante et al., "Long-term survival of Parkinson's disease: a population-based study," *Journal of Neurology*, vol. 253, no. 1, pp. 33–37, 2006.

[9] S. Pennington, K. Snell, M. Lee, and R. Walker, "The cause of death in idiopathic Parkinson's disease," *Parkinsonism and Related Disorders*, vol. 16, no. 7, pp. 434–437, 2010.

[10] A. D. Macleod, K. S. M. Taylor, and C. E. Counsell, "Mortality in Parkinson's disease: a systematic review and meta-analysis," *Movement Disorders*, vol. 29, no. 13, pp. 1615–1622, 2014.

[11] B. Pinter, A. Diem-Zangerl, G. K. Wenning et al., "Mortalidade em Parkinson's doença: Um estudo de seguimento de 38 anos," *Movement Disorders*, vol. 30, no. 2, pp. 266–269, 2014.

[12] V. N. Felix, S. M. A. Corrêa, and R. J. Soares, "A therapeutic maneuver for oropharyngeal dysphagia in patients with Parkinson's disease," *Clinics*, vol. 63, no. 5, pp. 661–666, 2008.

[13] Y. Manor, R. Mootanah, D. Freud, N. Giladi, and J. T. Cohen, "Video-assisted swallowing therapy for patients with Parkinson's disease," *Parkinsonism and Related Disorders*, vol. 19, no. 2, pp. 207–211, 2013.

[14] R. P. Athukorala, R. D. Jones, O. Sella, and M.-L. Huckabee, "Skill training for swallowing rehabilitation in patients with Parkinson's disease," *Archives of Physical Medicine and Rehabilitation*, vol. 95, no. 7, pp. 1374–1382, 2014.

[15] M. S. Troche, M. S. Okun, J. C. Rosenbek et al., "Aspiration and swallowing in Parkinson disease and rehabilitation with EMST: a randomized trial," *Neurology*, vol. 75, no. 21, pp. 1912–1919, 2010.

[16] L. W. J. Baijens, R. Speyer, V. L. Passos, W. Pilz, N. Roodenburg, and P. Clavé, "The effect of surface electrical stimulation on swallowing in dysphagic parkinson patients," *Dysphagia*, vol. 27, no. 4, pp. 528–537, 2012.

[17] N. Argolo, M. Sampaio, P. Pinho, A. Melo, and A. C. Nóbrega, "Do swallowing exercises improve swallowing dynamic and quality of life in Parkinson's disease?" *NeuroRehabilitation*, vol. 32, no. 4, pp. 949–955, 2013.

[18] K. F. Luchesi, S. Kitamura, and L. F. Mourão, "Dysphagia progression and swallowing management in Parkinson's disease: An Observational Study," *Brazilian Journal of Otorhinolaryngology*, vol. 81, no. 1, pp. 24–30, 2015.

[19] J. A. Russell, M. R. Ciucci, N. P. Connor, and T. Schallert, "Targeted exercise therapy for voice and swallow in persons with Parkinson's disease," *Brain Research*, vol. 1341, pp. 3–11, 2010.

[20] J. A. Logemann, G. Gensler, J. Robbins et al., "A randomized study of three interventions for aspiration of thin liquids in patients with dementia or Parkinson's disease," *Journal of Speech, Language, and Hearing Research*, vol. 51, no. 1, pp. 173–183, 2008.

[21] J. Robbins, G. Gensler, J. Hind et al., "Comparison of 2 interventions for liquid aspiration on pneumonia incidence: a randomized trial," *Annals of Internal Medicine*, vol. 148, pp. 509–518, 2008.

[22] A. J. Hughes, S. E. Daniel, L. Kilford, and A. J. Lees, "Accuracy of clinical diagnosis of idiopathic Parkinson's disease: a clinico-pathological study of 100 cases," *Journal of Neurology Neurosurgery and Psychiatry*, vol. 55, no. 3, pp. 181–184, 1992.

[23] P. P. Santoro, C. L. B. Furia, A. P. Forte et al., "Otolaryngology and speech therapy evaluation in the assessment of oropharyngeal dysphagia: a combined protocol proposal," *Brazilian Journal of Otorhinolaryngology*, vol. 77, no. 2, pp. 201–213, 2011.

[24] J. A. Logemann, S. Veis, and L. Colangelo, "A screening procedure for oropharyngeal dysphagia," *Dysphagia*, vol. 14, no. 1, pp. 44–51, 1999.

[25] M. A. Crary, G. D. Carnaby Mann, and M. E. Groher, "Initial psychometric assessment of a functional oral intake scale for dysphagia in stroke patients," *Archives of Physical Medicine and Rehabilitation*, vol. 86, no. 8, pp. 1516–1520, 2005.

[26] A. M. Furkim and A. B. Sacco, "Eficácia da fonoterapia em disfagia neurogênica usando a escala funcional de ingestão por via oral (FOIS) como marcador," *Revista CEFAC*, vol. 10, no. 4, pp. 503–512, 2008.

[27] J. G. Portas, *Validação para a língua portuguesa-brasileira dos questionários: qualidade de vida em disfagia (Swal-qol) e satisfação do paciente e qualidade do cuidado no tratamento da disfagia (Swal-care) [M.S. dissertation]*, Fundação Antônio Prudente, SP, 2009.

[28] K. F. Luchesi, S. Kitamura, and L. F. Mourão, "Management of dysphagia in Parkinson's disease and amyotrophic lateral sclerosis," *CoDAS*, vol. 25, no. 4, pp. 358–364, 2013.

[29] A. Ayres, G. P. Jotz, C. R. D. M. Rieder, A. F. S. Schuh, and M. R. Olchik, "The impact of dysphagia therapy on quality of life in patients with Parkinson's disease as measured by the swallowing quality of life questionnaire (SWALQOL)," *International Archives of Otorhinolaryngology*, vol. 20, no. 3, pp. 202–206, 2016.

[30] L. Mu, S. Sobotka, J. Chen et al., "Parkinson disease affects peripheral sensory nerves in the pharynx," *Journal of Neuropathology and Experimental Neurology*, vol. 72, no. 7, pp. 614–623, 2013.

[31] N. Kandiah, A. Zhang, A. R. Cenina, W. L. Au, N. Nadkarni, and L. C. Tan, "Montreal Cognitive Assessment for the screening and prediction of cognitive decline in early Parkinson's disease,"

21

Genetic Analysis of *LRRK2* R1628P in Parkinson's Disease in Asian Populations

Yuan Zhang,[1,2] Qiying Sun,[2,3,4] Minhan Yi,[5,6] Xun Zhou,[1] Jifeng Guo,[1,3,4,5] Qian Xu,[1] Beisha Tang,[1,3,4,5] and Xinxiang Yan[1,3,4]

[1] *Department of Neurology, Xiangya Hospital, Central South University, Changsha, Hunan 410008, China*
[2] *Department of Geriatrics, Xiangya Hospital, Central South University, Changsha, Hunan 410008, China*
[3] *National Clinical Research Center for Geriatric Diseases, Changsha, Hunan 410078, China*
[4] *Key Laboratory of Hunan Province in Neurodegenerative Disorders, Central South University, Changsha, Hunan 410008, China*
[5] *State Key Laboratory of Medical Genetics, Changsha, Hunan 410078, China*
[6] *Institute of Information Security and Big Data, Central South University, Changsha, Hunan 410083, China*

Correspondence should be addressed to Xinxiang Yan; xxyan1268@126.com

Academic Editor: Jan Aasly

Although the etiology of Parkinson's disease (PD) remains unclear, there is increasing evidence of genetic factors contributing to the onset of PD. Various mutations and risk variants of the gene *LRRK2* have been reported, but the association between *LRRK2* R1628P and PD is still inconsistent. Thus, we conducted a meta-analysis to determine the potential relationship between R1628P and PD. Our study sample was an aggregate of 17 publications, which in total consisted of 9,275 PD patients and 8,114 controls. All of these articles are of high quality according to NOS, and there was no obvious reporting bias or heterogeneity. In a general Asian population, the pooled OR of the risk genotype contrasts was 1.83 (95% CI: 1.57, 2.13). When stratified by ethnicity, the pooled ORs were 1.84 (95% CI: 1.56, 2.18) in a Chinese population and 1.79 (95% CI: 1.27, 2.52) in a non-Chinese population. Our study suggests that *LRRK2* R1628P appears to be a risk factor for PD in Asian populations, both Chinese and non-Chinese.

1. Introduction

Parkinson's disease (PD) is currently the second most common progressive neurodegenerative disorder in the world. Although current science has not been able to discern the exact causes of PD, there is an increasing evidence that genetic factors contribute to the etiology of PD [1].

Certain mutations and risk variants of the gene *leucine-rich repeat kinase 2* (*LRRK2*; PARK8) are very common in the PD-afflicted population, accounting for approximately 5–15% of familial and sporadic PD [2]. Besides, the prevalence differs among different populations [3, 4]. For instance, the reported proportion of G2019S carriers [5–7] in Ashkenazi Jews and North African Arabs is more than 30%, whereas it is nearly nonexistent in Asians. Likewise, in Asian populations, the mostly common variants are G2385R and R1628P [8, 9]. Between these two variants, it is the association between R1628P and PD; however, that is inconclusive. Other studies [10–13] have found that R1628P is a contributing factor to PD in mainland China, Taiwan, Malaysia, and Thailand. Conversely, a large multicenter study [14] and several other investigators [15–17] did not identify any associated risk of R1628P in either East Asian, Caucasian, or Arab-Berber cohorts.

In order to evaluate the association between R1628P and PD, we used meta-analytic methods to assess the possible role of R1628P in PD in a worldwide context.

2. Materials and Methods

2.1. Search Strategy. We searched electronic databases including Embase, PubMed, Cochrane Library, Web of knowledge, Wangfang database, and CNKI. We employed this search method until February 1st, 2017, using a combination of the following keywords, *LRRK2*, R1628P, PD, and Parkinso*, in both English and Chinese. Reference lists and personal communications of authors were also referred as sources to include articles cited elsewhere. All searched publications were imported to endnote for further management. Only one copy of the same papers, which were included in different databases, was kept to avoid duplication.

2.2. Selection Criteria. The following criteria were used to discern the eligibility of a study: (1) the article had to be a case-control study, with the exception of reviews, case reports, editorials, or functional research; (2) all PD patients were diagnosed according to UKBB or other accepted criteria with the exception that positive family history was not a part of the exclusion criteria; (3) all controls were free of symptoms suggestive of PD or other neurological disorders; (4) results of R1628P sequencing were reported both in patients and in controls. We excluded the following studies: (1) duplicate publications and articles which used an overlapping sample and (2) lack of original and sufficient data to calculate the OR.

2.3. Data Extraction and Quality Assessment. To select studies for further assessment, two authors independently scanned the abstracts, titles, or both sections of each retrieved record. All potentially relevant articles were investigated in full. For studies satisfying the aforesaid criteria, two authors independently extracted the following data: year of publication, first author's surname, ethnicity of participants, participant's country of origin, number of R1628P carriers, total number of PD patients and healthy controls, and finally the age and gender ratio for both PD patients and controls. The qualities of the included studies were evaluated by the Newcastle–Ottawa Scale (NOS) [18], of which the genotyping method was an essential part in quality rating process.

2.4. Statistical Analysis. In order to assess the strength of association between *LRRK2* R1628P and PD, the outcome was expressed as odds ratio (OR) along with a corresponding 95% confidence interval (CI). Heterogeneity across individual studies was identified using a standard Q test with a significance level of $\alpha = 0.1$ and I^2. If heterogeneity did not exist ($Q > 0.10$) or the severity of heterogeneity was accepted ($I^2 \leq 50\%$), then the fixed effect model was adopted to calculate the pooled OR value. Otherwise, the random effect model was used. Funnel-plot analysis was used to assess the reporting bias. All analyses were carried out by using the Review Manager software package v.5.3 (The Cochrane Collaboration, Oxford, England). In addition, subgroup analysis was performed according to ethnicity for all studies. In order to assess the stability of the results, sensitivity analysis was performed by removing each individual study from the combined total and then reanalyzing the remainder.

3. Results

3.1. Literature Selection and Study Characteristics. During the initial selection stage, we extracted 148 potentially relevant articles from databases stated above. First, we excluded 97 due to duplication in different databases. Then, 20 publications were excluded for irrelevance to both PD and R1628P, which was determined after screening the titles and abstracts. 14 papers were not included for lack of sequencing results of R1628P both in PD patients and in controls, or the data was not enough to calculate the OR. This process culminated to a total of 17 eligible studies included in qualitative analysis and 16 studies included in the further quantitative analysis. The flow chart illustrating the selection procedure is presented in Figure 1. The main characteristics of the included studies are summarized in Table 1. The NOS scores of the included publications were rated from 7 to 9 stars, which attested to their high quality.

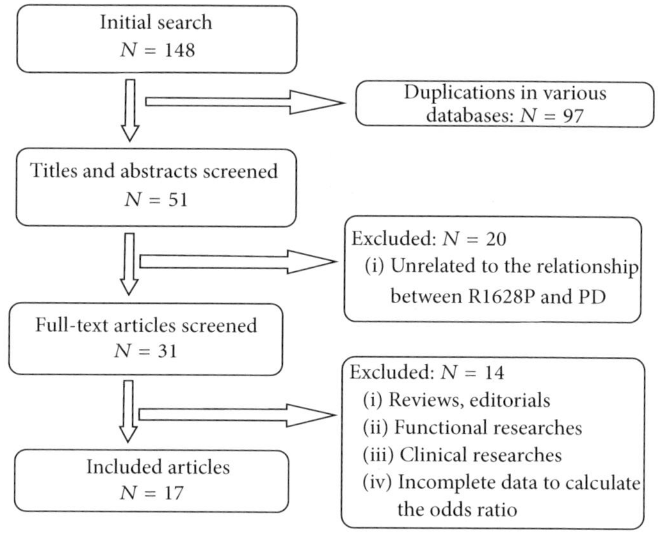

Figure 1: Flow chart of included publications.

3.2. Data Synthesis. All of the 17 included studies pertained to Asian populations. The pooled OR for R1628P in Asian was 1.83 (95% CI: 1.57, 2.13) (Figure 2). The funnel plot was symmetry (Figure 3). In a secondary analytic step, we divided all participants into Chinese and non-Chinese groups. Notably, among these chosen databases, the publication by Ross et al. [19] contained both Chinese and non-Chinese populations, which were analyzed individually. Within the Chinese population, there were 6738 cases of PD and 5767 controls. The pooled OR of the Chinese cohort demonstrates a significantly associated risk of R1628P, with the value of 1.84 (95% CI: 1.56, 2.18) (Figure 2). Among the non-Chinese subgroup, there were 2537 PD subjects and 2347 controls. Since no carriers were screened in Japanese [19–24], we conducted the meta-analysis using the other four publications. These publications were studied in Malaysian, Indian, Korean, and Thailand populations. While only the Thailand population demonstrated a significant, independent association, the pooled OR of R1628P in the combined non-Chinese group was 1.79 (95% CI: 1.27, 2.52) (Figure 2). During the sensitivity analysis, there were no significant changes to the outcomes.

TABLE 1: Attributes of all included studies.

Publications	Ethnicity	Region	Total number of cases/controls	R1628P carriers of case/control	Age of case/control	Male ratio of case/control	NOS
2008 Lu et al. [17]	Chinese	Taiwan	843/543	62/20	65.7 ± 11.8/51.9 ± 18.4	58.9/41.3	8
2008 Ross et al. [19]	Chinese	Taiwan and Singapore	1079/907	66/31	NA	NA	8
2008 Ross et al. [19]	Non-Chinese	Japan	151/95	0/0	NA	NA	8
2008 Tan et al. (2) [20]	Chinese	Singapore	246/243	21/8	66 ± 12/62 ± 10	56.0/54.0	8
2008 Tan et al. (1) [21]	Non-Chinese	Malaysia and Indian	192/265	3/6	60.3 ± 6.4/64.5 ± 3.7	NA	9
2009 Zhang et al. [22]	Chinese	China	600/459	43/11	NA/53.4 ± 13.4	57.0/56.0	7
2009 Yu et al. [23]	Chinese	China	328/300	17/6	NA/58.2 ± 10.3	54.3/57.7	9
2009 Zabetian et al. [24]	Non-Chinese	Japan	631/320	0/0	NA	NA	9
2010 Kim et al. [15]	Non-Chinese	Korea	383/379	3/1	NA	NA	8
2011 Pulkes et al. [25]	Thai/Chinese	Thai	154/156	15/5	NA	56.5/NA	8
2012 Zhou et al. [16]	Chinese	China	202/212	2/5	62.68 ± 10.69/62.87 ± 10.44	52.5/59.0	8
2013 Fu et al. [13]	Chinese	China	446/403	47/21	60.82±11.20/59.21±9.3	59.0/62.0	9
2013 Wu-Chou et al. [12]	Chinese	Taiwan	747/461	58/18	NA	NA	8
2013 Cai et al. [26]	Chinese	China	510/550	29/19	58.4 ± 11.0/59.34 ± 11.3	59.4/58.2	9
2013 Wu et al. [27]	Chinese	Taiwan	573/503	34/22	62.1 ± 11.5/59.4 ± 12.9	55.3/50.7	8
2014 Pulkes et al. [11]	Non-Chinese	Thai	485/480	54/29	65.0 ± 12.0/71.0 ± 7.0	46.0/61.0	9
2014 Gopalai et al. [10]	Non-Chinese	Malaysia	695/507	43/18	57.4 ± 11.8/59.3 ± 9.4	60.0/51.0	8
2015 Guo et al. [28]	Chinese	China	1019/1030	49/44	57.9 ± 12.3/57.2 ± 16.4	58.5/48.0	9

NOS: Newcastle–Ottawa Scale. NA: not available.

4. Discussion

In the meta-analysis, a combination of 9275 PD patients and 8114 controls was studied. All included publications were of high quality according to NOS and the results were stable during sensitive analysis. Furthermore, there was no publication reporting bias, as shown by the symmetric funnel plot. It is believed that the final results are credible. The included studies were conducted in mainland China, Taiwan, Singapore, Japan, Malaysia, India, Korea, and Thailand. We found that R1628P carriers were reported as simply being a part of the general Asian population and then subsequently divided them into Chinese and non-Chinese for further stratified analysis. Even though a variety of Asian countries were included, the heterogeneity of the sample was accepted with I^2 less than 50%. Therefore, based on the evidence, we found that *LRRK2* R1628P was a risk factor for PD in Asian, 'both Chinese and non-Chinese, populations.

Although the cause of PD is unclear, it is accepted that its etiology is the interaction of genetic and environmental factors, along with genetic insights which provide a way to explore the molecular causes of PD. As a result, more and more attention has been focused on the relationship between genetics and PD. *LRRK2*, one of the genes related to autosomal dominant form of PD, belongs to a member of the ROCO protein family [29] and has five major functional domains [30]: a leucine-rich repeat (LRR); a Roc domain (Ras in complex proteins); a COR domain (C-terminal of Roc); a TyrKc domain (tyrosine kinase catalytic), and WD40 domain. The variations of *LRRK2* account for approximately 5–15% of familial and sporadic PD [2]. Additionally, further studies show that various variants, such as G2019S and G2385R, have genetic correlations and heterogeneity. This means that different variations, including mutations and polymorphism, may play a diverse role depending on the given population.

R1628P, a substitution of a polar arginine (R) with a neutral nonproline (P), is located in the COR domain of LRRK2. This kind of substitution could change the secondary structure of LRRK2 and influence the interaction between the other domains of LRRK2 or different external proteins, which ultimately influences the kinase activity [31, 32]. In fact, a study in our team once reported that R1628P was not associated with PD risk in mainland China [28] (PD = 1019, $N = 1030$), which was consistent with [11, 27] or contrary to [12, 13, 22] other similar studies conducted. We suppose that a larger number of participants would be helpful for observing the actual results. To draw a comprehensive understanding, we performed a meta-analysis to evaluate the contribution of *LRRK2* R1628P to PD worldwide. And we found *LRRK2* R1628P was a risk factor in Asian ethnicities, which may help for further pathogenetic exploring of *LRKK2*, especially in the Asian population. Additionally, Shu's study identified that R1628P could be an example that explains the genetic-environmental interaction. Instead of upregulation of the

Study or subgroup	Experimental Events	Experimental Total	Control Events	Control Total	Weight	Odds ratio M-H, fixed, 95% CI
1.2.1 Chinese						
2008 Lu et al.	62	834	20	543	8.6%	2.10 [1.25, 3.52]
2008 Ross et al. (1)	66	1079	31	907	12.1%	1.84 [1.19, 2.85]
2008 Tan et al. (2)	21	246	8	243	2.8%	2.74 [1.19, 6.32]
2009 Yu et al.	17	328	6	300	2.3%	2.68 [1.04, 6.89]
2009 Zhang et al.	43	600	11	459	4.4%	3.14 [1.60, 6.17]
2011 Pulkes et al.	15	154	5	156	1.7%	3.26 [1.15, 9.20]
2012 Zhou et al.	2	202	5	212	1.9%	0.41 [0.08, 2.16]
2013 Cai et al.	29	510	19	550	6.6%	1.68 [0.93, 3.04]
2013 Fu et al.	47	446	21	403	7.6%	2.14 [1.26, 3.65]
2013 Wu et al.	34	573	22	503	8.4%	1.38 [0.80, 2.39]
2013 Wu-Chou et al.	58	747	18	461	7.9%	2.07 [1.20, 3.56]
2015 Guo et al.	49	1019	44	1030	16.0%	1.13 [0.75, 1.72]
Subtotal (95% CI)		*6738*		*5767*	*80.3%*	*1.84 [1.56, 2.18]*
Total events	443		210			
Heterogeneity: $\chi^2 = 15.33$, df = 11 ($P = 0.17$); $I^2 = 28\%$						
Test for overall effect: $Z = 7.08$ ($P < 0.00001$)						
1.2.2 Non-Chinese						
2008 Ross et al. (2)	0	151	0	95		Not estimable
2008 Tan et al. (1)	3	192	6	265	1.9%	0.69 [0.17, 2.77]
2009 Zabetian et al.	0	631	0	621		Not estimable
2010 Kim et al.	3	383	1	379	0.4%	2.98 [0.31, 28.82]
2014 Gopalai et al.	43	695	18	507	7.5%	1.79 [1.02, 3.14]
2014 Pulkes et al.	54	485	29	480	9.9%	1.95 [1.22, 3.12]
Subtotal (95% CI)		*2537*		*2347*	*19.7%*	*1.79 [1.27, 2.52]*
Total events	103		54			
Heterogeneity: $\chi^2 = 2.13$, df = 3 ($P = 0.55$); $I^2 = 0\%$						
Test for overall effect: $Z = 3.33$ ($P = 0.0009$)						
Total (95% CI)		*9275*		*8114*	*100.0%*	*1.83 [1.57, 2.13]*
Total events	546		264			
Heterogeneity: $\chi^2 = 17.46$, df = 15 ($P = 0.29$); $I^2 = 14\%$						
Test for overall effect: $Z = 7.82$ ($P < 0.00001$)						
Test for subgroup differences: $\chi^2 = 0.02$, df = 1 ($P = 0.88$), $I^2 = 0\%$						

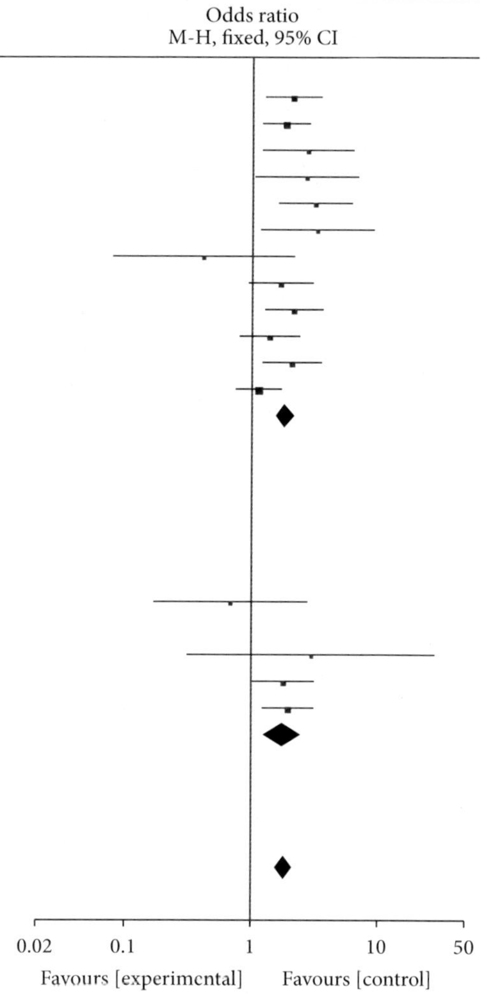

FIGURE 2: Forest plot of R1628P in PD.

kinase activity of LRRK2 directly, it was found that the status of R1628P in *LRRK2* provides a potential "two-hit" target: firstly environmentally toxic induced Cdk5 activation and then Cdk5 phosphorylating the adjacent amino residue S1627 of the R1628P mutation; thus LRRK2 kinase was activated which leads to the death of neurons.

The International Parkinson and Movement Disorder Society (MDS) Task Force proposed that PD should be divided into three stages [33]: preclinical PD, prodromal PD, and clinical PD. The stage of prodromal PD [34] refers to the presentation of symptoms or signs of PD neurodegeneration with absence of classic motor parkinsonism. Genetics findings, combined with age, environmental risk factors, and other diagnostic marker tests, play a vital role in the diagnosis of prodromal PD [34, 35]. We found *LRRK2* R1628P was a risk factor in Asian populations, both Chinese and non-Chinese. This may help for further exploring etiology and biomarker of PD, especially in Asian population.

A few limitations of this study should be acknowledged: firstly, as all data were extracted from previously published papers, we do not know the effects of the unpublished articles. Secondly, some articles [14, 36, 37], which otherwise met the eligibility criteria, were excluded for insufficient data. Thirdly, other confounding factors, like age, gender, and age at onset, may be affecting the outcomes and prevalence of PD.

In conclusion, our research showed a significant association between R1628P and the susceptibility to PD in the Asian population, both Chinese and non-Chinese. Further investigation of high quality, large cohort studies and function researches is needed to elaborate this relationship.

Acknowledgments

This work was supported by grants from the National Natural Science Foundation of China (no. 81401059, no. 31500999, and no. 81430023), the National Key Plan for Scientific Research and Development of China (no. 2016YFC1306000), and Hunan Provincial Innovation Foundation For Postgraduate (no. CX2017B066).

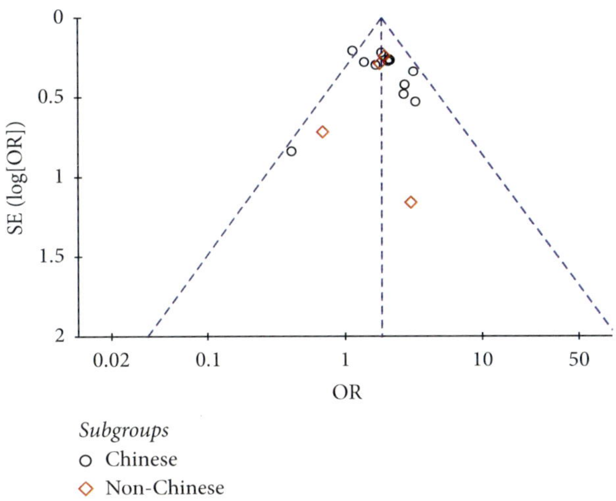

FIGURE 3: Funnel plot of R1628P in PD.

References

[1] L. V. Kalia and A. E. Lang, "Parkinson's disease," *The Lancet*, vol. 386, no. 9996, pp. 896–912, 2015.

[2] J. C. Dächsel and M. J. Farrer, "LRRK2 and Parkinson disease," *Archives of Neurology*, vol. 67, no. 5, pp. 542–547, 2010.

[3] A. Di Fonzo, C. Tassorelli, M. De Mari et al., "Comprehensive analysis of the LRRK2 gene in sixty families with Parkinson's disease," *European Journal of Human Genetics*, vol. 14, no. 3, pp. 322–331, 2006.

[4] C. Paisán-Ruíz, P. Nath, N. Washecka, J. R. Gibbs, and A. B. Singleton, "Comprehensive analysis of LRRK2 in publicly available Parkinson's disease cases and neurologically normal controls," *Human Mutation*, vol. 29, no. 4, pp. 485–490, 2008.

[5] S. Lesage, A. Dürr, M. Tazir et al., "LRRK2 G2019S as a cause of Parkinson's disease in North African Arabs," *The New England Journal of Medicine*, vol. 354, no. 4, pp. 422-423, 2006.

[6] M. M. Hulihan, L. Ishihara-Paul, J. Kachergus et al., "LRRK2 Gly2019Ser penetrance in Arab-Berber patients from Tunisia: a case-control genetic study," *The Lancet Neurology*, vol. 7, no. 7, pp. 591–594, 2008.

[7] T. Peeraully and E. K. Tan, "Genetic variants in sporadic parkinson's disease: East vs west," *Parkinsonism & Related Disorders*, vol. 18, supplement 1, pp. S63–S65, 2012.

[8] M. J. Farrer, J. T. Stone, C.-H. Lin et al., "Lrrk2 G2385R is an ancestral risk factor for Parkinson's disease in Asia," *Parkinsonism & Related Disorders*, vol. 13, no. 2, pp. 89–92, 2007.

[9] A. Di Fonzo, Y. H. Wu-Chou, C. S. Lu et al., "A common missense variant in the LRRK2 gene, Gly2385Arg, associated with Parkinson's disease risk in Taiwan," *neurogenetics*, vol. 7, no. 3, pp. 133–138, 2006.

[10] A. A. Gopalai, S.-Y. Lim, J. Y. Chua et al., "LRRK2 G2385R and R1628P Mutations Are Associated with an Increased Risk of Parkinson's Disease in the Malaysian Population," *BioMed Research International*, vol. 2014, Article ID 867321, 2014.

[11] T. Pulkes, C. Papsing, A. Thakkinstian et al., "Confirmation of the association between LRRK2 R1628P variant and susceptibility to Parkinson's disease in the Thai population," *Parkinsonism & Related Disorders*, vol. 20, no. 9, pp. 1018–1021, 2014.

[12] Y.-H. Wu-Chou, Y.-T. Chen, T.-H. Yeh et al., "Genetic variants of SNCA and LRRK2 genes are associated with sporadic PD susceptibility: a replication study in a Taiwanese cohort," *Parkinsonism & Related Disorders*, vol. 19, no. 2, pp. 251–255, 2013.

[13] X. Fu, Y. Zheng, H. Hong et al., "LRRK2 G2385R and LRRK2 R1628P increase risk of Parkinson's disease in a Han Chinese population from Southern Mainland China," *Parkinsonism & Related Disorders*, vol. 19, no. 3, pp. 397-398, 2013.

[14] O. A. Ross, A. I. Soto-Ortolaza, M. G. Heckman et al., "Association of LRRK2 exonic variants with susceptibility to Parkinson's disease: a case-control study," *The Lancet Neurology*, vol. 10, no. 10, pp. 898–908, 2011.

[15] J. M. Kim, J. Y. Lee, H. J. Kim et al., "The LRRK2 G2385R variant is a risk factor for sporadic Parkinson's disease in the Korean population," *Parkinsonism & Related Disorders*, vol. 16, no. 2, pp. 85–88, 2010.

[16] Y. Zhou, X. Luo, F. Li et al., "Association of Parkinson's disease with six single nucleotide polymorphisms located in four PARK genes in the northern Han Chinese population," *Journal of Clinical Neuroscience*, vol. 19, no. 7, pp. 1011–1015, 2012.

[17] C.-S. Lu, Y.-H. Wu-Chou, M. van Doeselaar et al., "The LRRK2 Arg1628Pro variant is a risk factor for Parkinson's disease in the Chinese population," *Neurogenetics*, vol. 9, no. 4, pp. 271–276, 2008.

[18] A. Stang, "Critical evaluation of the Newcastle-Ottawa scale for the assessment of the quality of nonrandomized studies in meta-analyses," *European Journal of Epidemiology*, vol. 25, no. 9, pp. 603–605, 2010.

[19] O. A. Ross, Y.-R. Wu, M.-C. Lee et al. et al., "Analysis of Lrrk2 R1628P as a risk factor for Parkinson's disease," *Annals of Neurology*, vol. 64, no. 1, pp. 88–92, 2008.

[20] E. K. Tan, M. Tang, L. C. Tan et al., "Lrrk2 R1628P in non-Chinese Asian races," *Annals of Neurology*, vol. 64, no. 4, pp. 472-473, 2008.

[21] E. K. Tan, L. C. Tan, H. Q. Lim et al., "LRRK2 R1628P increases risk of Parkinson's disease: replication evidence," *Human Genetics*, vol. 124, no. 3, pp. 287-288, 2008.

[22] Z. Zhang, J.-M. Burgunder, X. An et al., "LRRK2 R1628P variant is a risk factor of Parkinson's disease among Han-Chinese from mainland China," *Movement Disorders*, vol. 24, no. 13, pp. 1902–1905, 2009.

[23] L. Yu, F. Hu, X. Zou et al., "LRRK2 R1628P contributes to Parkinson's disease susceptibility in Chinese Han populations from mainland China," *Brain Research*, vol. 1296, pp. 113–116, 2009.

[24] C. P. Zabetian, M. Yamamoto, A. N. Lopez et al., "LRRK2 mutations and risk variants in Japanese patients with Parkinson's disease," *Movement Disorders*, vol. 24, no. 7, pp. 1034–1041, 2009.

[25] T. Pulkes, C. Papsing, S. Mahasirimongkol, M. Busabaratana, K. Kulkantrakorn, and S. Tiamkao, "Frequencies of LRRK2 variants in Thai patients with Parkinson's disease: evidence for an R1628P founder," *Journal of Neurology, Neurosurgery & Psychiatry*, vol. 82, no. 10, pp. 1179-1180, 2011.

[26] J. Cai, Y. Lin, W. Chen et al., "Association between G2385R and R1628P polymorphism of LRRK2 gene and sporadic Parkinson's disease in a Han-Chinese population in south-eastern China," *Neurological Sciences*, vol. 34, no. 11, pp. 2001–2006, 2013.

[27] Y.-R. Wu, K.-H. Chang, W.-T. Chang et al., "Genetic variants of LRRK2 in Taiwanese Parkinson's disease," *PLoS ONE*, vol. 8, no. 12, Article ID e82001, 2013.

[28] J.-F. Guo, K. Li, R.-L. Yu et al., "Polygenic determinants of Parkinson's disease in a Chinese population," *Neurobiology of Aging*, vol. 36, no. 4, pp. 1765.e1–1765.e6, 2015.

[29] L. Bosgraaf and P. J. M. van Haastert, "Roc, a Ras/GTPase domain in complex proteins," *Biochimica et Biophysica Acta*, vol. 1643, no. 1–3, pp. 5–10, 2003.

[30] A. Zimprich, S. Biskup, P. Leitner et al., "Mutations in LRRK2 cause autosomal-dominant parkinsonism with pleomorphic pathology," *Neuron*, vol. 44, no. 4, pp. 601–607, 2004.

[31] S. Saiki, S. Sato, and N. Hattori, "Molecular pathogenesis of Parkinson's disease: update," *Journal of Neurology, Neurosurgery & Psychiatry*, vol. 83, no. 4, pp. 430–436, 2012.

[32] S. L. Chan, D. C. Angeles, and E.-K. Tan, "Targeting leucine-rich repeat kinase 2 in Parkinson's disease," *Expert Opinion on Therapeutic Targets*, vol. 17, no. 12, pp. 1471–1482, 2013.

[33] D. Berg, R. B. Postuma, B. Bloem et al., "Time to redefine PD? Introductory statement of the MDS Task Force on the definition of Parkinson's disease," *Movement Disorders*, vol. 29, no. 4, pp. 454–462, 2014.

[34] D. Berg, R. B. Postuma, C. H. Adler et al., "MDS research criteria for prodromal Parkinson's disease," *Movement Disorders*, vol. 30, no. 12, pp. 1600–1611, 2015.

[35] M. A. Nalls, C. Y. McLean, J. Rick et al., "Diagnosis of Parkinson's disease on the basis of clinical and genetic classification: A population-based modelling study," *The Lancet Neurology*, vol. 14, no. 10, article no. 123, pp. 1002–1009, 2015.

[36] E. K. Tan, R. Peng, Y. Y. Teo et al., "Multiple LRRK2 variants modulate risk of Parkinson disease: a Chinese multicenter study," *Human Mutation*, vol. 31, no. 5, pp. 561–568, 2010.

[37] C. Wang, Y. Cai, Z. Zheng et al., "Penetrance of LRRK2 G2385R and R1628P is modified by common PD-associated genetic variants," *Parkinsonism & Related Disorders*, vol. 18, no. 8, pp. 958–963, 2012.

22

N-Acetylcysteine in Combination with IGF-1 Enhances Neuroprotection against Proteasome Dysfunction-Induced Neurotoxicity in SH-SY5Y Cells

Benxu Cheng,[1] Pinki Anand,[1] Anxiu Kuang,[2] Feroz Akhtar,[1] and Virginia L. Scofield[1]

[1]*Regional Academic Health Center, School of Medicine, University of Texas Rio Grande Valley, Edinburg, TX, USA*
[2]*Department of Biology, University of Texas Rio Grande Valley, Edinburg, TX, USA*

Correspondence should be addressed to Benxu Cheng; benxu.cheng@utrgv.edu

Academic Editor: Jan Aasly

Ubiquitin proteasome system (UPS) dysfunction has been implicated in the development of many neuronal disorders, including Parkinson's disease (PD). Previous studies focused on individual neuroprotective agents and their respective abilities to prevent neurotoxicity following a variety of toxic insults. However, the effects of the antioxidant N-acetylcysteine (NAC) on proteasome impairment-induced apoptosis have not been well characterized in human neuronal cells. The aim of this study was to determine whether cotreatment of NAC and insulin-like growth factor-1 (IGF-1) efficiently protected against proteasome inhibitor-induced cytotoxicity in SH-SY5Y cells. Our results demonstrate that the proteasome inhibitor, MG132, initiates poly(ADP-ribose) polymerase (PARP) cleavage, caspase 3 activation, and nuclear condensation and fragmentation. In addition, MG132 treatment leads to endoplasmic reticulum (ER) stress and autophagy-mediated cell death. All of these events can be attenuated without obvious reduction of MG132 induced protein ubiquitination by first treating the cells with NAC and IGF-1 separately or simultaneously prior to exposure to MG132. Moreover, our data demonstrated that the combination of the two proved to be significantly more effective for neuronal protection. Therefore, we conclude that the simultaneous use of growth/neurotrophic factors and a free radical scavenger may increase overall protection against UPS dysfunction-mediated cytotoxicity and neurodegeneration.

1. Introduction

In both sporadic and familial Parkinson's disease (PD), pathways leading to neuronal death are driven mainly by two key pathological events: aberrant protein homeostasis, including aggregation of proteins that normally would be disposed by the UPS system, and mitochondrial alterations secondary to proteinopathy-associated aggregation, which result from obligate mitochondrial Ca^{++} loading in response to this aggregation [1, 2]. A growing body of evidence implicates oxidative stress as an important intersection point between these two events [3]. Neurons are particularly vulnerable to proteinopathy (including abnormal aggregation of proteins) because of their long life span [4]. Death of dopaminergic neurons and accumulation of eosinophilic inclusions termed as Lewy bodies (LBs) in the substantia nigra pars compacta and other brain stem nuclei are the main pathological characteristics of PD [5]. During the development of PD, cellular defense mechanisms including antioxidants, the unfolded protein response (UPR), molecular chaperons, the ubiquitin-protease system (UPS), and autophagy are severely compromised [6]. Each of these defense systems offers therapeutic targets for intervention in the mechanism for their initiation and progression in the neurons.

In neurons, two particular protein clearance routes, the UPS and the autophagy pathways, are critical for the maintenance of cellular homeostasis, including ATP balance, amino-acid recycling, and protein quality control. Of these two mechanisms, UPS degradation of abnormal proteins is more important. The UPS process operates following "tagging" of abnormal proteins with ubiquitin, which in turn targets the tagged proteins to the proteasome for degradation [7]. However, treatment of cultured neurons with agents that cause proteasome inhibition results in compensatory autophagy, thereby preventing protein accumulation and cytotoxicity [7]. This suggests that clearance of proteins by the autophagy route correlates with their propensity to aggregate [8].

The LBs in substantia nigra neurons of PD patients are composed of a protein called α-synuclein, which is a substrate both for UPS degradation and for autophagy [7, 9]. Although neuronal autophagy appears primarily to be a protective process in the nervous system, it can also play a role in neuronal death because there is a limit to the number of autophagic vesicles (and their contained protein) that an individual cell can handle [8, 10].

The proteasome inhibitor MG132 (Carbobenzoxy-Leu-Leu-Leucinal), a membrane-permeable peptide aldehyde [11], effectively blocks the proteolytic activity of the proteosome complex. When the cell senses the buildup of aberrant proteins, its mitochondria begin to accumulate Ca^{++}, resulting in cytochrome c release and mitochondrial dysfunction [12], which initiates PARP mediated cell death. Aberrant proteins also initiate ER stress, as indicated by the induction of CCAAT/enhancer-binding protein homologous protein (CHOP) expression [13], and the unfolded protein response, which leads to apoptosis.

In eukaryotic cells, the UPS is the main system that degrades misfolded proteins exporting from the ER. However, ER stress, as part of the UPR pathway, can also activate autophagy by conjugation of LC3 (microtubule associated protein 1 light chain 3) to membrane lipids [14].

In many neuronal cell types and in the Central Nervous System (CNS), proteasome inhibition causes mitochondrial dysfunction, reduces glutathione levels, and increases generation of free radicals [15]. This leads to the elevation of intracellular reactive oxygen species (ROS), resulting in oxidative stress. Increase in the levels of free radicals increases protein oxidation and further compromises proteasomal degradative capacity. By these activities, oxidative stress may fuel a vicious cycle that links mitochondrial dysfunction to proteasomal inhibition and autophagy, both of which lead to neurodegeneration [16].

Previous research has shown that antioxidant treatment of PD patients can mitigate neuronal damage by uncoupling mitochondrial damage from cellular oxidative stress in neurotoxicity and autophagy [16]. N-Acetylcysteine (NAC) is a membrane-permeable antioxidant and free radical scavenger that increases intracellular GSH by delivering cysteine to cells and acting as a precursor for glutathione synthesis. Its neuroprotective effects have been established in animal models and cell culture studies of non-PD neurodegenerative disease [16–19], and it has been successfully used for the treatment of psychiatric disorders [20]. In the present study, we assessed the individual and combined efficacy of two classes of agents, an antioxidant and a neurotrophic factor, for their ability to prevent cell death in cultured neuronal cells following UPS impairment with the proteasome inhibitor MG132. NAC was chosen as the antioxidative component and insulin-like growth factor-1 (IGF-1) was chosen as the neurotrophic component. The latter compound is a 70-amino-acid-long polypeptide with known neurotrophic, neurogenic, neuroprotective, and antiapoptotic effects, and it is essential for the development of the nervous system where it regulates cell growth, differentiation, and survival of neurons and their supporting cells [21, 22]. The primary mechanism by which IGF-1 elicits these efforts is the PI3/AKT pathway [23]. To the best of our knowledge, NAC and IGF-1 have not been tested for their ability, in combination, to protect proteasome-inhibited human dopaminergic cell lines.

2. Materials and Methods

2.1. Reagents. N-Acetylcysteine, IGF-1, MG132, MTT [3-(4,5-dimethylthiazol-2-yl)-2,5-diphenyl tetrazolium bromide], and 3-methyladenine (3-MA) were purchased from Sigma-Aldrich (St. Louis, MO, USA) and Hoechst 33342 and 2′,7′-dichlorodihydrofluorescein diacetate (DCFDA) from Life Technologies (Eugene, OR, USA).

2.2. Cell Culture. Human SH-SY5Y cells and cell culture medium were purchased from the American Type Culture Collection (Manassas, VA, USA). The cells were cultured at 5% CO_2 at 37°C in EMEM: Ham's F-12K medium (1 : 1) containing 10% fetal bovine serum (FBS), penicillin (100 units/mL), and streptomycin (100 μg/mL). The cells were subcultured weekly in 60 mm or 100 mm cell culture dishes and used for experiments at 85–90% confluence. The culture medium was changed every 2-3 days. For Hoechst 33342 nucleic acid staining, cells were grown in 4-well chamber slides.

2.3. Inhibitor Treatments. The proteasome inhibitor MG132 was used to induce cytotoxicity in SH-SY5Y cultures. DMSO was used as a control vehicle, the final concentration of which was less than 0.1% in the cell culture medium. IGF-1 was suspended in sterile water, and NAC was dissolved in the culture medium. In neuroprotection experiments, SH-SY5Y cells were pretreated with IGF-1 (20 nM) and NAC (3 mM) alone, or with a combination of the two at the same concentration, for 18 h. The cells were then treated with MG132 (5 μM) for 24 h, unless otherwise indicated. To avoid any reversible action, the inhibitors were maintained throughout the duration of the experiment.

2.4. Cell Viability Assays. The cells were incubated in 24-well dishes, and cell viability data was determined using MTT assays, measuring the conversion of MTT [3-(4, 5-dimethylthiazol-2-yl)-2,5-diphenyl tetrazolium bromide] into formazan, as described in the previous study [24]. Thereafter, cells were treated with fresh media containing 0.25 mg/mL MTT for 2 h at 37°C. The medium was then removed and the purple formazan salt was solubilized with equal amounts of DMSO, and 100 μL of each sample was transferred to 96-well plates. The spectrophotometric densities were determined at absorption of 490 nm. At least 6 replicates of each treatment were used.

2.5. Immunoblot Assay. Changes in the amounts of protein expression were measured by Western blot analysis. For Western blotting, the cells were lysed in ice-cold RIPA lysis buffer containing freshly added protease and phosphatase inhibitors. The lysates were clarified by centrifugation at 4°C for 20 min at 13,000 rpm, and their protein concentrations were measured with a BCA Protein Assay Kit (Pierce, Rockford, IL, USA). Equal amounts of the protein samples (25–30 μg) were loaded and separated on 10% or 4–20% gradient polyacrylamide gels (Bio-Rad Laboratories, Hercules, CA, USA). The proteins were transferred to nitrocellulose membranes and blocked for either 1 h at room temperature or overnight at 4°C with Tris buffered saline containing 0.1% Tween 20 (TBST, pH 7.4) and 5% (w/v) skimmed dried milk.

Anti-PARP, anti-cleaved caspase 3, anti-CHOP and anti-LC3B antibodies were purchased from Cell Signaling (Beverly, MA, USA). Anti-ubiquitin antibody was obtained from Santa Cruz Biotechnology (Dallas, TX, USA). Anti β-actin was acquired from Sigma-Aldrich (St. Louis, MO, USA). The blotted membranes were incubated with primary antibodies for 1 h at room temperature or overnight at 4°C. They were then washed and incubated for 1 h with appropriate horseradish peroxidase-conjugated secondary antibodies. The protein bands were revealed using enhanced chemiluminescent (ECL) method, according to the manufacturer's instructions. Quantification of band densities was analyzed using one-way analysis of variance and Tukey's comparison test, using the Instat biostatistic program (GraphPad Software).

2.6. Cell Apoptotic Determination. An immunoblot assay was performed to assess PARP and caspase 3 cleavage for cells in the control and pretreated cultures. Nuclear morphological changes were assessed using Hoechst 33342 dye and visualized under a confocal microscope. For staining assays with the Hoechst 33342 nuclear dye, cells were cultured on glass-bottom dishes. After treatments, the cells were fixed with 3.7% paraformaldehyde for 20 min, washed with PBS three times, and stained with 1 μg/mL solution for 30 min. Stained cells were mounted using Vectashield Mounting Medium for Fluorescence (Vector Laboratories, Burlingame, CA, USA) and imaged with an Olympus FV1000 confocal microscope utilizing Olympus FV10-ASW3.1 software.

2.7. Oxidative Stress Assay. ROS production was detected using a cell-permeant fluorescent dye, 2′,7′-dichlorodihydrofluorescein diacetate (DCFDA), as previously described [25]. After treatment, cells were loaded with DCFDA (10 μM) and incubated for 30 min. The cells were then rinsed with PBS and fluorescence was measured immediately in a fluorescence microplate reader (SpectraMax, Molecular Devices). Wavelengths for excitation and emission were 485 and 520 nm, respectively.

2.8. Measurement of Reduced Glutathione. GSH levels were determined as previously described by Kamencic et al. 2000 [26]. Cells were cultured at 37°C in the presence or absence of the treatment reagents indicated above, washed with PBS, and incubated with monochlorobimane (MCB, 40 μmol/L) in the dark for 30 min at 37°C. After two washes with PBS, fluorescence was measured by spectrofluorophotometer (SpectraMax, Molecular Devices), with excitation

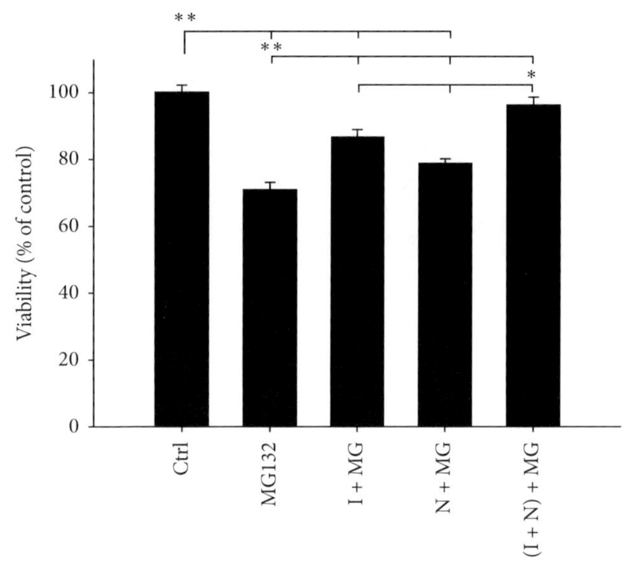

Figure 1: Pretreatment with IGF-1 and NAC increases cell viability after MG132 treatment. Cells were pretreated with vehicle (DMSO), IGF-1 (I), NAC (N), or both (I + N) for 18 h followed by the addition of MG132 (MG) (5 μM) for 24 h. Cell viability was determined by MTT assay as described in the Materials and Methods. The results are expressed as percentage means ± SEM of control and are representative of three independent experiments with five replicates. Level of significance is denoted as $^{*}p \leq 0.05$ and $^{**}p \leq 0.005$.

and emission wavelengths of 405 and 510 nm, respectively. Samples were assayed in triplicate.

2.9. Data Analysis. Our data was analyzed using one-way analysis of variance and Tukey comparison test, using GraphPad statistical software. Data is presented as the mean ± SEM of at least three independent experiments. In the figures, asterisks indicate the degree of significance for different treated cell cultures when compared to treatment controls or as specifically mentioned ($^{*}p \leq 0.05$–0.01, $^{**}p \leq 0.005$, resp.).

3. Results

3.1. The Combination of IGF-1 and NAC Increases SH-SY5Y Cells Protection against MG132 Induced Toxicity. The cells were treated either with 3 mM NAC or 20 nM IGF-1 or with the two in combination for 18 hours, followed by exposure to MG132 (5 μM) for 24 hours. The selection of dose and duration of exposure for IGF-1 and NAC were based on previously reported results [24] and preliminary dose effect data showing maximum protection, respectively.

As shown in Figure 1, MG132 treated cells showed significant reduction of cell viability, after 24-hour incubation, relative to untreated control cells ($p < 0.005$). In contrast, pretreatment of the cells with IGF-1 or NAC reduced MG132 induced cytotoxicity and promoted cell survival by 15.7% ± 2.26% and 7.82% ± 1.41%, respectively, compared to MG132 treated cells. Combined administration of NAC and IGF-1 produced the best protection of SH-SY5Y cells as evidenced by a 25.4% increase in cell viability ($p < 0.005$) (Figure 1).

3.2. The Combination of IGF-1 and NAC Attenuates MG132 Induced Apoptosis in SH-SY5Y Cells. Proteasome inhibition is known to be associated with induction of apoptosis [12]. To confirm and expand on the results from Figure 1, which suggested that NAC/IGF-1 are more effective together, Western blot analysis was used to detect two apoptotic markers, PARP cleavage and cleaved caspase 3 in treated and untreated cells. As shown in Figures 2(a) and 2(b), exposure of SH-SY5Y cells to MG132 for 24 hours resulted in significantly enhanced levels of both cleaved PARP and cleaved caspase 3 in comparison to control cells ($p < 0.005$). However, pretreatment of the cells with NAC or IGF-1 significantly reduced levels of both the markers ($p < 0.05$) in comparison to unprotected cells exposed to MG132. In agreement with Figure 1, the cells pretreated with both NAC and IGF-1 exerted complete protection against MG132 induced toxicity ($p < 0.005$) (Figures 2(a) and 2(b)).

In addition to the above apoptotic markers, we compared nuclear morphological changes between unprotected and protected cells. To visualize nuclear morphology, cells were stained with the DNA dye Hoechst 33342. Since lower doses of MG132, such as 5 μM, do not cause evident chromatin condensation after 24 hours, a higher MG132 concentration of 10 μM was employed. Cells incubated with MG132 alone exhibited extensive chromatin condensation and nuclear fragmentation, whereas relatively few of these structures were present in cells pretreated with NAC or IGF-1 alone. Furthermore, cotreatment with NAC and IGF-1 nearly completely prevented the appearance of apoptotic bodies in the cells (Figures 2(c) and 2(d)).

3.3. NAC and IGF-1 Alone or in Combination Attenuates MG132 Induced Reactive Oxygen Species (ROS) Generation and Depletion of Cellular GSH. SH-SY5Y cells were untreated or treated with NAC or IGF-1 alone or together for 18 hours followed by addition of 5 μM MG132 for an additional 24 hours as indicated in Figure 3. Thereafter the cells from all treatments were incubated with 10 μM DCFDA or 40 μM monochlorobimane (MCB) for 30 minutes, and their relative fluorescence was then measured. The results demonstrate that MG132 significantly reduced total intracellular GSH content ($p < 0.05$). However, MG132 induced depletion of GSH was attenuated by pretreatment with NAC or IGF-1, alone or in combination (Figure 3(a)). It was further noted that DCFDA intensity was elevated in cells treated with MG132 compared to the control. However, MG132 induced ROS production was significantly suppressed in cells pretreated with NAC ($p < 0.05$) or IGF-1 ($p < 0.005$) alone and was further reduced by the two together ($p < 0.005$) (Figure 3(a)).

3.4. Pretreatment with NAC and IGF-1 Does Not Reduce MG132 Induced Protein Ubiquitination, but It Inhibits Proteasome-Induced Autophagy. Proteasomal inhibition causes accumulation of ubiquitinated proteins in large amounts [24, 27] irrespective of protection afforded by pretreatment with retinoic acid or IGF-1. Therefore, in the present study we sought to determine whether NAC, used alone or in combination with IGF-1, can reduce protein ubiquitination or affect autophagy, which is the default protein disposal pathway used by neurons whose proteasomes are dysfunctional [8]. Figure 4(a) confirms our previous finding from studies with other protective agents showing that proteasome inhibitor-treated cells contain significantly increased levels of ubiquitinated protein regardless of the presence or absence of NAC or IGF-1. To determine whether autophagy is deployed in NAC/IGF-1 protected cells, we tested challenged cells, protected challenged cells, and untreated cells for their levels of the autophagosomal membrane (lipid-bound) form of LC3. This marker is a mammalian homolog of the autophagy-related gene 8 in yeast [28] and is one of the most reliable markers by which to monitor autophagy [29]. Figures 4(a) and 4(b) show that MG132-treated cells contain increased levels of lipid-bound LC3 ($p < 0.005$). Though not significant, a partial reduction in LC3 level resulted in cells pretreated with NAC or IGF-1 alone. However, cotreatment with NAC and IGF-1 reversed MG132 induced expression of LC3 ($p < 0.005$). Furthermore, compared to treatment with either IGF-1 or NAC alone, cotreatment with NAC and IGF-1, LC3-II was further decreased ($p < 0.05$). These results identify autophagy as a central player in protein quality control, and in the subsequent cell death versus cell survival, of NAC/IGF-1 protected cells.

3.5. Cotreatment with NAC and IGF-1 Attenuates Endoplasmic Reticulum Stress. The involvement of endoplasmic reticulum (ER) stress in PD neuronal damage has been well-established [30, 31]. Suppression of proteasome activity induces the accumulation of CCAAT/enhancer-binding protein homologous protein (CHOP) in the ER [32]. To assess the degree to which ER stress participates in MG132 induced cell death of SH-SY5Y cells, we evaluated the effect of NAC and IGF-1 on expression of CHOP. Figure 5(a) shows that exposure of the cells to MG132 results in the expression of CHOP. However, treatment of the cells with NAC, IGF-1, or both NAC and IGF-1 prior to MG132 exposure reduced its expression. In fact, cotreatment with both agents prior to MG132 exposure reduced the MG132 induced stress response to basal levels seen in the control. Densitometry analysis revealed CHOP levels significantly increased 14.5 ± 3 times ($p < 0.05$) in MG132 treated cells compared to the control, whereas the levels significantly decreased in cells pretreated with IGF-1, NAC, or both, respectively ($p < 0.05$) (Figure 5(b)).

3.6. Autophagy Inhibition Suppresses Apoptosis in SH-SY5Y Cells Treated with MG132. To investigate the contribution of autophagy to apoptosis, cell cultures were set up as described in Figures 1–5, but in the presence or absence of the autophagy inhibitor 3-methyladenine (3-MA), which blocks autophagosome formation via phosphatidylinositol 3-kinase (PI3K). As shown in Figure 6, MG132 induced apoptosis is indicated by the expression of cleaved PARP (Figure 6(b)) and cleaved caspase 3 (Figure 6(c)); however, when cells were treated with the autophagy inhibitor 3-MA, both PARP and caspase 3 cleavage were dramatically reduced, suggesting that

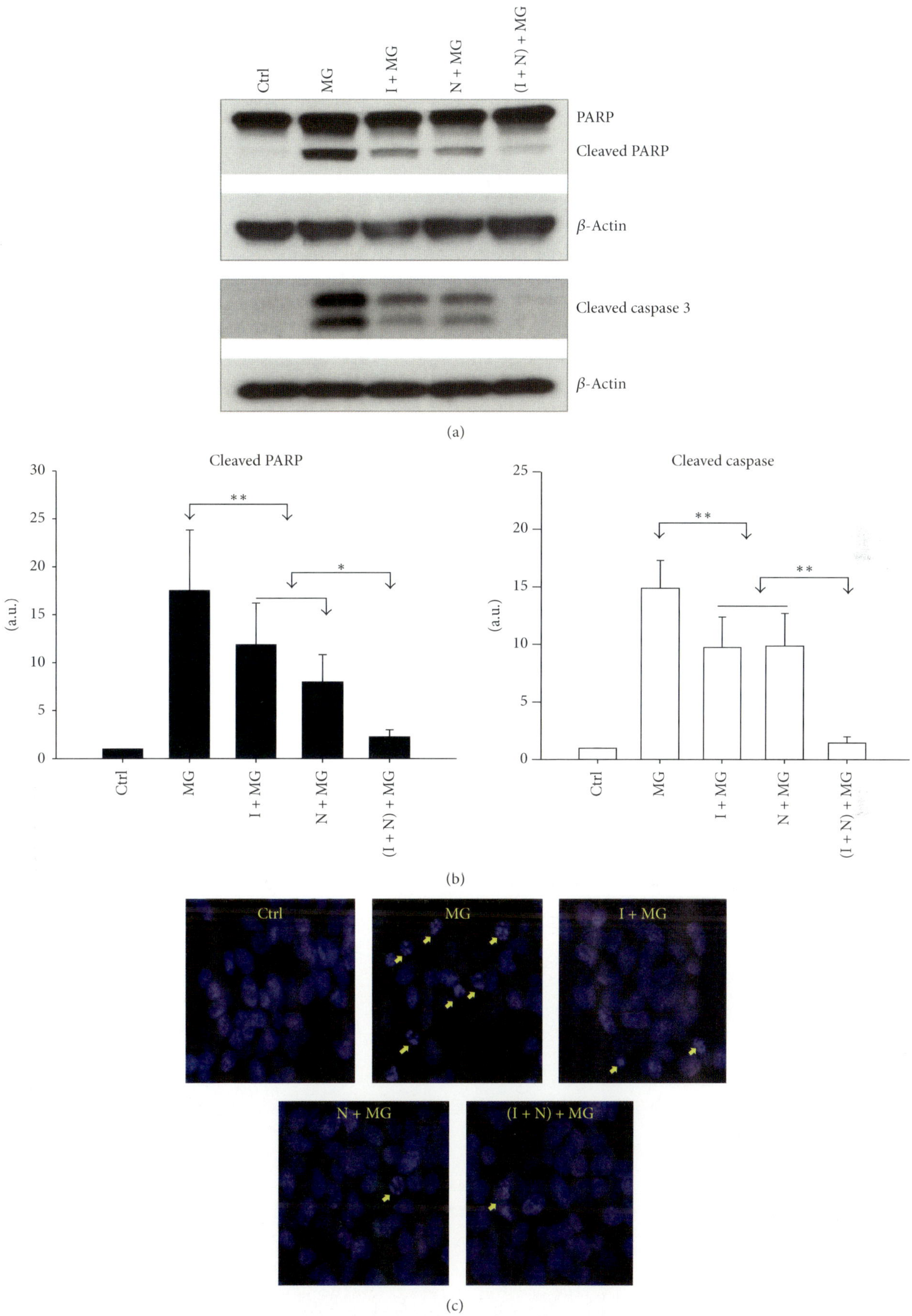

FIGURE 2: Continued.

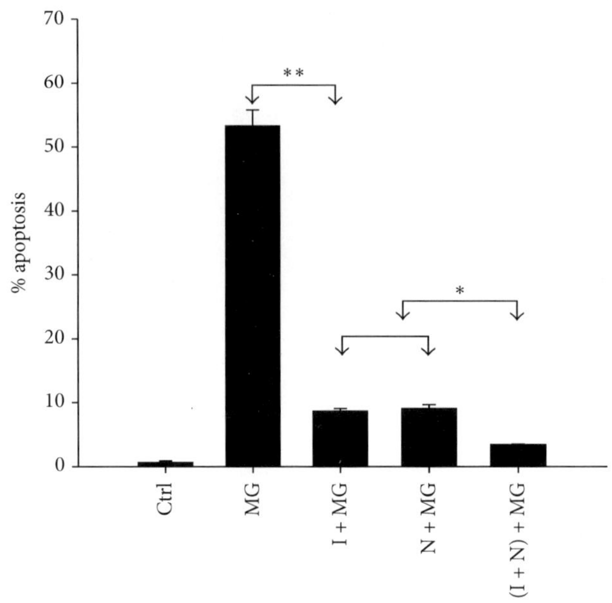

(d)

FIGURE 2: IGF-1 and NAC repress MG132 induced apoptosis. (a) Western blot analysis for two apoptotic markers: cleaved PARP and cleaved caspase 3. Results are representative of three independent experiments. (b) Densitometric analysis from three separate experiments. β-Actin served as the loading control. (c) IGF-1 and NAC prevent MG132 induced nuclear morphological changes. Cells were pretreated with IGF-1 (I), NAC (N), or both (I + N) for 18 h, followed by treatment with MG132 (MG) (10 μM) for 24 h, as indicated. The treated cells were then stained with the Hoechst reagent. Nuclear morphological changes were imaged using a confocal fluorescence microscope (arrows denote apoptotic nuclei). The photomicrographs shown are representative of three repeated experiments. (d) Quantification of cells with abnormal nuclei. Values are mean ± SEM ($n = 3$) ($^{*}p \leq 0.05$, $^{**}p \leq 0.005$).

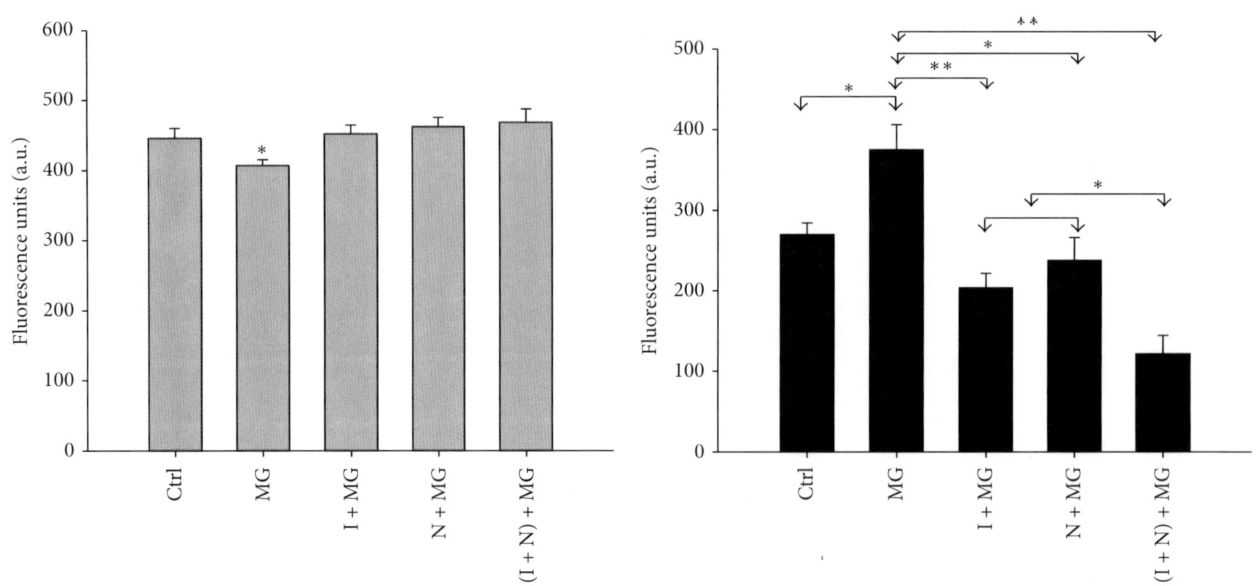

FIGURE 3: IGF-1 and NAC increase GSH production and reduce MG132 induced ROS generation in SH-SY5Y cells. Cell cultures were treated with NAC or IGF-1, separately or together, as described for Figure 1, followed by MG132 (5 μM). (a) Glutathione assay results for the control and treated cells versus MG132 treated cells only. (b) Intracellular ROS levels. Level of significance is denoted as $^{*}p \leq 0.05$ and $^{**}p \leq 0.005$.

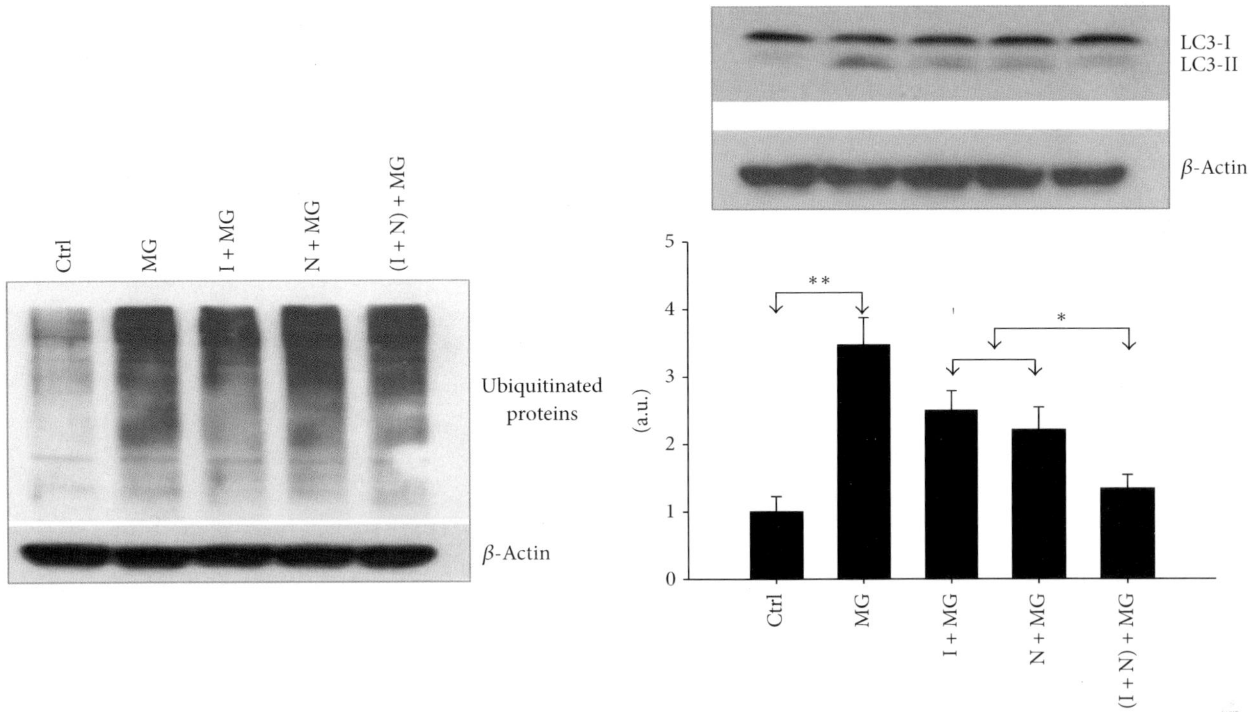

FIGURE 4: IGF-1 and NAC reduce MG132 induced autophagy without changing amounts of ubiquitinated proteins. After each treatment (indicated in the figure), total cell lysates were prepared for Western blot against ubiquitin and LC3B (an autophagy marker) antibodies. (a) Western blot for ubiquitinated protein. (b) Western blot analysis for LC3. β-Actin served as the loading control. Level of significance is denoted as $^*P \leq 0.05$ and $^{**}P \leq 0.005$.

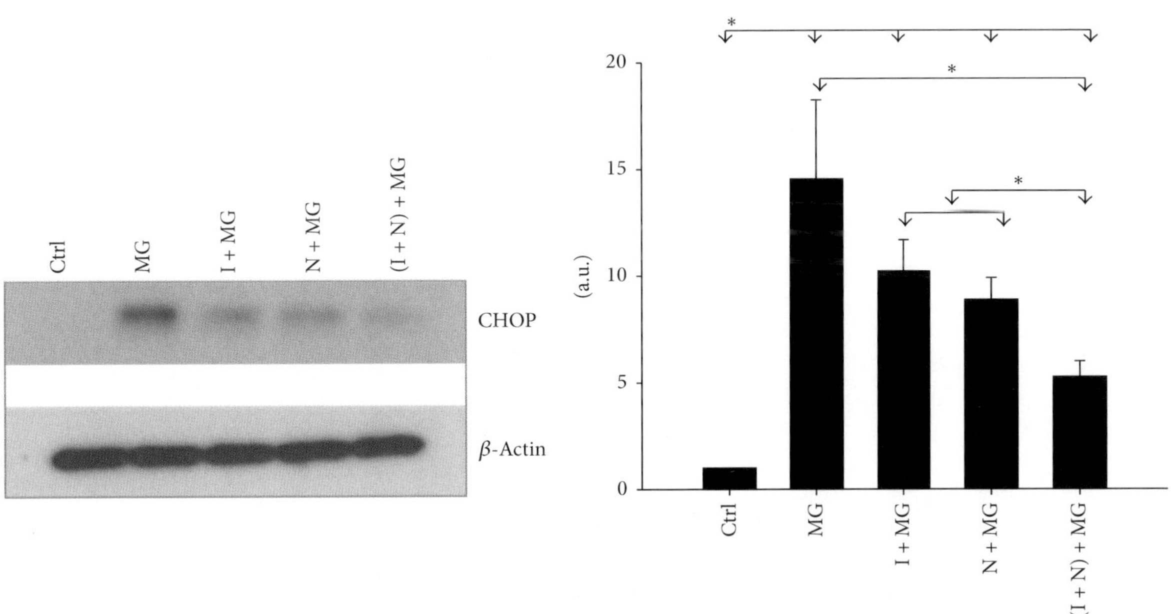

FIGURE 5: Pretreatment with IGF-1 and NAC represses MG132 induced ER stress. The cells were pretreated with IGF-1 and NAC, alone or together, for 18 h, followed by addition of MG132 (5 μM) for 24 h. (a) Western blot analysis for CHOP (an ER stress marker). Data are representative of three separate experiments. (b) Densitometric analysis of CHOP from three independent experiments. Level of significance is denoted as $^*P \leq 0.05$.

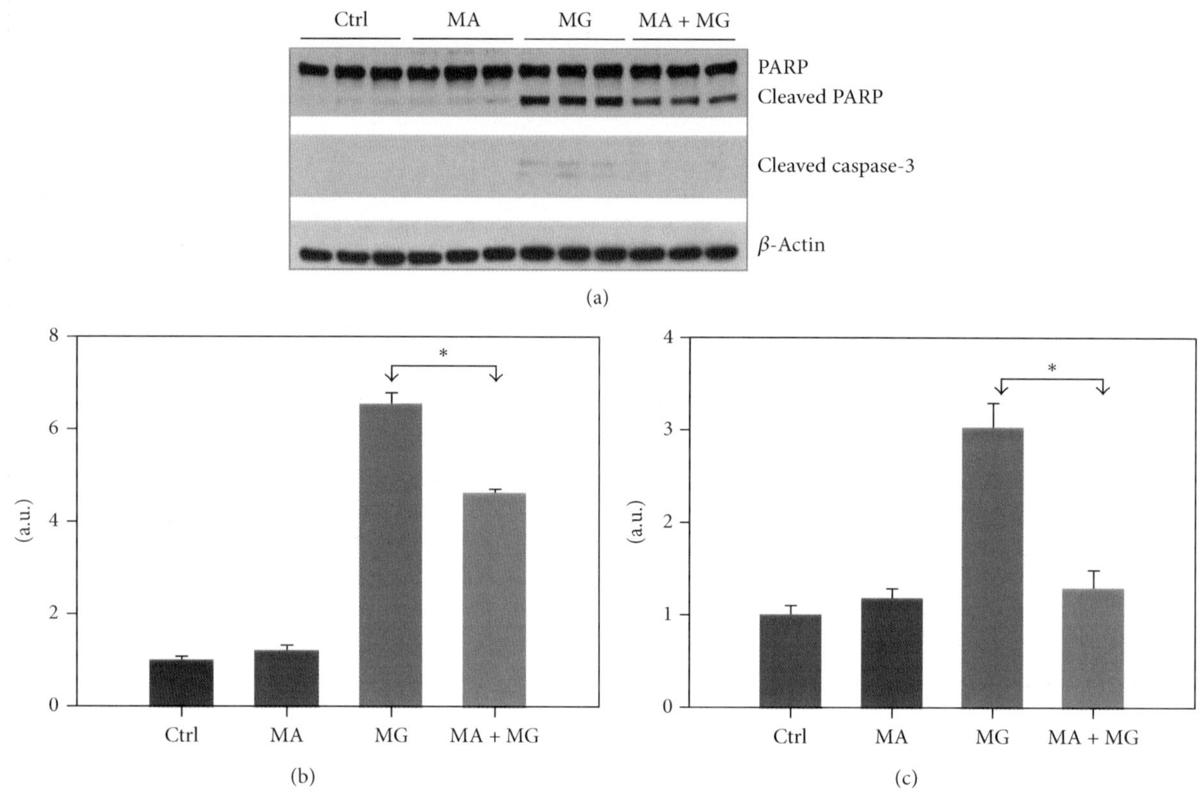

FIGURE 6: The autophagy inhibitor 3-methyladenine (3-MA) attenuates MG132 induced PARP and caspase 3 cleavage. The cells were pretreated with 3-MA (1 mM) for 1 h and then treated with MG132 for 24 h. (a) Western blot analysis for PARP, cleaved PARP, and cleaved caspase 3. Densitometric analysis for cleaved PARP (b) and cleaved caspase (c) from three independent experiments. Level of significance is denoted as $^{*}p \leq 0.01$.

autophagy is partially involved in MG132 induced apoptotic cell death of SH-SY5Y cells.

4. Discussion

The efficacy of combination therapy depends on the use of drugs with different but complimentary mechanisms of action. Since PD pathology is driven by multiple factors, concomitant neuroprotective treatments are likely to be more effective than treatment with a single agent. Some well-established anomalies associated with PD are aberrant protein homeostasis, oxidative stress, excitotoxicity, and inflammatory processes, which induce apoptosis in the nigral dopaminergic neurons [33, 34]. Therefore, agents that could prevent these events could be neuroprotective, and their effect on disease progression, or even prevention, may be substantially enhanced when combination therapies are used.

The present study evaluates the neuroprotective potential of monotherapy and combination therapy of NAC and IGF-1 on proteasome dysfunction-induced neurotoxicity in human neuroblastoma SH-SY5Y cells by exploring the relationship between oxidative stress, ER stress, autophagy, and apoptotic cell death following proteasome inhibition. The neuroprotective effect of NAC is mainly due to its ROS scavenging potential and its maintenance of cellular GSH [16], whereas IGF-1 protects neurons against cell death via intracellular pathways involving PI3k/Akt-mediated phosphorylation FKHRL1 (a subclass of winged-helix family of transcription factors) [24, 35, 36] and inhibition of oxidative stress [37, 38]. A combination of both agents may broaden the spectrum of protection by acting on multiple mechanisms involving oxidative stress and multiple antiapoptotic signaling pathways.

We find that MG132 treatment substantially reduced the viability of SH-SY5Y cells. Evaluation of various parameters such as nuclear condensation and fragmentation and activation of caspases and PARP cleavage clearly indicated a pronounced proapoptotic effect stimulated by MG132. This cell death pathway involved ROS formation, GSH depletion, ER stress, and induction of autophagy. This study confirms, once again, that treatment of SH-SY5Y cells with MG132 can be a reliable model that replicates all the neuropathological abnormalities of PD, such as mitochondrial dysfunction, oxidative stress, and loss of proteasomal function [15].

While MG132 had a significant cytotoxic effect on SH-SY5Y cells as demonstrated by MTT assay, pretreatment with either NAC or IGF-1 protected cells from MG132 induced damage. Cotreatment with both agents resulted in a striking increase in protection. This effect may be the result of mitigating apoptosis, enhancing intracellular GSH, reducing ROS, and/or attenuating ER stress and autophagy. The antiapoptotic potential of NAC has been established both *in vitro* [12, 39] and *in vivo* [40]. Although the protective effect of NAC against MG132 induced cell death has been reported

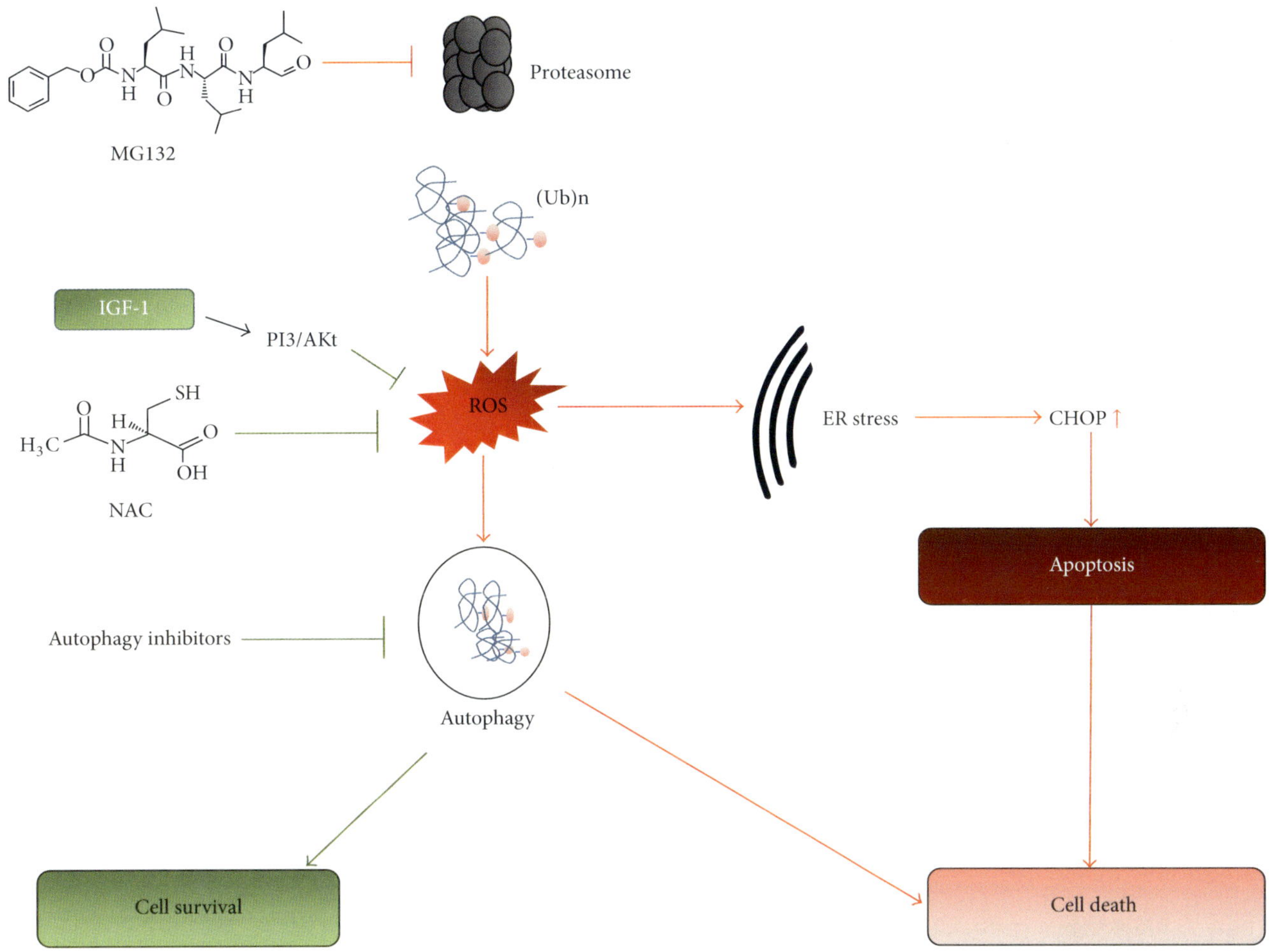

FIGURE 7: Schematic representation of molecular mechanisms of the proteasome inhibition induced cytotoxicity and its protection by NAC and IGF-1. Green lines represent cell survival pathways and red lines represent cell apoptotic and cell death pathways. Inhibition of proteasome by MG132 increases the aggregation of damaged and misfolded proteins. The accumulation of misfolded protein in the cytosol activates downstream ROS accumulation, ER stress, and cell death. Neuroprotective effect against MG132 of NAC and IGF-1 involves involvement of multiple protective pathways.

in various cell lines including neuronal cell lines, a similar *in vitro* dose of NAC did not attenuate the detrimental effect of MG132 in N27 cells [41]. This conflicting result may be attributed to the characteristic of the cell line used.

An important regulatory element in the protein ubiquitination pathway is the redox state of cellular GSH and its depletion may induce cell death [42]. MG132 induced cell death was preceded by pronounced depletion of GSH. Pretreatment of MG132 treated cells with either NAC, IGF-1, or both exerted similar effect of restoring the GSH levels. By acting as precursor to GSH and enhancing its biosynthesis NAC and IGF-1 maintain the reduced GSH content, respectively [43].

Pretreatment with NAC, IGF-1, or both significantly counteracted MG132 induced production of ROS. NAC acted as a direct scavenger and reduced more ROS in comparison to the individual treatments. Production of ROS is an intermediate step in MG132 induced apoptosis [44, 45] and thus protection of cells by NAC and IGF-1 pretreatment strongly highlights the key role of cellular redox status in the mechanism of neuroprotection by these two agents. Several lines of evidence also indicate the involvement of ROS and cellular redox status in the regulation of autophagy [46]. When we asked whether suppression of autophagy distinguishes protected, surviving MG132-treated cells from unprotected ones, we found that attenuation of autophagy is a defining feature of NAC/IGF-1-treated cells that survive MG132 challenge. While partial reduction of the autophagy marker LC3-II was detected in cells pretreated with either NAC or IGF-1, cotreatment of cells with both completely prevented MG132 induced autophagy, with the protective effects of either drug or both drugs being correlated with the degree to which the cells are protected.

Autophagy and ER stress are intimately related [47] and autophagy is accelerated in cells under ER stress [14]. In fact, impairment of autophagy by NAC or IGF-1 has been previously reported [16, 48]. Thus, the enhanced effect of NAC and IGF-1 demonstrates that combination treatment with these two agents has potential as a powerful therapeutic strategy against proteasome dysfunction-induced neurotoxicity.

Furthermore, by demonstrating that autophagy plays a role in NAC and IGF-1 neural protection, our study implies that autophagy is a potential therapeutic target for PD treatment.

Despite considerable recent advances, it is still debated whether autophagy is either a cytoprotective response triggered by cells to survive cellular stress or a cytotoxic phenomenon associated with cell death [49]. Dysregulation of autophagy has been described in neurodegenerative diseases including PD [50, 51]. However, depending upon the cellular milieu, autophagy may promote cell survival or death [52, 53]. To assess the effect of autophagy in our system from a different angle, we measured MG132 induced cell death in the presence of an inhibitor of autophagy, 3-methyladenine (3-MA). Treatment with 3-MA partially blocked MG132 induced apoptosis (Figure 5), suggesting the involvement of autophagy in MG132-mediated neurotoxicity within SH-SY5Y cells. In summary, inhibition of proteasome by MG132 increases the aggregation of damaged and misfolded proteins. Acting as the primary cytotoxic stressor, the aggregated proteins then trigger downstream ROS accumulation, ER stress, and cell death via the caspase cascade and/or autophagy (Figure 7). The complete inhibition of apoptosis by the NAC and IGF-1, which only partially reduces LC3-II, underscores the involvement of multiple protective pathways involving ROS formation and GSH depletion and ER stress and autophagy.

5. Conclusions

Proteasome inhibition in SH-SY5Y cells triggers apoptotic cell death. A drug combination therapy comprised of NAC and IGF-1 completely alleviates cytotoxicity associated with proteasome dysfunction. The neuroprotective effect relies on modulation of multiple pathways associated with apoptosis, which include reducing ROS, GSH depletion, lowering ER stress, and preventing autophagy (Figure 7). Thus a combination therapy employing a neurotrophic factor (IGF-1) and a free radical scavenger (NAC) may provide a novel and promising therapeutic strategy for UPS dysfunction-mediated neurocell degeneration.

Acknowledgments

This work was supported by funds from Innovative Research and Development Program (Texas State).

References

[1] H. E. Moon and S. H. Paek, "Mitochondrial dysfunction in Parkinson's disease," *Experimental Neurobiology*, vol. 24, no. 2, pp. 103–116, 2015.

[2] C. Henchcliffe and F. M. Beal, "Mitochondrial biology and oxidative stress in Parkinson disease pathogenesis," *Nature Clinical Practice Neurology*, vol. 4, no. 11, pp. 600–609, 2008.

[3] C. Chai and K.-L. Lim, "Genetic insights into sporadic Parkinson's disease pathogenesis," *Current Genomics*, vol. 14, no. 8, pp. 486–501, 2013.

[4] G. P. Meares, M. A. Mines, E. Beurel et al., "Glycogen synthase kinase-3 regulates endoplasmic reticulum (ER) stress-induced CHOP expression in neuronal cells," *Experimental Cell Research*, vol. 317, no. 11, pp. 1621–1628, 2011.

[5] W. Dauer and S. Przedborski, "Parkinson's disease: mechanisms and models," *Neuron*, vol. 39, no. 6, pp. 889–909, 2003.

[6] C. Cook, C. Stetler, and L. Petrucelli, "Disruption of protein quality control in Parkinson's disease," *Cold Spring Harbor Perspectives in Medicine*, vol. 2, no. 5, article a009423, 2012.

[7] A. Lilienbaum, "Relationship between the proteasomal system and autophagy," *International Journal of Biochemistry and Molecular Biology*, vol. 4, no. 1, pp. 1–26, 2013.

[8] A. M. Sánchez-Pérez, B. Claramonte-Clausell, J. V. Sánchez-Andrés, and M. T. Herrero, "Parkinson's disease and autophagy," *Parkinson's Disease*, vol. 2012, Article ID 429524, 6 pages, 2012.

[9] M. G. Spillantini, M. L. Schmidt, V. M.-Y. Lee, J. Q. Trojanowski, R. Jakes, and M. Goedert, "α-Synuclein in Lewy bodies," *Nature*, vol. 388, no. 6645, pp. 839–840, 1997.

[10] Y. Liu and B. Levine, "Autosis and autophagic cell death: the dark side of autophagy," *Cell Death and Differentiation*, vol. 22, no. 3, pp. 367–376, 2015.

[11] M. Jüllig, W. V. Zhang, A. Ferreira, and N. S. Stott, "MG132 induced apoptosis is associated with p53-independent induction of pro-apoptotic Noxa and transcriptional activity of β-catenin," *Apoptosis*, vol. 11, no. 4, pp. 627–641, 2006.

[12] Y. H. Han, Y. M. Yang, S. Z. Kim, and W. H. Park, "Attenuation of MG132-induced HeLa cell death by N-acetyl cysteine via reducing reactive oxygen species and preventing glutathione depletion," *Anticancer Research*, vol. 30, no. 6, pp. 2107–2112, 2010.

[13] S. Nakajima, H. Kato, S. Takahashi, H. Johno, and M. Kitamura, "Inhibition of NF-κB by MG132 through ER stress-mediated induction of LAP and LIP," *FEBS Letters*, vol. 585, no. 14, pp. 2249–2254, 2011.

[14] M. Ogata, S.-I. Hino, A. Saito et al., "Autophagy is activated for cell survival after endoplasmic reticulum stress," *Molecular and Cellular Biology*, vol. 26, no. 24, pp. 9220–9231, 2006.

[15] V. Dias, E. Junn, and M. M. Mouradian, "The role of oxidative stress in Parkinson's disease," *Journal of Parkinson's Disease*, vol. 3, no. 4, pp. 461–491, 2013.

[16] P. Chandramani Shivalingappa, H. Jin, V. Anantharam, A. Kanthasamy, and A. Kanthasamy, "N-acetyl cysteine protects against methamphetamine-induced dopaminergic neurodegeneration via modulation of redox status and autophagy in dopaminergic cells," *Parkinson's Disease*, vol. 2012, Article ID 424285, 11 pages, 2012.

[17] S. Alboni, L. Gibellini, C. Montanari et al., "*N*-acetyl-cysteine prevents toxic oxidative effects induced by IFN-α in human neurons," *International Journal of Neuropsychopharmacology*, vol. 16, no. 8, pp. 1849–1865, 2013.

[18] A. Cossarizza, C. Franceschi, D. Monti et al., "Protective effect of *N*-acetylcysteine in tumor necrosis factor-α-induced apoptosis in U937 cells: the role of mitochondria," *Experimental Cell Research*, vol. 220, no. 1, pp. 232–240, 1995.

[19] P. Watcharasit, S. Suntararuks, D. Visitnonthachai, A. Thiantanawat, and J. Satayavivad, "Acrylonitrile induced apoptosis via oxidative stress in neuroblastoma SH-SY5Y cell," *Journal of Applied Toxicology*, vol. 30, no. 7, pp. 649–655, 2010.

[20] M. Berk, D. L. Copolov, O. Dean et al., "N-acetyl cysteine for depressive symptoms in bipolar disorder-a double-blind randomized placebo-controlled trial," *Biological Psychiatry*, vol. 64, no. 6, pp. 468–475, 2008.

[21] Y. Kim, E. Li, and S. Park, "Insulin-like growth factor-1 inhibits 6-hydroxydopamine-mediated endoplasmic reticulum stress-induced apoptosis via regulation of heme oxygenase-1 and Nrf2 expression in PC12 cells," *International Journal of Neuroscience*, vol. 122, no. 11, pp. 641–649, 2012.

[22] V. C. Russo, P. D. Gluckman, E. L. Feldman, and G. A. Werther, "The insulin-like growth factor system and its pleiotropic functions in brain," *Endocrine Reviews*, vol. 26, no. 7, pp. 916–943, 2005.

[23] S. Humbert, E. A. Bryson, F. P. Cordelières et al., "The IGF-1/Akt pathway is neuroprotective in Huntington's disease and involves huntingtin phosphorylation by Akt," *Developmental Cell*, vol. 2, no. 6, pp. 831–837, 2002.

[24] B. Cheng, S. K. Maffi, A. A. Martinez, Y. P. V. Acosta, L. D. Morales, and J. L. Roberts, "Insulin-like growth factor-I mediates neuroprotection in proteasome inhibition-induced cytotoxicity in SH-SY5Y cells," *Molecular and Cellular Neuroscience*, vol. 47, no. 3, pp. 181–190, 2011.

[25] N. Cañas, T. Valero, M. Villarroya et al., "Chondroitin sulfate protects SH-SY5Y cells from oxidative stress by inducing heme oxygenase-1 via phosphatidylinositol 3-kinase/Akt," *Journal of Pharmacology and Experimental Therapeutics*, vol. 323, no. 3, pp. 946–953, 2007.

[26] H. Kamencic, A. Lyon, P. G. Paterson, and B. H. J. Juurlink, "Monochlorobimane fluorometric method to measure tissue glutathione," *Analytical Biochemistry*, vol. 286, no. 1, pp. 35–37, 2000.

[27] B. Cheng, A. A. Martinez, J. Morado, V. Scofield, J. L. Roberts, and S. K. Maffi, "Retinoic acid protects against proteasome inhibition associated cell death in SH-SY5Y cells via the AKT pathway," *Neurochemistry International*, vol. 62, no. 1, pp. 31–42, 2013.

[28] Y. Kabeya, N. Mizushima, T. Ueno et al., "LC3, a mammalian homologue of yeast Apg8p, is localized in autophagosome membranes after processing," *The EMBO Journal*, vol. 19, no. 21, pp. 5720–5728, 2000.

[29] T. Yoshimori, "Autophagy: a regulated bulk degradation process inside cells," *Biochemical and Biophysical Research Communications*, vol. 313, no. 2, pp. 453–458, 2004.

[30] W. A. Holtz and K. L. O'Malley, "Parkinsonian mimetics induce aspects of unfolded protein response in death of dopaminergic neurons," *The Journal of Biological Chemistry*, vol. 278, no. 21, pp. 19367–19377, 2003.

[31] E. J. Ryu, H. P. Harding, J. M. Angelastro, O. V. Vitolo, D. Ron, and L. A. Greene, "Endoplasmic reticulum stress and the unfolded protein response in cellular models of Parkinson's disease," *The Journal of Neuroscience*, vol. 22, no. 24, pp. 10690–10698, 2002.

[32] A.-H. Lee, N. N. Iwakoshi, K. C. Anderson, and L. H. Glimcher, "Proteasome inhibitors disrupt the unfolded protein response in myeloma cells," *Proceedings of the National Academy of Sciences of the United States of America*, vol. 100, no. 17, pp. 9946–9951, 2003.

[33] V. Licker, N. Turck, E. Kövari et al., "Proteomic analysis of human substantia nigra identifies novel candidates involved in Parkinson's disease pathogenesis," *Proteomics*, vol. 14, no. 6, pp. 784–794, 2014.

[34] A. M. Gorman, "Neuronal cell death in neurodegenerative diseases: recurring themes around protein handling," *Journal of Cellular and Molecular Medicine*, vol. 12, no. 6, pp. 2263–2280, 2008.

[35] Y. Cao, A. J. Gunn, L. Bennet et al., "Insulin-like growth factor (IGF)-1 suppresses oligodendrocyte caspase-3 activation and increases glial proliferation after ischemia in near-term fetal sheep," *Journal of Cerebral Blood Flow and Metabolism*, vol. 23, no. 6, pp. 739–747, 2003.

[36] W. H. Zheng, S. Kar, S. Dore, and R. Quirion, "Insulin-like growth factor-1 (IGF-1): a neuroprotective trophic factor acting via the Akt kinase pathway," *Journal of Neural Transmission. Supplementa*, no. 60, pp. 261–272, 2000.

[37] Y. Higashi, A. Pandey, B. Goodwin, and P. Delafontaine, "Insulin-like growth factor-1 regulates glutathione peroxidase expression and activity in vascular endothelial cells: implications for atheroprotective actions of insulin-like growth factor-1," *Biochimica et Biophysica Acta (BBA)—Molecular Basis of Disease*, vol. 1832, no. 3, pp. 391–399, 2013.

[38] Y.-G. Park, J.-K. Jeong, M.-H. Moon et al., "Insulin-like growth factor-1 protects against prion peptide-induced cell death in neuronal cells via inhibition of Bax translocation," *International Journal of Molecular Medicine*, vol. 30, no. 5, pp. 1069–1074, 2012.

[39] X. Zhang, A. Banerjee, W. A. Banks, and N. Ercal, "N-Acetylcysteine amide protects against methamphetamine-induced oxidative stress and neurotoxicity in immortalized human brain endothelial cells," *Brain Research*, vol. 1275, pp. 87–95, 2009.

[40] G. Fukami, K. Hashimoto, K. Koike, N. Okamura, E. Shimizu, and M. Iyo, "Effect of antioxidant N-acetyl-L-cysteine on behavioral changes and neurotoxicity in rats after administration of methamphetamine," *Brain Research*, vol. 1016, no. 1, pp. 90–95, 2004.

[41] K. S. Zafar, S. H. Inayat-Hussain, and D. Ross, "A comparative study of proteasomal inhibition and apoptosis induced in N27 mesencephalic cells by dopamine and MG132," *Journal of Neurochemistry*, vol. 102, no. 3, pp. 913–921, 2007.

[42] J. H. Qiu, A. Asai, S. Chi, N. Saito, H. Hamada, and T. Kirino, "Proteasome inhibitors induce cytochrome c-caspase-3-like protease- mediated apoptosis in cultured cortical neurons," *Journal of Neuroscience*, vol. 20, no. 1, pp. 259–265, 2000.

[43] S. Takahashi, A. Hisatsune, Y. Kurauchi, T. Seki, and H. Katsuki, "Insulin-like growth factor 1 specifically up-regulates expression of modifier subunit of glutamate-cysteine ligase and enhances glutathione synthesis in SH-SY5Y cells," *European Journal of Pharmacology*, vol. 771, pp. 99–106, 2016.

[44] W. H. Park and S. H. Kim, "MG132, a proteasome inhibitor, induces human pulmonary fibroblast cell death via increasing ROS levels and GSH depletion," *Oncology Reports*, vol. 27, no. 4, pp. 1284–1291, 2012.

[45] P. Pérez-Galán, G. Roue, N. Villamor, E. Montserrat, E. Campo, and D. Colomer, "The proteasome inhibitor bortezomib induces apoptosis in mantle-cell lymphoma through generation of ROS and Noxa activation independent of p53 status," *Blood*, vol. 107, no. 1, pp. 257–264, 2006.

[46] G. Filomeni, D. De Zio, and F. Cecconi, "Oxidative stress and autophagy: the clash between damage and metabolic needs," *Cell Death and Differentiation*, vol. 22, no. 3, pp. 377–388, 2015.

[47] G. Jia and J. R. Sowers, "Autophagy: a housekeeper in cardiorenal metabolic health and disease," *Biochimica et Biophysica Acta (BBA)—Molecular Basis of Disease*, vol. 1852, no. 2, pp. 219–224, 2015.

[48] G. Jia, G. Cheng, D. M. Gangahar, and D. K. Agrawal, "Insulin-like growth factor-1 and TNF-α regulate autophagy through c-jun N-terminal kinase and Akt pathways in human atherosclerotic vascular smooth cells," *Immunology and Cell Biology*, vol. 84, no. 5, pp. 448–454, 2006.

[49] Y.-F. Shen, Y. Tang, X.-J. Zhang, K.-X. Huang, and W.-D. Le, "Adaptive changes in autophagy after UPS impairment in Parkinson's disease," *Acta Pharmacologica Sinica*, vol. 34, no. 5, pp. 667–673, 2013.

[50] J. A. Lee, "Neuronal Autophagy: a housekeeper or a fighter in neuronal cell survival?" *Experimental Neurobiology*, vol. 21, pp. 1–8, 2012.

[51] S. Ghavami, S. Shojaei, B. Yeganeh et al., "Autophagy and apoptosis dysfunction in neurodegenerative disorders," *Progress in Neurobiology*, vol. 112, pp. 24–49, 2014.

[52] M. Salazar, A. Carracedo, Í. J. Salanueva et al., "Cannabinoid action induces autophagy-mediated cell death through stimulation of ER stress in human glioma cells," *Journal of Clinical Investigation*, vol. 119, no. 5, pp. 1359–1372, 2009.

[53] K. Arsikin, T. Kravic-Stevovic, M. Jovanovic et al., "Autophagy-dependent and -independent involvement of AMP-activated protein kinase in 6-hydroxydopamine toxicity to SH-SY5Y neuroblastoma cells," *Biochimica et Biophysica Acta—Molecular Basis of Disease*, vol. 1822, no. 11, pp. 1826–1836, 2012.

23

The Effects of Group-Based versus Individual-Based Tai Chi Training on Nonmotor Symptoms in Patients with Mild to Moderate Parkinson's Disease

Jing Hui Yang,[1] Ya Qun Wang,[1] Sai Qing Ye,[2] You Gen Cheng,[1] Yu Chen,[3] and Xiao Zhen Feng[1]

[1]*Department of Rehabilitation Medicine, Tongde Hospital of Zhejiang Province, Hangzhou, China*
[2]*Department of Rehabilitation Medicine, West China Hospital of Sichuan University, Chengdu, China*
[3]*Wuxi Tongren International Rehabilitation Hospital, Wuxi, China*

Correspondence should be addressed to Ya Qun Wang; tongde_kangfu@aliyun.com

Academic Editor: Antonio Pisani

Objective. To compare the effects of group-based and individual-based Tai Chi training on nonmotor symptoms in patients with mild to moderate Parkinson's disease. *Design*. Randomized controlled pilot study. *Methods*. 36 community-dwelling patients with Parkinson's disease (PD) were randomly assigned to either group-based training group ($n = 19$) or individual-based group ($n = 17$). Both groups received same content of Tai Chi training 3 times a week for 13 weeks. Participants were also asked to perform home exercises daily. The Non-Motor Symptoms Scale was used to assess global nonmotor symptoms change. Sleep quality, depression, and cognition were evaluated by Parkinson's Disease Sleep Scale, Hamilton Depression Scale, and Beijing version-Montreal Cognitive Assessment, respectively. Home exercise compliance was recorded. *Results*. There was no significant difference between two groups at baseline. After 13 weeks, there were no statistical significance between two groups. However, the within-group effect was different. Participants in group-based and individual-based groups showed a significant improvement on global nonmotor symptoms ($P < 0.001$, $P = 0.004$) and sleep ($P < 0.001$, $P < 0.001$). But only group-based training patients presented a significant improvement in cognitive impairment compared with baseline ($P = 0.002$, $P = 0.116$). For depression, no group gained a significant improvement($P = 0.123$, $P = 0.170$). Group-based participants had a higher home-exercise compliance rate (HeCR) than individual-based participants did ($P = 0.019$), and HeCR showed a moderate correlation with MoCA-BJ and NMSS scores changes in this study. *Conclusion*. Group-based Tai Chi training is considered to be a more effective and a more labor-saving method in the clinical settings, and patients tend to have a higher compliance rate in their home exercise program. This study is registered with ChiCTR-IPR-17010388.

1. Introduction

Idiopathic Parkinson's disease (PD) is a common neurodegenerative disorder affecting worldwide 1% of people over 55 years of age [1]. While PD is most commonly associated with motor symptoms, there are numerous nonmotor symptoms (NMS) associated with the condition as well, such as sleep disturbance, cognitive decline, anxiety, and depression [2]. NMS are found not only in the advanced stage but also in the early stage of the disease and may precede the onset of motor symptoms by several years [3]. Furthermore, some recent studies showed that NMS in PD patients could substantially reduce the quality of life to a greater extent than the motor symptoms [4, 5]. NMS in PD patients, especially sleeping disturbance, mood changes, and dysautonomia, can be caused by not only pathological alterations due to the disease itself but also the traditional dopaminergic treatments [6]. Therefore, a wide range of nonpharmaceutical therapies have now been delivered to PD patients. Many studies of different exercise models have been delivered to PD patients to evaluate the therapeutic effects on nonmotor symptoms, but the results are still controversial. In 2013, Shulman et al. [7] compared the efficacy of treadmill exercise and stretching and resistance exercise in improving gait speed, strength, fitness, and also nonmotor symptoms for patients with PD. Even though the three types of exercise demonstrated varied effectiveness in motor symptoms, no benefits were found in any nonmotor symptoms for any exercise group, including depression, fatigue, and quality of life. Some mind-body exercises were also applied to treat nonmotor symptoms in PD patients. Sharma et al. [8] reported a positive trend in the improvement of depression level after 24 sessions of yoga training. However, Schmitz-Hübsch et al. [9] showed insignificant findings of depression level after total of 6-month intervention of Qigong exercise.

Tai Chi is another option and seems to be a better choice. As a mind-body exercise intervention, Tai Chi consists of a series of slow and smooth movements with strict and mindful breathing and body control. A large-scale randomized trial conducted by Li and his colleagues in 2012 showed that Tai Chi training had better performance in reducing balance impairments, improving functional capacity, and reducing falls when compared to resistance training and stretching [10]. Besides improving motor function, Tai Chi had also been proved effective in relieving stress and thus improving the quality of life [11]. A recent study by Nocera et al. showed the positive changes on cognitive function and psychological wellbeing of patients with PD following 16-week Tai Chi exercise [12].

In China, the number of individuals with PD over age of 50 was approximately two million in 2005, and the population was expected to be nearly 4.94 million by the year 2030 [13]. The most frequently used approach is individual-based training, in which patients receive 1-on-1 training from a physiotherapist. With the rising number of PD patients and limited fiscal resources in the public health sector, China might face the dilemma of shortage of therapists for PD patients in near future. Furthermore, some researchers believed that different circumstances, such as a natural scenery, group-based exercise, and presence of family member, might have a positive training effect on NMS in PD patients [14]. Group settings could possibly contribute to aspects such as exercise frequency and involvement because of the peers' encouragement and the competition. So, we hypothesized that group-based training, as a more labor-saving option, may be an appealing approach if it can be proved to produce similar or even better outcomes. To date, there is no study that had directly compared the effects of group-based and individual-based Tai Chi training in this population.

This randomized controlled study aimed to compare the effects of group-based and individual-based Tai Chi training on NMS in PD patients. As this is a pilot study, the study designers also evaluated the compliance with home exercise during the study. Such information could provide useful insight in further development and implementation of Tai Chi training for the PD patients.

2. Methods

2.1. Ethics Statement. This pilot study was conducted at the Department of Rehabilitation Medicine of Tongde Hospital of Zhejiang Province in Hangzhou, China, between February 2016 and October 2016. It was conducted in strict accordance with the protocol approved by the Ethics Committee of Tongde Hospital of Zhejiang Province (Hangzhou, China). Written informed consent was obtained from all subjects (or their guardians) prior to enrolment.

2.2. Study Design. A randomized controlled pilot intervention trial was undertaken to evaluate the effects of 13-week Tai Chi training on NMS in patients with mild to moderate Parkinson's disease and compared the two delivery methods: group-based and individual-based training. The outcome assessors were blinded to the group allocation, making this a single-blinded study.

2.3. Subjects. A convenience sample of community-dwelling participants with idiopathic PD was recruited for this study. All the subjects recruited in this study had the membership of the *Parkinson's Disease Club*, which was established by Rehabilitation Medicine Department of Tongde Hospital in 2013. The club includes 113 registered PD patients, who regularly gather two times per month. PD patients in this club received suggestions about medication, diet, and exercise from doctors and therapists of the department. Psychological counselling is also provided by psychologists.

Evaluations and complete neurological examination were performed by experienced neurologists. Participants were included if they (1) were diagnosed of idiopathic PD by UK PD Brain Bank criteria, (2) had a disease rating of stages I to III on the Hoehn and Yahr (H&Y) scale, (3) were between 50 and 75 years old, (4) had stable medication usage, (5) could perform a whole circle of Tai Chi exercise without assistance, and (6) were willing to have Tai Chi exercise. Participants were excluded if they (1) had any history or evidence of neurological deficit other than PD, (2) had dementia (determined by a Beijing version-Montreal Cognitive Assessment less than 17), (3) suffered from significant depression (determined by a Hamilton Depression Scale larger than 20), (4) had somatic disease that could have a potential effect on NMS (e.g., pain syndromes, advanced diabetes mellitus), or (5) were on medications affecting balance or attention.

A total of 48 PD patients in the Parkinson's Disease Club met the criterion (Figure 1). Three of the 48 PD patients underwent another clinical study and were excluded from this study. The remaining patients were provided with detailed information regarding the purpose, procedure, interventions, and potential risks of the study by the research personnel. Six of the 45 PD patients refused to participate in the study because of the risk of fall or other considerations. Thus, 39 patients enrolled in this study.

2.4. Randomization. To ensure that the number of subjects in each group was approximately equal, each patient was given a random number following a random number table and ordered by their assigned numbers. The patients were

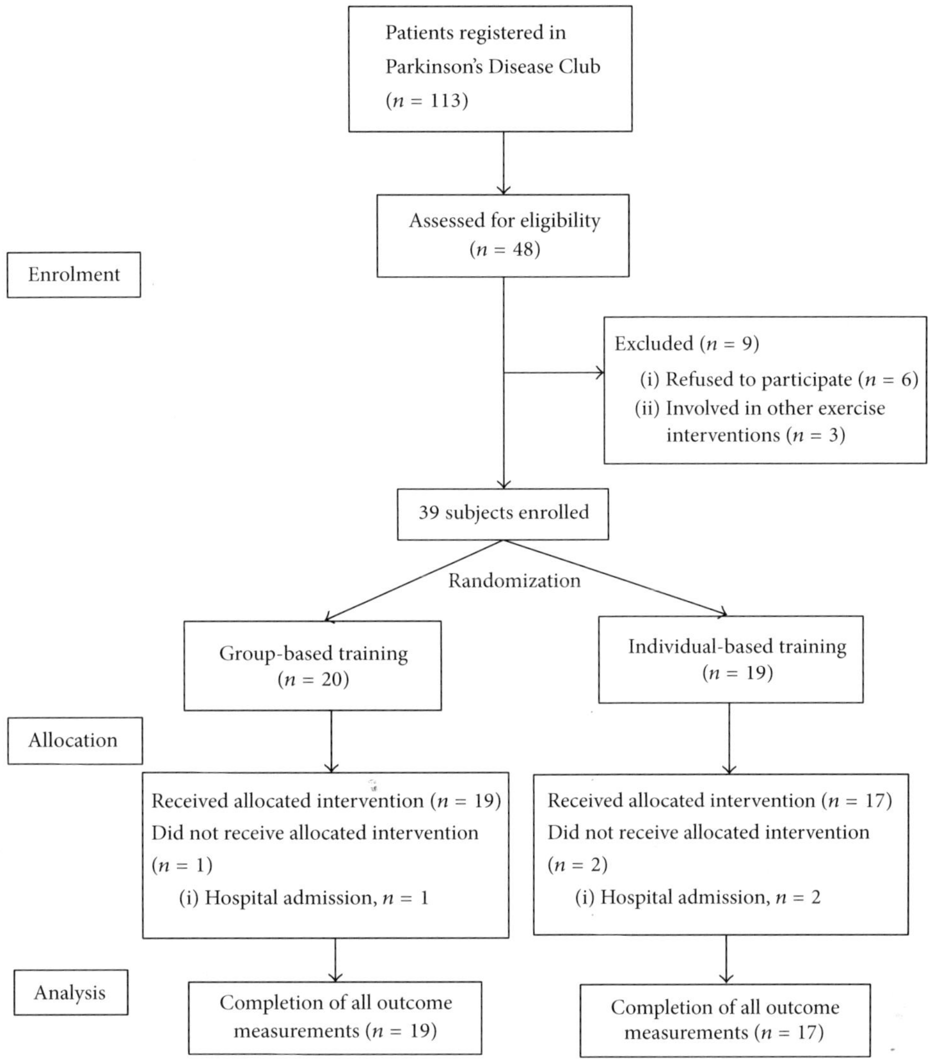

FIGURE 1: Patient flow diagram.

then assigned to groups by taking the first patient in the order list for group-based group (GbG), the next patient for the individual-based group (IbG), and so on until all were assigned. The randomization procedure was performed by a research therapist who was not involved in the assessment of the subjects. There were 20 patients in GbG and 19 patients in IbG at the start of the study.

2.5. Intervention. The Tai Chi classes were delivered by a 7-year experienced Tai Chi instructor who was specialized at 24-form Yang Style Tai Chi [15]. This style of Tai Chi is easy to learn and is the most popular form of Tai Chi in China. It emphasizes diagonal weight shifting, awareness of body position, and breathing. Every participant was taught in a one-on-one fashion to ensure they all understood and performed well before the beginning of the study.

Both groups received 39 sessions of 24-form Yang Style Tai Chi for 40~45 minutes each time, three times a week for 13 weeks. At the first 2 weeks, the training time was 20–25 minutes per session due to the bad endurance in these subjects, and the subjects could have a break when they reported any uncomfortable feelings, such as dizziness, tiredness, or nausea.

The patients to therapist ratio was 6~7 : 1 for the group-based training and 1 : 1 for individual-based training at the beginning. To maintain the consistency of the treatment approach, both group-based and individual-based training were conducted by the same Tai Chi instructor.

Every subject was suggested to do Tai Chi exercise at home every day (except for the days on which hospital training sessions took place) during the study period. A diary was used to record the home exercise date and duration for every patient. The home exercise content was the same as what they did in the hospital, but the patients did not need to repeat the whole session of the exercise. The home Tai Chi exercise would take approximately 20 to 25 min to be completed. The patients and their caregivers were provided with audiovisual material, and the caregivers were asked to be present to prevent falls and supervise accurate movement during the home exercise.

2.6. Outcome Measures

Nonmotor Symptoms. NMS may present in varied manifestations in PD patients. Chaudhuri et al. [15] have developed the Non-Motor Symptoms Scale (NMSS) for PD patients' evaluation. This scale is a reliable and valid tool for assessing the progress or potential response to treatment of NMS in PD patients. NMSS contains nine dimensions: cardiovascular (2 items), sleep/fatigue (4 items), mood/cognition (6 items), perceptual problems (3 items), attention/memory (3 items), gastrointestinal (3 items), urinary (3 items), sexual function (2 items), and miscellany (4 items). Score for each item is based on a multiple of severity (from 0 to 3) and frequency scores (from 1 to 4), and a higher score indicated more severer symptoms. NMSS was used to evaluate the global NMS changes in all subjects before and after the Tai Chi intervention in this study.

According to Song and other researchers, sleep dysfunction, mood problem, and cognition disorder are the most prevalent NMS in China's PD patients [16, 17], and these NMS are closely associated with the Health-Related Quality of Life of PD patients [18–20]. Therefore, we decided to use more specific measurement tools to assess these symptoms in these subjects. Sleep quality was assessed by Parkinson's Disease Sleep Scale (PDSS) [21]. Hamilton Depression Scale (HAMD) was used to assess the depression in PD patients. For cognitive impairment evaluation, Beijing version-Montreal Cognitive Assessment (MoCA-BJ) was used because it is more sensitive than the MMSE for detecting early cognitive decline and impairment change in nonmemory dysfunction in Chinese patients [22].

Each subjects' nonmotor symptoms were evaluated within five days of the initiation of the study and again within five days of the termination of the 13-week intervention. Both groups assessments were performed by the same independent assessor, who was an experienced physiotherapist and was blinded to the group assignment. The patients and their caregivers were instructed not to inform the assessor of the group allocation. The outcome assessor was also instructed not to ask the subjects which group they belonged to.

Home Exercise Compliance. A diary was used to record home exercise date and duration, and only when the exercise time was more than 20 min/day would it be regarded as ONE home exercise day. The home exercise compliance rate (% days) was calculated using the following formula: (number of days of home exercise participation) $*$ 100%/(total number of days).

2.7. Statistical Analysis. Descriptive statistics are reported as mean ± SD. Between-group differences in demographic and baseline variables were tested with a chi-square test for categorical variables and an independent t-test for continuous variables.

Independent t-test was used to compare the change scores between the groups. Paired t-test was used to examine within-group changes from baseline to 13 weeks. The Pearson's correlation coefficient was used to explore whether the changes of total NMSS scores and other measurement scores were associated with the home exercise compliance rate. All the statistical analyses were performed using the Statistical Package for the Social Sciences (SPSS Inc., Chicago, IL, USA) software program version 21.0. The level of significance was set at 0.05 (2-tailed). In addition, post hoc power analysis was performed. The effect size and power were calculated using G*Power (Faul and Erdfelder, Bonn University, Germany, 1992) statistical software version 3.1.9.2.

3. Result

48 PD patients were eligible for the study, 39 initiated the study, and 36 patients completed both pre- and postassessments. One participant and 2 participants withdrew from the group-based and individual-based group, respectively, because of hospital admission. As such, 19 group-based training participants and 17 individual-based training participants completed the study. No adverse event was reported during the study period.

There were no statistically significant differences between the 2 groups at baseline for all measures, including age, the proportion of male and female, height, weight, disease duration, age at onset, or the H&Y scale and UPDRS Total score (Table 1).

Pre- and postintervention results of the outcome measures were depicted in Table 2. After 13 weeks of Tai Chi training, both group-based and individual-based groups showed a significant improvement on global nonmotor symptoms (NMSS score: $P < 0.001$, $P = 0.002$) and sleep (PDSS score: $P < 0.001$, $P < 0.001$). However, only group-based group presented a significant improvement in cognitive impairment (MoCA-BJ score: $P = 0.002$, $P = 0.116$) after the intervention. And, for depression, no group gained a significant improvement after the intervention (HAMD score: $P = 0.123$, $P = 0.170$). Even though the mean changes of all outcome measures in group-based group were bigger than individual-based group, there were no statistical significance between two groups. For instance, the mean changes in MoCA-BJ score in group-based group were much bigger than individual-based group (1.63 versus 0.58), but no statistical difference ($P = 0.081$) showed. Similar results were found in NMSS score (9.94 versus 6.64, $P = 0.282$), PDSS score (10.73 versus 8.29, $P = 0.506$), and HAMD score (0.84 versus 0.76, $P = 0.918$) as well.

Home exercise compliance was significantly different between 2 groups (group-based: mean 64.84% (SD 13.99%); individual-based: mean 51.17% (SD 19.12%), $P = 0.019$). There was also a moderate correlation between the home exercise compliance rate and the change in MoCA-BJ scores and NMSS total scores following either group-based group ($r = 0.482$, $P = 0.036$; $r = -0.480$, $P = 0.038$) and individual-based group ($r = 0.535$, $P = 0.027$; $r = -0.541$, $P = 0.025$) (Figure 2). However, the data showed no significant correlation between home exercise compliance rate and the changes in PDSS score ($r = 0.380$, $P = 0.109$; $r = 0.195$, $P = 0.453$) and HAMD score ($r = 0.029$, $P = 0.907$; $r = 0.220$, $P = 0.397$) following two groups.

3.1. Post Hoc Power Analysis. The estimated effect size for NMSS, PDSS, HAMD, and MoCA-BJ was 0.40, 0.40, 0.04, and 0.72. These values represent a small-to-medium effect

Table 1: Baseline characteristics of participants in group-based and individual-based groups.

	Group-based group ($n = 19$)	Individual-based group ($n = 17$)	P value
Age	62.94 (5.45)	64.23 (5.72)	0.415
Gender (M/F)	11/8	9/8	0.765
Height (cm)	171.37 (5.63)	173.41 (4.14)	0.232
Weight (kg)	67.47 (5.95)	69.29 (6.29)	0.594
Disease duration (years)	4.89 (2.20)	4.47 (1.54)	0.531
Age at onset	58.05 (5.67)	59.76 (6.48)	0.379
H&Y scale	1–3	1–3	0.827
UPDRS total	31.10 (6.54)	31.52 (5.10)	0.900

Numbers in parentheses designate standard error. H&Y scale, Hoehn and Yahr scale; UPDRS, Unified Parkinson's Rating Scale.

Table 2: Comparison of mean changes before and after intervention.

Outcome measure	Group	Time: Baseline Mean (SD)	Time: After 13 weeks Mean (SD)	Changes Mean (SD)	P value
NMSS	Group-based	61.26 (19.86)	51.31 (20.72)	−9.94 (9.07)**	0.000
	Individual-based	68.82 (25.31)	62.17 (22.47)	−6.88 (7.54)**	0.002
	P value: GbG versus IbG	0.323		0.282	
PDSS	Group-based	97.42 (15.81)	108.15 (16.32)	10.21 (10.82)**	0.000
	Individual-based	96.82 (20.35)	105.11 (20.22)	8.29 (4.77)**	0.000
	P value: GbG versus IbG	0.923		0.506	
HAMD	Group-based	12.94 (3.59)	12.10 (3.05)	−0.84 (2.26)	0.123
	Individual-based	13.00 (3.35)	12.23 (3.68)	−0.76 (2.19)	0.170
	P value: GbG versus IbG	0.964		0.918	
MoCA-BJ	Group-based	21.26 (3.05)	22.89 (2.86)	1.63 (1.94)**	0.002
	Individual-based	22.00 (2.78)	22.58 (2.51)	0.58 (1.46)	0.116
	P value: GbG versus IbG	0.456		0.081	
HeCR	Group-based		64.84 (13.99)#		
	Individual-based		51.17 (19.12)		
	P value: GbG versus IbG		0.019		

Numbers in parentheses represent the standard error. $^{**}P < 0.01$ compared with baseline. $^{\#}P < 0.05$ group-based group (GbG) compared with individual-based group (IbG) after 13 weeks.. NMSS, Non-Motor Symptom Scale; PDSS, Parkinson's Disease Sleep Scale; HAMD, Hamilton Depression Scale; MoCA-BJ, Beijing version-Montreal Cognitive Assessment; HeCR, home exercise compliance rate.

size. With an alpha value of 0.05 and a sample size of 19 and 17 subjects in each group, the corresponding statistical power was calculated as 0.22, 0.21, 0.05, and 0.55, respectively.

4. Discussion

Nonmotor symptoms in PD patients can present at the very early stage and are highly impactful on quality of life. To date, most studies have investigated motor outcomes following Tai Chi exercise in patients with Parkinson's disease and many have demonstrated improvements [23]. However, most have ignored the potential additional benefits to NMS of this body-mind interaction activity. In this study, we compared group-based and individual-based Tai Chi training on NMS in patients with PD. After 13 weeks' intervention, the difference between two groups was not big, but we can still dig some interesting findings.

4.1. Group-Based versus Individual-Based Tai Chi Training. This present study compared the effects of 13 weeks' group-based and individual-based Tai Chi training on NMS in patients with mild to moderate PD. The results showed that both groups improved significantly in global NMS and sleep quality when compared to baseline. Even though the differences between two groups failed to reach the statistical significance level, the score changes in group-based group were larger than those in individual-based group. The possible explanation for the similar outcomes is that each approach we used in this study has a positive impact on NMS (except for depression), and the limited study duration could not show the superiority of the compared approaches. But for home exercise compliance rate (HeCR), group-based patients seem more likely to accomplish the home exercise (assigned by the study designer) than individual-based patients do. It may be impossible to distinguish whether the better

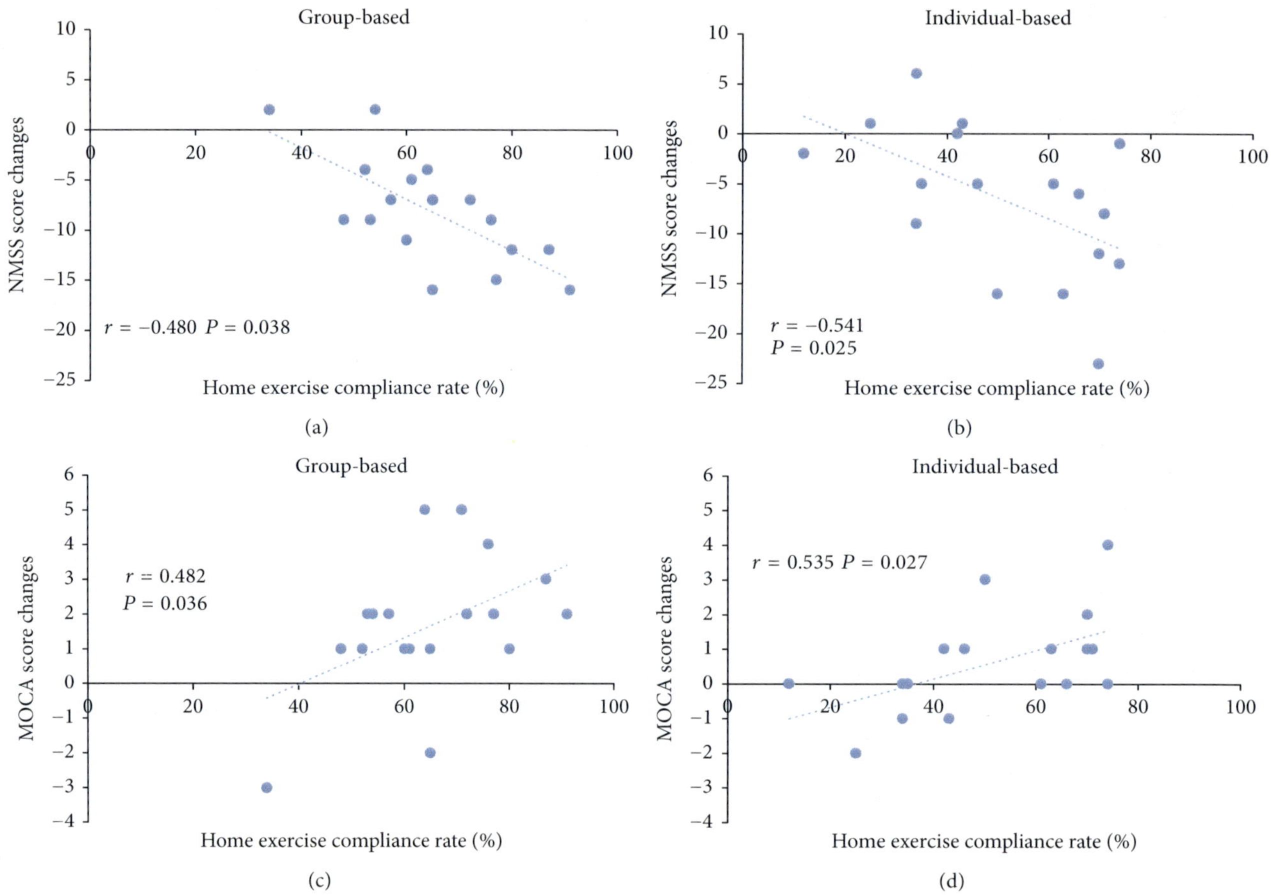

FIGURE 2: Significant correlation between the home exercise compliance rate (HeCR) and the changes in NMSS total scores and MOCA scores: (a) correlation between HeCR and the changes in NMSS total scores in group-based group; (b) correlation between HeCR and the changes in NMSS total scores in individual-based group; (c) correlation between HeCR and the changes in MOCA scores in group-based group; (d) correlation between HeCR and the changes in MOCA scores in individual-based group.

outcomes in group-based group are because of the group setting itself or the higher home exercise frequency. However, HeCR showed significant correlation with the global NMS and cognitive function. A higher HeCR may lead to a better outcome in a consistent way. So, we suppose that if we extend the study duration in the future, such as six months or one year, the patients in group-based setting may gain more obvious improvement on nonmotor symptoms.

The group-based patients have a higher home exercise frequency. The significantly higher HeCR may be due to more support and competitive motivations from his or her peers. First, the group-based training provides subjects more opportunities of social interaction and mind support. Secondly, group training makes participant more competitive, and this motivates them to perform better. Then, once they have a better performance in front of his or her groupmates, they may get more support and praise from the group. This virtuous circle may further encourage the subjects' participation in the training and home exercise [14]. In addition, a previous study found that social support networks were low in older adults compared with younger individuals, partly due to issues such as peers becoming less active and family fearing accidently falling or other injuries [24]. Thereby, group-based training could be more beneficial to the participants, especially for elders.

As a traditional Chinese exercise, Tai Chi is considered as an exercise requiring high level of attention and memory to learn and complete. In this study, we measured cognitive function changes before and after intervention. Both groups presented an increase of MoCA-BJ scores, but only group-based participants showed a significant improvement. We think the reason of this result is mainly because of the participant in group-based group did more Tai Chi exercise at home. Another explanation is exercise environment. According to Berman et al. [25], the interaction with natural environment could provide more cognitive function control when compared with urban environment. In this study, the participants usually chose community garden as the place to accomplish home exercise, which gives them more chance to expose themselves to the nature. This result also reminds us that if we want the patients to receive more cognitive control we should think about replacing the hospital training at a more natural environment in the future.

As for depression, neither of the group showed a significant improvement. Similar results for depression recovery were reported in studies using different type of exercise in PD patients. In 2013, Shulman et al. [7] compared the efficacy of 3 types of exercise (high intensity, low intensity, and resistant training) in PD patients. After 3-month intervention, all the participants in 3 groups did not show a significant improvement on depression. The same results could be seen in a tango exercise [26] and a dance intervention study [27] too. But a good result was shown in a formal exercise study [28] and a Nordic Waling program [29]. The participants in these 2 trials presented a significant improvement after intervention. The reasons for the conflicting results may due to the different exercise type, different measurement tools, and the study design, including training frequency and duration. Moreover, there was still not enough evidence on Tai Chi training in PD patient's depression issues.

4.2. Group Training and Home Exercise. Receiving exercise intervention in a group context may be particularly healthy for PD patients, which is at considerable risk of daily life and health care stigmatization and social isolation [30]. Also, PD patients' home exercise compliance is another issue that should be considered. In this study, we test the efficacy of group training plus home exercise program; the results showed a positive effect while compared to individual training. We believe that group training is a better option when facing the increasing number of clients, limited staffing,and budgetary cuts, the common issues nowadays. Besides, considering the inconvenient transportation for PD patients and the busy schedule of their caregivers, the implementation of home exercise program is an alternative method to increase the exercise frequency and duration without cost to the healthcare system.

4.3. Review Studies of Different Approaches on NMS in Parkinson's Disease. Some randomized controlled studies have examined the effect of different kind of nonpharmaceutical therapy on NMS in patients with PD. In a multicentre, randomized controlled clinical trial, Sturkenboom et al. [31] compared the efficacy of 10 weeks of home-based occupational therapy with usual care with no occupational therapy for patients with PD. The results showed that even though OT group gained a better self-perceived performance on prioritised activities (Canadian Occupational Performance Measure performance scale) at 3- and 6-month follow-up, the mean changes between two groups in quality of life (Visual Analogue Scale for QoL), fatigue (Fatigue Severity Scale), and depression (Beck Depression Inventory) were not significant. By contrast, Modugno et al. [32] found that PD patients (Hoehn and Yahr stages 2–4) who had undergone a theatre workshop rehabilitation program (6-h daily sessions, for a total of ~18 h/months, for 3 years) that was a combination of exercising basic skills and theatre performance skills (recreation of stage behaviours and emotions that could occur in real life) showed a very quick and significant improvement in the mood, quality of sleep, and perception of social support (as assessed by Hamilton Depression Rating Scale, Epworth Sleepiness Scale, and PDQ39 social support scale) compared with PD patients in the physiotherapy group. The authors believe that these remarkable results may be due to the combination of movements and stimulation of different sensory pathways and emotional involvement. In order to be an eligible "actor," PD patients have to control their movements and emotions simultaneously. In addition, theatre therapy asked patients to interact continuously, so they are forced to socialize. These features make theatre an ideal playground to motivate patients deeply. Some impressive benefits on NMS can also be found in a Nordic Waling study we mentioned before [29]. In this study, PD patients showed a significant improvement on all NMS that measured, including global NMS (NMSS), fatigue (PFS-16), depression (BDI), and apathy (SAS), after 12-week NW exercise. A study conducted by Foster et al. [33] in 2013 demonstrated that a community-based tango dance program (every PD patient was paired with a healthy caregiver as a group) could significantly increase the current activity participation, activity retention, and numbers of New Social activities after 12 months' intervention. Taken together, these findings indicate that we should pay more attention to other conditions when treating NMS in PD patients. These conditions may include natural environment (Nordic walking), group or paired exercise (Tai Chi, tango, and theatre training), novel and attractive intervention methods (theatre training), and other circumstances that may potentially increase the interactions with others or the activity participation.

5. Conclusion

Both group-based and individual-based Tai Chi training are effective in improving nonmotor symptoms in patients with mild to moderate Parkinson's disease. Group-based Tai Chi training is considered a more effective and a more labor-saving method in the clinical settings, and patients tend to have a higher compliance rate in their home exercise program. This may provide some insights for method of delivering Tai Chi training to PD patients in the future.

Additional Points

Limitations. The study has several limitations. First, as this was a pilot study, the sample size was relatively small. The results should thus be interpreted with caution, as the post hoc power analysis shown was low. Secondly, the intervention duration was relatively short. We think the results may be different if we have a 6-month or longer intervention based on the HeCR. Thirdly, we did not include a nontreatment control group. Thus, even though both groups showed an improvement after Tai Chi training, we cannot exclude the possibility that the good results in both groups were the consequence of normal medication treatment during the treatment period.

Ethical Approval

This study was conducted in strict accordance with the protocol approved by the Ethics Committee of Tongde Hospital of Zhejiang Province.

Disclosure

This study was conducted in strict accordance with the protocol approved by the Ethics Committee of Tongde Hospital of Zhejiang Province. The study was supported by a grant from Science Technology Department of Zhejiang Province (Grant no. 2015C33156). There are no financial benefits to the authors.

Acknowledgments

The authors gratefully acknowledge all the participants and staff who volunteered their time and efforts.

References

[1] A. J. Lees, J. Hardy, and T. Revesz, "Parkinson's disease," *The Lancet*, vol. 373, no. 9680, pp. 2055–2066, 2009.

[2] L. Kadastik-Eerme, M. Rosenthal, T. Paju, M. Muldmaa, and P. Taba, "Health-related quality of life in Parkinson's disease: a cross-sectional study focusing on non-motor symptoms," *Health and Quality of Life Outcomes*, vol. 13, no. 1, article 83, 2015.

[3] E. Tolosa, C. Gaig, J. Santamaría, and Y. Compta, "Diagnosis and the premotor phase of Parkinson disease," *Neurology*, vol. 72, no. 7, supplement 2, pp. S12–S20, 2009.

[4] G. W. Duncan, T. K. Khoo, A. J. Yarnall et al., "Health-related quality of life in early Parkinson's disease: the impact of nonmotor symptoms," *Movement Disorders*, vol. 29, no. 2, pp. 195–202, 2014.

[5] A. Cronin-Golomb, "Emergence of nonmotor symptoms as the focus of research and treatment of Parkinson's disease: Introduction to the special section on nonmotor dysfunctions in Parkinson's disease," *Behavioral Neuroscience*, vol. 127, no. 2, pp. 135–138, 2013.

[6] A. Park and M. Stacy, "Non-motor symptoms in Parkinson's disease," *Journal of Neurology*, vol. 256, no. 3, supplement, pp. 293–296, 2009.

[7] L. M. Shulman, L. I. Katzel, F. M. Ivey et al., "Randomized clinical trial of 3 types of physical exercise for patients with parkinson disease," *JAMA Neurology*, vol. 70, no. 2, pp. 183–190, 2013.

[8] N. K. Sharma, K. Robbins, K. Wagner, and Y. M. Colgrove, "A randomized controlled pilot study of the therapeutic effects of yoga in people with Parkinson's disease," *International Journal of Yoga*, vol. 8, no. 1, pp. 74–79, 2015.

[9] T. Schmitz-Hübsch, D. Pyfer, K. Kielwein, R. Fimmers, T. Klockgether, and U. Wüllner, "Qigong exercise for the symptoms of Parkinson's disease: A randomized, controlled pilot study," *Movement Disorders*, vol. 21, no. 4, pp. 543–548, 2006.

[10] F. Li, P. Harmer, K. Fitzgerald et al., "Tai chi and postural stability in patients with Parkinson's disease," *The New England Journal of Medicine*, vol. 366, no. 6, pp. 511–519, 2012.

[11] T. Esch, J. Duckstein, J. Welke et al., "Mind/body techniques for physiological and psychological stress reduction: stress management via Tai Chi training—a pilot study," *Medical Science Monitor*, vol. 13, no. 11, pp. CR488–CR497, 2007.

[12] J. R. Nocera, S. Amano, S. Vallabhajosula et al., "Tai Chi exercise to improve non-motor symptoms of Parkinson's disease," *Journal of Yoga & Physical Therapy*, vol. 3, article 137, 2013.

[13] E. R. Dorsey, R. Constantinescu, J. P. Thompson et al., "Projected number of people with Parkinson disease in the most populous nations, 2005 through 2030," *Neurology*, vol. 68, no. 5, pp. 384–386, 2007.

[14] M. E. Cusso, K. J. Donald, and T. K. Khoo, "The impact of physical activity on non-motor symptoms in parkinson's disease: a systematic review," *Frontiers in Medicine*, vol. 3, article 35, 2016.

[15] K. R. Chaudhuri, P. Martinez-Martin, R. G. Brown et al., "The metric properties of a novel non-motor symptoms scale for Parkinson's disease: results from an international pilot study," *Movement Disorders*, vol. 22, no. 13, pp. 1901–1911, 2007.

[16] W. Song, X. Guo, K. Chen et al., "The impact of non-motor symptoms on the Health-Related Quality of Life of Parkinson's disease patients from Southwest China," *Parkinsonism and Related Disorders*, vol. 20, no. 2, pp. 149–152, 2014.

[17] H. Li, M. Zhang, L. Chen et al., "Nonmotor symptoms are independently associated with impaired health-related quality of life in Chinese patients with Parkinson's disease," *Movement Disorders*, vol. 25, no. 16, pp. 2740–2746, 2010.

[18] S. Rahman, H. J. Griffin, N. P. Quinn, and M. Jahanshahi, "Quality of life in Parkinson's disease: the relative importance of the symptoms," *Movement Disorders*, vol. 23, no. 10, pp. 1428–1434, 2008.

[19] J. C. Gómez-Esteban, B. Tijero, J. Somme et al., "Impact of psychiatric symptoms and sleep disorders on the quality of life of patients with Parkinson's disease," *Journal of Neurology*, vol. 258, no. 3, pp. 494–499, 2011.

[20] P. Martinez-Martin, C. Rodriguez-Blazquez, M. M. Kurtis, and K. R. Chaudhuri, "The impact of non-motor symptoms on health-related quality of life of patients with Parkinson's disease," *Movement Disorders*, vol. 26, no. 3, pp. 399–406, 2011.

[21] G. Wang, Q. Cheng, J. Zeng et al., "Sleep disorders in Chinese patients with Parkinson's disease: validation study of a Chinese version of Parkinson's disease sleep scale," *Journal of the Neurological Sciences*, vol. 271, no. 1-2, pp. 153–157, 2008.

[22] L. Wang, K. Nie, Y. Zhang et al., "A pilot study of psychometric properties of the Beijing version of Montreal Cognitive Assessment in patients with idiopathic Parkinson's disease in China," *Journal of Clinical Neuroscience*, vol. 19, no. 11, pp. 1497–1500, 2012.

[23] J. Zhou, T. Yin, Q. Gao, and X. C. Yang, "A meta-analysis on the efficacy of tai chi in patients with parkinson?s disease between 2008 and 2014," *Evidence-Based Complementary and Alternative Medicine*, vol. 2015, 9 pages, 2015.

[24] R. E. Rhodes, A. D. Martin, J. E. Taunton, E. C. Rhodes, M. Donnelly, and J. Elliot, "Factors associated with exercise adherence among older adults. An individual perspective," *Sports Medicine*, vol. 28, no. 6, pp. 397–411, 1999.

[25] M. G. Berman, J. Jonides, and S. Kaplan, "The cognitive benefits of interacting with nature," *Psychological Science*, vol. 19, no. 12, pp. 1207–1212, 2008.

[26] S. R. Romenets, J. Anang, S. M. Fereshtehnejad, A. Pelletier, and R. Postuma, "Tango for treatment of motor and non-motor

manifestations in Parkinson's disease: a randomized control study," *Complementary Therapies in Medicine*, vol. 23, no. 2, pp. 175–184, 2015.

[27] R. P. Duncan and G. M. Earhart, "Randomized controlled trial of community-based dancing to modify disease progression in Parkinson disease," *Neurorehabilitation and Neural Repair*, vol. 26, no. 2, pp. 132–143, 2012.

[28] A. Park, D. Zid, J. Russell et al., "Effects of a formal exercise program on Parkinson's disease: A pilot study using a delayed start design," *Parkinsonism and Related Disorders*, vol. 20, no. 1, pp. 106–111, 2014.

[29] L. Cugusi, P. Solla, R. Serpe et al., "Effects of a Nordic Walking program on motor and non-motor symptoms, functional performance and body composition in patients with Parkinson's disease," *NeuroRehabilitation*, vol. 37, no. 2, pp. 245–254, 2015.

[30] L. Tickle-Degnen, L. A. Zebrowitz, and H.-I. Ma, "Culture, gender and health care stigma: Practitioners' response to facial masking experienced by people with Parkinson's disease," *Social Science and Medicine*, vol. 73, no. 1, pp. 95–102, 2011.

[31] I. H. Sturkenboom, M. J. Graff, J. C. Hendriks et al., "Efficacy of occupational therapy for patients with Parkinsons disease: a randomised controlled trial," *Lancet Neurol*, vol. 13, no. 6, pp. 577-566, 2014.

[32] N. Modugno, S. Iaconelli, M. Fiorilli, F. Lena, I. Kusch, and G. Mirabella, "Active theater as a complementary therapy for Parkinson's disease rehabilitation: A pilot study," *TheScientificWorldJournal*, vol. 10, pp. 2301–2313, 2010.

[33] E. R. Foster, L. Golden, R. P. Duncan, and G. M. Earhart, "Community-based argentine tango dance program is associated with increased activity participation among individuals with parkinson's disease," *Archives of Physical Medicine and Rehabilitation*, vol. 94, no. 2, pp. 240–249, 2013.

Evolution of Orofacial Symptoms and Disease Progression in Idiopathic Parkinson's Disease: Longitudinal Data from the Jönköping Parkinson Registry

Seyed-Mohammad Fereshtehnejad,[1,2] Örjan Skogar,[2,3] and Johan Lökk[2,4]

[1] *Department of Neurology and Neurosurgery, McGill University, Montreal, QC, Canada*
[2] *Division of Clinical Geriatrics, Department of Neurobiology, Care Sciences, and Society (NVS), Karolinska Institutet, Stockholm, Sweden*
[3] *FUTURUM, Academy for Health and Care, Jönköping, Sweden*
[4] *Department of Geriatric Medicine, Karolinska University Hospital, Stockholm, Sweden*

Correspondence should be addressed to Seyed-Mohammad Fereshtehnejad; sm.fereshtehnejad@ki.se

Academic Editor: Jan Aasly

Background. Orofacial symptoms are common in Parkinson's disease (PD) both as initial manifestations and late markers of disease complications. We aimed to investigate the evolution of orofacial manifestations and their prognostic value throughout PD progression. *Methods.* Data was obtained from "Jönköping Parkinson Registry" database on routine care visits of 314 people with idiopathic PD in southern Sweden. Information on baseline symptomatology, orofacial features, UPDRS, and medications was recorded at baseline and during each follow-up visit within an average of 4.2 (range: 1–12) years. *Results.* Hypomimia, affected speech, drooling, and impaired swallowing were present in 37.3%/91.6%, 14.1%/65.5%, 11.7%/55.3%, and 10.2%/34.5% at baseline/follow-up, respectively. Male sex [OR = 2.4 (95% CI: 1.0–5.9)], UPDRS motor scores [OR = 1.2 (95% CI: 1.1–1.3)], dominant rigidity [OR = 5.2 (95% CI: 1.4–19.1)], and autonomic disturbance [OR = 3.4 (95% CI: 1.1–10.9)] were risk factors for drooling. Individuals with more severe orofacial burden at baseline had shorter median time to develop UPDRS-Part III > 28 [3rd tertile = 4.7 yr, 2nd tertile = 6.2 yr, and 1st tertile = 7.8 yr; $p = 0.014$]. *Conclusions.* Majority of people with PD manifest orofacial manifestations at either early or late stages of the disease. PD severity, symmetry of motor disturbances, and autonomic disorders correlate with orofacial symptoms. Individuals with more severe orofacial burden at baseline progressed faster to more advanced stages.

1. Introduction

People with Parkinson's disease (PD) display a number of orofacial manifestations such as hypomimia, difficulties with speech, swallowing disturbances, and drooling of saliva. Cardinal motor features of PD, known as resting tremor, bradykinesia, and rigidity, could all potentially affect orofacial functions [1]. Neurophysiological studies show that, in PD, facial bradykinesia is primarily mediated by basal ganglia dysfunction [2], which reduces both the jaw mobility and the speed of jaw movements [3]. The process results in hypomimia, one of the most distinctive clinical features of PD. In parallel, rigidity and tremor complicate the formation and the placement of the food bolus as well as the chewing process [4, 5], which in turn induced food retention and dysphagia [1]. Drooling of saliva is another typical orofacial feature in PD caused by a combination of excessive spillover of saliva out of the oral cavity that brings various negative physical and psychosocial consequences for individuals with PD and their caregivers [6]. Several mechanisms including decreased frequency of swallowing, dysphagia, tongue tremor, diminished closure of the lips, and forward flexion of the head and neck known as antecollis contribute in the formation of sialorrhea in PD [7, 8].

Besides hypomimia as a clinical hallmark presented in almost all PD patients, other orofacial symptoms are also quite commonly occurred throughout the course of PD progression. Drooling and dysphagia, for instance, have been found in up to 78% [7] and 82% [9] of people with PD, respectively. Neuroepidemiologic studies have shown that orofacial manifestations can develop in mild to severe stages of PD [8] and their evolutionary trend varies from case to case. While in some individuals orofacial expressions represent early onset symptoms, for some others they happen in the late and potentially ominous states of PD. In addition to their psychosocial burden, orofacial dysfunctions, in particular dysphagia, was even once a major leading cause of mortality in PD through aspiration-induced pneumonia and choking in the pre-levodopa era [10]. Yet, due to the lack of true systematic prospective data collection in clinical practice, the knowledge in this field is insufficient. There is not enough comprehensive study on the evolution of orofacial dysfunctions and their contributing factors in PD. Furthermore, orofacial manifestations are usually easy to notice and feasible to track, which proposes them as suitable markers for disease progression.

Therefore, having access to a longitudinal cohort with rather long-term follow-up information, we aimed to investigate the following:

(1) Prevalence of different orofacial symptoms throughout the course of PD;

(2) Risk factors and determinants of different orofacial manifestations;

(3) Prognostic value of the occurrence and severity of orofacial symptoms to predict progression in PD.

2. Methods

This prospective study was performed using data from an ongoing registry of people with PD recruited from the outpatient department of Jönköping referral hospital in southern Sweden, during 1998–2014.

2.1. Jönköping Parkinson Registry. Since the end of the late 90s, outpatient individuals with parkinsonism have been asked for and given their permission for registration in the "*Jönköping Parkinson Registry.*" This was one of the first attempts in Sweden to continuously register specified variables dealing with PD and parkinsonism-related disorders. The database was manufactured by the computer engineering department at the *County Hospital Ryhov, Jönköpings läns landsting*, a region with about 150000 inhabitants, in order to register diagnosis, actual medication, the current symptom information, and status of patients with PD and other forms of parkinsonian syndrome who attended the outpatient visits at the "Clinic of Medicine" and the "Clinic of Geriatrics." Patients were primarily recruited from the primary care units of the region. After referral to the specialized clinics, they were routinely followed twice or at least once a year depending on the actual status of each individual. Data registration was performed during or immediately adjacent to each visit by the examining doctor. Some of the administrative data were collected and saved by the specialist nurse on duty. In total, five physicians, all with special interests in movement disorders, were involved in the registration of specific observations concerning orofacial symptoms.

The protocol for "*Jönköping Parkinson Registry*" and the access to the database was approved by the regional ethics committee. Participants were informed about the registration of their data and provided informed consent. Researchers followed all the sections, notes, and issues of the latest version of the Helsinki Declaration on research ethics. In order to ensure privacy, data were treated confidentially, protected from unauthorized access, and deidentified before analysis.

2.2. Study Population. In this study, we recruited 314 patients who fulfilled the clinical diagnosis of idiopathic Parkinson's disease (IPD) according to the UK Brain Bank Parkinson's Disease Criteria. Data from people with other parkinsonian syndromes were excluded.

2.3. Assessments. At baseline, demographic information, symptomatology, the Unified Parkinson's Disease Rating Scale (UPDRS) parts I–IV, and medications were recorded. A broad list of symptoms was assessed through self-reported answers or via basic physical examination by the attending neurologist at the clinic. The baseline symptoms consisted of resting tremor, bradykinesia, rigidity, fall, freezing, dyskinesia, wearing off, postural instability, visual impairment, hyposmia, urinary urgency, orthostatic hypotension, voice changes, and depression.

During each routine care visit, follow-up data consisting of UPDRS-Parts I–IV and change in antiparkinson drugs were also consecutively collected for each IPD patient over time. Follow-up data were available for 268 (85.4%) participants and the mean duration of follow-up time was 4.2 years ranging between >1 and 12 years. Using data from the UPDRS, scores were calculated for motor subtypes:

(i) *Tremor score*: mean of all UPDRS items on action and resting tremor on head and both left and right upper and lower extremities [11];

(ii) *Postural instability–gait difficulty (PIGD) score*: sum of UPDRS-Part III items concerning rise, gait, and postural instability [12];

(iii) *Asymmetry score*: absolute differences in UPDRS between left and right sides divided by the total UPDRS III (0 = perfect symmetry, 1 = absolute asymmetry) [13].

Orofacial manifestations were defined and assessed as follows:

(i) *Speech problems*: UPDRS-Part II-Item 5 score ≥2;

(ii) *Drooling of saliva*: UPDRS-Part II-Item 6 score ≥2;

(iii) *Swallowing difficulties*: UPDRS-Part II-Item 7 score ≥2;

(iv) *Facial expression (hypomimia)*: UPDRS-Part III-Item 19 score ≥2.

Furthermore, a new aggregate indicator was obtained to represent the entire orofacial burden/severity by summing the scores on UPDRS items 5, 6, 7, and 19. For the assessment of disease progression, three outcome variables were defined as follows:

(i) *Progression in motor symptoms*: follow-up UPDRS-Part II total score >10 (above median)

(ii) *Progression in motor signs*: follow-up UPDRS-Part III total score >28 (above median)

2.4. Statistical Analysis. Data were analyzed using SPSS software version 22 (IBM co., USA). To describe quantitative and qualitative variables mean [standard deviation (SD)] and frequency percentage (%) were reported, respectively. For univariate comparisons between the subgroups, Chi-square, Fisher's exact, and independent samples t tests were applied wherever appropriate. Multivariate binary logistic regression analyses were performed to investigate independent variables that associate with different orofacial symptoms after adjustment for sex, baseline age, duration of disease, and UPDRS-Part III (as the indicator of disease severity). For each orofacial manifestation, a multivariate regression model was created where, in addition to the list of control variables, other potential independent variables with a p value of <0.1 in univariate comparison were entered into the model. Multivariate Cox regression model was also applied to investigate the effects of baseline orofacial score on the progression of motor disability taking the time into account. Regarding the type of regression model, either odds' ratio (OR) or hazard ratio (HR) and their 95% confidence interval (CI) were reported.

Kaplan-Meier survival analysis was applied to calculate the mean and median time interval needed to develop certain outcomes of interest, namely, orofacial symptoms, UPDRS-Part I (>2), UPDRS-Part II (>10), and UPDRS-Part III (>28), of more than the median value of the maximum score during follow-up. In all analytical procedures, a two-tailed p value of less than 0.05 was considered to show statistical significant difference or association.

3. Results

3.1. Baseline Characteristics. A total number of 314 patients with IPD were recruited in this project. The study population consisted of 193 (61.5%) males and the average of age and disease duration was 64.7 (SD = 9.9) yr and 6.6 (SD = 5.5) yr at the time of registration. The average scores of the UPDRS-Part II, Part III, and entire scale at baseline were 9.3 (SD = 5.0), 21.7 (SD = 12.3), and 32.3 (SD = 15.0), respectively. More than 85% of the patients were under treatment with levodopa and dopamine agonists were prescribed in almost half of the study population. Other baseline and clinical characteristics are summarized in Table 1.

3.2. Prevalence and Time of Developing Orofacial Symptoms. Hypomimia, affected speech, drooling, and impaired swallowing were present in 37.3%, 14.1%, 11.7%, and 10.2% of the IPD patients at baseline. More patients developed orofacial symptoms during the follow-up period. Hypomimia (91.6%) followed by speech problems (65.5%) and drooling (55.3%) were the most common orofacial symptoms in this cohort (Figure 1). Descriptive Kaplan-Meier survival analysis demonstrated that the average time to develop hypomimia and speech problems was 0.9 (SE = 0.1) yr and 6.4 (SE = 0.4) yr, respectively. It took longer time to develop considerable drooling [7.4 (SE = 0.4) yr] and swallowing difficulties [8.3 (SE = 0.4) yr] in IPD patients following the baseline assessment.

Table 1: Baseline, demographic, and clinical characteristics of the study population with idiopathic Parkinson's disease (IPD) (n = 314).

Characteristic	Value
Sex-male (%)	61.5%
Age (at baseline) (yr) mean (SD)	64.7 (9.9)
Disease duration (yr) mean (SD)	6.6 (5.5)
Follow-up time (yr) mean (SD)	3.5 (2.9)
Baseline symptoms (%)	
Resting tremor	76.9%
Bradykinesia	73.4%
Rigidity	76.2%
Fall	18.2%
Freezing	13.3%
Dyskinesia	23.8%
Wearing off	14.7%
Postural instability	8.4%
Visual impairment	19.6%
Hyposmia	9.1%
Urinary urgency	21.7%
Orthostatic hypotension	12.6%
Voice changes	16.8%
Depression	18.2%
UPDRS score (at baseline) mean (SD)	
Part I	0.8 (1.3)
Part II	9.3 (5.0)
Part III	21.7 (12.3)
Part IV	0.5 (1.7)
Total	32.3 (15.0)
Type of medication (%)	
Levodopa	85.3%
Dopamine agonist	49.2%
MAO-B inhibitor	13.2%
Other dopaminergics	5.6%
Orofacial symptoms (during follow-up) (%)	
Drooling	55.3%
Speech problems	65.5%
Swallowing difficulties	34.5%
Facial expression	91.6%

SD: standard deviation; UPDRS: Unified Parkinson's Disease Rating Scale.

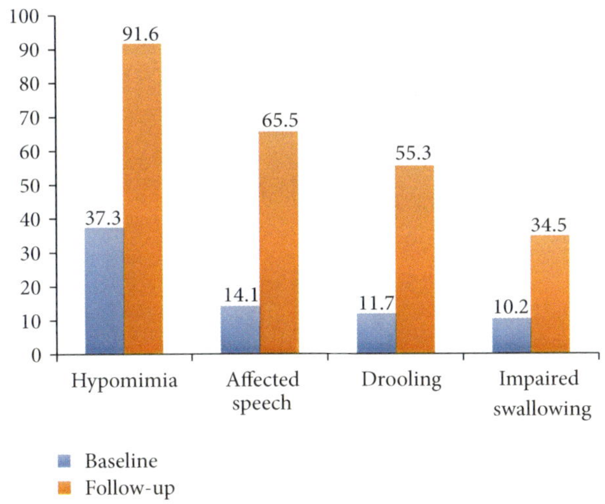

FIGURE 1: Prevalence rate (%) of different orofacial symptoms in study participants with idiopathic Parkinson's disease (IPD) at baseline and at the end of follow-up.

3.3. Determinant Factors of Orofacial Symptoms. Results from univariate comparison of baseline demographic and clinical characteristics between IPD patients with and without different orofacial symptoms are summarized in Table 2. At baseline, voice changes were more commonly presented in IPD patients who further developed speech problems (46.4% versus 9.3%, $p < 0.001$). Asymmetry index was significantly lower in this subgroup of participants as well as the ones with drooling, swallowing difficulties, and hypomimia (all $p < 0.05$). Orthostatic hypotension was more prevalent in patients with drooling (23.8% versus 6.6%, $p = 0.044$). IPD patients with prominent hypomimia had significantly higher prevalence of rigidity (83.0% versus 60.5%, $p = 0.004$), dyskinesia (30.0% versus 9.3%, $p = 0.009$), and urinary urgency (29.0% versus 4.7%, $p = 0.001$) compared to those who did not develop hypomimia (Table 2). As shown in Table 2, administration of different medications including levodopa, dopamine agonist, MAO-B inhibitor, and other dopaminergic drugs was not significantly different between IPD patients with and without orofacial symptoms (all $p > 0.05$). However, levodopa was in general more commonly used among those who developed orofacial symptoms (Table 2). We also analyzed whether medications correlate with the progression of orofacial symptoms over time. After adjusting by disease duration, administration of MAO-B inhibitor significantly lessened the progression of drooling over time ($p = 0.011$).

Multivariate analysis was performed to explore the factors that independently associated with the development of orofacial symptoms after adjustment for sex, baseline age, duration, and severity of the disease (measured by UPDRS-Part III). As shown in Table 3, except for swallowing difficulties, male sex was a risk factor for developing speech problems [OR = 2.3 (95% CI: 1.0–4.9)], drooling [OR = 2.4 (95% CI: 1.0–5.9)], and hypomimia [OR = 2.0 (95% CI: 1.1–3.6)]. More asymmetric manifestation [OR = 0.2 (95% CI: 0.1–0.8)] and higher tremor score [OR = 0.3 (95% CI: 0.1–0.7)] were found to be protective factors for speech impairment. Participants with dominant rigidity [OR = 5.2 (95% CI: 1.4–19.1)] and autonomic disturbances [OR = 3.4 (95% CI: 1.1–10.9)] at baseline were more likely to develop drooling. Urinary urgency was a strong determinant factor for considerable hypomimia during follow-up [OR = 6.7 (95% CI: 1.5–30.7)].

3.4. Prognostic Value of Orofacial Symptoms for Disease Progression. Kaplan-Meier analysis showed that IPD patients with speech impairments [4.4 (SE = 0.6) yr versus 8.5 (SE = 0.4) yr; $p = 0.006$] and drooling [5.0 (SE = 1.6) yr versus 8.1 (SE = 0.8) yr; $p = 0.018$] more quickly progressed to the UPDRS-Part II score of >10. In addition, participants with hypomimia [5.4 (SE = 0.6) yr versus 12.5 (SE = 3.2) yr; $p = 0.001$] and drooling [4.9 (SE = 1.0) yr versus 7.2 (SE = 0.9) yr; $p = 0.030$] had worse prognosis by more rapid progression to the UPDRS-Part III score of >28. As illustrated in Figure 2, further analysis was performed dividing study population into three tertiles based on the sum of the baseline UPDRS scores on orofacial items. IPD patients with more severe orofacial symptoms at baseline had a shorter median time to develop into a worse motor disability status showed by UPDRS-Part II > 10 [3rd tertile = 0.8 yr (SE = 0.6), 2nd tertile = 8.0 yr (SE = 1.3), and 1st tertile = 8.5 yr (SE = 1.4); $p < 0.001$] and UPDRS-Part III > 28 [3rd tertile = 4.7 (SE = 2.2) yr, 2nd tertile = 6.2 (SE = 0.9) yr, and 1st tertile = 7.8 (SE = 1.0) yr; $p = 0.014$]. Finally, results from a multivariate Cox regression model showed that baseline orofacial burden score [HR = 1.10 (95% CI: 1.01–1.20)] was a stronger predictor of hazard of developing UPDRS-Part III > 28 when compared to baseline PIGD score [1.08 (95% CI: 0.92–1.28)]. Similarly, baseline orofacial score [HR = 1.20 (95% CI: 1.10–1.31)] significantly associated with hazard of UPDRS-Part II > 10, whereas baseline PIGD score failed [HR = 0.75 (95% CI: 0.56–1.00)].

4. Discussion

Capitalizing upon the collection of longitudinal data from routine clinical practice of a PD cohort, our study is one of the few to extensively explore the picture of orofacial symptoms in people with IPD. Hypomimia was found to be the most common orofacial manifestation both at the baseline and throughout the course of progression followed, respectively, by speech problems, drooling of saliva, and impaired swallowing. More symmetric involvement, autonomic disturbances, and male gender were found to be significant determinants of developing different orofacial symptoms in PD. We also created a new single indicator to represent orofacial burden by adding up the scores of all orofacial manifestations. The indicator was significantly correlated to disease prognosis after an average of 4.2 years. The more severe orofacial burden was at baseline, the more rapidly individuals progressed into a more severe motor disability state. Interestingly, the single indicator, orofacial burden, showed more promising results in prediction of PD progression compared to the PIGD score at baseline.

Table 2: Univariate comparison of the baseline, demographic, and clinical characteristics of Parkinson's disease patients regarding orofacial symptoms.

Characteristic	Speech			Salivation			Swallowing			Facial expression		
	Normal ($n = 141$)	Affected ($n = 65$)	p value	Normal ($n = 158$)	Affected ($n = 48$)	p value	Normal ($n = 170$)	Affected ($n = 36$)	p value	Normal ($n = 116$)	Affected ($n = 195$)	p value
Sex-male (%)	60.3%	73.8%	0.059	62.0%	72.9%	0.167	62.9%	72.2%	0.290	55.2%	65.6%	0.066
Age (at baseline) (yr) mean (SD)	61.7 (8.7)	62.9 (10.0)	0.388	61.7 (9.1)	63.3 (9.2)	0.279	62.4 (8.8)	60.4 (10.4)	0.213	64.0 (10.6)	65.1 (9.6)	0.359
Disease duration (yr) mean (SD)	7.0 (5.7)	7.6 (5.7)	0.556	7.1 (5.8)	7.4 (5.5)	0.768	6.7 (5.5)	9.2 (5.8)	**0.032**	5.8 (5.6)	7.0 (5.4)	0.144
Baseline symptoms (%)												
Resting tremor	79.6%	67.9%	0.239	77.0%	71.4%	0.605	73.1%	86.7%	0.339	86.0%	73.0%	0.090
Bradykinesia	81.5%	75.0%	0.492	75.4%	90.5%	0.214	83.6%	60.0%	**0.042**	62.8%	78.0%	0.059
Rigidity	77.8%	85.7%	0.559	75.4%	95.2%	0.058	80.6%	80.0%	1	60.5%	83.0%	**0.004**
Fall	20.4%	14.3%	0.563	16.4%	23.8%	0.448	14.9%	33.3%	0.096	18.6%	18.0%	0.931
Freezing	16.7%	14.3%	1	18.0%	9.5%	0.498	16.4%	13.3%	1	7.0%	16.0%	0.185
Dyskinesia	31.5%	28.6%	0.786	34.4%	19.0%	0.273	26.9%	46.7%	0.132	9.3%	30.0%	**0.009**
Wearing off	24.1%	10.7%	0.239	21.3%	14.3%	0.750	16.4%	33.3%	0.135	9.3%	17.0%	0.307
Postural instability	7.4%	10.7%	0.686	8.2%	9.5%	1	6.0%	20.0%	0.111	4.7%	10.0%	0.511
Visual impairment	31.5%	17.9%	0.187	27.9%	23.8%	0.717	28.4%	20.0%	0.748	11.6%	23.0%	0.116
Hyposmia	13.0%	10.7%	1	9.8%	19.0%	0.269	13.4%	6.7%	0.680	9.3%	9.0%	0.954
Urinary urgency	20.4%	28.6%	0.404	18.0%	38.1%	0.060	25.4%	13.3%	0.501	4.7%	29.0%	**0.001**
Orthostatic hypotension	7.4%	17.9%	0.262	6.6%	23.8%	**0.044**	10.4%	13.3%	0.666	11.6%	13.0%	0.821
Voice changes	9.3%	46.4%	**<0.001**	21.3%	23.8%	0.811	20.9%	26.7%	0.731	9.3%	20.0%	0.146
Depression	16.7%	21.4%	0.597	18.0%	19.0%	1	17.9%	20.0%	1	14.0%	20.0%	0.390
UPDRS score (at baseline) mean (SD)												
Part I	1.1 (1.5)	1.0 (1.4)	0.558	1.1 (1.5)	1.2 (1.6)	0.756	1.1 (1.5)	1.1 (1.6)	0.890	0.6 (1.1)	0.9 (1.5)	**0.028**
Part II	8.6 (5.1)	11.0 (4.3)	**0.011**	8.4 (4.3)	12.2 (5.9)	**<0.001**	9.2 (5.2)	9.6 (4.1)	0.735	7.4 (3.8)	9.9 (4.5)	**0.002**
Part III	18.6 (9.5)	22.0 (10.9)	**0.027**	18.2 (9.5)	24.4 (10.3)	**<0.001**	19.2 (9.7)	21.5 (11.4)	0.212	17.3 (10.8)	24.4 (12.4)	**<0.001**
Part IV	0.7 (1.9)	0.7 (1.9)	0.801	0.7 (1.9)	0.8 (2.1)	0.840	0.8 (2.0)	0.6 (1.3)	0.633	0.2 (1.1)	0.7 (1.9)	**0.013**
Total	30.1 (14.2)	37.9 (15.9)	**0.010**	29.4 (13.8)	41.1 (15.5)	**<0.001**	31.9 (14.4)	34.0 (17.8)	0.567	25.2 (13.4)	35.9 (14.6)	**<0.001**
Type of medication (%)												
Levodopa	78.8%	90.9%	0.137	81.4%	87.5%	0.590	80.8%	92.0%	0.243	78.0%	88.4%	0.058
Dopamine agonist	49.4%	61.4%	0.197	55.7%	46.9%	0.387	54.8%	48.0%	0.540	54.2%	47.1%	0.359
MAO-B inhibitor	15.3%	9.1%	0.416	11.3%	18.8%	0.283	13.5%	12.0%	1	10.2%	14.5%	0.412
Other dopaminergics	7.1%	4.5%	0.715	6.2%	6.3%	1	6.7%	4.0%	1	5.1%	5.8%	1
Disease parameters mean (SD)												
Tremor score	0.5 (0.5)	0.4 (0.4)	0.063	0.5 (0.4)	0.5 (0.5)	0.731	0.5 (0.4)	0.6 (0.5)	0.296	0.4 (0.4)	0.5 (0.5)	0.072
PIGD score	0.6 (0.6)	0.7 (0.5)	0.207	0.6 (0.5)	0.8 (0.7)	0.069	0.6 (0.6)	0.6 (0.6)	0.728	0.7 (0.7)	0.8 (0.8)	0.203
Asymmetry index	0.6 (0.4)	0.4 (0.3)	**0.001**	0.6 (0.4)	0.4 (0.3)	**0.004**	0.6 (0.4)	0.4 (0.3)	**0.035**	0.6 (0.4)	0.4 (0.3)	**<0.001**

SD: standard deviation; UPDRS: Unified Parkinson's Disease Rating Scale; PIGD: postural instability/gait difficulty; all orofacial symptoms were considered present if a score of at least 2 in the UPDRS-Part II or III was recorded at any time during the follow-up period.

TABLE 3: Multivariate regression models for significant independent determinant factors of different orofacial symptoms in patients with idiopathic Parkinson's disease (IPD).

Orofacial symptom	Significant determinants (*Logistic regression model*)
Speech	Male sex: OR = 2.3 (95% CI: 1.0–4.9)
	UPDRS-Part III: OR = 1.1 (95% CI: 1.0–1.1)
	Voice changes: OR = 9.4 (95% CI: 2.6–33.2)
	Tremor score: OR = 0.3 (95% CI: 0.1–0.7)
	Asymmetry index: OR = 0.2 (95% CI: 0.1–0.8)
Salivation	Male sex: OR = 2.4 (95% CI: 1.0–5.9)
	UPDRS-Part II: OR = 1.2 (95% CI: 1.1–1.3)
	UPDRS-Part III: OR = 1.1 (95% CI: 1.0–1.1)
	Dominant rigidity: OR = 5.2 (95% CI: 1.4–19.1)
	Autonomic disturbance: OR = 3.4 (95% CI: 1.1–10.9)
Swallowing	Disease duration: OR = 1.1 (95% CI: 1.0–1.2)
Facial expression	Male sex: OR = 2.0 (95% CI: 1.1–3.6)
	UPDRS-Part III: OR = 1.1 (95% CI: 1.0–1.1)
	Dominant rigidity: OR = 2.8 (95% CI: 1.1–6.6)
	Dyskinesia: OR = 5.7 (95% CI: 1.6–19.8)
	Urinary urgency: OR = 6.7 (95% CI: 1.5–30.7)

OR: odds' ratio; UPDRS: Unified Parkinson's Disease Rating Scale; all orofacial symptoms were considered present if a score of at least 2 in the UPDRS-Part II or III was recorded at any time during the follow-up period; all variables with a p value of <0.1 in univariate comparisons were checked for an independent effect in multivariate regression models; all regression models have been adjusted at least for sex, baseline age, duration of disease, and UPDRS-Part III (as the indicator of disease severity either as score or tertile); all presented determinant factors showed a p value of <0.05 in each multivariate regression model.

Having gathered data on an orofacial screening test consisting of masticatory performance and oral health, Bakke et al. showed consistent correlation between the severity of PD (measured by Hoehn and Yahr and UPDRS score) and orofacial manifestations [1]. As also shown by our study, it is demonstrated that, in general, severity of orofacial symptoms is a reflection of the severity of motor disability in PD. In line with our results, another study showed that drooling of saliva more commonly occurred in males and those with a more advanced PD, though it could also happen as early as in Hoehn and Yahr stages 1 and 2, too [8, 14]. Kalf et al., in an investigation on 104 consecutive outpatients showed that people with PD who complained of drooling were significantly older and had longer disease duration and more severe PD [15]. While we also found higher UPDRS score as a significant determinant of drooling, disease duration and age failed to be strong associates of drooling in our cohort. The lack of a prominent association between disease duration and drooling has been recently shown by Ou et al. in another large cohort of 518 Chinese PD patients [16], too. However, this study also demonstrated higher UPDRS-Part-III as a significant determinant for drooling [16]. The fact that drooling is mostly associated with higher motor disability but not necessarily with disease duration indicates that drooling could be a manifestation of a more rapidly progressing phenotype of PD.

Our study is one of the few to report an association between autonomic dysfunction and more symmetric pattern with drooling. This connection was shown by few other studies [14, 17] and is consistent with the theory on the involvement of the vagus nerve in the pathophysiologic pathway of drooling via controlling deglutition and esophageal motility [18].

Impaired swallowing or dysphagia, as another common orofacial manifestation of PD, was present in 34.5% of our cohort during the follow-up. A recent systematic review revealed that a wide range of prevalence from 11% to 81% has been reported for dysphagia in different PD populations [19]. Our findings showed that swallowing ability is more likely to be impaired in individuals with longer duration of PD and a more symmetric phenotype. Another study found that dysphasia progression is closely associated with age at onset and severity of motor disability in PD [20]. Other determinants of dysphagia in PD reported in the literature are low body weight, drooling of saliva, and dementia [21]. Prevalence of speech problems increased by 4-5 times from baseline and reached up to 65% within the course of PD progression in our study. It has been estimated that as high as 89% of PD populations eventually experience speech impairment [22]. In line with our findings, Dias et al. also found that speech impairment does not correlate with the age of onset, but it is more likely to happen in people with more severe PD [23]. Moreover, according to our findings, speech problems were also more common among males, and those with a more symmetric PD. Our findings of higher burden of orofacial manifestations in people with more symmetric PD are consistent with a recent longitudinal investigation showing more symmetric distribution of motor symptoms in PD accompanies with a poorer prognosis in general [24]. Even though this association is thought to be entirely explained by the confounding effect of higher age and longer disease duration [24], our multivariate analysis showed that symmetric PD correlates with higher prevalence of orofacial features independent of disease duration and severity.

To our knowledge, our study is one of the few to comprehensively explore the evolution of orofacial symptoms in PD and the first to investigate the prognostic value of the aggregated orofacial burden for PD prognosis with longitudinal follow-up. Nevertheless, we acknowledge the limitations of our study. First, due to the real-world registry-based nature of our database and the time limitation during each visit, we did not have information on various other manifestations of PD such as cognition, sleep problems, full autonomic assessment, and psychiatric features. Second, based on the same reasons, we used subjective self-reported data for some symptoms (i.e., depression, hyposmia) and not validated batteries, questionnaires, and instruments. Yet, all examinations and assessments were done by expert neurologists and even self-reported data are quite commonly and reliably used in register-based settings. Lastly, detailed information on treatment options, in particular the specific interventions for drooling such as botulinum toxin, was not available.

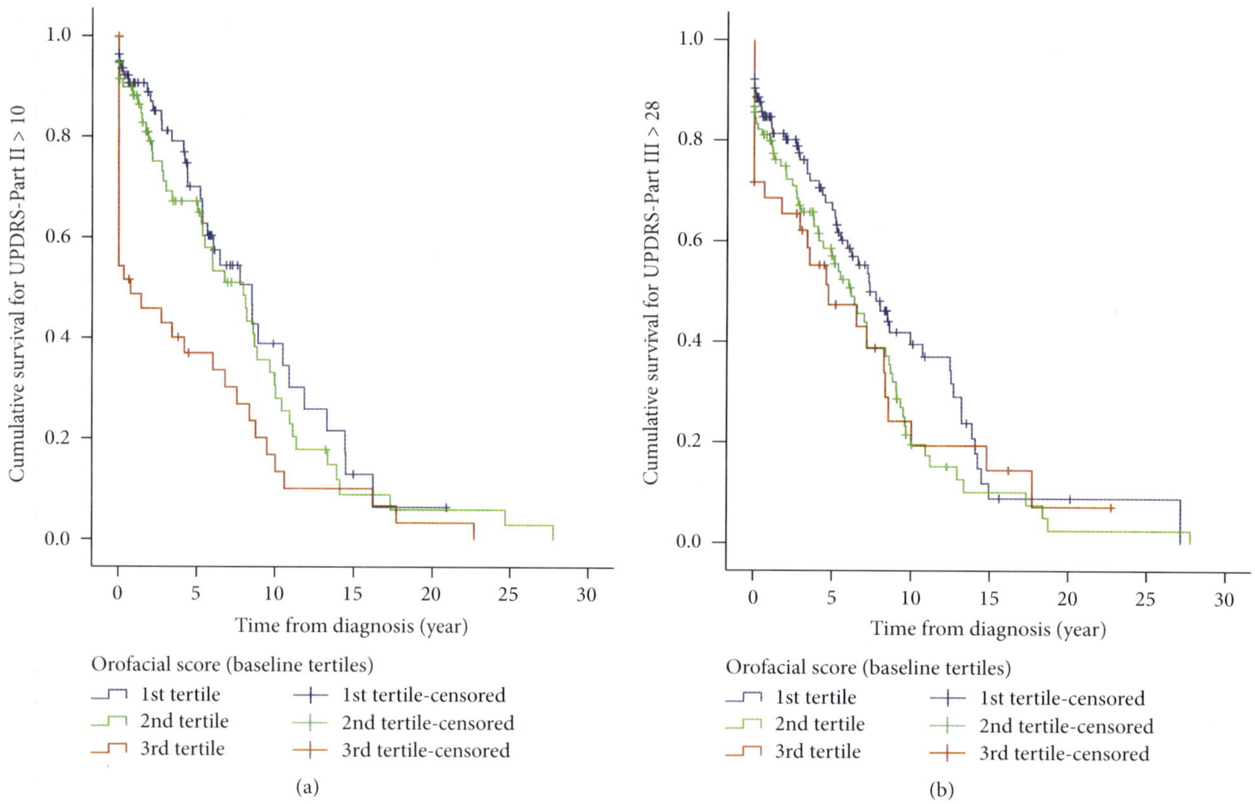

FIGURE 2: Survival curve to progress into the more than median value of the maximum UPDRS scores during the follow-up in patients with idiopathic Parkinson's disease with different severities of orofacial symptoms at baseline: (a) UPDRS-Part II: 1st tertile [median survival time = 8.5 yr (SE = 1.4)], 2nd tertile [median survival time = 8.0 yr (SE = 1.3)], and 3rd tertile [median survival time = 0.8 yr (SE = 0.6)] (Breslow p value < 0.001). (b) UPDRS-Part III: 1st tertile [median survival time = 7.8 yr (SE = 1.0)], 2nd tertile [median survival time = 6.2 yr (SE = 0.9)], and 3rd tertile [median survival time = 4.7 yr (SE = 2.2)] (Breslow p value = 0.014).

In conclusion, orofacial manifestations are important components of PD phenotyping. Majority of people with PD evolve orofacial problems such as hypomimia, speech problems, drooling of saliva, and impaired swallowing. Measures of disease severity, symmetry, and autonomic disturbance correlate with orofacial manifestations. Individuals with more severe orofacial burden at baseline progressed faster to the advanced stages of PD with further motor disability. This prognostic value could be an applicable finding bearing in mind that orofacial manifestations are quite visible and easy to recognize. In addition, orofacial symptoms such as drooling and speech problems may potentially cause embarrassment, suffering, and increased disease burden [18]. Nevertheless, orofacial features of PD have not been fully addressed and are frequently neglected by the patients, their caregivers, and their clinicians. Greater awareness of the importance of orofacial features in PD is needed to optimize their management and potentially slow down the rate of disease progression.

From another perspective, our study highlights the usefulness of data registration in PD outpatient clinics. Having collected data from clinical practice, such real-world information could be a great reflection of what is routinely happening in people with PD, what is the natural course of progression, and what are its predictors. Of note, the "*Jönköping Parkinson Registry*" is now a part of the national PD register in Sweden launched in 2011.

Acknowledgments

The authors are grateful to all patients, care givers, physicians, data administrators, and reporting units for their contribution in the "*Jönköping Parkinson Registry.*" Special thanks are due to Sven-Erik Pålhagen, M.D., Ph.D., who was the promotor of this register.

References

[1] M. Bakke, S. L. Larsen, C. Lautrup, and M. Karlsborg, "Orofacial function and oral health in patients with Parkinson's disease," *European Journal of Oral Sciences*, vol. 119, no. 1, pp. 27–32, 2011.

[2] M. Bologna, G. Fabbrini, L. Marsili, G. Defazio, P. D. Thompson, and A. Berardelli, "Facial bradykinesia," *Journal of Neurology, Neurosurgery and Psychiatry*, vol. 84, no. 6, pp. 681–685, 2013.

[3] L. T. Robertson and J. P. Hammerstad, "Jaw movement dysfunction related to Parkinson's disease and partially modified

by levodopa," *Journal of Neurology Neurosurgery and Psychiatry*, vol. 60, no. 1, pp. 41–50, 1996.

[4] S. Karlsson, M. Persson, and B. Johnels, "Levodopa induced on-off motor fluctuations in Parkinson's disease related to rhythmical masticatory jaw movements," *Journal of Neurology Neurosurgery and Psychiatry*, vol. 55, no. 4, pp. 304–307, 1992.

[5] N. A. Leopold and M. C. Kagel, "Prepharyngeal dysphagia in Parkinson's disease," *Dysphagia*, vol. 11, no. 1, pp. 14–22, 1996.

[6] P. Srivanitchapoom, S. Pandey, and M. Hallett, "Drooling in Parkinson's disease: a review," *Parkinsonism and Related Disorders*, vol. 20, no. 11, pp. 1109–1118, 2014.

[7] K. L. Chou, M. Evatt, V. Hinson, and K. Kompoliti, "Sialorrhea in Parkinson's disease: a review," *Movement Disorders*, vol. 22, no. 16, pp. 2306–2313, 2007.

[8] A. Q. Rana, M. S. Yousuf, N. Awan, and A. Fattah, "Impact of progression of Parkinson's disease on drooling in various ethnic groups," *European Neurology*, vol. 67, no. 5, pp. 312–314, 2012.

[9] J. G. Kalf, B. J. M. de Swart, B. R. Bloem, and M. Munneke, "Prevalence of oropharyngeal dysphagia in Parkinson's disease: a meta-analysis," *Parkinsonism and Related Disorders*, vol. 18, no. 4, pp. 311–315, 2012.

[10] J. P. Sutton, "Dysphagia in Parkinson's disease is responsive to levodopa," *Parkinsonism and Related Disorders*, vol. 19, no. 3, pp. 282–284, 2013.

[11] M. C. Schiess, H. Zheng, V. M. Soukup, J. G. Bonnen, and H. J. W. Nauta, "Parkinson's disease subtypes: Clinical classification and ventricular cerebrospinal fluid analysis," *Parkinsonism and Related Disorders*, vol. 6, no. 2, pp. 69–76, 2000.

[12] S. M. Van Rooden, F. Colas, P. Martínez-Martín et al., "Clinical subtypes of Parkinson's disease," *Movement Disorders*, vol. 26, no. 1, pp. 51–58, 2011.

[13] A. J. Espay, J.-Y. Li, L. Johnston, R. Chen, and A. E. Lang, "Mirror movements in parkinsonism: Evaluation of a new clinical sign," *Journal of Neurology, Neurosurgery and Psychiatry*, vol. 76, no. 10, pp. 1355–1358, 2005.

[14] D. Verbaan, J. Marinus, M. Visser, S. M. Van Rooden, A. M. Stiggelbout, and J. J. Van Hilten, "Patient-reported autonomic symptoms in Parkinson disease," *Neurology*, vol. 69, no. 4, pp. 333–341, 2007.

[15] J. G. Kalf, B. R. Bloem, and M. Munneke, "Diurnal and nocturnal drooling in Parkinson's disease," *Journal of Neurology*, vol. 259, no. 1, pp. 119–123, 2012.

[16] R. Ou, X. Guo, Q. Wei et al., "Prevalence and clinical correlates of drooling in Parkinson disease: A study on 518 Chinese patients," *Parkinsonism and Related Disorders*, vol. 21, no. 3, pp. 211–215, 2015.

[17] M. F. Siddiqui, S. Rast, M. J. Lynn, A. P. Auchus, and R. F. Pfeiffer, "Autonomic dysfunction in Parkinson's disease: a comprehensive symptom survey," *Parkinsonism and Related Disorders*, vol. 8, no. 4, pp. 277–284, 2002.

[18] Y. Zlotnik, Y. Balash, A. D. Korczyn, N. Giladi, and T. Gurevich, "Disorders of the oral cavity in parkinson's disease and parkinsonian syndromes," *Parkinson's Disease*, vol. 2015, Article ID 379482, 6 pages, 2015.

[19] C. Takizawa, E. Gemmell, J. Kenworthy, and R. Speyer, "A Systematic Review of the Prevalence of Oropharyngeal Dysphagia in Stroke, Parkinson's Disease, Alzheimer's Disease, Head Injury, and Pneumonia," *Dysphagia*, vol. 31, no. 3, pp. 434–441, 2016.

[20] L. Liu, X.-G. Luo, C.-L. Dy et al., "Characteristics of language impairment in Parkinson's disease and its influencing factors," *Translational Neurodegeneration*, vol. 4, no. 1, article 2, 2015.

[21] I. Suttrup and T. Warnecke, "Dysphagia in Parkinson's Disease," *Dysphagia*, vol. 31, no. 1, pp. 24–32, 2016.

[22] J. R. Duffy, *Motor Speech Disorders: Substrates, Differential Diagnosis, and Management*, Mosby, St. Louis, Mo, USA, 2nd edition, 2005.

[23] A. E. Dias, M. T. Barbosa, J. C. P. Limongi, and E. R. Barbosa, "Speech disorders did not correlate with age at onset of Parkinson's disease," *Arquivos de Neuro-Psiquiatria*, vol. 74, no. 2, pp. 117–121, 2016.

[24] J. Marinus and J. J. van Hilten, "The significance of motor (A)symmetry in Parkinson's disease," *Movement Disorders*, vol. 30, no. 3, pp. 379–385, 2015.

25

Pisa Syndrome in Parkinson's Disease: Evidence for Bilateral Vestibulospinal Dysfunction

Giulia Di Lazzaro,[1] Tommaso Schirinzi,[1] Maria Pia Giambrone,[1] Roberta Di Mauro,[2] Maria Giuseppina Palmieri,[1] Camilla Rocchi,[1] Michele Tinazzi,[3] Nicola Biagio Mercuri,[1,4] Stefano Di Girolamo,[2] and Antonio Pisani[1,4]

[1]*Department of Systems Medicine, University of Rome Tor Vergata, Rome, Italy*
[2]*Department of Otorhinolaryngology, University of Rome Tor Vergata, Rome, Italy*
[3]*Department of Neuroscience, Biomedicine and Movement Sciences, University of Verona, Verona, Italy*
[4]*Fondazione Santa Lucia IRCCS, Rome, Italy*

Correspondence should be addressed to Antonio Pisani; pisani@uniroma2.it

Academic Editor: Pablo Mir

Introduction. Pisa syndrome (PS) is a postural complication of Parkinson's disease (PD). Yet, its pathophysiology remains unclear, although a multifactorial component is probable. Cervical vestibular evoked myogenic potentials (cVEMPs) explore vestibulospinal pathway, but they have not been measured yet in PD patients with PS (PDPS) to assess a potential vestibular impairment. *Materials and Methods.* We enrolled 15 PD patients, 15 PDPS patients, and 30 healthy controls (HCs). They underwent neurological examination and were examined with Unified Parkinson's Disease Rating Scale II-III (UPDRSII-III), audiovestibular workup, and cVEMP recordings. Data were analysed with Chi-square, one-way ANOVA, multinomial regression, nonparametric, and Spearman's tests. *Results.* cVEMPs were significantly impaired in both PD and PDPS compared with HCs. PDPS exhibited more severe cVEMP abnormalities with prevalent bilateral loss of potentials, compared with the PD group, in which a prevalent unilateral loss was instead observed. No clinical-neurophysiological correlations emerged. *Conclusions.* Differently from HC, cVEMPs are altered in PD. Severity of cVEMPs alterations increases from PD without PS to PDPS, suggesting an involvement of vestibulospinal pathway in the pathophysiology of PS. Our results provide evidence for a significant impairment of cVEMPs in PDPS patients and encourage further studies to test validity of cVEMPs as diagnostic and prognostic biomarkers of PD progression.

1. Introduction

Parkinson's disease (PD) is a common neurodegenerative disease characterized by both motor and nonmotor features. While motor signs (tremor, rigidity, and bradykinesia) mainly originate from the loss of dopaminergic neurons of *substantia nigra pars compacta* (SNpc) [1, 2], the pathophysiology of the large cohort of symptoms complicating the disease course, such as postural impairment, remains unclear, although it has been ascribed to the progressive degeneration of other cortical and subcortical structures [1].

Pisa syndrome (PS) is a peculiar postural complication, consisting in a persistent lateral trunk flexion (LTF) of more than 10° that can be reduced by passive mobilization or supine positioning, occurring throughout the disease course but favoured by the longer disease duration and responsible for severe disability [3–5]. Neurochemical imbalance in the basal ganglia homeostasis, defective sensory-motor integration, abnormal body scheme perception, together with a peripheral involvement consisting in myopathy, and other musculoskeletal affections have been proposed to contribute to the pathophysiology of PS [3, 6, 7]. However, the precise mechanisms have not been clarified yet.

Recently, a renewed interest emerged for vestibular evoked myogenic potentials (VEMPs), utilized for testing short-latency myogenic responses evoked by sound stimulation of vestibular system [8]. Specifically, cervical vestibular evoked myogenic potentials (cVEMPs) represent the sternocleidomastoid (SCM) muscle response to sound activation of saccule and signal transmission via the vestibulospinal tract. Thus, cVEMPs are a simple and reliable tool to explore the activity of the vestibulocollic reflex, linking the VIII and XI cranial nuclei, thereby representing an index of brainstem integrity [9–12]. Indeed, the vestibular system has been involved in the pathophysiology of PS [13], as well as in falls and other motor complications of advanced PD [13–15].

In spite of such evidence, to date, few studies addressed these issues in PD population. Evidence has been provided for the loss of muscular potentials, in the absence of clear correlations with relevant clinical features, such as disease duration and severity, gait, or sleep disturbances [15–17]. However, cVEMPs measurement has not been utilized yet to evaluate vestibular involvement in PS.

In this study, we recorded cVEMPs to assess vestibular integrity in PD patients with PS (PDPS) compared with both PD patients without PS and healthy controls (HCs).

2. Materials and Methods

2.1. Materials. A total of 60 subjects were consecutively recruited at the movement disorders outpatient service, Tor Vergata University Hospital, Rome, Italy, between 2015 and 2017. Subjects were divided into 3 groups: PD patients ($n = 15$), PD patients with PS (PDPS, $n = 15$), and healthy controls (HC, $n = 30$). Idiopathic PD was diagnosed according to the British Parkinson's Disease Society Brain Bank criteria and confirmed by DaTscan [18]; PDPS patients showed trunk lateral flexion of at least 10°measured with a wall goniometer, alleviated by passive mobilization or supine positioning, according to recent diagnostic criteria [3]. HCs were healthy age-matched control subjects recruited from nonblood relatives of PD patients who did not show any neurological sign.

Exclusion criteria included dementia (MMSE score <24), cervical herniation, history of orthopaedic diseases (such as scoliosis), major spinal surgery, improper neck movements that could alter audiological assessment, middle ear diseases, hearing thresholds exceeding 50 dBHL, and medical therapy potentially interfering with vestibular function or potentially able to induce PS (e.g., neuroleptics).

All patients were evaluated by a movement disorder specialist, with Unified Parkinson's Disease Rating Scale (UPDRS) Sections II and III and Hoehn and Yahr scale (H & Y). Medical therapy was accurately recorded, and total levodopa equivalent daily dose (LEDD) was calculated for each patient.

All enrolled subjects underwent audiological workup to exclude hearing impairment, which could alter VEMPs recording. Then, cVEMPs were recorded, as described below. The entire assessment was performed in "on-therapy" state.

The study was conducted in agreement with ethical principles of Helsinki declaration. Informed consent was obtained from all participants.

2.2. Procedures

2.2.1. cVEMPs Recording. The test was performed in a hypoechoic room, with the patient lying down on an examination bed, head positioned at 30°. Five surface electrodes were placed, the negative ones on the medium third of SCM muscles bilaterally, the positive ones in the centre of claviculae, and the ground electrode on the sternum. While maintaining tonic contraction of SCM, a bilateral acoustic stimulation (alternate click) was given to the subject continuously for 30 s, at a frequency of 4 Hz, duration of 100 μs and at an intensity of 135 dB SPL, similarly in the three groups. The compound muscle action potentials (CMAPs) were then recorded as described [9].

Although muscle tonic activation was not measured, it was continuously monitored by visual feedback to assist the subject in maintaining the task. The recorded signals were amplified, averaged, and band-pass filtered (10–500 Hz). The procedure was performed at least twice to ensure reproducibility; grand average was analysed. CMAPs were evaluated qualitatively (present/absent) and quantitatively, measuring wave latencies and peak amplitudes from stimulus onset to the peak of the initial positivity (P13) and subsequent negativity (N23) [9]; interpeak latencies were also calculated [11] (Figure 1).

2.2.2. Audiological Workup. Each subject underwent an otolaryngologic evaluation, including otoscopic examination, acoustic impedance test and pure-tone audiometry (PTA) to exclude middle ear disorders. Hearing loss was estimated bilaterally and for each pure-tone frequency stimulation (from 125 to 8000 Hz). The intensity threshold of the acoustic reflex was determined for each ear using 500 Hz, 1000 Hz, 2000 Hz, and 4000 Hz stimulus tones. The stimulus was presented either to the same ear as the compliance probe (ipsilateral reflex) or to the opposite ear (contralateral reflex).

For the Brainstem Auditory Evoked Responses (BAER) assessment, the active electrode was mounted to the middle of the forehead "Fpz," the reference electrode to the ipsilateral mastoid "M1," and the ground to the contralateral one "M2." The test procedures followed the Sininger protocol [19]. Analysis of BAER was done quantitatively to assess the absolute latencies of waves I, III, and V and interpeak latencies of these waves (I–III, III–V, and I–V). Qualitative analysis of the waveform morphology included the subjective judgment on the shape and the quality of the waveforms.

2.3. Statistical Analysis. Differences among groups in categorical variables were calculated using the Chi-square test. Audiometric data were assessed separately by Kruskal–Wallis test for multiple comparisons and Wilcoxon test for repeated measures, as they were nonnormally distributed.

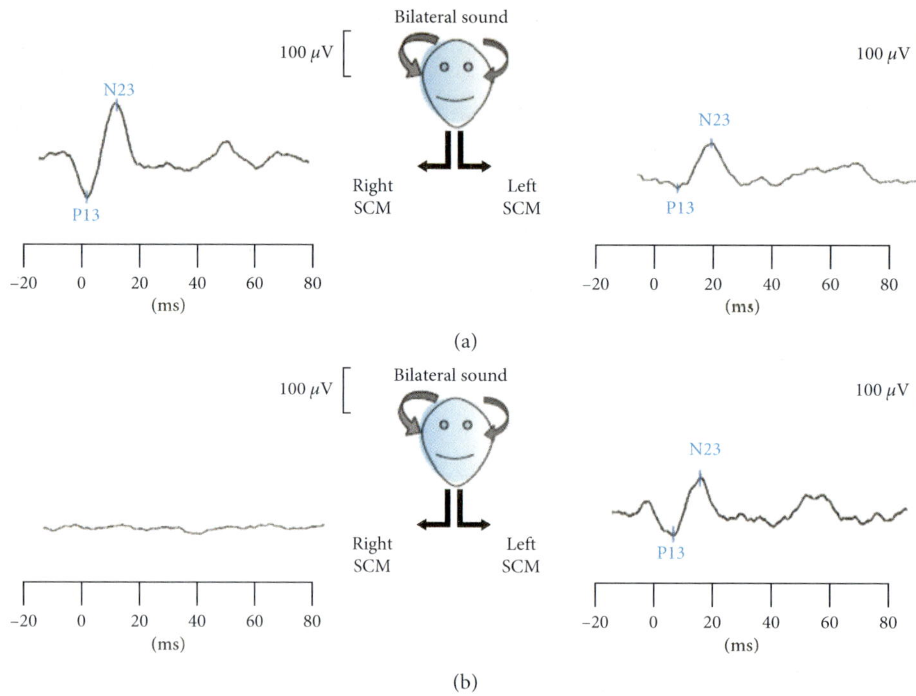

FIGURE 1: cVEMP recording in normal (a) and altered (b) conditions. In both (a) and (b) boxes, the two traces correspond, respectively, to right and left SCM muscle potential evoked by bilateral sound stimulation. P13 represents the potential's first peak of positivity, N23 the subsequent peak of negativity. In (a), cVEMPs are present bilaterally; in (b), cVEMP is lost on the right side.

The one-way ANOVA test with Bonferroni correction was performed for cVEMPs amplitude and latencies analysis among groups.

Correlations between neurophysiological parameters (unilateral or bilateral absence of cVEMPs, their amplitudes and latencies) and clinical features (disease duration, age of onset, UPDRS II-III as total scores and single subitems, degrees of LTF, and bending side) were assessed with Spearman's test. Moreover, after testing differences in cVEMPs alterations within the groups, the association between vestibular dysfunction and clinical presentation of PD was further assessed by means of multinomial logistic regression, using disease duration as covariate.

The level of statistical significance (p value) was set at 0.05. Statistical analyses were performed using the SPSS version 21 for Mac (SPSS Inc., Chicago).

3. Results

Main demographic, clinical, and neurophysiological data are summarized in Table 1.

Groups did not significantly differ in age, gender, and auditory testing (auditory thresholds and BAER latencies, data not shown). Disease duration, UPDRS part II-III scores, and LEDD were significantly higher in PDPS than in PD (respectively, $p < 0.001$, $p < 0.001$, $p < 0.001$, and $p = 0.013$). Conversely, no difference emerged in the prevalence of dopaminergic medications used in PD and PDPS groups; specifically, 11/15 PD patients and 9/15 PDPS patients were on dopamine agonists, 10/15 PD and 9/15 PDPS were on MAO-B inhibitors, and 12/15 PD and 13/15 PDPS were on levodopa.

Consistent with previous findings, the main alteration we observed in cVEMPs within the PD groups was the unilateral or bilateral absence of evoked potentials (Figure 1); even if PDPS and PD patients had longer P13 and N23 latencies, no significant differences emerged among other analysed variables.

Table 1 shows, for each group, the percentage of "normal," "unilateral absence," and "bilateral absence" of cVEMPs. Chi-square analysis demonstrated that normal cVEMPs were significantly reduced in both PD and PDPS compared with HC (respectively, $p < 0.001$ and $p < 0.001$). However, the pattern of cVEMP abnormalities significantly differed between PDPS and PD ($p < 0.0001$), with PDPS showing lower normal responses ($p < 0.05$) and more frequent "bilateral absence" ($p < 0.001$); otherwise "unilateral absence" was more common in PD than in PDPS ($p < 0.05$) (Figure 2).

Multinomial logistic regression showed that "unilateral absence" of cVEMPs but not "bilateral absence" is significantly associated with pure PD condition ($T = 21.9$, $p < 0.001$), independently from disease duration. Moreover, either "unilateral" or "bilateral" cVEMPs absence are directly associated with PDPS condition (respectively, $T = 3.4$, $p = 0.02$ $p = 0.02$ and $T = 21.2$, $p < 0.001$), as well as disease duration ($T = 0.4$, $p = 0.004$).

Finally, correlation analysis between neurophysiological and clinical parameters did not provide any significant result among the groups.

TABLE 1: Clinical and electrophysiological data (y = years; M = males; F = females; mg = milligrams; ms = millisecond; mcV = microVolt; LTF = lateral trunk flexion; R = right; L = left; LEDD = levodopa equivalent daily dose; n.s. = statistically nonsignificant). Data are expressed as mean ± standard deviation (SD).

	PDPS ($n = 15$)	PD ($n = 15$)	HC ($n = 30$)	
Age (y)	73.3 ± 3.6	69.6 ± 7.11	69.36 ± 6.67	n.s.
Gender (M/F)	8/7	7/8	15/15	n.s.
Disease duration (y)	8.7 ± 4.4	4.6 ± 3.83	—	$p < 0.001$
UPDRS II	12.4 ± 2.8	6.2 ± 3	—	$p < 0.001$
UPDRS III	30 ± 6.1	18.9 ± 6.1	—	$p < 0.001$
LTF (°)	21 ± 9	—	—	
Side of LTF (R/L)	7/8	—	—	
LEDD (mg)	814 ± 275	369 ± 202	—	$p = 0.013$
Normal cVEMPs	48%	68%	97%	$p < 0.001$
Unilateral absence of cVEMPs	12%	26%	0%	$p < 0.001$
Bilateral absence of cVEMPs	40%	6%	3%	$p < 0.001$
P13 latencies (ms)	17.8 ± 10.82	14.32 ± 3.3	16.07 ± 8.97	n.s.
N23 latencies (ms)	26.53 ± 10.28	22.68 ± 4.2	25.77 ± 10.48	n.s.
P13 amplitudes (mcV)	46.18 ± 29.88	41.92 ± 37.75	40.57 ± 26.1	n.s.
N23 amplitudes (mcV)	−44.9 ± 35.26	−54.6 ± 34.01	−63.16 ± 42.31	n.s.
Interpeak latencies (ms)	8.6 ± 2.5	8.5 ± 2.3	9.6 ± 3.4	n.s.

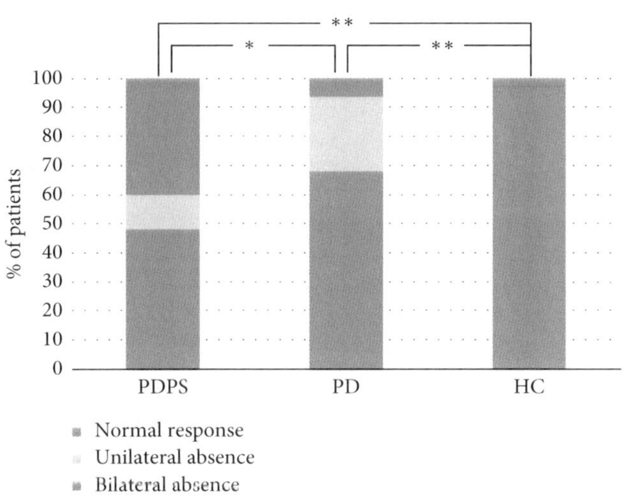

FIGURE 2: The plot summarizes the percentage of different cVEMPs responses in the three groups. Significance markers (* = $p < 0.05$; ** = $p < 0.001$) refer to the presence of "normal responses." Other data are expressed in the text.

4. Discussion

The neuropathological hallmark of PD is the ascending accumulation of α-synuclein immunoreactive Lewy bodies (LB) from SNpc and other brainstem structures to superior brain areas; however, LB deposition has been recently demonstrated in all brainstem fiber tracts and cranial nerve nuclei, including the vestibular system [20]. Of note, dopamine, whose levels are critically reduced in PD, is a fundamental modulator of vestibular nuclei function [21]. cVEMPs are now considered a reliable tool to assess vestibular and brainstem functions in distinct neurological disorders, including neuroaudiological, demyelinating and cerebrovascular diseases, migraine, and CNS tumours [8, 22]. Conversely, few studies examined the potential utilization of cVEMPs as a tool to monitor neurodegenerative diseases, particularly PD [15].

In our cross-sectional analysis of cVEMPs among PDPS, PD patients without PS and HCs without neurodegenerative conditions, we demonstrate that PD patients, compared with the latter group, have significantly abnormal vestibular evoked responses, consisting in unilateral or bilateral loss of cVEMPs. Furthermore, our findings indicate that the neurophysiological profile differs between PD patients with and without PS. The PD group mostly exhibits the unilateral absence of cVEMPs, whereas the PDPS group shows prevalently bilateral loss of responses. Our data on vestibular dysfunction may thus reflect the progression of brainstem neurodegeneration along disease course, with a progressive worsening in advanced stages, when postural complications are more frequently observed [23].

Despite the absence of significant correlations between neurophysiological parameters and specific clinical features, our results show a peculiar alteration of vestibular functioning in PS. While a previous study demonstrated unilateral peripheral vestibular hypofunction, ipsilateral to the LTF side [13], we observed a higher prevalence of bilateral alterations in PDPS patients here. A note of caution in the interpretation of our data is required, as our study lacks peripheral testing, which might have been useful in the anatomoclinical correlation. However, combining existing data with our novel observations, we hypothesize that central vestibular impairment might concur with peripheral dysfunction in patients with PS [13], suggesting the specific frailty of the vestibular system in this condition, even if longer disease duration might also play a role.

The study also included an audiometric examination of the three groups, which showed no significant differences in the hearing thresholds of subjects with PD, PDPS, and HCs. This finding partially disagrees with evidence by Vitale and colleagues [24, 25], instead demonstrating the occurrence of neurosensory hearing impairment in PD patients. The exclusion, in our study, of subjects with hearing thresholds over 50 dBHL even at a single frequency and additionally the smaller sample size and the different clinical-demographic features of the cohorts may account for this discrepancy.

5. Conclusions

cVEMPs are a noninvasive and inexpensive test exploring vestibulospinal tract, a crucial pathway for postural control. Despite the small sample size, here we observed that vestibulospinal dysfunction progresses in PD, with a milder involvement (unilateral loss of cVEMPs) in the absence of postural disabilities and more severe alterations (bilateral loss of cVEMPs) in the presence of PS. Therefore, we suggest that a major impairment of vestibular system might be involved in pathophysiology of PS, probably mirroring more advanced brainstem pathology in parallel with a longer disease duration. Further prospective studies on larger samples are mandatory to understand the associations between audiovestibular dysfunction and clinical progression of PD, allowing to establish the potential usefulness of cVEMPs as diagnostic and prognostic biomarkers for PD.

Disclosure

The abstract has been presented at the 4th Congress of Accademia LIMPE-DISMOV in May 2018.

References

[1] L. V. Kalia and A. E. Lang, "Parkinson's disease," *The Lancet*, vol. 386, no. 9996, pp. 896–912, 2015.

[2] T. Schirinzi, G. Madeo, G. Martella et al., "Early synaptic dysfunction in Parkinson's disease: insights from animal models," *Movement Disorders*, vol. 31, no. 6, pp. 802–813, 2016.

[3] M. Tinazzi, C. Geroin, M. Gandolfi et al., "Pisa syndrome in Parkinson's disease: an integrated approach from pathophysiology to management," *Movement Disorders*, vol. 31, no. 12, pp. 1785–1795, 2016.

[4] M. Tinazzi, A. Fasano, C. Geroin et al., "Pisa syndrome in Parkinson disease: an observational multicenter Italian study," *Neurology*, vol. 85, no. 20, pp. 1769–1779, 2015.

[5] M. Alwardat, G. Di Lazzaro, T. Schirinzi, P. Sinibaldi Salime, N. B. Mercuri, and A. Pisani, "Does pisa syndrome affect upper limb function in patients with Parkinson's disease? an observational cross-sectional study," *NeuroRehabilitation*, vol. 42, no. 2, pp. 143–148, 2018.

[6] K. M. Doherty, B. P. van de Warrenburg, M. C. Peralta et al., "Postural deformities in Parkinson's disease," *The Lancet Neurology*, vol. 10, no. 6, pp. 538–549, 2011.

[7] P. Barone, G. Santangelo, M. Amboni, M. T. Pellecchia, and C. Vitale, "Pisa syndrome in Parkinson's disease and parkinsonism: clinical features, pathophysiology, and treatment," *Lancet Neurology*, vol. 15, no. 10, pp. 1063–1074, 2016.

[8] T. D. Fife, J. G. Colebatch, K. A. Kerber et al., "Practice guideline: cervical and ocular vestibular evoked myogenic potential testing," *Neurology*, vol. 89, no. 22, pp. 2288–2296, 2017.

[9] J. G. Colebatch, G. M. Halmagyi, and N. F. Skuse, "Myogenic potentials generated by a click-evoked vestibulocollic reflex," *Journal of Neurology, Neurosurgery and Psychiatry*, vol. 57, no. 2, pp. 190–197, 1994.

[10] E. R. de Natale, F. Ginatempo, K. S. Paulus et al., "Paired neurophysiological and clinical study of the brainstem at different stages of Parkinson's disease," *Clinical Neurophysiology*, vol. 126, no. 10, pp. 1871–1878, 2015.

[11] S. M. Rosengren, M. S. Welgampola, and J. G. Colebatch, "Vestibular evoked myogenic potentials: past, present and future," *Clinical Neurophysiology*, vol. 121, no. 5, pp. 636–651, 2010.

[12] M. Pötter-Nerger, S. Govender, G. Deuschl, J. Volkmann, and J. G. Colebatch, "Selective changes of ocular vestibular myogenic potentials in Parkinson's disease," *Movement Disorders*, vol. 30, no. 4, pp. 584–589, 2015.

[13] C. Vitale, V. Marcelli, T. Furia et al., "Vestibular impairment and adaptive postural imbalance in parkinsonian patients with lateral trunk flexion," *Movement Disorders*, vol. 26, no. 8, pp. 1458–1463, 2011.

[14] P. A. Pahapill and A. M. Lozano, "The pedunculopontine nucleus and Parkinson's disease," *Brain*, vol. 123, no. 9, pp. 1767–1783, 2000.

[15] E. R. de Natale, F. Ginatempo, K. S. Paulus et al., "Abnormalities of vestibular-evoked myogenic potentials in idiopathic Parkinson's disease are associated with clinical evidence of brainstem involvement," *Neurological Sciences*, vol. 36, no. 6, pp. 995–1001, 2015.

[16] L. Pollak, T. Prohorov, M. Kushnir, and M. Rabey, "Vestibulocervical reflexes in idiopathic Parkinson disease," *Neurophysiologie Clinique/Clinical Neurophysiology*, vol. 39, no. 4-5, pp. 235–240, 2009.

[17] J. Venhovens, J. Meulstee, B. R. Bloem, W. I. M. Verhagen, and J. Foxe, "Neurovestibular analysis and falls in Parkinson's disease and atypical parkinsonism," *European Journal of Neuroscience*, vol. 43, no. 12, pp. 1636–1646, 2016.

[18] A. J. Hughes, S. E. Daniel, L. Kilford, and A. J. Lees, "Accuracy of clinical diagnosis of idiopathic Parkinson's disease: a clinico-pathological study of 100 cases," *Journal of Neurology, Neurosurgery and Psychiatry*, vol. 55, no. 3, pp. 181–184, 1992.

[19] Y. S. Sininger, "Auditory brain stem response for objective measures of hearing," *Ear and Hearing*, vol. 14, no. 1, pp. 23–30, 1993.

[20] K. Seidel, J. Mahlke, S. Siswanto et al., "The brainstem pathologies of Parkinson's disease and dementia with lewy bodies," *Brain Pathology*, vol. 25, no. 2, pp. 121–135, 2015.

[21] P. F. Smith, "Age-related neurochemical changes in the vestibular nuclei," *Frontiers in Neurology*, vol. 7, pp. 1–9, 2016.

[22] J. Venhovens, J. Meulstee, and W. I. M. Verhagen, "Vestibular evoked myogenic potentials (VEMPs) in central neurological disorders," *Clinical Neurophysiology*, vol. 127, no. 1, pp. 40–49, 2016.

[23] H. Braak, E. Ghebremedhin, U. Rüb, H. Bratzke, and K. Del Tredici, "Stages in the development of Parkinson's disease-related pathology," *Cell and Tissue Research*, vol. 318, no. 1, pp. 121–134, 2004.

[24] C. Vitale, V. Marcelli, R. Allocca et al., "Hearing impairment in Parkinson's disease: expanding the nonmotor phenotype," *Movement Disorders*, vol. 27, no. 12, pp. 1530–1535, 2012.

[25] C. Vitale, V. Marcelli, T. Abate et al., "Speech discrimination is impaired in parkinsonian patients: expanding the audiologic findings of Parkinson's disease," *Parkinsonism and Related Disorders*, vol. 22, pp. S138–S143, 2016.

26

Impact of Combined Subthalamic Nucleus and Substantia Nigra Stimulation on Neuropsychiatric Symptoms in Parkinson's Disease Patients

U. Hidding,[1] A. Gulberti,[1,2] A. Horn,[1] C. Buhmann,[1] W. Hamel,[3] J. A. Koeppen,[3] M. Westphal,[3] A. K. Engel,[2] C. Gerloff,[1] D. Weiss,[4] C. K. E. Moll,[2] and M. Pötter-Nerger[1]

[1]*Department of Neurology, University Medical Center Hamburg-Eppendorf, 20246 Hamburg, Germany*
[2]*Department of Neurophysiology and Pathophysiology, University Medical Center Hamburg-Eppendorf, 20246 Hamburg, Germany*
[3]*Department of Neurosurgery, University Medical Center Hamburg-Eppendorf, 20246 Hamburg, Germany*
[4]*Department for Neurodegenerative Diseases and Hertie Institute for Clinical Brain Research, University of Tübingen, 72076 Tübingen, Germany*

Correspondence should be addressed to M. Pötter-Nerger; m.poetter-nerger@uke.de

Academic Editor: Zoltan Mari

The goal of the study was to compare the tolerability and the effects of conventional subthalamic nucleus (STN) and combined subthalamic nucleus and substantia nigra (STN+SNr) high-frequency stimulation in regard to neuropsychiatric symptoms in Parkinson's disease patients. In this single center, randomized, double-blind, cross-over clinical trial, twelve patients with advanced Parkinson's disease (1 female; age: 61.3±7.3 years; disease duration: 12.3±5.4 years; Hoehn and Yahr stage: 2.2±0.39) were included. Apathy, fatigue, depression, and impulse control disorder were assessed using a comprehensive set of standardized rating scales and questionnaires such as the Lille Apathy Rating Scale (LARS), Modified Fatigue Impact Scale (MFIS), Becks Depression Inventory (BDI-I), Questionnaire for Impulsive-Compulsive Disorders in Parkinson's Disease Rating Scale (QUIP-RS), and Parkinson's Disease Questionnaire (PDQ-39). Three patients that were initially assigned to the STN+SNr stimulation mode withdrew from the study within the first week due to discomfort. Statistical comparison of data retrieved from patients who completed the study revealed no significant differences between both stimulation conditions in terms of mean scores of scales measuring apathy, fatigue, depression, impulse control disorder, and quality of life. Individual cases showed an improvement of apathy under combined STN+SNr stimulation. In general, combined STN+SNr stimulation seems to be safe in terms of neuropsychiatric side effects, although careful patient selection and monitoring in the short-term period after changing stimulation settings are recommended.

1. Introduction

Neuropsychiatric symptoms in Parkinson's disease (PD) represent a common, disabling, occasionally socially disruptive condition; they are difficult to treat and have a major impact on quality of life [1, 2]. Emotional neuropsychiatric symptoms represent a spectrum of various phenomena including apathy, fatigue, and depression on the one hand and impulse control disorder and mania on the other hand [1, 3]. Emotional symptoms are related to several factors such as environmental and cultural influences or personality traits. Of particular importance is the relation of neuropsychiatric symptoms to the disease itself, as in the case of apathy and depression, and the relation to the antiparkinsonian treatment observed for impulse control disorder [1, 4]. Apathy, fatigue, and depression are common and disabling symptoms preceding the onset of motor symptoms by several years [5]. In the pathophysiological understanding of neuropsychiatric symptoms, observations of early alpha synuclein pathology of nondopaminergic brainstem nuclei such as the locus coeruleus (LC) and the raphe nuclei have shed new light on the role of brainstem nuclei and basal ganglia-brainstem projections [6, 7]. Particularly, the noradrenergic LC moved into the focus of interest, since the LC is interconnected via widespread ascending projections to cortical, subcortical, cerebellar, brainstem, and spinal cord circuits [8]. According to this broad efferent linking, the LC is involved in numerous functions, such as arousal, regulation of the sleep-wake-cycle, attention, behavioral flexibility, memory, posture, gait and balance, and emotions [9, 10]. The LC might therefore represent an important structure in the pathogenesis of certain neuropsychiatric symptoms such as apathy, fatigue, or depression.

Some neuropsychiatric symptoms might represent a contraindication for deep brain stimulation (DBS) in the subthalamic nucleus (STN) such as severe depression. Despite contradictory observations [11–13], some symptoms such as impulse control disorder have the chance to ameliorate with STN-DBS in well selected patients [14, 15].

Preoperatively, it has to be differentiated whether the neuropsychiatric symptom is mainly due to the disease itself or due to the dopaminergic medication [4]. After STN-DBS surgery, the reduction of dopaminergic medication, including dopamine agonists, might worsen certain hypodopaminergic neuropsychiatric symptoms such as apathy or depression or improve hyperdopaminergic symptoms such as impulse control disorders. Still, the effect of DBS on neuropsychiatric symptoms is varied and complex in the literature indicating a challenging interaction of DBS and emotional symptoms [4, 16].

Recently, increased interest has been focused on the basal ganglia-brainstem projections in the mediation of STN-DBS beneficial effects [17, 18]. In the current basal ganglia model of PD, it is assumed that the pathologically "overactive" STN induces an increased inhibition of subcortical basal ganglia routes to brainstem centers via increased activation of the inhibitory globus pallidus internus (GPi) and substantia nigra pars reticulata (SNr) [17, 19]. It has been proposed that STN-DBS normalizes the efferent basal ganglia output and results in disinhibition of brainstem activity (see Figure 1) [20, 21]. In view of apparently untreatable, residual, mainly brainstem-mediated symptoms such as axial symptoms and gait disorders under STN-DBS, efforts have been made to costimulate the substantia nigra [22]. The assumption of an additional benefit of SNr stimulation is based on the hypothesis that there might be still residual overactivity of SNr in PD with STN-DBS resulting in ongoing increased GABAergic inhibition of brainstem nuclei which would be supplementarily suppressed by simultaneous high-frequency stimulation within the SNr. The substantia nigra pars reticulata is of particular interest since animal data suggest dense reciprocal GABAergic interconnections between the SNr and mesencephalic brainstem centers such as the pedunculopontine nucleus [23, 24] and consecutively the LC in the downstream. In a recent double-blinded cross-over study, costimulation of the STN and SNr induced an improvement of freezing of gait without effects on depression (assessed by BDI) and impulsiveness (assessed by Barrett Impulsiveness Scale) [22]. Other neuropsychiatric symptoms such as apathy and fatigue were not yet systematically investigated.

The aim of the current study was to compare the costimulation of STN and SNr to conventional STN stimulation in terms of certain LC associated neuropsychiatric symptoms such as apathy, fatigue, and depression. In particular, we intended to demonstrate the safety of a combined STN+SNr stimulation, namely, that STN+SNr stimulation would not worsen neuropsychiatric symptoms in PD patients treated with DBS.

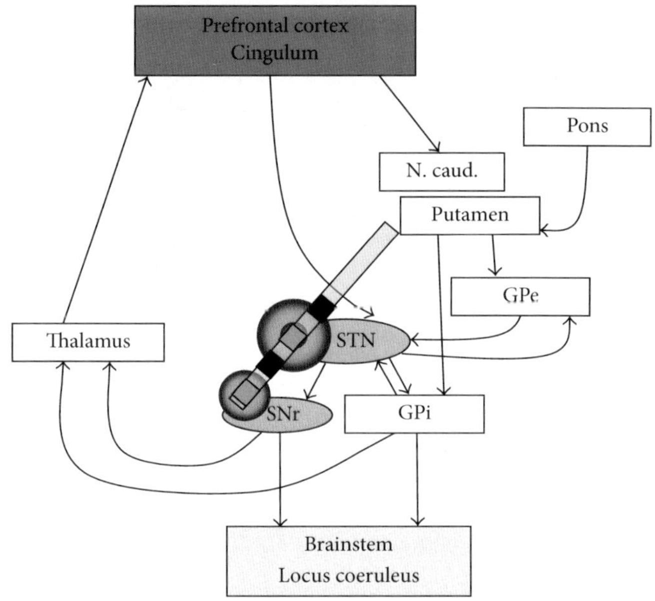

Figure 1: Simplified model of DBS induced modulation of the limbic basal ganglia loops including brainstem projections. N. caud.: nucleus caudatus; GPe: globus pallidus externus; GPi: globus pallidus internus; STN: nucleus subthalamicus; SNr: substantia nigra pars reticulata.

2. Materials and Methods

All statistical values in this section are given as mean ± standard deviation (SD).

2.1. Participants. Twelve patients (1 female; age: 61.3 ± 7.3 years) suffering from advanced idiopathic PD (disease duration: 12.3 ± 5.4 years; Hoehn and Yahr stage: 2.2 ± 0.39 in the MED-ON and STN-DBS-ON condition [25]) participated in the study (see Table 1). The inclusion criteria for this study were the following: (1) PD patients with bilateral electrode implantation in the STN for DBS for at least 3 months; (2) the deepest contacts of the implanted electrodes having to be positioned within the dorsal aspect of the SNr (see below for stereotactic reconstruction technique); (3) unchanged dopaminergic medication in the preceding 4 weeks; (4) MoCA score at baseline ≥ 20 [26]; (5) good effect of conventional STN stimulation on motor symptoms (response to STN stimulation > 30%). There was no further stratification of PD patients, for example, in terms of severity of freezing of gait or neuropsychiatric parameters except dementia.

Preoperatively, all PD patients were screened and selected for DBS surgery in accordance with common guidelines [27]. Patients showed a significant improvement of the motor

TABLE 1: Clinical and demographic characteristics of PD patients.

Case, gender, age	Disease duration [years]	Time with DBS [months]	LEDD [mg]	MoCA score at baseline	DBS System	STN-DBS parameters Left electrode Right electrode	Combined STN+SNr-DBS parameters Left electrode Right electrode	X, Y, Z coordinates Left electrode Right electrode
1, M, 61	23	54	1150	30	ME	Left: 1– 2– G+, 3.5 V, 60 μs, 125 Hz Right: 9– 10– G+, 2.7 V, 60 μs, 125 Hz	Left: 1– 2– G+, 3.5 V, 60 μs, 125 Hz; 0– G+, 2.0 V, 60 μs, 125 Hz Right: 9– 10– G+, 2.7 V, 60 μs, 125 Hz; 8– G+, 2.0 V, 60 μs, 125 Hz	Left: 10.9, 2.2, 4.7 Right: 10.5, 3.8, 4.7
2, M, 63	23	105	860	26	ME	Left: 1– G+, 1.9 V, 60 μs, 125 Hz; 2– G+, 2.9 V, 60 μs, 125 Hz Right: 9– G+, 1.9 V, 60 μs, 125 Hz; 10– G+, 3.3 V, 60 μs, 125 Hz	Left: 2– G+, 2.9 V, 60 μs, 125 Hz; 1– 0– G+, 1.9 V (1.5 V), 60 μs, 125 Hz Right: 10– G+, 3.3 V, 60 μs, 125 Hz; 8– 9– G+, 1.9 V (1.5 V) 60 μs, 125 Hz	Left: 11.2, 1.9, 5.6 Right: 8.3, 5.5, 4
3, M, 56	9	36	880	25	ME	Left: 1+ 2– G+, 2.2 V, 60 μs, 125 Hz Right: 10– G+, 4.3 V, 60 μs, 125 Hz	Left: 2– G+, 2.2 V, 60 μs, 125 Hz; 0– G+, 1.0 V, 60 μs, 125 Hz Right: 10– G+, 4.3 V, 60 μs, 125 Hz, 8– G+, 1.0 V, 60 μs, 125 Hz	Left: 9.5, 2.8, 6.4 Right: 11.2, 1.4, 7.2
4, M, 67	16	60	600	23	ME	Left: 1– G+, 1.5 V, 60 μ, 125 Hz Right: 9– 10– G+, 3.9 V, 60 μs, 125 Hz	Left: 1– G+, 1.5 V, 60 μ, 125 Hz; 0– G+, 2.0 V, 60 μs, 125 Hz Right: 9– 10– G+, 3.9 V, 60 μs, 125 Hz; 8– G+, 2.0 V, 60 μs, 125 Hz	Left: 9.6, 4.7, 6.6 Right: 11.7, 3.1, 3.2
5, M, 65	9	9	300	28	ME	Left: 1– G+, 2.8 V, 60 μs, 125 Hz Right: 9– G+, 3.0 V, 60 μs, 125 Hz	Left: 1– G+, 2.8 V, 60 μs, 125 Hz; 0– G+, 1.5 V, 60 μs, 125 Hz Right: 9– G+, 3.0 V, 60 μs, 125 Hz; 8– G+, 1.5 V, 60 μs, 125 Hz	Left: 10.9, 1.4, 7.7 Right: 11.1, 2.7, 6.7
6, M, 74	9	9	360	22	ME	Left: 1– G+, 2.7 V, 130 Hz Right: 9– G+, 2.6 V, 60 μs, 130 Hz	Left: 1– G+, 2.7 V, 60 μs, 125 Hz; 0– G+, 1.5 V, 60 μs, 125 Hz Right: 9– G+, 2.9 V, 60 μs, 125 Hz; 8– G+, 1.5 V, 60 μs, 125 Hz	Left: 10.7, 2.6, 4.9 Right: 10.2, 2.5, 4.5
7, M, 51	9	15	900	27	BS	Left: 2– 30%, 3– 70%, 3.4 mA, 60 μs, 125 Hz Right: 10– 20%, 11– 80%, 4.0 mA, 60 μs, 125 Hz	Left: 1– 23%, 2– 23%, 3– 54%, 4.4 mA, 60 μs, 125 Hz Right: 9– 20%, 10– 16%, 11– 64%, 5.0 mA, 60 μs, 125 Hz	Left: 8.81, 3.38, 7.37 Right: 7.04, 4.28, 6.41

Table 1: Continued.

Case, gender, age	Disease duration [years]	Time with DBS [months]	LEDD [mg]	MoCA score at baseline	DBS System	STN-DBS parameters Left electrode Right electrode	Combined STN+SNr-DBS parameters Left electrode Right electrode	X, Y, Z coordinates Left electrode Right electrode
8, M, 57	7	18	580	27	BS	Left: 3– 70%, 4– 30%, 4.5 mA, 60 μs, 130 Hz Right: 12– 100%, 3.8 mA, 60 μs, 130 Hz	Left: 3– 61%, 4– 26%, 1– 13%, 5.2 mA, 60 μs, 130 Hz Right: 12– 85%, 9– 15%, 4.5 mA, 60 μs, 130 Hz	Left: 11.85, 3.37, 6.09 Right: 11.63, 2.69, 5.9
9, M, 71	11	13	600	27	ME	Left: 1– G+, 3.5 V, 60 μs, 125 Hz Right: 9– G+, 2.7 V, 60 μs, 125 Hz	Left: 1– G+, 3.5 V, 60 μs, 125 Hz; 0– G+, 1.0 V, 60 μs, 125 Hz Right: 9– G+, 2.7 V, 60 μs, 125 Hz; 8– G+, 1.0 V, 60 μs, 125 Hz	Left: 11.34, 2.18, 6.24 Right: 12.23, 0.2, 5.22
10, F, 66	9	5	700	25	ME	Withdrawal, experimental phase not performed	Left: 2– G+, 2.4 V, 60 μs, 125 Hz; 0– G+, 0.7 V, 60 μs, 125 Hz Right: 11– G+, 2.5 V, 60 μs, 125 Hz; 8– G+, 0.7 V, 60 μs, 125 Hz	Left: 10.2, 0.9, 5.2 Right: 9, 0.6, 7.8
11, M, 55	13	23	700	28	ME	Withdrawal, experimental phase not performed	Left: 3– G+, 2.9 V, 60 μs, 125 Hz; 0– G+, 0.7 V, 60 μs, 125 Hz Right: 10– G+, 2.9 V, 60 μs, 125 Hz; 8– G+, 0.7 V, 60 μs, 125 Hz	Left: 9.2, 2.8, 7.7 Right: 10.2, 2.4, 6
12, M, 53	10	16	860	24	BS	Withdrawal, experimental phase not performed	Left: 3– G+, 2,7 mA, 60 μs, 119 Hz; 1– G+, 0.7 mA, 60 μs, 119 Hz Right: 12–/13– G+, 4,7 mA, 60 μs, 119 Hz; 9– G+, 0.7 mA, 60 μs, 119 Hz	Left: 10.73, 5.34, 6.87 Right: 7.72, 3.14, 6.82

"Disease duration [years]" is calculated from the date of the first diagnosis to the date of baseline measurement of the experiment. "DBS parameters" include active contacts, amplitude (volts or mA), pulse width (microseconds), and stimulation frequency (Hz), for the left and right electrode, respectively. Electrode coordinates are given as mm lateral to the midline (X), posterior to the midcommissural point (Y), and inferior to the intercommissural plane (Z). Note that the deepest contacts were contacts 0 and 8 (Medtronic) or contacts 1 and 9 (Boston Scientific). LEDD: levodopa equivalent daily dose; ME: Medtronic; BS: Boston Scientific.

subscore (III) of the Movement Disorder Society Unified Parkinson's Disease Rating Scale (MDS-UPDRS) after intake of soluble levodopa (MED-OFF 39.0 ± 17.3, MED-ON 10.5 ± 6.3, improvement of 72%). Preoperatively, the levodopa equivalent daily dose (LEDD) was 921.0 ± 348.5 mg (conversion factors used for the calculation of LEDD according to Tomlinson et al. 2010 [28]). Neuropsychiatric or medical comorbidities as well as MRI abnormalities were preoperatively excluded. Postoperatively, at the time of baseline measurement, the motor subscore (III) of MDS-UPDRS in "Dopa-on" with STN-DBS-OFF was 34.4 ± 6.7. The postoperative LEDD was 707.5 ± 240.3 mg. Further clinical details are summarized in Table 1. All participants had to read and sign an information consent before participation into the study. The study was approved by the local ethics committee and was conducted in agreement with the Code of Ethics of the World Medical Association (Declaration of Helsinki, 1967).

2.2. Electrode Implantation and Contact-Position Reconstruction. Surgical details and a precise description of the microelectrode (MER) guided mapping procedure of the subthalamic region are given elsewhere [29, 30]. Briefly, the dorsal STN was targeted 11-12 mm lateral to midline, 0–3 mm posterior to the midcommissural point, and 1–3 mm inferior to the intercommissural plane. Preoperative high-resolution T2-weighted magnetic resonance images (fused with stereotactic computed tomography (CT) scans) were used to adjust target coordinates in individual patients. The majority of patients ($n = 9$) were awake during stereotactic DBS electrode placement. In three cases, DBS surgery was carried out under general anesthesia with propofol and remifentanil [31]. In all cases, final electrode placement was guided by the results of intraoperative MER and test stimulation. To this end, up to five parallel tracks (3 ± 1) were used to map the subthalamic region with sharp tungsten electrodes (AlphaOmega, Nazareth, Israel; impedance, 595 ± 167 kOhm). Unit activity was amplified and high-pass-filtered between 300 Hz and 6 kHz and stored for offline analysis (NeurOmega, AlphaOmega, Nazareth, Israel). The sensorimotor STN was identified by cell responses to passive and active movements and a high prevalence of oscillating unit activities in the range between 10 and 30 Hz. Differentiation of STN from SNr was based on established electrophysiological criteria. Specifically, the decrease of background noise and the replacement of irregular STN unit activity by tonic regular high-frequency spiking of SNr neurons marked the ventral exit of the STN and dorsal aspect of the SNr, respectively. For all tracks that traversed the target nuclei, we first reconstructed the 3D location of the ventral STN border and the dorsal SNr relative to the midcommissural point. Then we determined the Euclidean distance of these positions to the ventral DBS electrode contact. The localization of the implanted electrode contacts (model 3389, Medtronic, Minneapolis, Minnesota, USA, in 8 cases, and 8-poled electrode model, Boston Scientific, Valencia, CA, USA, in 2 cases) was determined by coregistration of the preoperative T1 magnetic resonance imaging (MRI) scans and postoperative CT scans using commercially available software (iPlan stereotaxy; Brainlab, Feldkirchen, Germany). A detailed description of the reconstruction of single electrode contacts is provided elsewhere [32, 33]. According to stereotactic atlases, high-resolution MRI, and MER-guided mapping, the upper border of the SNr is positioned 4.5–6 mm below the plane in between anterior and posterior commissure [22].

2.3. Design. The study design was a single center, randomized, double-blind, cross-over clinical trial to compare the effects of STN stimulation versus combined STN+SNr stimulation as described previously [22]. Blinded patients were investigated at three visits with a time interval of three weeks in between (baseline recording, phase I and phase II, see Figure 2). All visits were performed in a medication-on condition and included motor tests and questionnaires concerning different aspects of everyday life during the preceding 3 weeks. Motor tests and questionnaires were performed by blinded investigators. After testing thresholds for side effects in the SNr, defined stimulation settings for the STN and STN+SNr stimulation were fixed for the course of the experiment. The STN settings were not different from those before the study. Afterwards, stimulation of the STN or combined STN+SNr was set by a nonblinded investigator in a randomized manner for the following three weeks; that is, 5 of 12 PD patients received first a conventional STN stimulation (the control stimulation for placebo effects) and after three weeks the combined STN+SNr stimulation, while the other 7 patients received first the combined STN+SNr stimulation followed by conventional STN stimulation (see Figure 2). After completion of phase I, the second visit was performed with reprogramming of stimulation parameters in a cross-over manner for the following three weeks (starting phase II). The third visit was performed after six weeks when phase II was completed. Patients were unblinded and the preferred stimulation mode was programmed as permanent therapeutic stimulation. Medication and stimulation parameters were held constant during phase I and phase II of the study. Only in one case did the stimulation amplitude in the SNr have to be reduced after two days due to dyskinesias.

2.4. Questionnaires and Outcome Measures. The goal of the study was to investigate the tolerability and the effect of a combined STN+SNr stimulation with regard to neuropsychiatric issues like apathy, fatigue, depression, and impulse control disorders (ICDs). For this aim, we used the Lille Apathy Rating Scale (LARS [34]), Modified Fatigue Impact Scale (MFIS [35, 36]), Becks Depression Inventory (BDI-I [37]), and the Questionnaire for Impulsive-Compulsive Disorders in Parkinson's Disease Rating Scale (QUIP-RS [38, 39]). To evaluate a possible impact of different stimulation settings on the quality of life of the patients, the Parkinson's Disease Questionnaire (PDQ-39) was applied [40].

The LARS is designed to diagnose and measure severity of apathy symptoms. The score is based on a structured interview including 33 items divided into 9 domains (everyday productivity, interests, taking the initiative, novelty seeking, motivation, voluntary actions, emotional responses, concern, social life, and self-awareness, each domain ranging from −4

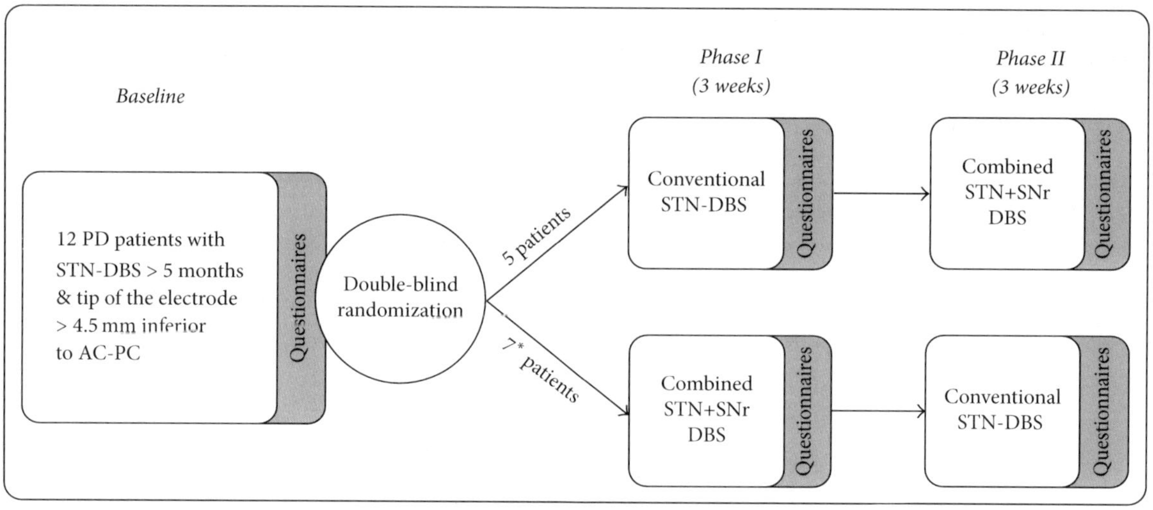

FIGURE 2: Study design: randomized cross-over trial over 6 weeks. After baseline assessment, PD patients were assigned in phase I to either conventional STN-DBS or combined STN+SNr stimulation. After 3 weeks, patients were switched to the other stimulation mode. (∗) Three of the 7 patients starting the phase I with a combined STN+SNr-DBS withdrew within the first week.

to 4 points). The global score ranges from −36 to +36, with higher scores indicating a higher degree of apathy. Cut-off values range from −36 to −22 for nonapathetic, from −21 to −17 for slightly apathetic, and from −16 to −10 and from −9 to +36 for moderate and severely apathetic patients, respectively [34]. To the best of our knowledge, at the moment there is no study assessing the LARS sensitivity to changes in apathy over a shorter interval of time than 3 months [34, 41–43].

The MFIS consists of 21 items and provides an assessment of the global effects of fatigue expressed as a total score and, more specifically, in terms of physical, cognitive, and psychosocial functioning as subscores. In particular, all items are scaled so that higher scores indicate a greater impact of fatigue on personal activities. The total MFIS score ranges from 0 to 84, while the physical subscale can range from 0 to 36, the cognitive subscale from 0 to 40, and psychosocial subscale from 0 to 8. Schiehser et al. (2013) tested 100 nondemented PD patients at mild-moderate stages with the MFIS, collecting a mean total score of 32 points [44]. To the best of our knowledge, a specific cut-off score for the MFIS in PD patients could not be established yet [44].

The BDI-I is a 21-item questionnaire to assess depressive symptoms with scoring of 0–3 for each item. A maximum of 63 points can be achieved (higher score indicating worse symptoms). A score of 16 is considered the cut-off for mild depression in PD [45].

The QUIP-RS is a standardized instrument for detecting and assessing impulse control disorders. It has four main questions (concerning frequently reported thoughts, urges/desires, and behaviors related to ICDs), each applied to four ICDs (compulsive gambling, buying, eating, and sexual behavior) and 3 related disorders (medication use, punding, and hobbyism). It displays a five-point Likert scale (score of 0–4 for each question) to assess the frequency of behaviors. The total QUIP-RS score can range from a minimum of 0 to a maximum of 112 points. The cut-off points for individual ICDs (possible score of 0–16 for each ICD) are as follows: gambling ≥ 6; buying ≥ 8; sex ≥ 8; and eating ≥ 7. For combined ICDs (possible score of 0–64), a QUIP-ICD score can be calculated and the cut-off point is ≥10. Hobbyism-punding (possible score of 0–32) has a cut-off point of ≥7 [39].

The Parkinson's Disease Questionnaire (PDQ-39) is a 39-item self-report questionnaire, which records frequent and specific health-related problems over the last month and reproduces reliably the quality of life of Parkinson patients [40]. Besides, the Parkinson's disease summary index (PDSI) provides an index of the global impact of PD on health status of the patients. The PDQ-39 assesses how often PD patients experience difficulties across 8 different dimensions of quality of life: mobility, activities of daily living, emotional well-being, stigma, social support, cognition, communication, and bodily discomfort. The PDSI is derived by the sum of the eight PDQ-39 scale scores divided by eight (the number of subscales), which yields a score between 0 and 100 (higher scores indicating impaired quality of life). This is equivalent to expressing the sum of all 39 item responses as a percentage score [46].

2.5. Statistics. Since three patients withdrew from the study due to intolerance of combined STN+SNr-DBS, ANOVAs were calculated for the 9 patients that completed the study. This number of patients is in line with analog DBS studies with similar intends, limitations, and approaches [14, 22, 47–49]. The scores as collected at the three experimental visits were compared: (1) baseline, (2) standard STN-DBS, and (3) combined STN+SNr-DBS. Repeated measures ANOVAs with the within-subjects factor DBS (baseline, STN-DBS, and STN+SNr-DBS) were performed separately for each test (BDI-I, LARS, QUIP-RS, QUIP-ICD, MFIS, and PDQ39) with PASW Statistics (PASW Statistics for Mac, version 18.0, SPSS Inc., Chicago, IL, USA). For interaction effects, Greenhouse–Geisser corrected p values were calculated if sphericity was violated (Mauchly's sphericity test). Alpha level was set at 0.05. Post hoc comparisons were performed with Wilcoxon signed rank test (Matlab 7.10 and associated toolboxes, MathWorks, Natick, MA). For scales with validated cut-off levels for PD (i.e., BDI-I, LARS, and QUIP-ICD), Fisher's exact tests were performed on a 2 × 2 contingency table with categories "kind of DBS-stimulation" × "symptomaticity."

3. Results

Descriptive statistics in the main text include mean ± standard deviation (SD) of the mean, while in the boxplots median, interquartile range (IQR), whiskers (highest/lowest values of the dataset within 1.5 times the IQR), and outliers (<1st percentile and the >99th percentile) are illustrated.

3.1. Stereotactic Reconstruction of Recording Positions and Electrode Contacts. For this study, MER data was successfully retrieved from 23/24 hemispheres (due to technical reasons, MER could not be performed on the left hemisphere of one patient). 59/71 tracks (83%) traversed the STN. SNr unit activity was recorded on 52/71 tracks (73%). In most cases, either the central (15/24, 63%) or the anterior trajectory (7/24, 29%) was chosen for permanent implantation of DBS electrodes. The remaining two electrodes were implanted in the posterior and lateral trajectory, respectively.

Figure 3 shows the localization of the reconstructed most ventral DBS contacts (squares), which were used for combined STN+SNr stimulation, in relation to the MER-defined ventral STN border (circles) and nigral recording sites (diamonds) for every patient.

The ventral DBS electrode contact was located significantly closer to the dorsal SNr (1.9 ± 1 mm) compared to the ventral border of the STN (2.4 ± 1.4 mm; paired t-test, p = 0.02). The stereotactic coordinates of the most ventral DBS contact relative to the midcommissural point (MCP; mean + SD in mm) were $x = 10.4 \pm 0.9$, $y = 2.8 \pm 1.3$, and $z = 6.3 \pm 1.0$ for the left hemisphere and $x = 10.1 \pm 1.7$, $y = 2.7 \pm 1.5$, and $z = 5.7 \pm 1.4$ for the right side (x: lateral to midline; y: posterior to MCP; z: inferior to AC-PC level). Furthermore, in the majority of the cases studied here (16/23, 70%), the depth (z-axis) of the ventral DBS electrode contact was located below the MER-defined dorsal level of the substantia nigra. This quite deep position of the electrode occurred as part of the normal variation during routine care.

3.2. Stimulation Effects on Apathy. PD patients of the investigated cohort were slightly apathetic at baseline as measured by the LARS (−20.56 ± 7.73 for the nine patients completing the study; −23.33 ± 3.79 for the three withdrawals). The mean degree of apathy of PD patients was not significantly modulated by factor DBS [$F(2, 16) = 0.491$; $p = 0.621$]. The scores during conventional STN-DBS (−19.00 ± 6.32) and combined STN+SNr-DBS (−20.89 ± 7.78) remained in a similar range (see Figure 4). Post hoc comparisons did not reveal any significant significance between the stimulation conditions.

According to the cut-off criteria for the LARS, at baseline, six patients of twelve patients were nonapathetic, three patients showed a slight apathy, two patients were moderately apathetic, and one was severely apathetic. During conventional STN-DBS in the study, four of nine patients were nonapathetic, while three patients showed a slight apathy, one a moderate apathy, and one a severe apathy. With the combined STN+SNr-DBS-stimulation, six of nine patients were nonapathetic, one patient was slight apathetic, one patient was moderately apathetic, and one patient was severely apathetic. Fisher's exact tests performed on a 2 × 2 contingency table with categories "kind of DBS-stimulation" × "apathy" did not show any significant change in terms of apathy between the different stimulation modes ($p = 1$ for baseline versus STN-DBS alone; $p = 0.637$ for baseline versus combined STN+SNr-DBS; $p = 0.637$ for STN-DBS alone versus combined STN+SNr-DBS, Fisher's exact tests). Thus, there was no significant change of overall mean apathy scores considering the total cohort, although single cases might have had benefit. A nonparametric Spearman's correlation performed with the MoCA scores and the LARS scores at baseline did not reveal a possible interplay between apathy and the cognitive state of the patients (rho = −0.297; p = 0.437).

3.3. Stimulation Effects on Fatigue. Fatigue represents sometimes the only symptom that apathetic patients complain about [1]; these two symptoms seem to be closely associated.

For the nine patients completing the study, the mean MFIS score at baseline was 28.89 ± 16.05 (24.33 ± 5.03 for the three withdrawals). The general level of fatigue was not significantly influenced by DBS [$F(2, 16) = 0.607$; $p = 0.557$] (Figure 5). Compared to conventional STN-DBS (27.00 ± 17.23) there was a slight reduction of fatigue with combined STN+SNr-DBS (23.22 ± 21.02), which was not significant in post hoc analyses. Further ANOVAs performed separately for the three MFIS subscales (i.e., physical, cognitive, and psychosocial fatigue) did also not reveal any significant modulation of fatigue subscores due to different DBS modes (for all ANOVAs performed on the above-mentioned 3 subscales [$F(2, 16) \leq 1.020$; $p \geq 0.383$]).

3.4. Stimulation Effects on Depression. The recruited PD patients did not reveal depressive symptoms at baseline (three withdrawals: 8.67 ± 4.04; nine patients completing the study: 6.67 ± 4.77). The BDI-I score was not modulated by factor DBS [$F(2, 16) = 0.378$; $p = 0.691$] meaning that neither STN-DBS (6.22 ± 4.57), nor STN+SNr stimulation (7.33 ± 6.26) worsened depressive symptoms (Figure 6). Post hoc comparisons did not reveal any significant difference between the two stimulation conditions.

Fisher's exact tests performed on a 2 × 2 contingency table with categories "kind of DBS-stimulation" × "depression" did not show any significant change in terms of symptoms at the three experimental time points ($p = 1$ for all three comparisons).

3.5. Stimulation Effect on Impulse Control Disorders. To measure the impact of the different DBS conditions on impulse

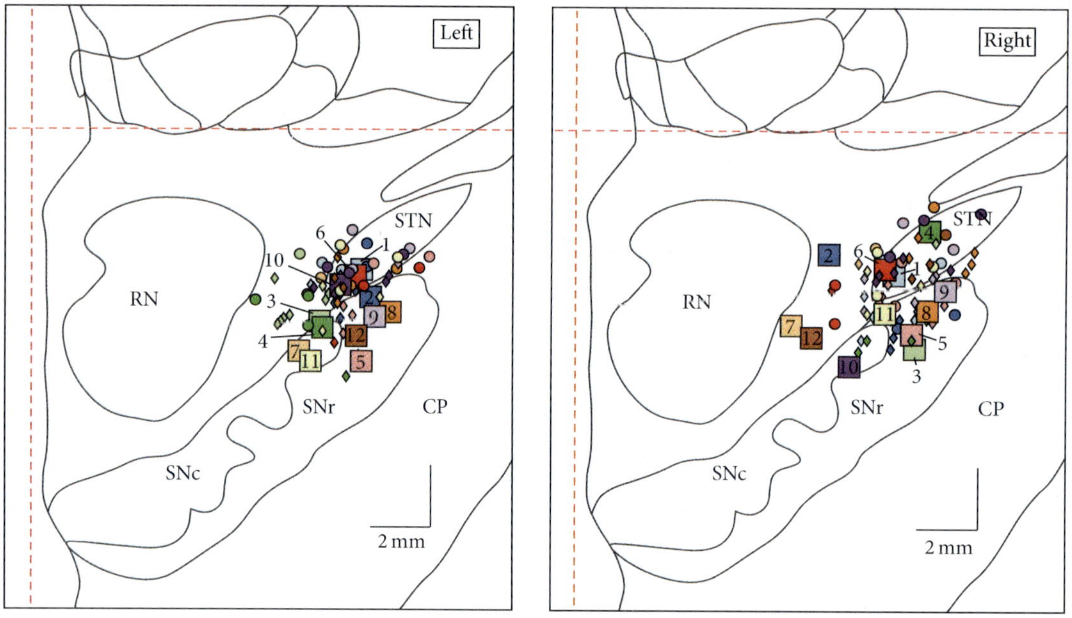

FIGURE 3: Stereotactic reconstruction: squares indicate the localization of the most ventral DBS electrode contacts, superimposed on frontal sections of the stereotactic atlas of Morel, at a level 5 mm behind midcommissural point [50]. Circles indicate the ventral STN border as defined by standard electrophysiological criteria. Diamonds indicate the presence of unambiguous SNr cell activity on MER tracks. Colors represent individual patients. The dashed red lines denote midline and AC-PC level, respectively. STN: subthalamic nucleus; SNr: substantia nigra pars reticulata; SNc: substantia nigra pars compacta; CP: cerebral peduncle; RN, red nucleus.

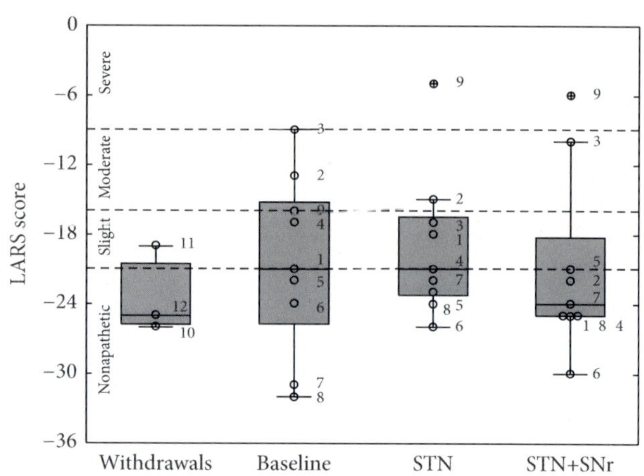

FIGURE 4: Boxplots of LARS scores: the box plot depicted on the left represents the baseline values of the three patients who withdrew. The other three box plots represent the values of the 9 PD patients who have completed the study at the three experimental time points: (1) baseline, (2) STN alone, and (3) combined STN+SNr-DBS. The numbered circles represent the single patients as listed in Table 1. The dashed horizontal lines represent the cut-offs as previously described.

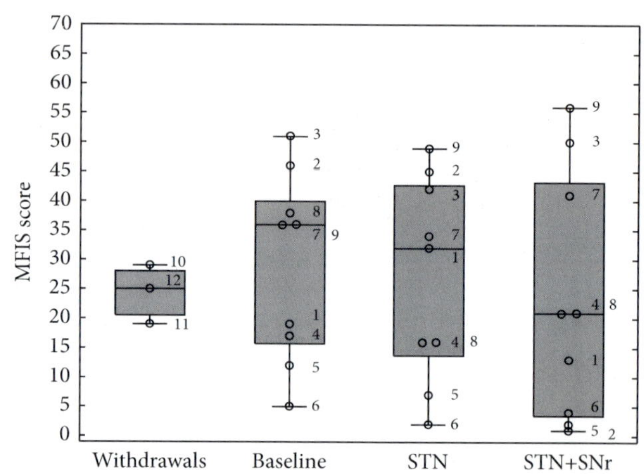

FIGURE 5: Boxplots of MFIS scores: the box plot depicted on the left represents the baseline values of the three patients who withdrew. The other three box plots represent the values of the 9 PD patients who have completed the study at the three experimental time points: (1) baseline, (2) STN alone, and (3) combined STN+SNr-DBS. The numbered circles represent the single patients as listed in Table 1.

control disorders, both the QUIP-RS total score (Figure 7) and the combined QUIP-ICD score (Figure 8) have been analysed.

The QUIP-RS total score at baseline was 11.22 ± 12.11 (for the three withdrawals 17.00 ± 3.61), while at control STN stimulation was 12.22 ± 18.25. The QUIP-RS total score with the combined STN+SNr-DBS was 13.33 ± 14.41. ANOVA testing of QUIP scores did not reveal any modulation due to the DBS mode [$F(2, 16) = 0.065$; $p = 0.850$]. Planned post hoc comparisons did also not reveal any significant contrast between stimulation conditions.

Regarding the combined QUIP-ICD score (Figure 8), PD patients did also not reveal any modulation of scores for impulse control disorders due to the DBS mode, as measured

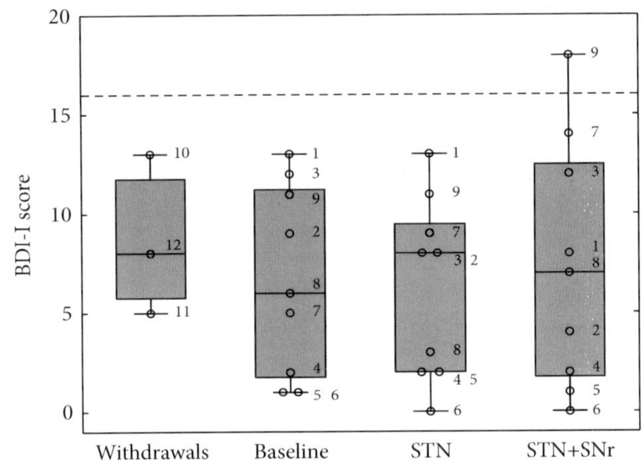

FIGURE 6: Boxplots of BDI-I scores: the box plot depicted on the left represents the baseline values of the three patients who withdrew. The other three box plots represent the values of the 9 PD patients who have completed the study at the three experimental time points: (1) baseline, (2) STN alone, and (3) combined STN+SNr-DBS. The numbered circles represent the single patients as listed in Table 1. The dashed horizontal line represents the cut-off for PD patients as previously discussed in Material and Methods.

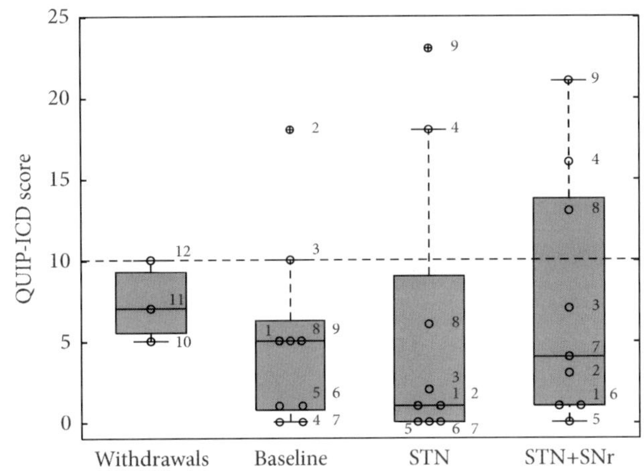

FIGURE 8: Boxplots of combined QUIP-ICD scores: the box plot depicted on the left represents the baseline values of the three patients who withdrew. The other three box plots represent the values of the 9 PD patients who have completed the study at the three experimental time points: (1) baseline, (2) STN alone, and (3) combined STN+SNr-DBS. The numbered circles represent the single patients as listed in Table 1. For the combined QUIP-ICD score the cut-off point is ≥10.

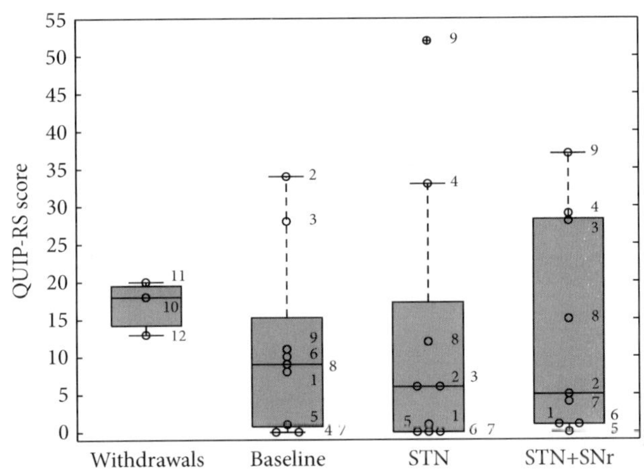

FIGURE 7: Boxplots of QUIP-RS scores: the box plot depicted on the left represents the baseline values of the three patients who withdrew. The other three box plots represent the values of the 9 PD patients who have completed the study at the three visits: (1) baseline, (2) STN alone, and (3) combined STN+SNr-DBS. The numbered circles represent the single patients as listed in Table 1. A cut-off for the total QUIP-RS score is not available.

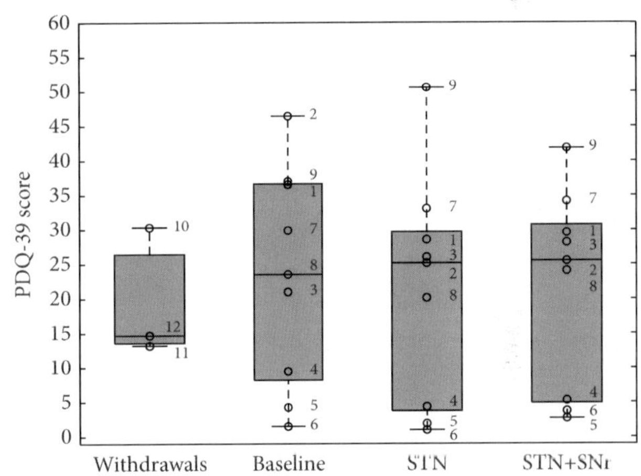

FIGURE 9: Boxplots of PDQ-39 scores expressed as Parkinson's disease summary index (PDSI) scores: the box plot depicted on the left represents the baseline values of the three patients who withdrew. The other three box plots represent the values of the 9 PD patients who have completed the study at the three experimental time points: (1) baseline, (2) STN alone, and (3) combined STN+SNr-DBS. The numbered circles represent the single patients as listed in Table 1.

at the three experimental visits [$F(2, 16) = 0.331$; $p = 0.602$]. The QUIP-ICD score at baseline was 5.00 ± 5.87 (7.3 ± 2.52 for the three withdrawals), while at control STN stimulation was 5.67 ± 8.7. The QUIP-ICD score with the combined STN+SNr-DBS was 7.33 ± 7.57. Fisher's exact tests performed on a 2 × 2 contingency table with categories "kind of DBS-stimulation" × "ICD" did not show any significant change in terms of ICD behaviors between the different stimulation modes ($p = 1$ for all three comparisons). Also for the QUIP-ICD score, as for the QUIP-RS total score, planned post hoc comparisons did not reveal any significant score modulation due to different stimulation regimes.

3.6. Stimulation Effects on Quality of Life. As measured by means of PDQ-39 (Figure 9), quality of life was not significantly influenced by DBS modes in the PD cohort [$F(2, 16) = 0.374$; $p = 0.596$] with scores of 23.33 ± 15.70 (19.46 ± 9.46 for the three withdrawals) at baseline, 21.21 ± 16.42 with STN stimulation, and 21.68 ± 14.30 with STN+SNr-DBS. Planned comparisons by means of the Wilcoxon signed rank test showed nonsignificant differences for the PDSI scores at the different visits. Further ANOVAs separately performed on the different 8 PDQ-39 subscales for STN-DBS versus the combined STN+SNr-DBS did not reveal significant differences (for all ANOVAs performed for the 8 subscores [$F(2, 16) \leq 2.519$; $p \geq 0.112$]).

4. Discussion

In this study, combined STN+SNr stimulation was noninferior compared to STN stimulation in terms of neuropsychiatric symptoms assessed in this study in PD patients. There were no significant differences between these two stimulation conditions in terms of mean scores of apathy, fatigue, depression, impulse control disorder, and quality of life, although individual cases profited from the combined stimulation mode in terms of apathy. In PD patients with low neuropsychiatric morbidity in terms of apathy, fatigue, depression, and impulsivity at baseline, the combined STN+SNr stimulation mode did not induce or deteriorate emotional symptoms in accordance with previous reports [22]. Currently, STN+SNr stimulation is predominantly applied in PD patients with specific motor symptoms to improve freezing of gait [22, 51]. The results confirm safety and good tolerability of combined STN+SNr stimulation applied in otherwise neuropsychologically healthy, carefully selected PD patients who are treated with this stimulation mode for improvement of freezing of gait, for instance.

Three patients withdrew from the study prematurely due to side effects. All three patients terminated the study under a combined STN+SNr-DBS regime, suggesting that for these patients this stimulation mode was not adequate or even disadvantageous. In detail, side effects were worsening of motor functions as well as a lack of beneficial effects of levodopa (case 10), akathisia (case 11), and increased confusion and hallucinations (case 12). From baseline neuropsychiatric measurements and electrode position, these three patients did not differ from the other PD patients who completed the study. In the interpretation of the results, one needs to consider the limits of the study with a small number of patients, gender disparity, and the lack of comparison to controls. Another constraint may be represented by a nonsensitivity of the LARS to changes in apathy over a short period of 3 weeks [34, 41–43]. Further investigations with a larger, controlled patient cohort need to evaluate whether certain neuropsychiatric characteristics of PD patients may be red flags to select or not select patients to undergo combined STN+SNr stimulation.

There are some rare and selected reports of stimulation induced neuropsychiatric side effects of ventral limbic STN stimulation [52] or SNr stimulation [53, 54] such as stimulation induced mania or even depression. In a recent trial, combined interleaving STN+SNr stimulation with application of different, adapted amplitudes in both nuclei was safe in terms of neuropsychiatric side effects [22]. This finding could be reproduced in our cohort of PD patients which completed the study. The stimulation associated neuropsychiatric effects are divergent and are proposed to be dependent on the preexisting medical and psychiatric condition [53], the exact electrode position within the nuclei, and the voltage used for stimulation. High-amplitude stimulation might be associated with some overlapping effects on the limbic part of the STN and the dorsal SNr due to the extended electrical field, so adjustment of amplitudes, for example, in the interleaving stimulation mode seems to be favorable for the combined stimulation.

Recent work has focused on the description and analyses of postoperative apathy, fatigue, and depression [1–3]. Apathy is one of the most common and disabling neuropsychiatric symptoms in PD with a prevalence of 15–70% depending on disease severity [55, 56]. It can be defined as a lack of motivation, interests, and emotions resulting in decreased goal-directed behaviors. Several studies in early PD have shown that apathy correlates with more severe motor impairment, suggesting an underlying common mechanism such as hypodopaminergic drive [56]. It has been proposed that, in the spectrum of dopamine-dependent symptoms, apathy is a neuropsychiatric correlate of the motor symptom akinesia, impulse control disorder, a nonmotor counterpart of dyskinesia [3].

Certain neuropsychiatric symptoms are differentially associated with specific domains of cognitive decline in PD [57–59]. The cohort of enrolled PD patients was predominantly cognitively normal in screening tests at baseline and had low scores in regard of apathy, depression, fatigue, and impulsivity. In this cohort of patients, we did not find specific, significant effects of combined STN+SNr stimulation.

Postoperatively after STN-DBS, the reduction of the dopaminergic medication differentially influenced hypo- and hyperdopaminergic symptoms [3]. While akinesia is sufficiently improved with STN-DBS with low L-Dopa dosage [60–63], apathy and depression are not. Dyskinesias and impulse control disorders might improve both with postoperative LEDD reduction. Apathy might be difficult to treat, since there is insufficient response to antidepressants [39] and increase of postoperative LEDD for apathy treatment might tilt the "dopaminergic scale" and reinforce dyskinesia and impulse control disorder.

Dopamine seems to be a key player in the pathogenesis of Parkinsonian apathy, but it is probably not the only neurotransmitter involved. In a recent study, beside dopaminergic denervation, serotonergic involvement within the basal ganglia network was detected in apathetic de novo PD patients [64]. Noradrenergic involvement might be also involved in emotional and cognitive domains in Parkinson's disease [65]. Such observations justify the attempt to facilitate nondopaminergic brainstem nuclei such as the LC to improve neuropsychiatric symptoms in PD.

In some individual cases, apathy was slightly improved by the combined STN+SNr stimulation mode, but there was no comparable trend for depression, fatigue, or impulse control disorder. This divergent effect might be due to different underlying anatomical loops mediating diverse emotional manifestations [1]. PET and structural and functional MRT studies revealed in depressed PD patients anatomical changes of the temporal lobe, orbitofrontal cortex, and anterior cingulate cortex [66] associated with reduced connectivity in cortico-subcortical loops reflecting a disturbed top-down regulation of cortico-limbic emotional loops [67, 68]. In apathetic PD patients, there are anatomical changes of several cortical areas such as the precentral gyrus, inferior parietal gyrus, inferior frontal gyrus, insula, cingulum, and precuneus [69] as well as the nucleus accumbens [70]. Functional connectivity reductions were detected in left-sided circuits, predominantly involving limbic striatal and frontal territories [71]. Further brain structures might be involved in the complex nature of apathy with bottom up- and downregulation as derived from observations in health and disease [3, 72]. Those limbic circuits were demonstrated to be influenced by STN-DBS as shown for, for example, the right frontal gyri in PET studies [73]. Thus, STN+SNr stimulation might differentially modulate different cortico-subcortical loops.

Brainstem and probably the LC might be involved in the pathophysiology of apathy, fatigue, and depression [8, 74, 75]. It is suggested that SNr stimulation might increase the drive of basal ganglia-brainstem projections by the release of pathological inhibition of brainstem centers such as LC activity (Figure 1). This model focuses on direct basal ganglia output structures such as the brainstem which are predominantly modulated by DBS. The constraint of this model is the neglect of large-scale remote circuits which might be also involved in the pathogenesis of apathy or depression. Further evaluation of DBS effects on those remote circuits needs to be assessed in PD patients with neuropsychiatric complications.

It remains to be investigated in a larger cohort of apathetic, depressed PD patients with fatigue whether costimulation of STN and SNr might be superior to STN stimulation in impacting LC associated neuropsychiatric symptoms such as apathy, fatigue, and depression by additional "pushing" basal ganglia-brainstem projections without the need to change the postoperative LEDD. If so, the combined STN+SNr stimulation mode represented a routinely applicable therapeutic option to overcome postoperative hypodopaminergic neuropsychiatric complications to improve quality of life.

Authors' Contributions

The work presented here was carried out in collaboration between all authors. (1) Research project: (A) U. Hidding, A. Gulberti, A. Horn, C. Buhmann, W. Hamel, J. A. Koeppen, M. Westphal, A. K. Engel, C. Gerloff, D. Weiss, C. K. E. Moll and M. Pötter-Nerger designed methods and assessments and conceived the study. (B) U. Hidding, A. Gulberti, A. Horn, C. K. E. Moll, and M. Pötter-Nerger organized the study. (C) U. Hidding, A. Gulberti, A. Horn, C. K. E. Moll, and M. Pötter-Nerger executed the study. (2) Statistical Analysis: U. Hidding, A. Gulberti, A. Horn, and M. Pötter-Nerger carried out statistical analysis. (3) U. Hidding, A. Gulberti, A. Horn, C. Buhmann, W. Hamel, J. A. Koeppen, M. Westphal, A. K. Engel, C. Gerloff, D. Weiss, C. K. E. Moll, and M. Pötter-Nerger were responsible for the manuscript. All authors have contributed to, seen, and approved the manuscript. U. Hidding and A. Gulberti as first authors as well as C. K. E. Moll and M. Pötter-Nerger as last authors contributed equally to this paper.

Acknowledgments

The authors are indebted to all the patients who participated to this long-term study. They are grateful to Beate Schönwald and Bianca Müller for technical assistance. This study was supported by funding from the DFG (SFB936/C8).

References

[1] A. Castrioto, S. Thobois, S. Carnicella, A. Maillet, and P. Krack, "Emotional manifestations of PD: neurobiological basis," *Movement Disorders*, vol. 31, no. 8, pp. 1103–1113, 2016.

[2] R. Martinez-Fernandez, P. Pelissier, J.-L. Quesada et al., "Postoperative apathy can neutralise benefits in quality of life after subthalamic stimulation for Parkinson's disease," *Journal of Neurology, Neurosurgery and Psychiatry*, vol. 87, no. 3, pp. 311–318, 2016.

[3] M. Sierra, S. Carnicella, A. P. Strafella et al., "Apathy and impulse control disorders: yin & yang of dopamine dependent behaviors," *Journal of Parkinson's Disease*, vol. 5, no. 3, pp. 625–636, 2015.

[4] D. Weintraub and D. J. Burn, "Parkinson's disease: the quintessential neuropsychiatric disorder," *Movement Disorders*, vol. 26, no. 6, pp. 1022–1031, 2011.

[5] C. Pont-Sunyer, A. Hotter, C. Gaig et al., "The onset of nonmotor symptoms in parkinson's disease (The ONSET PD Study)," *Movement Disorders*, vol. 30, no. 2, pp. 229–237, 2015.

[6] K. Del Tredici and H. Braak, "Dysfunction of the locus coeruleus-norepinephrine system and related circuitry in Parkinson's disease-related dementia," *Journal of Neurology, Neurosurgery & Psychiatry*, vol. 84, no. 7, pp. 774–783, 2013.

[7] H. Braak, K. Del Tredici, H. Bratzke, J. Hamm-Clement, D. Sandmann-Keil, and U. Rüb, "Staging of the intracerebral inclusion body pathology associated with idiopathic Parkinson's disease (preclinical and clinical stages)," *Journal of Neurology, Supplement*, vol. 249, supplement 3, pp. III/1–III/5, 2002.

[8] S. L. Foote, F. E. Bloom, and G. Aston-Jones, "Nucleus locus ceruleus: new evidence of anatomical and physiological specificity," *Physiological Reviews*, vol. 63, no. 3, pp. 844–914, 1983.

[9] G. Aston-Jones, "Brain structures and receptors involved in alertness," *Sleep Medicine*, vol. 6, no. 1, pp. S3–S7, 2005.

[10] E. E. Benarroch, "The locus ceruleus norepinephrine system: functional organization and potential clinical significance," *Neurology*, vol. 73, no. 20, pp. 1699–1704, 2009.

[11] P. J. Rossi, A. Gunduz, and M. S. Okun, "The Subthalamic Nucleus, Limbic Function, and Impulse Control," *Neuropsychology Review*, vol. 25, no. 4, pp. 398–410, 2015.

[12] T. D. Hälbig, W. Tse, P. G. Frisina et al., "Subthalamic deep brain stimulation and impulse control in Parkinson's disease," *European Journal of Neurology*, vol. 16, no. 4, pp. 493–497, 2009.

[13] H. M. M. Smeding, A. E. Goudriaan, E. M. J. Foncke, P. R. Schuurman, J. D. Speelman, and B. Schmand, "Pathological gambling after bilateral subthalamic nucleus stimulation in Parkinson disease," *Journal of Neurology, Neurosurgery and Psychiatry*, vol. 78, no. 5, pp. 517–519, 2007.

[14] L. Gee, H. Smith, P. De La Cruz et al., "The influence of bilateral subthalamic nucleus deep brain stimulation on impulsivity and prepulse inhibition in Parkinson's disease patients," *Stereotactic and Functional Neurosurgery*, vol. 93, no. 4, pp. 265–270, 2015.

[15] P. Pollak, "Deep brain stimulation for Parkinson's disease—

patient selection," *Handbook of Clinical Neurology*, vol. 116, pp. 97–105, 2013.

[16] J. L. Houeto, V. Mesnage, L. Mallet et al., "Behavioural disorders, Parkinson's disease and subthalamic stimulation," *Journal of Neurology Neurosurgery and Psychiatry*, vol. 72, no. 6, pp. 701–707, 2002.

[17] D. Nandi, T. Z. Aziz, X. Liu, and J. F. Stein, "Brainstem motor loops in the control of movement," *Movement Disorders*, vol. 17, no. 3, pp. S22–S27, 2002.

[18] P. A. Pahapill and A. M. Lozano, "The pedunculopontine nucleus and Parkinson's disease," *Brain*, vol. 123, no. 9, pp. 1767–1783, 2000.

[19] G. E. Alexander, M. D. Crutcher, and M. R. DeLong, "Basal ganglia-thalamocortical circuits: parallel substrates for motor, oculomotor, "prefrontal" and "limbic" functions," *Progress in Brain Research*, vol. 85, pp. 119–146, 1990.

[20] M. Pötter, J. Herzog, H. R. Siebner et al., "Subthalamic nucleus stimulation modulates audiospinal reactions in Parkinson disease," *Neurology*, vol. 70, no. 16, pp. 1445–1451, 2008.

[21] M. Pötter, M. Illert, R. Wenzelburger, G. Deuschl, and J. Volkmann, "The effect of subthalamic nucleus stimulation on autogenic inhibition in Parkinson disease," *Neurology*, vol. 63, no. 7, pp. 1234–1239, 2004.

[22] D. Weiss, M. Walach, C. Meisner et al., "Nigral stimulation for resistant axial motor impairment in Parkinson's disease? A randomized controlled trial," *Brain*, vol. 136, no. 7, pp. 2098–2108, 2013.

[23] S. Breit, R. Bouali-Benazzouz, A.-L. Benabid, and A. Benazzouz, "Unilateral lesion of the nigrostriatal pathway induces an increase of neuronal activity of the pedunculopontine nucleus, which is reversed by the lesion of the subthalamic nucleus in the rat," *European Journal of Neuroscience*, vol. 14, no. 11, pp. 1833–1842, 2001.

[24] S. Breit, L. Lessmann, A. Benazzouz, and J. B. Schulz, "Unilateral lesion of the pedunculopontine nucleus induces hyperactivity in the subthalamic nucleus and substantia nigra in the rat," *European Journal of Neuroscience*, vol. 22, no. 9, pp. 2283–2294, 2005.

[25] M. M. Hoehn and M. D. Yahr, "Parkinsonism: onset, progression, and mortality," *Neurology*, vol. 17, no. 5, pp. 427–442, 1967.

[26] D. J. Gill, A. Freshman, J. A. Blender, and B. Ravina, "The montreal cognitive assessment as a screening tool for cognitive impairment in Parkinson's disease," *Movement Disorders*, vol. 23, no. 7, pp. 1043–1046, 2008.

[27] J. M. Bronstein, M. Tagliati, R. L. Alterman et al., "Deep brain stimulation for Parkinson disease an expert consensus and review of key issues," *Archives of Neurology*, vol. 68, no. 2, pp. 165–171, 2011.

[28] C. L. Tomlinson, R. Stowe, S. Patel, C. Rick, R. Gray, and C. E. Clarke, "Systematic review of levodopa dose equivalency reporting in Parkinson's disease," *Movement Disorders*, vol. 25, no. 15, pp. 2649–2653, 2010.

[29] A. Sharott, A. Gulberti, S. Zittel et al., "Activity parameters of subthalamic nucleus neurons selectively predict motor symptom severity in Parkinson's disease," *Journal of Neuroscience*, vol. 34, no. 18, pp. 6273–6285, 2014.

[30] C. K. E. Moll, E. Galindo-Leon, A. Sharott et al., "Asymmetric pallidal neuronal activity in patients with cervical dystonia," *Frontiers in Systems Neuroscience*, vol. 8, article no. 15, 2014.

[31] C. K. E. Moll, S. Payer, A. Gulberti et al., "STN stimulation in general anaesthesia: evidence beyond 'evidence-based medicine'," *Acta Neurochirurgica. Supplement*, no. 117, pp. 19–25, 2013.

[32] W. Hamel, U. Fietzek, A. Morsnowski et al., "Deep brain stimulation of the subthalamic nucleus in Parkinson's disease: evaluation of active electrode contacts," *Journal of Neurology Neurosurgery and Psychiatry*, vol. 74, no. 8, pp. 1036–1046, 2003.

[33] P. Fischer, J. P. Ossandón, J. Keyser et al., "STN-DBS reduces saccadic hypometria but not visuospatial bias in Parkinson's disease patients," *Frontiers in Behavioral Neuroscience*, vol. 10, article no. 85, 2016.

[34] P. Sockeel, K. Dujardin, D. Devos, C. Denève, A. Destée, and L. Defebvre, "The Lille apathy rating scale (LARS), a new instrument for detecting and quantifying apathy: validation in Parkinson's disease," *Journal of Neurology, Neurosurgery and Psychiatry*, vol. 77, no. 5, pp. 579–584, 2006.

[35] J. D. Fisk, P. G. Ritvo, L. Ross, D. A. Haase, T. J. Marrie, and W. F. Schlech, "Measuring the functional impact of fatigue: initial validation of the fatigue impact scale," *Clinical Infectious Diseases*, vol. 18, pp. S79–S83, 1994.

[36] P. Flachenecker, T. Kümpfel, B. Kallmann et al., "Fatigue in multiple sclerosis: a comparison of different rating scales and correlation to clinical parameters," *Multiple Sclerosis*, vol. 8, no. 6, pp. 523–526, 2002.

[37] A. T. Beck, C. H. Ward, M. Mendelson, J. Mock, and J. Erbaugh, "An inventory for measuring depression," *Archives of General Psychiatry*, vol. 4, no. 6, pp. 561–571, 1961.

[38] C. C. Probst, L. M. Winter, B. Möller et al., "Validation of the questionnaire for impulsive-compulsive disorders in Parkinson's disease (QUIP) and the QUIP-rating scale in a German speaking sample," *Journal of Neurology*, vol. 261, no. 5, pp. 936–942, 2014.

[39] D. Weintraub, E. Mamikonyan, K. Papay, J. A. Shea, S. X. Xie, and A. Siderowf, "Questionnaire for impulsive-compulsive disorders in Parkinson's Disease-Rating Scale," *Movement Disorders*, vol. 27, no. 2, pp. 242–247, 2012.

[40] C. Jenkinson, R. Fitzpatrick, V. Peto, R. Greenhall, and N. Hyman, "The Parkinson's disease questionnaire (PDQ-39): development and validation of a Parkinson's disease summary index score," *Age and Ageing*, vol. 26, no. 5, pp. 353–357, 1997.

[41] D. Devos, C. Moreau, D. Maltête et al., "Rivastigmine in apathetic but dementia and depression-free patients with Parkinson's disease: a double-blind, placebo-controlled, randomised clinical trial," *Journal of Neurology, Neurosurgery and Psychiatry*, vol. 85, no. 6, pp. 668–674, 2014.

[42] D. E. Clarke, J. Y. Ko, E. A. Kuhl, R. van Reekum, R. Salvador, and R. S. Marin, "Are the available apathy measures reliable and valid? A review of the psychometric evidence," *Journal of Psychosomatic Research*, vol. 70, no. 1, pp. 73–97, 2011.

[43] A. Schrag, "Apathy and depression scales in Parkinson's disease: are they good enough?" *Journal of the Neurological Sciences*, vol. 310, no. 1-2, pp. 216–219, 2011.

[44] D. M. Schiehser, C. R. Ayers, L. Liu, S. Lessig, D. S. Song, and J. V. Filoteo, "Validation of the modified fatigue impact scale in Parkinson's disease," *Parkinsonism and Related Disorders*, vol. 19, no. 3, pp. 335–338, 2013.

[45] A. F. G. Leentjens, F. R. J. Verhey, G.-J. Luijckx, and J. Troost, "The validity of the Beck depression inventory as a screening and diagnostic instrument for depression in patients with Parkinson's disease," *Movement Disorders*, vol. 15, no. 6, pp. 1221–1224, 2000.

[46] P. Hagell and M. H. Nilsson, "The 39-item Parkinson's Disease

Questionnaire (PDQ-39): is it a unidimensional construct?" *Therapeutic Advances in Neurological Disorders*, vol. 2, no. 4, pp. 205–214, 2009.

[47] D. Weiss, T. Wachter, C. Meisner et al., "Combined STN/SNr-DBS for the treatment of refractory gait disturbances in Parkinson's disease: study protocol for a randomized controlled trial," *Trials*, vol. 12, article 222, 2011.

[48] L. L. Trépanier, R. Kumar, A. M. Lozano, A. E. Lang, and J. A. Saint-Cyr, "Neuropsychological outcome of GPi pallidotomy and GPi or STN deep brain stimulation in Parkinson's disease," *Brain and Cognition*, vol. 42, no. 3, pp. 324–347, 2000.

[49] M. Ulla, S. Thobois, P.-M. Llorca et al., "Contact dependent reproducible hypomania induced by deep brain stimulation in Parkinson's disease: clinical, anatomical and functional imaging study," *Journal of Neurology, Neurosurgery and Psychiatry*, vol. 82, no. 6, pp. 607–614, 2011.

[50] A. Morel, *Stereotactic Atlas of the Human Thalamus and Basal Ganglia*, 2007.

[51] D. Weiss, S. Breit, T. Wächter, C. Plewnia, A. Gharabaghi, and R. Krüger, "Combined stimulation of the substantia nigra pars reticulata and the subthalamic nucleus is effective in hypokinetic gait disturbance in Parkinson's disease," *Journal of Neurology*, vol. 258, no. 6, pp. 1183–1185, 2011.

[52] A. Chopra, S. J. Tye, K. H. Lee et al., "Underlying neurobiology and clinical correlates of mania status after subthalamic nucleus deep brain stimulation in Parkinson's disease: a review of the literature," *Journal of Neuropsychiatry and Clinical Neurosciences*, vol. 24, no. 1, pp. 102–110, 2012.

[53] M. Ulla, S. Thobois, J.-J. Lemaire et al., "Manic behaviour induced by deep-brain stimulation in Parkinson's disease: evidence of substantia nigra implication?" *Journal of Neurology, Neurosurgery and Psychiatry*, vol. 77, no. 12, pp. 1363–1366, 2006.

[54] B.-P. Bejjani, P. Damier, I. Arnulf et al., "Transient acute depression induced by high-frequency deep-brain stimulation," *New England Journal of Medicine*, vol. 340, no. 19, pp. 1476–1480, 1999.

[55] K. Dujardin, C. Langlois, L. Plomhause et al., "Apathy in untreated early-stage Parkinson disease: relationship with other non-motor symptoms," *Movement Disorders*, vol. 29, no. 14, pp. 1796–1801, 2014.

[56] J. Pagonabarraga, J. Kulisevsky, A. P. Strafella, and P. Krack, "Apathy in Parkinson's disease: clinical features, neural substrates, diagnosis, and treatment," *The Lancet Neurology*, vol. 14, no. 5, pp. 518–531, 2015.

[57] H. Alzahrani and A. Venneri, "Cognitive and neuroanatomical correlates of neuropsychiatric symptoms in Parkinson's disease: a systematic review," *Journal of the Neurological Sciences*, vol. 356, no. 1-2, pp. 32–44, 2015.

[58] G. Santangelo, C. Vitale, L. Trojano et al., "Relationship between apathy and cognitive dysfunctions in de novo untreated Parkinson's disease: a prospective longitudinal study," *European Journal of Neurology*, vol. 22, no. 2, pp. 253–260, 2015.

[59] Y. Bogdanova and A. Cronin-Golomb, "Neurocognitive correlates of apathy and anxiety in parkinson's disease," *Parkinson's Disease*, vol. 2012, Article ID 793076, 9 pages, 2012.

[60] G. Deuschl, C. Schade-Brittinger, P. Krack et al., "A randomized trial of deep-brain stimulation for Parkinson's disease," *New England Journal of Medicine*, vol. 355, no. 9, pp. 896–908, 2006.

[61] A. Williams, S. Gill, T. Varma et al., "Deep brain stimulation plus best medical therapy versus best medical therapy alone for advanced Parkinson's disease (PD SURG trial): a randomised, open-label trial," *The Lancet Neurology*, vol. 9, no. 6, pp. 581–591, 2010.

[62] K. A. Follett, F. M. Weaver, M. Stern et al., "Pallidal versus subthalamic deep-brain stimulation for Parkinson's disease," *New England Journal of Medicine*, vol. 362, no. 22, pp. 2077–2091, 2010.

[63] M. S. Okun, B. V. Gallo, G. Mandybur et al., "Subthalamic deep brain stimulation with a constant-current device in Parkinson's disease: an open-label randomised controlled trial," *The Lancet Neurology*, vol. 11, no. 2, pp. 140–149, 2012.

[64] A. Maillet, P. Krack, E. Lhommée et al., "The prominent role of serotonergic degeneration in apathy, anxiety and depression in de novo Parkinson's disease," *Brain*, vol. 139, no. 9, pp. 2486–2502, 2016.

[65] L. Loued-Khenissi and K. Preuschoff, "Apathy and noradrenaline: silent partners to mild cognitive impairment in Parkinson's disease?" *Current Opinion in Neurology*, vol. 28, no. 4, pp. 344–350, 2015.

[66] A. Feldmann, Z. Illes, P. Kosztolanyi et al., "Morphometric changes of gray matter in Parkinson's disease with depression: a voxel-based morphometry study," *Movement Disorders*, vol. 23, no. 1, pp. 42–46, 2008.

[67] C. Luo, Q. Chen, W. Song et al., "Resting-state fMRI study on drug-naive patients with Parkinson's disease and with depression," *Journal of Neurology, Neurosurgery & Psychiatry*, vol. 85, no. 6, pp. 675–683, 2014.

[68] X. Hu, X. Song, Y. Yuan et al., "Abnormal functional connectivity of the amygdala is associated with depression in Parkinson's disease," *Movement Disorders*, vol. 30, no. 2, pp. 238–244, 2015.

[69] J. S. A. M. Reijnders, B. Scholtissen, W. E. J. Weber, P. Aalten, F. R. J. Verhey, and A. F. G. Leentjens, "Neuroanatomical correlates of apathy in Parkinson's disease: a magnetic resonance imaging study using voxel-based morphometry," *Movement Disorders* vol. 25, no. 14, pp. 2318–2325, 2010.

[70] N. Carriere, P. Besson, K. Dujardin et al., "Apathy in Parkinson's disease is associated with nucleus accumbens atrophy: a magnetic resonance imaging shape analysis," *Movement Disorders* vol. 29, no. 7, pp. 897–903, 2014.

[71] H. C. Baggio, B. Segura, J. L. Garrido-Millan et al., "Resting-state frontostriatal functional connectivity in Parkinson's disease-related apathy," *Movement Disorders*, vol. 30, no. 5, pp. 671–679, 2015.

[72] K. N. Ochsner, R. R. Ray, B. Hughes et al., "Bottom-up and top-down processes in emotion generation: common and distinct neural mechanisms," *Psychological Science*, vol. 20, no. 11, pp. 1322–1331, 2009.

[73] F. Le Jeune, D. Drapier, A. Bourguignon et al., "Subthalamic nucleus stimulation in Parkinson disease induces apathy: a PET study," *Neurology*, vol. 73, no. 21, pp. 1746–1751, 2009.

[74] G. Aston-Jones, J. Rajkowski, and J. Cohen, "Locus coeruleus and regulation of behavioral flexibility and attention," *Progress in Brain Research*, vol. 126, pp. 165–182, 2000.

[75] G. Aston-Jones, J. Rajkowski, P. Kubiak, R. J. Valentino, and M. T. Shipley, "Role of the locus coeruleus in emotional activation," *Progress in Brain Research*, vol. 107, pp. 379–402, 1996.

27

Evidence of Oropharyngeal Dysfunction in Feeding in the Rat Rotenone Model of Parkinson's Disease

François D. H. Gould,[1] Andrew Gross,[1] Rebecca Z. German,[1] and Jason R. Richardson[2]

[1]*Department of Anatomy and Neurobiology, Northeast Ohio Medical University, Rootstown, OH, USA*
[2]*Department of Pharmaceutical Science, Northeast Ohio Medical University, Rootstown, OH, USA*

Correspondence should be addressed to François D. H. Gould; fgould@neomed.edu

Academic Editor: Giovanni Mirabella

Swallowing disorders in Parkinson's disease are not responsive to dopamine depletion therapy and contribute to morbidity. They are poorly understood owing to a lack of adequate models. We present the first evidence of oropharyngeal changes in a rotenone toxicity model of Parkinson's disease. Rats were recorded while feeding before and after daily rotenone injections at two different doses (2.75 mg/kg and 3 mg/kg). The higher dose had a much more severe parkinsonian phenotype than the low dose. Timing and amplitude of chewing changed, as did the coordination of chewing and swallowing. Dose-dependent effects were evident. These preliminary results indicate that future research in toxicological models of Parkinson's disease should incorporate the study of oropharyngeal dysfunction. A better understanding of nongenetic models of Parkinson's disease in feeding may open new avenues for research into the neurological and behavioral bases for swallowing dysfunction in Parkinson's disease.

1. Introduction

Parkinson's disease is the second most common primary neurodegenerative disorder worldwide, with both genetic and environmental etiologies [1–3]. The characteristic signs of Parkinson's disease—bradykinesia, rigidity, and tremor—have been linked to dopamine loss resulting from neuronal death in the substantia nigra [2, 4, 5]. However, it is becoming clear that damage occurs on a larger scale, throughout the nervous system in PD, and that many symptoms are not responsive to treatments targeting dopamine loss [6], including problems with eating and swallowing [7, 8]. Such problems are frequent in patients with Parkinson's disease. In one study, 68% of late-stage Parkinson's disease patients reported subjective dysphagia symptoms [9]. Using objective diagnostic tools such as videofluoroscopy, another study reported that over half the early stage patients in the study had objective signs of dysphagia without reporting symptoms [10]. Feeding parameters respond inconsistently to current treatments for Parkinson's diseases, deep brain stimulation, and L-dopa. Certain aspects may show improvement while others do not within the same study [11]. In other studies, responses do not improve [12, 13] or even get worse [14] with L-dopa or deep brain stimulation. As well as presenting a challenge for effective, consistent treatment of dysphagia in Parkinson's disease, these conflicting results indicate that the neurological basis for dysphagia in Parkinson's disease is probably complex and poorly understood. These significant problems constitute a major medical challenge for PD patients, severely reducing the quality of life [15]. Further, aspiration pneumonia, a complication of chronic dysphagia (pathological swallowing), has an incidence rate four times that of the general population in Parkinson's disease [16, 17] and is the leading cause of death in long-term studies [18]. The etiology, progression, and neurological basis of swallowing dysfunction in PD remain poorly understood [19, 20], owing in part to the lack of animal models addressing this question specifically [21].

The complex 1 inhibitor rotenone, a commercially available pesticide, has become established as a compound which, when administered to rats, reproduces many of the neurodegenerative and behavioral phenotypes of Parkinson's disease [22–24]. These include nigrostriatal dopamine loss, alpha synuclein aggregation, polyubiquitin formation, and evidence of inflammation and microglial activation. Behaviorally, rats with rotenone-induced parkinsonism display rigidity, bradykinesia, reduced mobility, and reduced performance in a number of tasks associated with locomotion and limb use. However, the effect of rotenone injection on swallowing and feeding function has not been assessed. In fact, so far only very limited animal model work has focused on the swallowing dysfunction component of Parkinson's disease, including studies on a single genetic variant, the Pink1 rat [25, 26], and some work on chewing in nonhuman primate models. Work on the Pink1 rat has indicated that oropharyngeal dysfunction in Parkinson's disease may appear as an early onset sign [25]; thus, by the time it is diagnosed in patients, dysphagia may be well advanced. This progression, combined with the complex nature of the neurological control of feeding and swallowing, means that little is known about the neurological basis and time of onset of swallowing dysfunction in Parkinson's disease generally and in toxin-based models of the disease specifically. The purpose of this study was to begin to establish how oropharyngeal function is affected in rotenone models of Parkinson's disease. We demonstrate and characterize disruption of the different oropharyngeal behaviors that compose feeding and swallowing in an aggressive, fast-acting rotenone model of idiopathic PD [22], as a first attempt at documenting the effects of rotenone on swallowing and feeding physiology and function. Our null hypothesis for all variables is that there is no effect of rotenone treatment. Our alternative hypotheses are as follows:

(i) We hypothesize that range of motion during chewing of the tongue and jaw will increase in the dorsoventral axis and decrease in the rostrocaudal axis, as a result of dyskinesia affecting the complex palynal chewing stroke of rodents.

(ii) We hypothesize that all measurements of duration in chewing (duration of chewing cycle, duration of jaw closing, duration of power stroke, time of tongue rostralmost position, and relative time of tongue and jaw movement) will increase due to bradykinesia caused by rotenone.

(iii) We hypothesize that measurements of timing in swallowing (swallow onset delay, pharyngeal transit time, interswallow interval, and swallow rate) will increase following rotenone injections.

2. Methods

2.1. Rotenone Administrations Protocol. The methods followed Cannon et al. [22]. Rotenone crystals were diluted into a stock solution of DMSO and emulsified in Miglyol to produce an injectable solution. 12 adult Lewis rats (Charles River, Wilmington, MA) (6 females and 6 males, 14 weeks of age) were divided into two groups that received daily IP injections of the rotenone emulsification at either 2.75 mg/kg or 3 mg/kg. These doses represent the extremes of the range for which permanent loss of dopaminergic neurons, and associated decrease of motor function, was seen in the original study on which this work is based. As the study by Cannon et al. [22] documented phenotypic variation in the progression of parkinsonian symptoms under these two dose regimes, both doses were used here. Injections were administered daily until the rats showed significant weight loss, or significant debilitative behaviors (akinesia, poor grooming, and lack of feeding). Qualitative observation confirmed the development of parkinsonian symptoms (tail and limb rigidity, akinesia, and bradykinesia), as detailed in the results. All animal studies were approved by the NEOMED IACUC (protocol number 16-002) and followed NIH guidelines for the care and use of laboratory animals. In the high-dose group, animals were euthanized when they showed severely impaired locomotion and lack of feeding drive. In the low-dose group, animals were euthanized when the animals had lost 18% of their preinjection body mass.

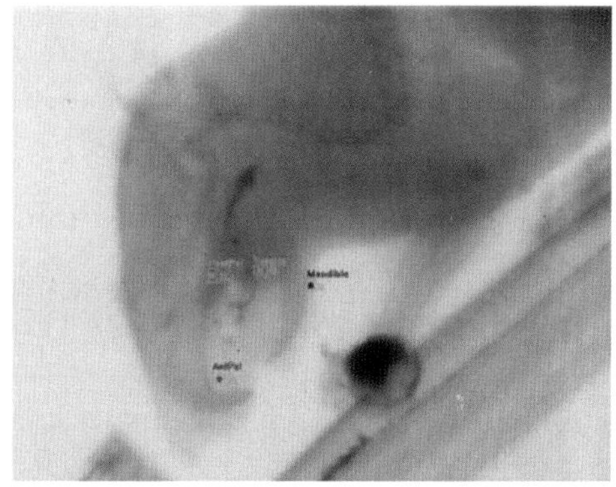

FIGURE 1: Videofluroscopic still from marker-tracking software, showing marker positions. PostPal: posterior palate; AntPal: anterior palate; Tongue: tongue; Mandible: mandible.

2.2. Radio Opaque Marker Implantation and Videofluoroscopy. Prior to recording of behavior or injection of rotenone, the rats were trained to feed on breakfast cereal (Fruit Loops, Kellogg's, Battle Creek, MI) coated with radio opaque barium powder. Once the training was complete, the rats were anesthetized with isoflurane, and radio opaque markers were implanted into the tongue, palatal gingiva, and mandibular gingiva using a 22 gauge needle and a fine wire as a plunger (Figure 1). Rats were then recorded feeding using techniques adapted from pig [27, 28] and rodent [29] models of swallowing function. Feeding was recorded at 200 frames/second (MA: 4.0, kVp: 90) until 20–25 swallows had occurred in each session. X-rays were activated using a foot pedal when the animal began feeding and were turned off once twenty to twenty-five swallows had been counted on a monitor. This reduced radiation exposure and size of the recordings. Each recording was about 50 to 100 seconds long. The methods and dosage used for this study are standard and have been tested and validated in over 30 years of studies [30, 31]. No radiation damage to animals has been observed in that time. Two preinjection sessions were recorded and then once daily from the day of the first injection until the end of the experiment.

TABLE 1: Variables measured in this study: chewing variables.

Variable	Description
Mandible: dorsoventral range	Within a chewing cycle, maximum distance travelled in the dorsoventral (y) axis by the mandibular marker.
Mandible: rostrocaudal range	Within a chewing cycle, maximum distance travelled in the rostrocaudal (x) axis by the mandibular marker.
Duration of chewing cycle	Time elapsed from maximum gape to maximum gape.
Duration of jaw closing	Time elapsed from maximum gape to mimimum gape within a cycle.
Duration of power stroke	Time from minimum gape to rostralmost position of the mandible.
Tongue: dorsoventral range	Within a chewing cycle, maximum distance travelled in the dorsoventral (y) axis by the tongue marker.
Tongue: rostrocaudal range	Within a chewing cycle, maximum distance travelled in the rostrocaudal (x) axis by the tongue marker.
Time of tongue rostralmost position	Time from beginning of chewing cycle to tongue reaching its rostralmost position.
Relative timing of tongue and jaw	Time from the mandible reaching occlusion to the tongue reaching its rostralmost position.

TABLE 2: Variables measured in this study: swallowing variables.

Variable	Description
Pharyngeal transit time	Time from first frame of movement of the bolus into the oropharynx to when the tail of the bolus passes the level of cervical vertebra 4.
Interswallow interval	Time between the onset of two consecutive swallows.
Swallow rate	Ratio of number of swallows to duration of feeding bout.
Swallow onset delay	Time between maximum gape of previous jaw cycle and onset of swallow inserted within that cycle. Categorised by jaw cycle type (chewing or biting/ingestion).

2.3. Data Collection. Feeding parameters were calculated for both chewing and swallowing. For chewing, multiple video segments comprising 5–7 consecutive chewing cycles (defined as cycles in which full molar occlusion could be seen in the video) were isolated from longer feeding videos, for a total of 15 to 20 chewing cycles per feeding bout. For each video segment, the position of the palatal, tongue, and mandibular markers was digitized using automated tracking software (ProAnalyst, Excitex, MA). These (x, y) coordinates were then scaled, rotated, and translated using the palate markers as reference points, following an established protocol [27]. This procedure removes elements of movement due to whole head movements and allows between sequence comparisons of the feeding kinematics. From these scaled, rotated, and translated data, we calculated a series of time and distance-based chewing variables (Table 1). As there were no markers in the pharynx, we were unable to extend the approach used for chewing to measure swallowing. Therefore, we measured the duration of several events directly from observation of the videos (Table 2). Summary statistics are reported in Supplementary Table 1. These variables were adapted from other studies of swallowing function in rodent models [32, 33]. Error studies were performed to assess the repeatability of these video scored events [34].

2.4. Statistical Analysis. Data were analyzed using linear mixed model multifactorial ANOVA with pre/postinjection dose, and their interaction as fixed factors, and individual as a random factor to account for interindividual variation. The units of analysis were the chewing cycle for all chewing variables. For pharyngeal transit time and swallow onset delay, the unit of analysis was the swallow. For swallow rate and interswallow interval, the unit of analysis was the feeding sequence. Although longitudinal data were collected, for this preliminary analysis, only the last time point of the rotenone pre/postinjection was included, as the focus was to document the presence of oropharyngeal dysfunction in this model. Significance level was set at 0.05. Where the interaction was significant, independent contrasts were used to test the specific effect of rotenone injection in high- and low-dose groups. For swallow onset delay, the inclusion of the extra factor (jaw cycle type) meant that there were

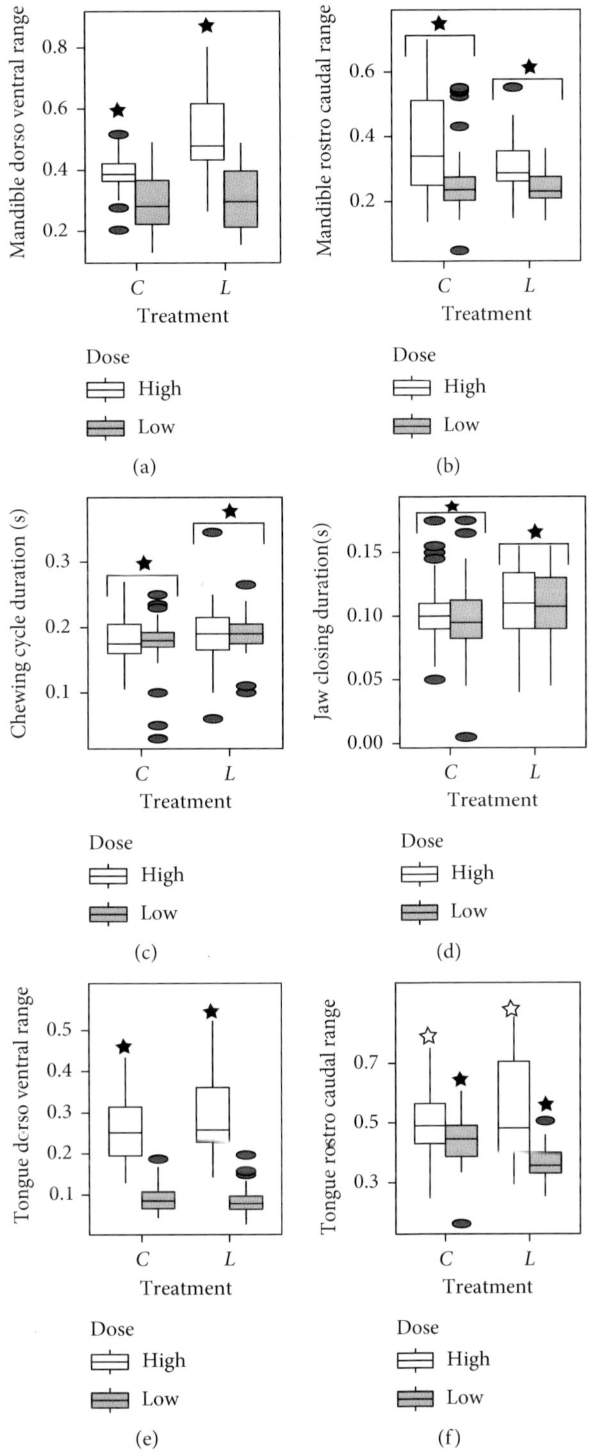

Figure 2: Boxplots of the chewing variables for which significant injection or injection-dose interactions were found. Stars indicate pairwise differences that were significant ($p < 0.005$). $n = 188$ chew cycles. C: preinjection measurements and L: last day postinjection measurements.

insufficient degrees of freedom to perform a full model with pre/postinjection, dose, cycle type, and all potential interactions. Thus, high- and low-dose groups were analyzed separately, with pre/postinjection, jaw cycle type, and their interaction as factors in the model. All statistics and calculations were performed in R [35].

3. Results

3.1. Effects of Rotenone Injection on Weight and General Motor Behavior. In the high-dose group, weight loss was recorded in all rats within 48 h of the first injection and continued throughout the course of injection until the end of the

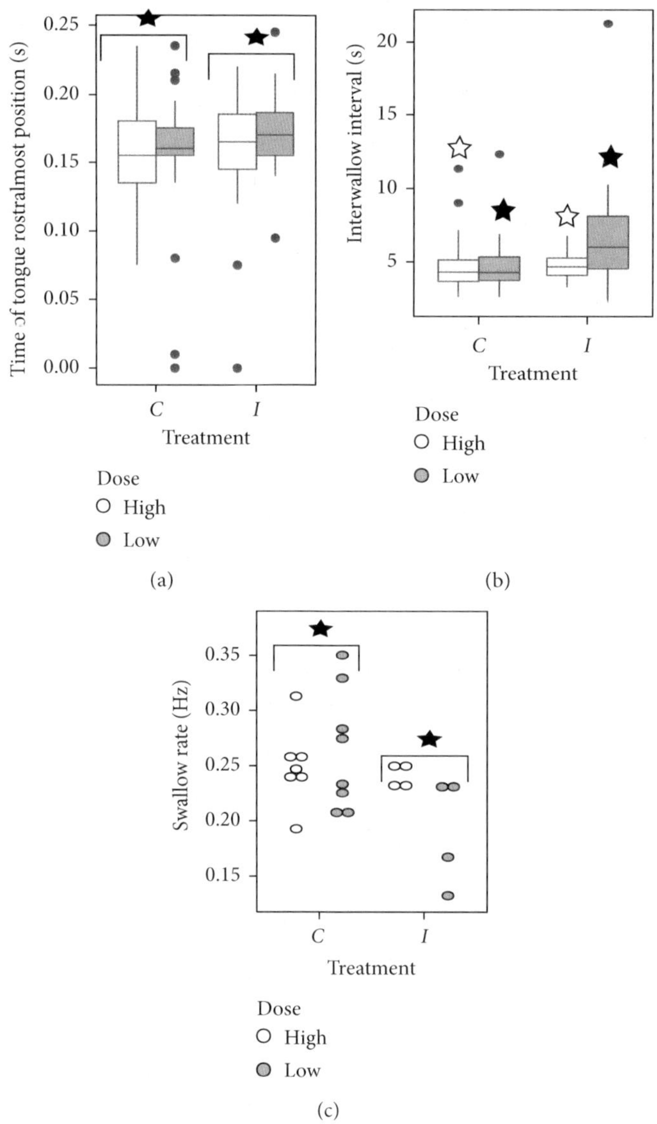

FIGURE 3: Boxplot and doplot of tongue and swallowing variables for which significant injection or injection-dose interactions were found. Stars indicate significant pairwise differences ($p < 0.05$). $n = 188$ chews (time of tongue rostralmost position). $n = 199$ swallows (interswallow interval). $n = 20$ sequences (swallow rate). C: preinjection measurements, L: last day postinjection measurements.

experiments. Porphyrin buildup and poor pelage condition, indicating impaired grooming ability, were visible in most rats from day three. Reduced to absent feeding drive is manifested from day 4. Hypokinesis, manifesting as limited motion around the cage and limited use of hindlimbs (resulting in a twisted posture when feeding), was evident from day 4. Rats in this group reached complete immobility with inability to locomote or maintain posture by day five.

In the low-dose group, weight loss began after the first injection, and by day 7 postinjection had all lost 18% of the initial body weight, the IACUC approved the end point of the study. In this group, tail rigidity, mild postural changes, and reduction in pelage condition were noted from day four. Phenotypic progression was much less than that in the high-dose group and did not progress to complete immobility.

3.2. Effects of Rotenone on Chewing and Swallowing Variables. Statistical results for the chewing variables are summarized in Supplementary Table 2(a). A significant effect of injection with rotenone, regardless of dose level, was found for rostrocaudal mandibular range of motion ($F(1,184) = 16.49$, $p < 0.001$), duration of chewing cycle ($F(1,184) = 5.25$, $p = 0.023$), duration of jaw closing ($F(1,183) = 6.95$, $p = 0.009$), and time of tongue rostralmost movement ($F(1,183) = 4.67$, $p = 0.032$). The hypothesis of longer duration of movements posttreatment is supported for chewing cycle duration, jaw closing duration, and time of rostralmost tongue position. In the high-dose rats, there was an effect of injection on dorsoventral mandibular range of motion ($p < 0.001$), tongue dorsoventral range of motion ($p = 0.049$), and tongue rostrocaudal range of motion ($p < 0.001$). In the low-dose rats, there was an effect of injection on tongue rostrocaudal range of motion ($p < 0.001$) (Figure 2). Effects of injection on swallowing variables were less pervasive than that on chewing variables (Supplementary Tables 2(b) and 2(c)). There was an effect of injection on the rate of swallowing ($F(1,13) = 5.67$, $p = 0.033$). In both the low- and high-dose injection groups, interswallow interval was longer (low dose $p < 0.001$, high dose $p < 0.001$). In the low-dose group, there was a significant effect of the interaction of injection and jaw cycle type on the delay between start of the previous jaw cycle and start of the swallow ($F(1,55) = 7.94$, $p = 0.007$). However, there is no significant difference between swallow start delay pre- and postinjection in either ingestion or chewing cycles (Figure 3).

4. Discussion

The null hypothesis of no effect could not be rejected for duration of power stroke, relative timing of tongue and jaw movement, pharyngeal transit time, and swallow onset delay. For the tongue and jaw range of motion in chewing, the alternative hypothesis of increased dorsoventral and decreased rostrocaudal range of motion was supported. For timing variables where the null hypothesis was rejected (chewing cycle duration, jaw closing time, time of tongue rostralmost position, interswallow interval, and chewing rate), the alternative hypothesis that durations increased, indicating a slowing down of movement, was supported.

The most consistent perturbations are found in chewing movement speed and range of motion changing. Chewing is affected in parkinsonian patients [36–38]. In our study, pharyngeal swallowing duration is not affected and swallowing rate decreases. This is informative neurologically and anatomically, as the embryonic origins and neural systems controlling the jaw and the pharynx are distinct [39–41]. Although these results suggest that dysphagia results from chewing deficits leading to inadequate bolus formation prior to swallow, previous work cautions against this interpretation. Chewing responds to L-dopa [36], yet this treatment does not improve dysphagia outcomes in PD patients in studies using both qualitative assessments and videofluoroscopic swallow studies [14].

Although central nervous system degeneration hypotheses could explain these patterns, peripheral neural and even muscular changes in patients with Parkinson's disease, affecting the function of nerves and muscles outside the central nervous system [42, 43], may also lie behind some of these differences.

These preliminary findings support further research into the rotenone model of Parkinson's disease to study dysphagia and oropharyngeal dysfunction in Parkinson's disease. If verified in models of Parkinson's disease that more closely reflect the clinical progression of the disease, such research may indicate new avenues for neurological and behavioral research into these debilitating conditions. General slowing down of the entire feeding process, changes in chewing kinematics, and limited effect on the pharyngeal transit time of swallowing are consistent with results from the Pink1 rat model of genetic PD [25]. We deliberately chose a fast-acting, aggressive model, yet we found differences between the two groups. Some of these may be due to the fact that the high-dose group did not receive injections for as long (the high-dose group on average survived three days of injections, the low-dose group seven). With the accelerated toxicity seen in the high-dose group, not all musculoskeletal functions may be impaired to the same degree. Given the known role of environmental toxicant exposure in Parkinson's disease, and the variability of such exposure, dosage dependency may be clinically important regarding underlying variability of Parkinson's [1, 44]. Further studies are necessary to explicitly and systematically investigate dose-dependent effects. The variation in the presence and severity of dysphagia in Parkinson's disease [20] may reflect differences in the etiology of the disease, some of which may be due to duration and severity of environmental toxin exposure, which we can model in animal systems.

This study is a preliminary attempt at documenting oropharyngeal dysfunction in a well-characterized toxicological model of Parkinson's disease. We chose to use an aggressive, fast-acting model of rotenone-induced Parkinson's disease, which limits the immediate applicability to feeding dysfunction in the human disease by omitting the gradual, progressive nature of Parkinson's disease. Future work with newer, more gradual models of rotenone-induced neurodegeneration will bridge this gap. We acknowledge limitations of this study. The study was preliminary and focused on establishing changes in oropharyngeal function in a well-validated, reliable model of pesticide-induced Parkinson's disease. As such, important data, including quantitative measurements of limb discoordination and neurodegeneration, were not included. Future studies will incorporate a more complete view of behavioral and neural degradation, including neuron damage in regions outside the nigrostriatal complex. As a result, some caution is warranted in overinterpreting these results with regard to their significance for clinical cases of Parkinson's-induced dysphagia. We only compared the end points reached by each animal relative to preinjection control recordings, so there are no results on progression. Owing to individual variation in response to toxicity and difficulties in obtaining behavioral data towards the end of the experiment, the individual animal end points vary by up to 48 hours within each dosage group. The large variances seen in our measurements may reflect different degrees of impairment at the date of last recording. Some animals for which we did not obtain later recordings may have still been able to feed but have been unwilling due to suppressed feeding drive. Thus we have a weak control for similarity in the degree of impairment. A major challenge of adopting rodent models of neurological disease for the study of dysphagia lies in the highly derived feeding behavior and anatomy of rodents, such that they rarely aspirate (take food into the airway). Thus, the main diagnostic criterion of clinical dysphagia in human patients is not transferable to rodents. However, general changes in oropharyngeal function in rodents are informative about neurological mechanisms specific to feeding that are affected in Parkinson's disease and affect the general quality of life of patients in the broader context of eating as a complex motor behavior. The usefulness of rodent models for studying these diseases is spurring research into the development of rodent-specific measures of feeding efficiency that are explicitly tied to measurable physiological changes in neuromotor function [32, 33, 45].

Acknowledgments

The authors would like to thank members of the Richardson and German labs for help in running these experiments and the staff at the NEOMED Comparative Medicine Unit for Animal Care. This work was supported in part by NIH R01ES021800. Additional support was provided by private support from the Glenn and Karen Leppo, the Richard Nicely, and the Alan and Janice Woll Parkinson's Research Funds, as well as NEOMED funds to R. Z. German. The content of this article is solely the responsibility of the authors and does not necessarily represent the official views of the National Institutes of Health or any other funding source.

References

[1] L. M. de Lau and M. M. Breteler, "Epidemiology of Parkinson's disease," *The Lancet Neurology*, vol. 5, no. 6, pp. 525–535, 2006.

[2] S. J. Kish, K. Shannak, and O. Hornykiewicz, "Uneven pattern of dopamine loss in the striatum of patients with idiopathic Parkinson's disease," *New England Journal of Medicine*, vol. 318, no. 14, pp. 876–880, 1988.

[3] W. Dauer and S. Przedborski, "Parkinson's disease: mechanisms and models," *Neuron*, vol. 39, no. 6, pp. 889–909, 2003.

[4] J. M. Fearnley and A. J. Lees, "Ageing and Parkinson's disease: substantia nigra regional selectivity," *Brain*, vol. 114, no. 5, pp. 2283–2301, 1991.

[5] D. Sulzer, "Multiple hit hypotheses for dopamine neuron loss in Parkinson's disease," *Trends in Neurosciences*, vol. 30, no. 5, pp. 244–250, 2007.

[6] M. A. Hely, J. G. L. Morris, W. G. J. Reid, and R. Trafficante, "Sydney multicenter study of Parkinson's disease: non-L-dopa-responsive problems dominate at 15 years," *Movement Disorders*, vol. 20, no. 2, pp. 190–199, 2005.

[7] G. Umemoto, Y. Tsuboi, A. Kitashima, H. Furuya, and T. Kikuta, "Impaired food transportation in Parkinson's disease related to lingual bradykinesia," *Dysphagia*, vol. 26, no. 3, pp. 250–255, 2011.

[8] J. S. Kim, J. Youn, M. K. Suh et al., "Cognitive and motor aspects of Parkinson's disease associated with dysphagia," *Canadian Journal of Neurological Sciences*, vol. 42, no. 6, pp. 395–400, 2015.

[9] M. Coelho, M. J. Marti, E. Tolosa et al., "Late-stage Parkinson's disease: the Barcelona and Lisbon cohort," *Journal of Neurology*, vol. 257, no. 9, pp. 1524–1532, 2010.

[10] J.-L. Fuh, R.-C. Lee, S.-J. Wang et al., "Swallowing difficulty in Parkinson's disease," *Clinical Neurology and Neurosurgery*, vol. 99, no. 2, pp. 106–112, 1997.

[11] M. R. Ciucci, J. M. Barkmeier-Kraemer, and S. J. Sherman, "Subthalamic nucleus deep brain stimulation improves deglutition in Parkinson's disease," *Movement Disorders*, vol. 23, no. 5, pp. 676–683, 2008.

[12] M. S. Troche, A. E. Brandimore, K. D. Foote et al., "Swallowing outcomes following unilateral STN vs. GPi surgery: a retrospective analysis," *Dysphagia*, vol. 29, no. 4, pp. 425–431, 2014.

[13] S. Lengerer, J. Kipping, N. Rommel et al., "Deep-brain-stimulation does not impair deglutition in Parkinson's disease," *Parkinsonism and Related Disorders*, vol. 18, no. 7, pp. 847–853, 2012.

[14] E. Michou, S. Hamdy, M. Harris et al., "Characterization of corticobulbar pharyngeal neurophysiology in dysphagic patients with Parkinson's disease," *Clinical Gastroenterology and Hepatology*, vol. 12, no. 12, pp. 2037.e4–2045.e4, 2014.

[15] E. K. Plowman-Prine, C. M. Sapienza, M. S. Okun et al., "The relationship between quality of life and swallowing in Parkinson's disease," *Movement Disorders*, vol. 24, no. 9, pp. 1352–1358, 2009.

[16] U. Akbar, B. Dham, Y. He et al., "Incidence and mortality trends of aspiration pneumonia in Parkinson's disease in the United States, 1979–2010," *Parkinsonism and Related Disorders*, vol. 21, no. 9, pp. 1082–1086, 2015.

[17] L. Morgante, G. Salemi, F. Meneghini et al., "Parkinson disease survival: a population-based study," *Archives of Neurology*, vol. 57, no. 4, pp. 507–512, 2000.

[18] M. A. Hely, J. G. L. Morris, R. Traficante, W. G. J. Reid, D. J. O'Sullivan, and P. M. Williamson, "The Sydney multicentre study of Parkinson's disease: progression and mortality at 10 years," *Journal of Neurology, Neurosurgery and Psychiatry*, vol. 67, no. 3, pp. 300–307, 1999.

[19] E. Michou and S. Hamdy, "Dysphagia in Parkinson's disease: a therapeutic challenge?," *Expert Review of Neurotherapeutics*, vol. 10, no. 6, pp. 875–878, 2010.

[20] I. Suttrup and T. Warnecke, "Dysphagia in Parkinson's disease," *Dysphagia*, vol. 31, no. 1, pp. 24–32, 2016.

[21] R. Z. German, A. W. Crompton, F. D. H. Gould, and A. J. Thexton, "Animal models for dysphagia studies: what have we learnt so far," *Dysphagia*, vol. 32, no. 1, pp. 73–77, 2017.

[22] J. R. Cannon, V. Tapias, H. M. Na, A. S. Honick, R. E. Drolet, and J. T. Greenamyre, "A highly reproducible rotenone model of Parkinson's disease," *Neurobiology of Disease*, vol. 34, no. 2, pp. 279–290, 2009.

[23] J. T. Greenamyre, R. Betarbet, and T. B. Sherer, "The rotenone model of Parkinson's disease: genes, environment and mitochondria," *Parkinsonism and Related Disorders*, vol. 9, no. 2, pp. 59–64, 2003.

[24] J. Blesa and S. Przedborski, "Parkinson's disease: animal models and dopaminergic cell vulnerability," *Frontiers in Neuroanatomy*, vol. 8, 2014.

[25] L. M. Grant, C. A. Kelm-Nelson, B. L. Hilby et al., "Evidence for early and progressive ultrasonic vocalization and oromotor deficits in a *PINK1* gene knockout rat model of Parkinson's disease: cranial-sensorimotor pathology in *PINK1* rats," *Journal of Neuroscience Research*, vol. 93, no. 11, pp. 1713–1727, 2015.

[26] M. R. Ciucci, S. T. Ma, J. R. Kane, A. M. Ahrens, and T. Schallert, "Limb use and complex ultrasonic vocalization in a rat model of Parkinson's disease: deficit-targeted training," *Parkinsonism and Related Disorders*, vol. 14, no. 2, pp. S172–S175, 2008.

[27] F. D. H. Gould, J. Ohlemacher, A. R. Lammers et al., "Central nervous system integration of sensorimotor signals in oral and pharyngeal structures: oropharyngeal kinematics response to recurrent laryngeal nerve lesion," *Journal of Applied Physiology*, vol. 120, no. 5, pp. 495–502, 2016.

[28] S. D. Holman, R. Campbell-Malone, P. Ding et al., "Swallowing kinematics and airway protection after palatal local anesthesia in infant pigs: swallowing after palatal anesthesia,"

The Laryngoscope, vol. 124, no. 2, pp. 436–445, 2014.

[29] T. E. Lever, S. M. Braun, R. T. Brooks et al., "Adapting human videofluoroscopic swallow study methods to detect and characterize dysphagia in murine disease models," *Journal of Visualized Experiments*, vol. 97, 2015.

[30] H. A. Franks, R. Z. German, A. W. Crompton, and K. M. Hiiemae, "Mechanism of intra-oral transport in a herbivore, the hyrax (Procavia syriacus)," *Archives of Oral Biology*, vol. 30, no. 7, pp. 539–544, 1985.

[31] R. Z. German, A. W. Crompton, L. C. Levitch, and A. J. Thexton, "The mechanism of suckling in two species of infant mammal: miniature pigs and long-tailed macaques," *Journal of Experimental Zoology*, vol. 261, no. 3, pp. 322–330, 1992.

[32] J. A. Russell, M. R. Ciucci, M. J. Hammer, and N. P. Connor, "Videofluorographic assessment of deglutitive behaviors in a rat model of aging and Parkinson disease," *Dysphagia*, vol. 28, no. 1, pp. 95–104, 2013.

[33] T. E. Lever, R. T. Brooks, L. A. Thombs et al., "Videofluoroscopic validation of a translational murine model of presbyphagia," *Dysphagia*, vol. 30, no. 3, pp. 328–342, 2015.

[34] R. C. Bailey and J. Byrnes, "A new, old method for assessing measurement error in both univariate and multivariate morphometric studies," *Systematic Zoology*, vol. 39, no. 2, pp. 124–130, 1990.

[35] R Core Team, *R: A Language and Environment for Statistical Computing*, R Foundation for Statistical Computing, Vienna, Austria, 2015.

[36] L. T. Robertson and J. P. Hammerstad, "Jaw movement dysfunction related to Parkinson's disease and partially modified by levodopa," *Journal of Neurology, Neurosurgery and Psychiatry*, vol. 60, no. 1, pp. 41–50, 1996.

[37] N. A. Leopold and M. C. Kagel, "Prepharyngeal dysphagia in Parkinson's disease," *Dysphagia*, vol. 11, no. 1, pp. 14–22, 1996.

[38] M. Bakke, S. L. Larsen, C. Lautrup, and M. Karlsborg, "Orofacial function and oral health in patients with Parkinson's disease," *European Journal of Oral Sciences*, vol. 119, no. 1, pp. 27–32, 2011.

[39] R. Z. German and A. W. Crompton, "The ontogeny of feeding in mammals," in *Feeding: Form, Function and Evolution in Tetrapod Vertebrates*, K. Schwenk, Ed., p. 537, Academic Press, San Diego, CA, USA, 2000.

[40] A. J. Miller, "Oral and pharyngeal reflexes in the mammalian nervous system: their diverse range in complexity and the pivotal role of the tongue," *Critical Reviews in Oral Biology and Medicine*, vol. 13, no. 5, pp. 409–425, 2002.

[41] K. Naganuma, M. Inoue, K. Yamamura, K. Hanada, and Y. Yamada, "Tongue and jaw muscle activities during chewing and swallowing in freely behaving rabbits," *Brain Research*, vol. 915, no. 2, pp. 185–194, 2001.

[42] L. Mu, S. Sobotka, J. Chen et al., "Arizona Parkinson's disease consortium, Parkinson disease affects peripheral sensory nerves in the pharynx," *Journal of Neuropathology and Experimental Neurology*, vol. 72, no. 7, pp. 614–623, 2013.

[43] L. Mu, S. Sobotka, J. Chen et al., "Arizona Parkinson's disease consortium, altered pharyngeal muscles in Parkinson disease," *Journal of Neuropathology and Experimental Neurology*, vol. 71, no. 6, pp. 520–530, 2012.

[44] D. A. Di Monte, "The role of environmental agents in Parkinson's disease," *Clinical Neuroscience Research*, vol. 1, no. 6, pp. 419–426, 2001.

[45] T. E. Lever, E. Simon, K. T. Cox et al., "A mouse model of pharyngeal dysphagia in amyotrophic lateral sclerosis," *Dysphagia*, vol. 25, no. 2, pp. 112–126, 2009.

28

Complexity Analysis of Electroencephalogram Dynamics in Patients with Parkinson's Disease

Guotao Liu,[1] Yanping Zhang,[1] Zhenghui Hu,[2] Xiuquan Du,[1] Wanqing Wu,[3] Chenchu Xu,[1] Xiangyang Wang,[4] and Shuo Li[5]

[1]*School of Computer Science and Technology, Anhui University, Hefei 230601, China*
[2]*Center for Optics and Optoelectronics Research, College of Science, Zhejiang University of Technology, Pingfeng Campus, Liuhe Road 288, Xihu District, Hangzhou 310023, China*
[3]*Shenzhen Institutes of Advanced Technology, Chinese Academy of Sciences, Shenzhen 518055, China*
[4]*Anhui Electrical Engineering Professional Technique College, Hefei 230051, China*
[5]*Department of Medical Imaging, Schulich School of Medicine and Dentistry, University of Western Ontario, 1151 Richmond St, London, ON, Canada*

Correspondence should be addressed to Xiuquan Du; dxqllp@163.com and Wanqing Wu; wq.wu@siat.ac.cn

Academic Editor: Peipeng Liang

In this study, a new combination scheme has been proposed for detecting Parkinson's disease (PD) from electroencephalogram (EEG) signal recorded from normal subjects and PD patients. The scheme is based on discrete wavelet transform (DWT), sample entropy (SampEn), and the three-way decision model in analysis of EEG signal. The EEG signal is noisy and nonstationary, and, as a consequence, it becomes difficult to distinguish it visually. However, the scheme is a well-established methodology in analysis of EEG signal in three stages. In the first stage, the DWT was applied to acquire the split frequency information; here, we use three-level DWT to decompose EEG signal into approximation and detail coefficients; in this stage, we aim to remove the useless and noise information and acquire the effective information. In the second stage, as the SampEn has advantage in analyzing the EEG signal, we use the approximation coefficient to compute the SampEn values. Finally, we detect the PD patients using three-way decision based on optimal center constructive covering algorithm (O_CCA) with the accuracy about 92.86%. Without DWT as preprocessing step, the detection rate reduces to 88.10%. Overall, the combination scheme we proposed is suitable and efficient in analyzing the EEG signal with higher accuracy.

1. Introduction

Parkinson's disease (PD) is a physical disorder that occurs in the brain and affects the motor system. It is the second most common neurodegenerative disease after Alzheimer's disease. 1% to 2% of the elderly are affected because the incidence increases above the age of 50 [1]. Most cases of PD are sporadic and known as idiopathic. However, the causes of PD are unknown; several possible mechanisms have been proposed, such as exogenous toxins, inflammation, genetic mutations, and the combinations of these factors [2]. A generally accepted hypothesis is that PD is related to genetic and environmental factors most. In PD patients, there are three cardinal motor symptoms, such as bradykinesia, rigidity, and tremor. Some statistics about PD indicate that tremor is its most visible signature. Tremor is the predominant symptom in some PD patients, while, in others patients, the tremor is absent or mild. The gait problems are another spectrum of PD symptoms, characterized by shuffling, small steps, decreased arm swing, and a forward bended posture. Furthermore, freezing of gait (FOG) occurs in 30–60% of the PD patients [3]. Serious damage to multiple neuronal systems causing complex biochemical changes explained the severity of PD. Through the study of the PD pathology, researchers have put forward a variety of effective detecting PD methods, including resting state functional magnetic resonance imaging and the EEG signal analysis. However, on the one hand, the accuracy of detection rate is still not satisfactory, and, on the other hand, the methods used are complex and not efficient in detecting PD.

The German psychiatrist, Hans Berger, recorded the electrical currents in the brain which was discovered by Richard Canton, and he named them the electroencephalogram (EEG) [4]. The clinical EEG signal is a time series of electrical potentials representing the sum of a very large number of neuronal dendritic potentials in the brain. It contains a lot of useful information relating to the different physiological states of the brain. In other words, the EEG signal is a useful way in understanding the complex dynamical behavior of the brain. Since EEG signal can be in a noninvasive way to record a long time spacing, we can exclude contingency and the monitoring incidental disorders under some conditions.

EEG records the brain electrical signals, and PD is a central nervous system dementia in which EEG signal abnormalities are more frequently shown [5]. For these reasons, it is necessary to promote EEG signal detection techniques that help to identify PD clinically. In 2012, a method for detection of freezing of gait (FOG) in PD patients using EEG signals has been proposed by Handojoseno et al. [6]. FOG is one of the symptom in PD patients; and their method used discrete wavelet transform (DWT) to decompose the EEG signal into EEG subbands, Wavelet Energy and Total Wavelet Entropy. Then, the features of PD patients' EEG signal would be identified by the backpropagation neural network classifier, and the accuracy is around 75%. Later on, they found that the frequency domain information was better than time domain information in discrimination EEG signals. In this case, they used the two domains in PD detection, acquiring the combination accuracy of 80.2% [7]. Hansen et al. researched the idiopathic rapid eye movement (REM) sleep behavior disorder (iRBD) in early prediction of Parkinson's disease [8]. They classified the subjects into two classes by the EEG similarity. The classical K-means and Bayesian classifier were the classification. The study demonstrated that the sensitivity and specificity will reach 80% and 90% from the classifiers above. Another two novel and effective methods were shown in the next. One of the methods is to characterize alterations in directional brain connectivity unique to PD with depression using the resting state functional magnetic resonance imaging (rs-fMRI) [9]. Another method is, though, the changes of amplitude of low-frequency fluctuations (ALFF) in patients with PD [10], and the rs-fMRI has been considered for development as a biomarker and analytical tool for evaluation of PD [11]. The proposed methods could detect the significant alterations of ALFF in the subcortical regions and prefrontal cortex in PD patients.

Few studies have been applied EEG in PD patients; they found differences in the EEG signals recorded from PD patients and normal subjects. To make the detection method developed in this study much more fit to people's decision-making rules, three-way decision model was proposed in rough set theory, and it is very suitable in dealing with decision or classifying issue. In this study, we proposed a new combination scheme to detect the PD EEG signal in normal subject and PD patients. The discrete wavelet transform (DWT) decomposed the EEG into subbands. Then, using the sample entropy (SampEn), we analyzed these subbands and obtained the SampEn values. At last, the three-way decision model based on optimal center constructive covering algorithm (O_CCA) was designed to detect the EEG signal. The O_CCA was a classifier in the scheme, and it used the SampEn values as its condition attributes in classification. In the experiment, it is shown that the scheme we proposed is able to detect the PD EEG signal with a high accuracy.

This paper is organized as follows. Section 2 describes the data acquirement and its format that we used in this work, describes the combination methods, respectively, gives the features that are in subbands decomposed by DWT, then describes SampEn method and SampEn values in detail (these methods aim to extract the features from EEG signal), and defines the attributes and O_CCA classifier that were used. Section 3 presents the classification results, reviews the scheme, and discusses the results obtained in this study. In the end, Section 4 gives the conclusions.

2. Materials and Methods

2.1. Data. This study is designed according to the principles of the Declaration of Helsinki and approved by the Ethics Committee of the Second People's Hospital of Shenzhen in China. The EEG data are from 42 participants aged 63 to 78 years. All participants had been notified that we will take their EEG signal recording in this study. The participants include two cases: 25 healthy subjects that include 15 male (aged 65 to 73) and 10 female (aged 63 to 74) and 17 PD patients that include 10 male (aged 68 to 76) and 7 female (aged 70 to 78). All the participants do not have other diseases (such as insomnia, heart disease, and chronic obstructive pulmonary disease) which influence EEG signal in this study. The experiment of this study was performed in Matlab (R2014b, 64 bits).

The clinical EEG signal data we used in this study is recorded by 10-channel EEG time series, and the recordings were made under awake and relaxed conditions. All subjects closed their eyes to reduce the nictation noise interference, and each recording continues 40 seconds at a sampling rate of 250 Hz. The 10-channel EEG electrode placement was shown in Figure 1, F3 and F4 channels were measured on the frontal region, C3 and C4 channels on the central region, T3 and T4 channels on the temporal region, P3 and P4 channels on the parietal region, and O1 and O2 channels on the occipital region.

2.2. Methodology. In this work, the EEG signals analysis procedures are composed of four main steps, boxed in Figure 2. We first apply DWT to decompose the EEG signal into subbands and then analyze these subbands which was significant part and compute the sample entropy. Use the SampEn as condition attributes in three-way decision model based on the optimal center constructive covering algorithm (O_CCA). At last, we use the three-way decision rules to analyze the EEG signal that belongs to PD patient or not. These methods are explained in detail below. DWT and

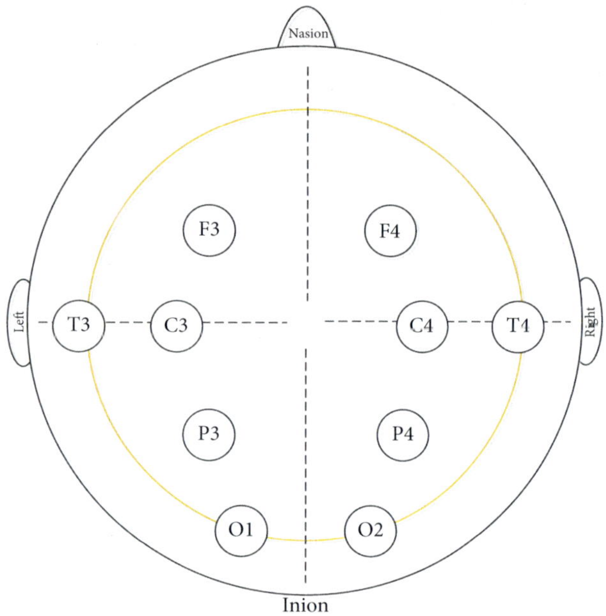

FIGURE 1: 10-channel EEG electrode placement.

SampEn methods are the feature extraction methods; three-way decision model is the classifier in this scheme, and also we compare the accuracy rate with other binary classifiers such as SVM and KNN in the end.

2.2.1. Discrete Wavelet Transform. Wavelet transform (WT) and Fourier transform (FT) are widely applied to solve various problems in many research fields, respectively. The Fourier transform of a signal contains the frequency domain, but it lacks the time domain over the analysis window. The FT coefficient does not change with time and it is constant in the majority of situations [12]. In this case, it cannot analyze the nonstationary signal with a minimum error. Besides, the FT coefficient is the global region and the time localization information cannot reflect very clearly. The short-time Fourier transform (STFT) is proposed to divide signal into sort time interval and then acquire time and frequency domain in the localization analysis windows. STFT could only give the fixed time and frequency analysis window with the entire signal. Over the past few decades, wavelet transform analysis has been developed as an improvement on Fourier transform especially in the STFT. Its main advantage in analyzing physiological systems is its capability to detect and analyze nonstationarity in signals and its related aspect like trends, breakdown points, and discontinuity. Wavelets are well localized in both time and frequency domain [13]. In WT, we could get better low-frequency information in long time window and get high frequency in short-time window. Unlike Fourier transform, WT could generate sensitivity frequency information in a low frequency and provide sensitivity time detailed information in a high frequency.

Contrary to Fourier transforms, the continuous wavelet transform (CWT) [14] on the basis of wavelet function ψ, scaled (a) and shifted (b) and the signal $x(t)$, is defined by

$$\mathrm{CWT}(a,b) = \int_{-\infty}^{\infty} x(t) \frac{1}{\sqrt{|a|}} \psi^{*}\left(\frac{t-b}{a}\right) dt, \qquad (1)$$

where $(*)$ denotes the complex conjugation, a is called scaling or reciprocal of frequency parameters, and b is called shifting or time localization parameters. The parameters of CWT were complicated in calculate. Therefore, the more efficient and brief wavelet analysis was present with the changed time scaled parameters (a, b), so that the correlation called discrete wavelet transform (DWT), such wavelet analysis, could be written as

$$\mathrm{DWT}(j,k) = \frac{1}{\sqrt{|2^j|}} \int_{-\infty}^{\infty} x(t) \psi\left(\frac{t-2^j k}{2^j}\right) dt, \qquad (2)$$

with 2^j replacing a and $2^j k$ replacing b. In the multiresolution signal analysis, Mallat proposed efficient methods to analyze the signal through a series of quadrature mirror filters which contains high-pass (HP) and low-pass (LP) filter.

In DWT algorithm, the signal passed through HP and LP filters to acquire the split frequency information [15]. According to the basic theory of Nyquist sampling theorem [16], the frequency information from the HP filter is referred to as detail coefficient; it has reserved the high frequency bandwidth of the original signal. Similarly, the frequency information from the LP filter is referred to as approximation coefficient; it has reserved the low-frequency bandwidth of the original signal. After the first-level filter, the detail and approximation coefficients are called D_1 and A_1, respectively. The structure of this wavelet decomposition with the corresponding EEG signal and its approximation and detail coefficients at each level are shown in Figure 3.

In this study, DWT is the first stage in feature extraction. As the EEG signals have been noised by the movements of eyes and contractions of facial muscles in collecting process, we employed the three-level DWT to analyze EEG signal of both normal and PD patients [17]. D_1, A_1, D_2, A_2, D_3, and A_3 represent each level detail and approximation coefficients. Here, we used f to represent the sampling frequency 250 Hz of original EEG signal, and the corresponding frequency bands of each detail and approximation coefficients are $f/2 - f, 0 - f/2, f/4 - f/2, 0 - f/4, f/8 - f/4, 0 - f/8$. The original EEG signal and its detail and approximation coefficients that applied the three-level DWT are shown in Figure 4. It has illustrated the amplitude and frequency alterations of the normal subject C4 channel of the signal.

2.2.2. Sample Entropy. SampEn is a measure that quantifies the regularity or predictability of experimental EEG and biological time series. It is also a parameter to analyze the time series [18]. SampEn was proposed by Richman and Moorman [19]; it is a measure of signal regularity and complexity like approximate entropy (ApEn). The sample and approximate entropy both measure the data regularity of the data patterns of each other. Pincus proposed the ApEn algorithm [20]; it is

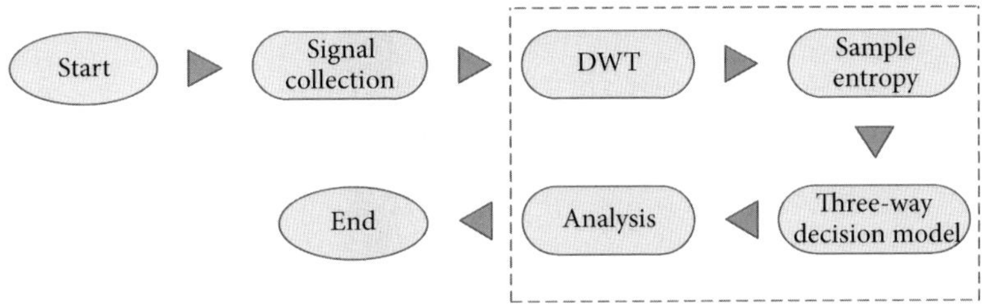

FIGURE 2: Overall EEG signals analysis procedure.

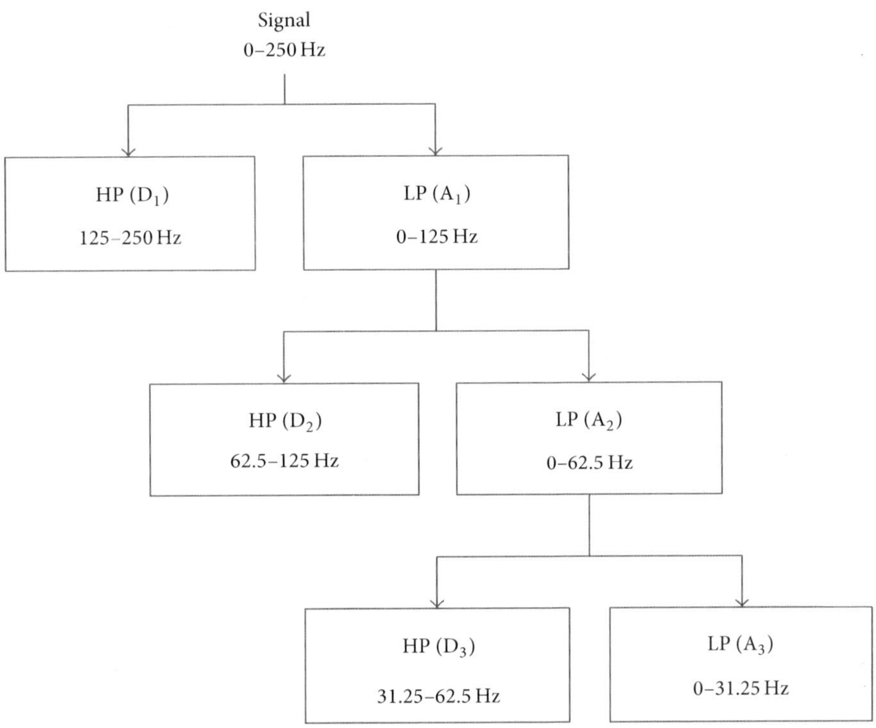

FIGURE 3: The structure of the three-level DWT of EEG signal.

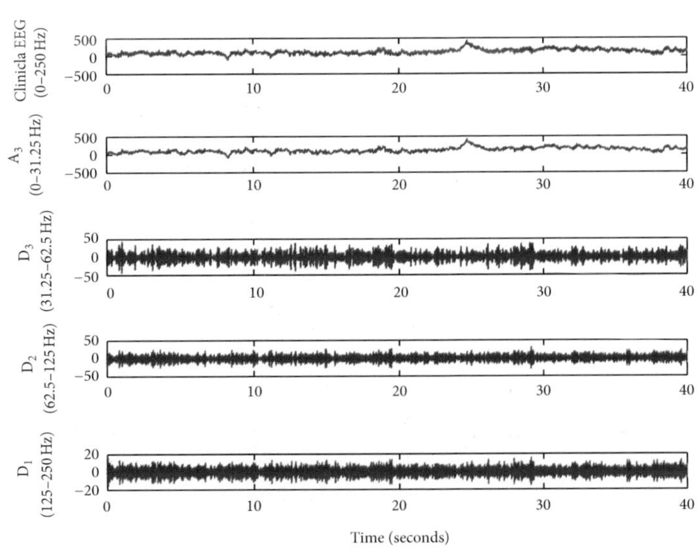

FIGURE 4: Applied three-level DWT of a clinical EEG signal.

a stability and independent model. The detail of computing ApEn is shown in the following. Consider the time series of EEG signal, $x(n)$, $n = 1, 2, \ldots, N$. A data pattern length m, which is also called embedding dimension, is used to construct the state vectors $u(i)$ in the embedding space R^m, $u(i) = [x(i), x(i+1), \ldots, x(i+m-1)]$, for each i, $1 \le i \le N - m + 1$, and next

$$C_i^m(r) = \frac{1}{N-m+1} \sum_{j=1}^{N-m+1} \theta(r - d(u(i), u(j))), \quad (3)$$

with θ is the Heaviside function, $\theta(x) = 1$ if $x \ge 0$ and $\theta(x) = 0$; otherwise, r is the signal comparison distance vector and $d(u(i), u(j))$ is distance measure written as

$$d(u(i), u(j)) = \max_{k=1,2,\ldots,m} (|x(i+k) - x(j+k)|), \quad (4)$$

with $1 \le k \le m-1$; $1 \le i, j \le N - m + 1$, $i \ne j$. Then, define $\Phi^m(r)$ as

$$\Phi^m(r) = \frac{1}{N-m+1} \sum_{i=1}^{N-m+1} \log C_i^m(r). \quad (5)$$

We have the ApEn formulation defined by

$$\text{ApEn}(m, r, N) = \Phi^m(r) - \Phi^{m+1}(r), \quad (6)$$

where the ApEn basically measures the logarithmic likelihood that runs of patterns close to length m within the same tolerance within r which will remain close on next incremental comparisons. To compute the ApEn, we should specify the two input parameters, m and r; it is also set to fixed values.

SampEn is largely independent of record length and displays relative consistencies under circumstances where ApEn does not [21]. SampEn is an improved algorithm based on ApEn, which is a novel measure that quantifies the regularity or predictability of a time series. To calculate the SampEn, there is some similarity to ApEn, as the time series of data is $x(n)$, $n = 1, 2, \ldots, N$, the other condition and $d(u(i), u(j))$ are similar to ApEn algorithm, and, next, for each i, $1 \le i \le N - m$, $i \ne j$,

$$B^m(r) = \frac{1}{N-m} \sum_{i=1}^{N-m} \theta(r - d(u(i), u(j))), \quad (7)$$

and, for the same for the embedding dimension $M = m + 1$, we define $A_i^M(r)$ as

$$A^M(r) = \frac{1}{N-m} \sum_{i=1}^{N-m} \theta(r - d(u_M(i), u_M(j))), \quad (8)$$

where

$$d(u_M(i), u_M(j)) = \max_{k=1,2,\ldots,m} (|x(i+k) - x(j+k)|), \quad (9)$$

with $1 \le k \le M - 1$; $1 \le i, j \le N - M + 1$, $i \ne j$.

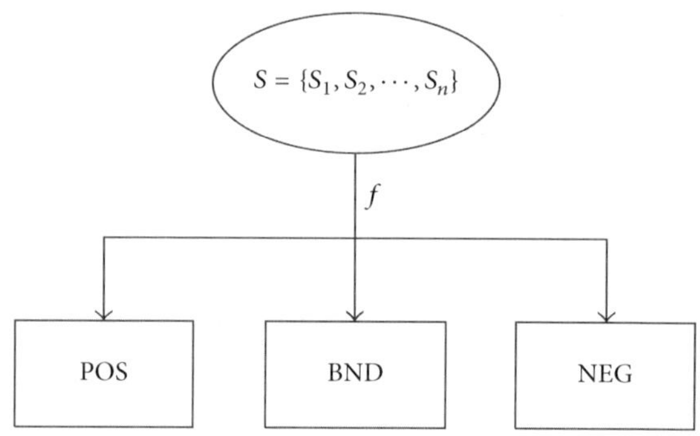

FIGURE 5: Three-way decisions model.

For fixed m, r, SampEn is given by the following formula:

$$\text{SampEn}(m, r, N) = -\ln\left[\frac{A^M(r)}{B^m(r)}\right], \quad (10)$$

where m and r are the two input parameters, m means the length of time series that will be compared, and r represents the similarity criterion, and N is the length of the time series. It is imperative that parameters should be carefully chosen; in this study, we have calculated SampEn (m, r, N) for all signals with $m = 2$ and $r = 20\%$ of the standard deviation of the specific individual subject's time series [22] and N as 10000. The signal length of each channel is fixed value.

Comparing (6) and (10), there are two major differences between ApEn and SampEn algorithm; SampEn does not statistics self-matches and does not use a template-wise approach when estimating conditional probabilities. It also shown that SampEn algorithm is of much less space complexity and time complexity. Hence, in this work, we use SampEn instead of ApEn to analyze the complexity and regularity of EEG signal in each channel. Then, the SampEn features were fed to the classifier three-way decisions model.

2.2.3. Three-Way Decisions Model. The theory of three-way decisions is proposed by Yao and used to interpret the three regions in rough set [23], and it is constructed based on the notions of acceptance, rejection, and noncommitment [24]. It is an extension of the traditional used binary-decision model with an added third option. The model is widely used in the uncertain or incomplete information areas, commonly used in everyday life, and widely applied in many fields. Based on the thresholds, it divides the universe into three regions as positive region (POS), boundary region (BND), and negative region (NEG) [25], as shown in Figure 5. However, a challenge of the early study of three-way decision model based on the rough set, such as Decision Theoretic of Rough Set Model (DTRSM), is how to compute the thresholds [26]. In most cases, the thresholds are calculated from given loss functions based on the experience of experts. In this case, the model cannot avoid artificial disturbance in selection of loss functions, as they could lead to a subjective result. In this paper, we applied the three-way decision model in detecting PD patients by the EEG features. So we should

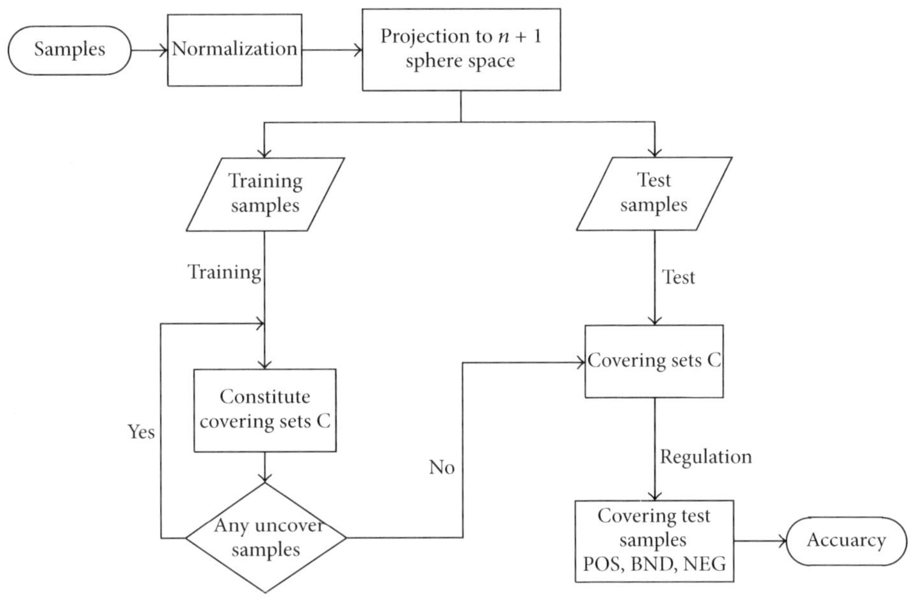

FIGURE 6: The O_CCA algorithm.

make the data analysis in objective way and decrease artificial disturbance.

We propose a novel three-way decision model based on the optimal center in constructive covering algorithm (O_CCA). It is the development of the CCA by exactly finding out the center of the covering regions [27]. The O_CCA could produce three regions automatically according to the data; it not necessary to give parameters by the a priori knowledge. We classify the data based on the three regions. The realization steps of model based on O_CCA were introduced in the following.

We begin from the work by giving the data set $U = \{(x_1, y_1), (x_2, y_2), \ldots, (x_p, y_p)\}$, where $x_i = (x_i^1, x_i^2, \ldots, x_i^n)$, $(i = 1, 2, \ldots, p)$ represents the dimensional condition attribute of the sample and y_i is the decision attribute.

The first step of processing data is normalization, and then map data to $(n+1)$ dimensional sphere S^{n+1} by $T : U \rightarrow S^{n+1}, T(x) = (x, \sqrt{R^2 - |x|^2})$, where $R \geq \max\{|x|,\ x \in U\}$. We project the samples onto $n+1$-dimensional sphere to make the length of each of the samples equal. And, then, we divided samples to training and testing based on the 10-fold cross-validation. For the training samples, we first select all the not covered samples belonging to the same class to constitute covering sets C_{set} and then compute x^{mean} from condition attributes. According to the nearest mean [28] and Euclidean distance, we select the most closest sample x_i to x^{mean} from the C_{set} as the center of a cover. Compute the cover radius θ [29]. Based on the center x_i and radius θ, get the covering sets C on S^{n+1}. Execute the steps above until all the training samples are covered. At the end, we acquire a set of covers $C = \{C_1, C_2, \ldots, C_m\}$, where $C_i = \{C_i^1, C_i^2, \ldots, C_i^{m_i}\}$, representing that cover C_i has at least one subcover and includes all of the ith training samples.

According to the definition of three regions [30] based on O_CCA, we can make three-way decisions on the test samples. We assume (c_1^k, θ_1^k) as the center and radius of $C_1^k \in C_1$, (c_2^l, θ_2^l) is the center and radius of $C_2^l \in C_2$. The rules of three-way decision of the test sample x_t are shown as follows:

(1) $x_t \in \text{POS}(C_1)$, where the condition is $\text{dist}(x_t, c_1^k) \leq \theta_1^k$ and $\text{dist}(x_t, c_2^l) > \theta_2^l$, meaning that x_t has the same decision attribute with the cover sets C_1, and we have the right classification.

(2) $x_t \in \text{NEG}(C_1)$, where the condition is $\text{dist}(x_t, c_1^k) > \theta_1^k$ and $\text{dist}(x_t, c_2^l) \leq \theta_2^l$, meaning that x_t has the different decision attribute with the cover sets C_1, and we did not classify it correctly.

(3) $x_t \in \text{BND}(C_1)$, otherwise, it means that, under the judgment condition of the current, we cannot give its category directly. We need much more evidence to classify the samples in this cover.

All the steps could be got from Figure 6 briefly. In this model, the three regions are formed automatically based on the distribution of the samples without any parameters. At the end, according to the decision rules, we can classify the test samples directly.

3. Result and Discussion

Detecting the PD patients' EEG signal from normal subjects and PD patients is a hard task for a trained professional visually. In our study, we used the DWT as the preprocessing step, as it provides the time-frequency localization information of signal and then uses sample entropy theory to acquire the SampEn of each of the channels. At last, we use the three-way decision model based on the optimal center constructive covering algorithm (O_CCA) as the classifier to distinguish the EEG signal.

TABLE 1: Results of classification from the O_CCA classifier model.

EEG signal (SI)	DWT (yes/no)	Classifier	ECI	BI	CCI	Err (%)	Bnd (%)	Acc (%)
42	Yes	O_CCA	2	1	39	4.76	2.38	92.86
42	No	O_CCA	3	2	37	7.14	4.76	88.10

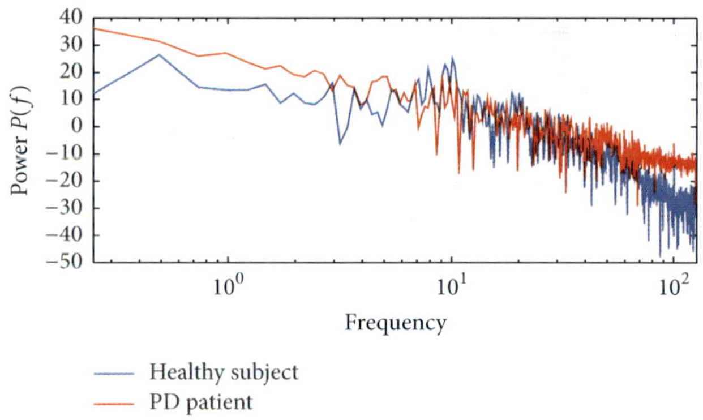

FIGURE 7: Power spectra (the occipital region O2-channel signal; the blue is healthy subject and red is PD patient).

Three-level DWT was applied to the clinical EEG signal for both normal subject and PD patients. The structure for this DWT along with the corresponding frequency bands of the approximations and detail coefficients at each level is in Figure 3. In Figure 4, the approximation and detail coefficients of channel C4 measured on the central region are shown.

Power spectra can provide information about the excitability of EEG signals [31]. The composition of frequency of the different EEG frequency states is well-established. Figure 7 shows the power spectra of channel O2 measured on the occipital region. Blue means the normal subject power spectra, and red means the power spectra of PD patient EEG signal. Comparing the two power spectra, a difference in the clinical EEG signal has been indicated, and it shows some understanding of the relationship between spectral information and SampEn. The significant difference of the two power spectra is in the 0–110 Hz, so the DWT of the EEG signal is necessary.

In the three-way decision model based on O_CCA, each instance used in the model contains 11 attributes, which consist of 10 condition attributes and one decision attribute. The 10 condition attributes are the SampEn of the 10 channels of one subject. The decision attributes are set by 0 to normal objects and 1 to PD patients. In order to detect the validity of the classification model, we have established three evaluation criteria, which are Acc = CCI/SI, Err = ECI/SI, Bnd = BI/SI, where SI means all EEG signal instances; CCI means the number of instances correctly classified in the POS regions; ECI means the number of instances mistakenly classified in the NEG regions; BI means the number of instances classified in the boundary regions. We compute the two forms of the data; they were originated in two types of SampEn, one that applied the DWT of clinical EEG signal.

TABLE 2: The data applied DWT of results in binary classifier.

EEG signal (SI)	Classifier	ECI	CCI	Err (%)	Acc (%)
42	SVM	1	41	2.38	97.62
42	KNN	4	38	9.52	90.48
42	NB	5	37	11.90	88.10
42	RF	7	35	19.67	83.33

The results of classifying subjects with three-way decision model based on O_CCA with two types of data are shown in Table 1. From the table, we can see that, in the same classifier, the data that applied DWT provided well performing results. The classification accuracy which applied DWT is 92.86%. It is higher than the accuracy 88.10% without DWT. This indicates that the DWT is an absolutely necessary part of analysis of EEG signal. Although applying DWT increases the complexity, the accuracy of classifier has improved obviously. We choose three-way decision model as classifier instead of the numerous binary classifiers; three-way decision model has boundary region compared to binary classifier. In detection of Parkinson's disease, the classifier we applied should not only have a high accuracy but also be suitable to analyze biomedical information. The instances in the boundary region mean delay decision; that is, by the present information, the model being unable to detect this instance is PD subject or normal. We need much more information to detect it. In the practical life, the boundary region represents the subject that needs further investigation.

To compare this classifier model efficiently, we use the applied DWT EEG data in the binary classifier and in common use binary classifier. Table 2 shows that only classical SVM has higher accuracy than our model, but all these binary classifiers cannot provide the boundary region. It is arbitrary decision in diagnosis. Overall, the three-way decision model based on O_CCA has a high accuracy and gives a boundary region; these classification methods are much more suitable in detecting PD EEG signal than binary classifier. In this study, we have proposed a complexity analysis of EEG signal scheme, which combines three methods as follows: DWT, SampEn as the feature extraction methods, and O_CCA as the classifier method. As a combination scheme, DWT is necessary in clinical EEG signal preprocessing step; the study also demonstrated that choosing the SampEn for the classification condition attributes is sensible. In our study, we can infer from the classification accuracy that the three-way decision model based on O_CCA is suitable and efficient in analyzing the EEG signal.

In this study, in the feature, we need more subjects in order to generalize the results obtained in analysis. Simultaneously, we will abide by the standard of choosing participants, and we will also extract more data related to PD features in the following study. Possibly only some channels related to PD, not all channels, attribute reduction maybe improve the sensitivity in the detection of PD.

4. Conclusion

The clinical EEG signal can be used to detect normal subjects and PD patients by suitable methods. In this study, PD patients' EEG state detection has been proposed based on the DWT, sample entropy, and O_CCA. We have shown that the three-way decision model based on O_CCA via the SampEn as condition attributes could differentiate the EEG signal with clinically significant classification accuracy of 92.86. As a result of the experiment, the O_CCA is a suitable and efficient method in EEG signal analysis. Hence, the proposed scheme methodology is appropriate for the complexity analysis of the EEG dynamics in patients with Parkinson's disease.

Authors' Contributions

In this manuscript, author Xiangyang Wang contributes in the three-way decision model analysis of the new combination scheme. As we can see from the manuscript, the new combination scheme we proposed contains DWT, SampEn, and three-way decision model. Wang is responsible for the data analysis based on three-way decision model and chooses parameters in the classifier model.

Acknowledgments

This study is supported by the National Natural Science Foundation of China (no. 61673020, no. 61602003, and no. 61402006), supported by Provincial Natural Science Research Program of Higher Education Institutions of Anhui Province (no. KJ2013A016), supported by Open Funding Project of Co-Innovation Center for Information Supply & Assurance Technology of Anhui University (no. ADXXBZ201410), supported by the Provincial Natural Science Foundation of Anhui Province (no. 1508085MF113), supported by Grants CXZZ20140909004122087 and JCYJ20150529164154046, Guangdong Image-Guided Therapy Innovation Team (2011S013), and supported by the Guangzhou Science and Technology Planning Project (no. 2016A030310129).

References

[1] A. L. Bartels and K. L. Leenders, "Parkinson's disease: the syndrome, the pathogenesis and pathophysiology," *Cortex*, vol. 45, no. 8, pp. 915–921, 2009.

[2] A. J. Angwin, D. A. Copland, H. J. Chenery, B. E. Murdoch, and P. A. Silburn, "The influence of dopamine on semantic activation in Parkinson's disease: evidence from a multipriming task," *Neuropsychology*, vol. 20, no. 3, pp. 299–306, 2006.

[3] N. Giladi, R. Kao, and S. Fahn, "Freezing phenomenon in patients with parkinsonian syndromes," *Movement Disorders*, vol. 12, no. 3, pp. 302–305, 1997.

[4] H. Berger, "Über das elektrenkephalogramm des menschen," *Archiv für Psychiatrie und Nervenkrankheiten*, vol. 87, no. 1, pp. 527–570, 1929.

[5] N. Yahia, *The Clinical, Electroencephalographic and MRI Findings in Patients with Temporal Lobe Epilepsy*, UOFK, 2015.

[6] A. M. A. Handojoseno, J. M. Shine, T. N. Nguyen et al., "The detection of Freezing of Gait in Parkinson's disease patients using EEG signals based on Wavelet decomposition," in *Proceedings of the IEEE Annual International Conference of the IEEE Engineering in Medicine and Biology Society*, pp. 69–72, San Diego, Calif, USA, August 2012.

[7] A. M. A. Handojoseno, J. M. Shine, T. N. Nguyen, Y. Tran, S. J. G. Lewis, and H. T. Nguyen, "Analysis and prediction of the freezing of gait using EEG brain dynamics," *IEEE Transactions on Neural Systems and Rehabilitation Engineering*, vol. 23, no. 5, pp. 887–896, 2015.

[8] I. H. Hansen, M. Marcussen, J. A. E. Christensen, P. Jennum, and H. B. D. Sorensen, "Detection of a sleep disorder predicting Parkinson's disease," in *Proceedings of the 35th Annual International Conference of the IEEE Engineering in Medicine and Biology Society (EMBC '13)*, pp. 5793–5796, IEEE, Osaka, Japan, July 2013.

[9] P. Liang, G. Deshpande, S. Zhao, J. Liu, X. Hu, and K. Li, "Altered directional connectivity between emotion network and motor network in Parkinson's disease with depression," *Medicine*, vol. 95, no. 30, article no. e4222, 2016.

[10] J. Xiang, X. Jia, H. Li, J. Qin, P. Liang, and K. Li, "Altered spontaneous brain activity in cortical and subcortical regions in Parkinson's disease," *Parkinson's Disease*, vol. 2016, Article ID 5246021, 6 pages, 2016.

[11] J. Zhang, L. Wei, X. Hu et al., "Specific frequency band of amplitude low-frequency flligatureuctuation predicts Parkinson's disease," *Behavioural Brain Research*, vol. 252, pp. 18–23, 2013.

[12] M. K. Kiymik, M. Akin, and A. Subasi, "Automatic recognition of alertness level by using wavelet transform and artificial neural network," *Journal of Neuroscience Methods*, vol. 139, no. 2, pp. 231–240, 2004.

[13] A. M. Ardi Handojoseno, J. M. Shine, T. N. Nguyen, Y. Tran, S. J. G. Lewis, and H. T. Nguyen, "Analysis and prediction of the freezing of gait using EEG brain dynamics," *IEEE Transactions on Neural Systems and Rehabilitation Engineering*, vol. 23, no. 5, pp. 887–896, 2015.

[14] Y. U. Khan and J. Gotman, "Wavelet based automatic seizure detection in intracerebral electroencephalogram," *Clinical Neurophysiology*, vol. 114, no. 5, pp. 898–908, 2003.

[15] S. G. Mallat, "A theory for multiresolution signal decomposition: the wavelet representation," *IEEE Transactions on Pattern Analysis and Machine Intelligence*, vol. 11, no. 7, pp. 674–693, 1989.

[16] H. Ocak, "Automatic detection of epileptic seizures in EEG using discrete wavelet transform and approximate entropy," *Expert Systems with Applications*, vol. 36, no. 2, pp. 2027–2036, 2009.

[17] S. Sanei and J. A. Chambers, *EEG Signal Processing*, John Wiley & Sons, 2013.

[18] N. Kannathal, M. L. Choo, U. R. Acharya, and P. K. Sadasivan, "Entropies for detection of epilepsy in EEG," *Computer Methods and Programs in Biomedicine*, vol. 80, no. 3, pp. 187–194, 2005.

[19] J. S. Richman and J. R. Moorman, "Physiological time-series analysis using approximate and sample entropy," *American Journal of Physiology—Heart and Circulatory Physiology*, vol. 278, no. 6, pp. H2039–H2049, 2000.

[20] S. M. Pincus, "Approximate entropy as a measure of system complexity," *Proceedings of the National Academy of Sciences of the United States of America*, vol. 88, no. 6, pp. 2297–2301, 1991.

[21] J. S. Richman and J. R. Moorman, "Physiological time-series analysis using approximate entropy and sample entropy," *American Journal of Physiology—Heart and Circulatory Physiology*, vol. 278, no. 6, pp. H2039–H2049, 2000.

[22] J. M. Yentes, N. Hunt, K. K. Schmid, J. P. Kaipust, D. McGrath, and N. Stergiou, "The appropriate use of approximate entropy and sample entropy with short data sets," *Annals of Biomedical Engineering*, vol. 41, no. 2, pp. 349–365, 2013.

[23] Y. Yao, "An outline of a theory of three-way decisions," in *Proceedings of the International Conference on Rough Sets and Current Trends in Computing*, pp. 1–17, Springer, Chengdu, China, August 2012.

[24] H. Yu and Y. Wang, "Three-way decisions method for overlapping clustering," in *Rough Sets and Current Trends in Computing: 8th International Conference, RSCTC 2012, Chengdu, China, August 17–20, 2012.Proceedings*, vol. 7413 of *Lecture Notes in Computer Science*, pp. 277–286, Springer, Berlin, Germany, 2012.

[25] Y. Yao, "The superiority of three-way decisions in probabilistic rough set models," *Information Sciences*, vol. 181, no. 6, pp. 1080–1096, 2011.

[26] X. Deng and Y. Yao, "An information-theoretic interpretation of thresholds in probabilistic rough sets," in *Proceedings of the International Conference on Rough Sets and Knowledge Technology*, pp. 369–378, Springer, Chengdu, China, August 2012.

[27] Y. Zhang, H. Xing, H. Zou et al., "A three-way decisions model based on constructive covering algorithm," in *Proceedings of the International Conference on Rough Sets and Knowledge Technology*, pp. 346–353, Springer, Halifax, Canada, October 2013.

[28] M. Skurıchina, L. I. Kuncheva, and R. P. W. Duin, "Bagging and boosting for the nearest mean classifier: effects of sample size on diversity and accuracy," in *Proceedings of the International Workshop on Multiple Classifier Systems*, pp. 62–71, Springer, Cagliari, Italy, June 2002.

[29] J. Chen, S. Zhao, and Y. Zhang, "A multi-view decision model based on CCA," in *Rough Sets and Knowledge Technology: Book Subtitle 10th International Conference, RSKT 2015, Held as Part of the International Joint Conference on Rough Sets, IJCRS 2015, Tianjin, China, November 20–23, 2015, Proceedings*, vol. 9436 of *Lecture Notes in Computer Science*, pp. 266–274, Springer, Berlin, Germany, 2015.

[30] J. Chen, Y.-P. Zhang, and S. Zhao, "Multi-granular mining for boundary regions in three-way decision theory," *Knowledge-Based Systems*, vol. 91, pp. 287–292, 2016.

[31] C. H. Bastien, M. LeBlanc, J. Carrier, and C. M. Morin, "Sleep EEG power spectra, insomnia, and chronic use of benzodiazepines," *Sleep*, vol. 26, no. 3, pp. 313–317, 2003.

Correlation of MRI Visual Scales with Neuropsychological Profile in Mild Cognitive Impairment of Parkinson's Disease

Luiz Felipe Vasconcellos,[1] João Santos Pereira,[1] Marcelo Adachi,[2] Denise Greca,[3] Manuela Cruz,[3] Ana Lara Malak,[3] Helenice Charchat-Fichman,[3] and Mariana Spitz[1]

[1]*Movement Disorders Unit, Neurology Service, Pedro Ernesto University Hospital, State University of Rio de Janeiro, Rio de Janeiro, RJ, Brazil*
[2]*Radiology Department, Hospital Central da Polícia Militar, Rio de Janeiro, RJ, Brazil*
[3]*Psychology Department, Pontifical Catholic University of Rio de Janeiro (PUC-Rio), Rio de Janeiro, RJ, Brazil*

Correspondence should be addressed to Luiz Felipe Vasconcellos; luizneurol@terra.com.br

Academic Editor: Carlo Colosimo

Few studies have evaluated magnetic resonance imaging (MRI) visual scales in Parkinson's disease-Mild Cognitive Impairment (PD-MCI). We selected 79 PD patients and 92 controls (CO) to perform neurologic and neuropsychological evaluation. Brain MRI was performed to evaluate the following scales: Global Cortical Atrophy (GCA), Fazekas, and medial temporal atrophy (MTA). The analysis revealed that both PD groups (amnestic and nonamnestic) showed worse performance on several tests when compared to CO. Memory, executive function, and attention impairment were more severe in amnestic PD-MCI group. Overall analysis of frequency of MRI visual scales by MCI subtype did not reveal any statistically significant result. Statistically significant inverse correlation was observed between GCA scale and Mini-Mental Status Examination (MMSE), Montreal Cognitive Assessment (MoCA), semantic verbal fluency, Stroop test, figure memory test, trail making test (TMT) B, and Rey Auditory Verbal Learning Test (RAVLT). The MTA scale correlated with Stroop test and Fazekas scale with figure memory test, digit span, and Stroop test according to the subgroup evaluated. Visual scales by MRI in MCI should be evaluated by cognitive domain and might be more useful in more severely impaired MCI or dementia patients.

1. Introduction

Parkinson's disease (PD) is characterized by motor and nonmotor features. Among nonmotor symptoms, cognitive impairment results in significant morbidity and mortality; therefore early diagnosis is essential for appropriate treatment and subsequent reduction of the disease burden [1]. Some variables related to increased risk of cognitive decline have been suggested, such as rigid-akinetic phenotype, aging, female gender, anticholinergic use, and mild cognitive impairment [2]. Neuropsychological risk factors to PD dementia (PDD) are impaired, semantic fluency and visuospatial and executive function [2, 3].

PD-Mild Cognitive Impairment (PD-MCI) represents a cognitive impairment not severe as to interfere in daily activities and does not fulfill criteria for dementia in a patient with clinically established PD. MCI can be classified, according to the main area of impairment, as amnestic (memory primarily affected) or nonamnestic (other cognitive function). These differences are beyond the main cognitive domain as well prognosis (higher risk for conversion to dementia) [3, 4].

Movement Disorders Society (MDS) criteria for PD-MCI and PDD seem to be the most suitable to diagnose such conditions. These criteria can be rated as level 1 or 2 depending on cognitive assessment. Level 2 (which has a higher specificity) requires neuropsychological testing of multiple domains [4, 5].

PD patients have increased risk for developing cognitive impairment and it is recommended to periodically perform a neuropsychological assessment in these patients. It is important to emphasize that executive function could worsen in OFF phase, so use of levodopa is mandatory preceding neuropsychological assessment [6].

Structural abnormalities revealed by brain magnetic resonance imaging (MRI) may be related to cognitive impairment in PD-MCI or PDD. Besides MRI, other neuroimaging tools used for this purpose include PET or SPECT, available only in specialized centers at a high cost. Conventional MRI is widely available, cost-effective, and easy to perform despite limited sensitivity and specificity. MRI visual rating scales which are useful in cognitive impairment include global cortical atrophy (GCA), medial temporal atrophy (MTA), and Fazekas scale [7]. Atrophy of several brain structures has been associated with cognitive impairment in PD, as memory with MTA and dysexecutive syndrome with cortical-subcortical structures. Comparing PDD with Alzheimer's disease (AD), abnormalities of MTA can be detected in both conditions, but with more expressive reduction in AD. A lesser degree of MTA in PD-MCI has also reported, even in cognitively intact PD patients. Possibly the association of PD-MCI and MTA represents a higher risk to develop PDD [8, 9]. One important factor to consider when analyzing previous MRI studies correlating PD-MCI with visual scales is how the diagnosis of MCI was established, as more specific criteria for PD-MCI have been recently defined. Therefore, a patient formerly diagnosed with MCI could in fact have PDD.

Studies with GCA, MTA, and white matter hyperintensity (WMH) evaluated by the Fazekas scale in PD-MCI are rare and present doubtful results.

We evaluated in the present study if these structural changes detected by MRI could be related to MCI subtype and its frequency in PD patients comparing with control group (CO).

2. Methods

PD patients were sequentially and prospectively recruited from 3 outpatient Movement Disorders Clinics during 18 months. All fulfilled UK Brain Bank Criteria for PD [10]. Control group (CO) consisted of individuals without any neurologic or psychiatric diagnoses being family members of patients or hospital employees. All patients and controls were between 50 and 75 years old and had more than 4 years of education. Both groups consisted of individuals with MCI according to neuropsychology evaluation. They underwent blood screening exams, including thyroid hormones, B12 vitamin, folic acid, and venereal disease research test and brain MRI. They were excluded in the case of any abnormality in the exams, for example, any kind of stroke in the MRI. The use of benzodiazepine and anticholinergic was another exclusion criterion. Subjects previously diagnosed with dementia and depression were also excluded.

The assessment consisted of neurologic examination with several clinical scales:

(i) Motor assessment: Hoehn-Yahr Scale and Unified Parkinson's Disease Rating Scale (UPDRS).
(ii) Quality of life: PDQ-39.
(iii) Activities of daily living: Schwab-England.
(iv) Total medication: levodopa equivalent dose (LED).
(v) Criteria for depression and anxiety: DSM IV.

PD patients were classified according to the predominant motor sign: tremulous, akinetic-rigid, or mixed.

Neuropsychology evaluation with the following tests was performed:

(i) Mini-Mental Status Examination (MMSE).
(ii) Montreal Cognitive Assessment (MoCA).
(iii) Clock Drawing Test.
(iv) Verbal fluency: semantic (animals) and phonemic (letters F, A, and S).
(v) Stroop test.
(vi) Figure memory test (FMT).
(vii) Trail making test (TMT).
(viii) Digit span (WAIS-III).
(ix) Rey Auditory Verbal Learning Test (RAVLT).
(x) Hooper Visual Organization Test.
(xi) Beck Depression Inventory (BDI).

PD-MCI was classified according to MDS criteria (Level 2) and CO-MCI according to Forlenza et al., both with −1.5 standard deviation (SD) below the mean [4, 11]. Memory impairment characterized amnestic MCI and impairment of one or more non-memory cognitive domains, including executive function, attention, language and visuospatial skills, characterized nonamnestic MCI.

The medium time lapse between neuropsychological evaluation and MRI was 2 months. MRI scans were performed on a Siemens 1.5-Tesla device. Three-dimensional T1-weighted images were acquired in sagittal orientation employing a 3D-SPGR sequence [TR = 8.8 ms, TE = 4 ms, and matrix = 240 × 240]; 170 slices were collected with 1.0 mm thickness without gap. Axial *FLAIR* images with 5.0 mm thickness [TR = 11.000 ms, TE = 140 ms, and matrix = 512 × 512] were obtained for WM analysis. The radiologist was blinded to the sex, age, and diagnosis of the subjects. The scales evaluated were as follows.

(i) Global Cortical Atrophy (GCA) or Pasquier scale: scored on FLAIR sequence [12].

Score:

(0) no cortical atrophy;
(1) mild atrophy (opening of sulci);
(2) moderate atrophy (volume loss of gyri);
(3) severe (end-stage) atrophy ("knife blade" atrophy).

(ii) Medial Temporal Lobe Atrophy (MTA) or Scheltens scale: rated on coronal T1-weighted slice through the corpus of the hippocampus, at the level of the anterior pons [13]. In the case of asymmetry, the highest score is the one to consider.

Score:

(0) no atrophy;
(1) only widening of choroid fissure;
(2) also widening of temporal horn of lateral ventricle;

(3) moderate loss of hippocampal volume (decrease in height);

(4) severe volume loss of hippocampus;

<75 years old: score (2) or more is abnormal;

>75 years old: score (3) or more is abnormal.

(iii) Fazekas scale for WMH lesions: scored on axial FLAIR or T2-weighted images [14].

Score:

(0) none or a single punctate WMH lesion;

(1) multiple punctate lesions;

(2) beginning confluency of lesions (bridging);

(3) large confluent lesions;

<70 years old: score (2) or more is considered abnormal;

>70 years old: score (3) is abnormal.

This study was approved by the ethical committee of all institutions involved, and written informed consent was obtained from all subjects.

2.1. Statistical Analysis. Mann–Whitney test was used to compare groups in terms of disease duration, L-dopa equivalent dose, UPDRS-III, PDQ-39 and Schwab-England scores, and Kruskal-Wallis test for demographics characteristics.

The neuropsychological performance of patients and controls was compared by using Kruskal-Wallis test. Spearman correlation was conducted between MRI analysis and neuropsychological tests scores.

Statistical significance was set at $p < 0.05$ for all analyses.

3. Results

Seventy-nine PD patients and 92 controls (CO) with MCI were evaluated as potential candidates. Thirty-five PD patients and 48 CO had one or more findings that could be responsible for another cause of cognitive impairment (exclusion criteria). Both groups (44 PD and 44 CO) were classified by neuropsychological profile as MCI amnestic ($n = 23$) or nonamnestic ($n = 21$). The sample was homogeneous on most of demographic data (Table 1) as no significant differences were observed between amnestic × nonamnestic groups of PD and CO for age, education level, MMSE, MoCA, and BDI. Higher scores of UPDRS, Schwab-England, and LED were documented in nonamnestic PD-MCI group without significance. PD group consisted mainly of men, whereas the controls were predominantly women. The majority of amnestic PD-MCI, nonamnestic PD-MCI, and amnestic CO-MCI did not have vascular risk factor (Table 1).

Neuropsychological data with statistical significance are shown in Table 1. Both PD groups (amnestic and nonamnestic) showed worse performance on several tests when compared to CO. Memory (RAVLT and FMT), attention (RAVLT- trail A1, FMT-incidental memory, and TMT), and executive function (TMT and RAVLT-retroactive interference) impairment were more severe in amnestic PD-MCI group. Nonamnestic PD-MCI presented more severe impairment of executive function (TMT and RAVLT-retroactive interference) when compared with nonamnestic CO-MCI. No differences were observed in language and visuospatial function between the 4 groups.

The data of visual scale score according to MCI subgroup did not allow any logical correlation between PD × CO groups or amnestic × nonamnestic subgroups (Table 1). Table 2 shows the variables with statistical correlation between MRI visual scales, clinical data, and neuropsychology tests. The following inverse correlations with $p < 0.05$ were observed in the different groups: (a) *amnestic PD-MCI*: (1) GCA scale with age, MoCA, memory (learning FMT and long-term memory FMT), and executive function (learning FMT), (2) MTA scale with UPDRS, and (3) Fazekas scale with memory (learning FMT) and executive function (learning FMT and T1 Stroop); (b) *nonamnestic PD-MCI*: (1) GCA scale with MMSE, executive function (T1 and T2 Stroop), and semantic memory/language (verbal semantic fluency); (c) *amnestic CO-MCI*: (1) GCA scale with executive function and attention (error 3 Stroop), (2) MTA scale with age and executive function (T2 Stroop), and (3) Fazekas scale with executive function (T1 Stroop); (d) *nonamnestic CO-MCI*: (1) GCA scale with education level, MoCA, and memory (recognition memory RAVLT).

4. Discussion

Our objective was to evaluate if clinical variables and MRI findings could have some peculiarities in amnestic and nonamnestic MCI in PD comparing with CO group.

An overall assessment of the frequency (descriptive statistic) of MRI visual scales changes according to each MCI subtype (Table 1) did not reveal consistent results. The analysis of each test score relative to the visual scales (statistical inference) provided several correlations (Table 2). Statistically significant inverse correlation was observed between GCA scale and the following neuropsychology scores: MMSE, MoCA, verbal semantic fluency (semantic memory/language), Stroop test (executive function and attention), FMT (memory and executive function), TMT-B (executive function), and RAVLT (memory). The MTA scale correlated with Stroop (executive function) and the Fazekas scale with FMT (memory and executive function) and Stroop test (executive function), according to the subgroup evaluated as described in Table 2.

WMH, evaluated by Fazekas scale, damages cholinergic pathways and results in impairment of cognitive functions. WMH in PD-MCI with attention deficit has already been reported and can be considered a risk factor for MCI in PD patients [15, 16]. The impact of white matter lesions in our study was documented by a correlation between Fazekas scale with memory and executive function in amnestic PD and executive function in amnestic CO.

Cortical gray matter atrophy (CGMA) also has been related to lower neuropsychological scores and as a predictor of dementia in PD-MCI [3]. The CGMA could be related to GCA as cerebral cortex is composed of gray matter. In our sample lower memory score was documented in amnestic PD

TABLE 1: Sample characteristics and performance in the neuropsychological tests (raw scores).

Variables	PD-MCI (n = 44) Amnestic (n = 23) Mean (sd)	PD-MCI (n = 44) Nonamnestic (n = 21) Mean (sd)	CO-MCI (n = 44) Amnestic (n = 23) Mean (sd)	CO-MCI (n = 44) Nonamnestic (n = 21) Mean (sd)	$p^{(a)}$
Age (years)	61.61 (6.867)	61.62 (8.047)	61.48 (6.901)	61.24 (6.549)	0.999
Education level (years)	9.61 (4.153)	10.62 (3.556)	11.43 (3.501)	11.24 (4.300)	0.385
Sex% (male/female)	56.5/43.5	71.4/28.6	30.4/69.6	28.6/71.4	—
Vascular risk factor% (yes/no)	40.0/60.0	21.4/78.6	37.5/62.5	54.5/45.5	—
MMSE	27.13 (2.201)	27.81 (1.401)	27.39 (1.158)	27.76 (1.221)	0.559
MoCA	22.0 (3.849)	22.86 (3.410)	21.35 (3.725)	22.67 (3.596)	0.619
BDI	9.52 (6.186)	5.67 (4.386)	8.35 (4.978)	7.10 (4.679)	0.168
Duration of symptoms (months)	76.17 (35.006)	73.14 (38.681)	—	—	$0.634^{(b)}$
L-dopa equivalent dose (mg)	673.09 (295.904)	1284.76 (3072.005)	—	—	$0.715^{(b)}$
UPDRS-III	25.96 (34.458)	67.62 (86.098)	—	—	$0.495^{(b)}$
PDQ39 (total)	31.29 (13.768)	21.89 (13.547)	—	—	$0.018^{(b)}$
Schwab-England scale	82.17 (7.359)	87.14 (5.606)	—	—	$0.014^{(b)}$
$MI^{(c;1)}$	4.65 (1.152)	5.67 (1.653)	5.26 (1.054)	5.81 (1.250)	0.025
$M1^{(c;2)}$	7.13 (1.140)	8.14 (1.108)	8.09 (0.996)	9.00 (0.949)	<0.001
$M2^{(c;3)}$	8.35 (1.071)	9.05 (1.024)	8.43 (1.376)	9.57 (0.598)	<0.001
$M5^{(c;4)}$	6.74 (1.888)	8.10 (1.640)	8.26 (1.137)	8.95 (0.973)	<0.001
$A1^{(d;5)}$	4.04 (0.976)	4.62 (1.322)	4.57 (1.647)	5.76 (1868)	0.010
$B1^{(d;6)}$	3.83 (1.466)	5.19 (1.601)	4.65 (1.824)	5.33 (2.129)	0.015
$A6^{(d;7)}$	3.96 (2.440)	7.71 (2.704)	6.57 (3.273)	8.71 (2.704)	<0.001
$A7^{(d;8)}$	3.87 (2.181)	8.10 (2.948)	6.52 (3.475)	10.0 (2.588)	<0.001
$LOT^{(d;9)}$	10.57 (5.558)	18.90 (7.516)	17.48 (7.609)	17.90 (5.957)	<0.001
$RI^{(d;10)}$	0.50 (0.261)	0.71 (0.172)	0.70 (0.298)	0.75 (0.167)	0.008
$Recognition^{(d;11)}$	4.13 (3.912)	10.71 (2.883)	5.09 (4.709)	11.14 (2.833)	<0.001
TMT $A^{(e;12)}$	68.75 (20.914)	66.71 (19.587)	55.82 (18.213)	49.64 (21.135)	0.003
TMT $B^{(e;13)}$	231.12 (128.926)	186.83 (79.737)	168.16 (99.767)	147.59 (66.065)	0.028
GCA% ((0) = none/(1) = mild/(2) = moderate/(3) = severe)	30.4/52.2/17.4/0	38.1/57.1/4.8/0	26.1/60.9/13/0	33.3/57.1/9.5/0	—
MTA% ((0) = none/(1) = ↑ of choroid fissure/(2) = ↑ of temporal horn/(3) = ↓ hippocampus/(4) = ↓↓ hippocampus)	52.2/39.1/8.7/0/0	57.1/42.9/0/0/0	56.5/30.4/8.7/4.3/0	57.1/42.9/0/0/0	—
FAZEKAS% ((0) = none or single punctate lesion/(1) = multiple punctate lesions /(2) = confluency lesions/(3) = large confluent)	39.1/34.8/17.4/8.7	38.1/47.6/9.5/4.8	26.1/52.2/13.0/8.7	9.5/52.4/33.3/4.8	—

(a) Kruskal-Wallis test; (b) Mann-Whitney; (c) Figures Memory Test; (1) Incidental memory; (2) Learning; (3) Number of figures recalled after 1-minute visualization; (4) Recall of memorized figures after 5 minutes; (d) Rey Auditory Verbal Learning Test; (5) Retrieval of words presented in a list of 15 substantives; (6) Retrieval of words included in the interference list of 15 new substantives; (7) Number of words memorized from list A without reread; (8) Number of words memorized from list A, without reread, after 20-minute interval; (9) Leaning curve of the words during attempts A1 to A5; (10) Retroactive Interference (A6/A5); (11) Correct answers in recognition list; (e) Trail making test; (12) trail A (time in seconds); (13) trail B (time in seconds).

TABLE 2: Spearman correlation.

	PD-MCI amnestic $n = 23$ (p value)	PD-MCI nonamnestic $n = 21$ (p value)	CO-MCI amnestic $n = 23$ (p value)	CO-MCI nonamnestic $n = 21$ (p value)
GCA × age	0.467 (0.025)			
GCA × education Level				−0.460 (0.036)
GCA × MMSE(1)		−0.516 (0.017)		
GCA × learning FMT(2)	−0.440 (0.035)			
GCA × long-term memory FMT(2)	−0.485 (0.019)			
GCA × verbal semantic fluency test		−0.454 (0.38)		
GCA × recognition memory RAVLT(3)				−0.549 (0.010)
GCA × T1 Stroop(4)		0.442 (0.045)		
GCA × T2 Stroop(5)		0.614 (0.003)		
GCA × error 3 Stroop(6)			0.450 (0.036)	
GCA × TMT-B(7)	0.439 (0.036)			
GCA × MoCA(8)	−0.521 (0.011)			−0.440 (0.046)
MTA × Age			0.482 (0.020)	
MTA × T2 Stroop(5)			0.499 (0.015)	
MTA × UPDRS-III	0.446 (0.033)			
MTA × UPDRS-total	0.454 (0.030)			
FAZEKAS scale × learning FMT(2)	−0.446 (0.033)			
FAZEKAS scale × T1 Stroop(4)			0.532 (0.009)	

(1)Mini-Mental Status Examination; (2)Figures Memory Test; (3)Rey Auditory Verbal Learning Test; (4)naming time (seconds) card 1, Stroop test; (5)naming time (seconds) card 2, Stroop test; (6)number of errors card 3, Stroop test; (7)trail B (seconds), trail making test; (8)Montreal Cognitive Assessment.

which presented correlation with GCA; therefore more severe memory impairment could be related to GCA.

The medial temporal lobe is the main structure related to memory, a wide cognitive process [13]. In PD the pathophysiology of memory problems seems to be more complex with impairment retrieval (frontostriatal dysfunction), learning, and recognition deficits [1, 6, 16]. We did not find a correlation between memory impairment and MTA. Probably the MTA scale has a low sensitivity for memory impairment in PD-MCI due to the aforementioned pathophysiology.

We excluded almost 50% of individuals with MCI initially selected due to posterior detection of secondary causes that could justify the cognitive impairment, hence avoiding bias. The use of benzodiazepine and silent stroke in the elderly population is relatively common and these two are the main causes of exclusion in our sample. As a result, there were a relative low number of participants, which can be considered a limitation of the study.

When we prospectively analyzed our data, we might conclude which scales abnormalities in MCI could be a risk factor for developing dementia, and if this is higher in PD group, as such individuals are more prone to develop an unfavorable cognitive outcome.

5. Conclusion

Structural abnormalities in MRI were found in PD-MCI and CO-MCI. Evaluation of frequency according to PD-MCI or CO-MCI did not reveal any consistent result. Analyzing each neuropsychological test score with MRI visual scales revealed an inverse correlation with the following cognitive domain: memory, attention, executive function, and language. Visual scales by MRI in MCI should be evaluated by cognitive domain and might be more useful in more severely impaired MCI or dementia patients.

Acknowledgments

This study was conducted in the Movement Disorders Unit, Neurology Service, Pedro Ernesto University Hospital, Rio de Janeiro State University, Brazil, with the support of the Carlos Chagas Filho Research Foundation of the State of Rio de Janeiro (FAPERJ).

References

[1] P. Svenningsson, E. Westman, C. Ballard, and D. Aarsland, "Cognitive impairment in patients with Parkinson's disease: diagnosis, biomarkers, and treatment," *The Lancet Neurology*, vol. 11, no. 8, pp. 697–707, 2012.

[2] C. H. Williams-Gray, T. Foltynie, C. E. G. Brayne, T. W. Robbins, and R. A. Barker, "Evolution of cognitive dysfunction in an incident Parkinson's disease cohort," *Brain*, vol. 130, no. 7, pp. 1787–1798, 2007.

[3] J. E. Lee, K. H. Cho, S. K. Song et al., "Exploratory analysis of neuropsychological and neuroanatomical correlates of progressive mild cognitive impairment in Parkinson's disease," *Journal of Neurology, Neurosurgery and Psychiatry*, vol. 85, no. 1, pp. 7–16, 2014.

[4] I. Litvan, J. G. Goldman, A. I. Tröster et al., "Diagnostic criteria for mild cognitive impairment in Parkinson's disease: movement Disorder Society Task Force guidelines," *Movement Disorders*, vol. 27, no. 3, pp. 349–356, 2012.

[5] B. Dubois, D. Burn, C. Goetz et al., "Diagnostic procedures for Parkinson's disease dementia: recommendations from the movement disorder society task force," *Movement Disorders*, vol. 22, no. 16, pp. 2314–2324, 2007.

[6] N. Sawamoto, P. Piccini, G. Hotton, N. Pavese, K. Thielemans, and D. J. Brooks, "Cognitive deficits and striato-frontal dopamine release in Parkinson's disease," *Brain*, vol. 131, no. 5, pp. 1294–1302, 2008.

[7] L. Harper, F. Barkhof, N. C. Fox, and J. M. Schott, "Using visual rating to diagnose dementia: a critical evaluation of MRI atrophy scales," *Journal of Neurology, Neurosurgery and Psychiatry*, vol. 86, no. 11, pp. 1225–1233, 2015.

[8] C. W. C. Tam, E. J. Burton, I. G. McKeith, D. J. Burn, and J. T. O'Brien, "Temporal lobe atrophy on MRI in Parkinson disease with dementia: a comparison with Alzheimer disease and dementia with Lewy bodies," *Neurology*, vol. 64, no. 5, pp. 861–865, 2005.

[9] N. Ibarretxe-Bilbao, C. Junque, M. J. Marti, and E. Tolosa, "Brain structural MRI correlates of cognitive dysfunctions in Parkinson's disease," *Journal of the Neurological Sciences*, vol. 310, no. 1-2, pp. 70–74, 2011.

[10] A. J. Hughes, S. E. Daniel, L. Kilford, and A. J. Lees, "Accuracy of clinical diagnosis of idiopathic Parkinson's disease: a clinico-pathological study of 100 cases," *Journal of Neurology Neurosurgery and Psychiatry*, vol. 55, no. 3, pp. 181–184, 1992.

[11] O. V. Forlenza, B. S. Diniz, F. Stella, A. L. Teixeira, and W. F. Gattaz, "Mild cognitive impairment (part 1): clinical characteristics and predictors of dementia," *Revista Brasileira de Psiquiatria*, vol. 35, no. 2, pp. 178–185, 2013.

[12] F. Pasquer, D. Leys, J. G. E. Weerts, F. Mounier, F. Barkhof, and P. Scheltens, "Inter- and intraobserver reproducibility of cerebral atrophy assessment on MRI scans with hemispheric infarcts," *European Neurology*, vol. 36, no. 5, pp. 268–272, 1996.

[13] P. Scheltens, M. Kuiper, E. Ch Wolters et al., "Atrophy of medial temporal lobes on MRI in 'probable' Alzheimer's disease and normal ageing: diagnostic value and neuropsychological correlates," *Journal of Neurology, Neurosurgery and Psychiatry*, vol. 55, no. 10, pp. 967–972, 1992.

[14] F. Fazekas, J. B. Chawluk, A. Alavi, H. I. Hurtig, and R. A. Zimmerman, "MR signal abnormalities at 1.5 T in Alzheimer's dementia and normal aging," *American Journal of Roentgenology*, vol. 149, no. 2, pp. 351–356, 1987.

[15] J. Shin, S. Choi, J. E. Lee, H. S. Lee, Y. H. Sohn, and P. H. Lee, "Subcortical white matter hyperintensities within the cholinergic pathways of Parkinson's disease patients according to cognitive status," *Journal of Neurology, Neurosurgery and Psychiatry*, vol. 83, no. 3, pp. 315–321, 2012.

[16] N. Kandiah, E. Mak, A. Ng et al., "Cerebral white matter hyperintensity in Parkinson's disease: a major risk factor for mild cognitive impairment," *Parkinsonism and Related Disorders*, vol. 19, no. 7, pp. 680–683, 2013.

Patients' Views on a Combined Action Observation and Motor Imagery Intervention for Parkinson's Disease

Judith Bek,[1] Jordan Webb,[1] Emma Gowen,[1] Stefan Vogt,[2] Trevor J. Crawford,[2] Matthew S. Sullivan,[3] and Ellen Poliakoff[1]

[1] *University of Manchester, Manchester, UK*
[2] *Lancaster University, Lancaster, UK*
[3] *Manchester Metropolitan University, Manchester, UK*

Correspondence should be addressed to Judith Bek; judith.bek@manchester.ac.uk

Academic Editor: Ivan Bodis-Wollner

Background. Action observation and motor imagery activate neural structures involved in action execution, thereby facilitating movement and learning. Although some benefits of action observation and motor imagery have been reported in Parkinson's disease (PD), methods have been based on stroke rehabilitation and may be less suitable for PD. Moreover, previous studies have focused on either observation or imagery, yet combining these enhances effects in healthy participants. The present study explores the feasibility of a PD-specific home-based intervention combining observation, imagery, and imitation of meaningful everyday actions. *Methods.* A focus group was conducted with six people with mild to moderate PD and two companions, exploring topics relating to the utility and feasibility of a home-based observation and imagery intervention. *Results.* Five themes were identified. Participants reported their experiences of exercise and use of action observation and motor imagery in everyday activities, and the need for strategies to improve movement was expressed. Motivational factors including feedback, challenge, and social support were identified as key issues. The importance of offering a broad range of actions and flexible training was also highlighted. *Conclusions.* A home-based intervention utilising action observation and motor imagery would be useful and feasible in mild to moderate PD.

1. Introduction

People with PD often have difficulty in initiating movements, and movements can be slower and reduced in size. External cueing can be effective in facilitating movement in PD [1, 2]; for example, lines on the floor or laser pointers can help to improve initiation of gait and maintain appropriate step length. Observation of human movement may provide another form of cueing, and researchers have recently begun to investigate the therapeutic potential of action observation (AO) in rehabilitation for PD (for reviews see [3, 4]).

Observing another person's movement activates neural structures involved in performing the same movement [5, 6], facilitating subsequent action. Imitation involves both the observation and execution of an action, thereby offering a particularly effective means of priming movement [7, 8], while motor imagery (MI) is the imagination of a movement in the absence of action execution. MI involves visual and kinaesthetic (sensorimotor) representations and also activates the motor system [9, 10]. AO, MI, and imitation have been shown to improve movement and increase learning in healthy individuals (e.g., [11–13]).

Previous research has shown benefits of AO and MI in stroke rehabilitation, with improvements in activities of daily living found after training with AO and imitation [14–16], as well as MI interventions [17]. Increased neural activation in the motor system has also been reported following AO training in stroke [14]. The evidence base documenting the effects of such interventions in PD is comparatively sparse, although some encouraging results have been reported. For example, AO has been found to improve sequential movements, increase self-reported mobility, and reduce freezing of gait [18–20], and MI has also been shown to reduce freezing of gait [21]. Although no large-scale studies of AO or MI training have been reported in PD, a pilot randomised controlled study found improvements in functional independence following training with AO and imitation alongside conventional physiotherapy, compared with physiotherapy alone [22]. Training with MI has also been found to improve timed motor performance when combined with physical practice [23].

Although imitation ability may be affected in PD [24, 25], the above findings suggest that it can nonetheless be applied successfully in rehabilitation. MI has also been shown to be preserved in PD [26–28], although compensatory mechanisms may be involved [28, 29]. Previous studies in PD have focused on either AO or MI, but behavioural [12, 30] and neuroimaging [31–33] findings indicate that combining these processes can enhance effects and increase activation of the motor system in healthy individuals (for review, see [34]). Based on these findings, we sought to obtain patients' views on the development of a PD-specific intervention utilising principles of AO, MI, and imitation.

Importantly, while benefits of AO interventions for everyday actions have been demonstrated in stroke patients, different objectives must be considered in designing a PD-specific intervention. Whereas stroke rehabilitation aims to restore or compensate for lost function, therapies for PD should be targeted at improving or maintaining control of movement, such as facilitating initiation and increasing amplitude or speed. Thus, it is important to consult with people with PD and those working with PD patients to identify appropriate training goals, as well as consulting potential users on issues relating to feasibility and design of interventions [35, 36]. An initial concept for an AO + MI intervention for PD has been informed by researchers with expertise in PD and AO, as well as physiotherapists, clinicians, and PD representatives. The proposed intervention will be delivered via mobile technology in the user's home (using a tablet PC, although other devices could potentially also be used), with suggested daily practice of approximately 30 minutes, allowing flexibility to accommodate other commitments and fluctuations in symptoms. Training consists of observing videos of actions, engaging in motor imagery, and then performing the target action. Users will be provided with a set of personally selected training videos, working with a researcher or therapist to devise an individualised training programme. The aim of the present study was to conduct a focus group to explore the views of people with PD and their carers or companions on the proposed intervention.

2. Method

Ethical approval for the study was obtained from a UK National Health Service Research Ethics Committee (NRES Committee North West, Greater Manchester South), and written informed consent was obtained from all participants.

2.1. Participants. Participant demographics are reported in Table 1. Six people with idiopathic PD (4 males and 2 females) presenting with mild to moderate symptoms (Hoehn & Yahr stages 1–3 [37]) were recruited from a panel of research volunteers who had taken part in previous studies at the University of Manchester. All but one of the participants were taking dopaminergic medication. Companions (1 male and 1 female) of two of the PD participants (spouses of P2 and P5, resp.) also contributed to the focus group discussions. The present sample size is typical of focus group studies and based on recommendations in the literature [38].

2.2. Procedure. Demographic information and disease history were obtained prior to the session, and motor examination scores from the Unified Parkinson's Disease Rating Scale (UPDRS [39]) were obtained within a period of 8 weeks prior to the focus group as part of a previous study. Participants also completed a short form of the Parkinson's Disease Questionnaire (PDQ-8 [40]) on the day of the focus group to provide a general measure of functioning and well-being.

To assess the ability of participants to engage in motor imagery, we analysed data collected as part of a previous study using a short form of the Kinaesthetic and Visual Imagery Questionnaire (KVIQ [41]). The KVIQ was devised to measure MI in people both with and without disabilities and has been validated for use in PD patients [42]. Participants are asked to perform and then imagine performing simple movements of the head, shoulders, trunk, upper limbs, and lower limbs. The clarity of the image (visual imagery) and intensity of the sensations (kinaesthetic imagery) are rated on a 5-point scale, with higher scores representing stronger imagery.

The focus group took place at the University of Manchester and lasted approximately 1 hour and 20 minutes. The session was chaired by one researcher and facilitated by two others, and a schedule of topics was used to guide discussions. Open-ended questions were used with prompts to elicit further information where needed, and visual aids were used to help explain concepts underlying the proposed therapy.

Participants were first asked about their general experience of physical activity or physiotherapy and their thoughts on a home-based intervention to improve movement. The concepts of action observation, motor imagery, and imitation were then introduced (some advance information had also been provided in a participant information sheet) and participants were asked if they had any experience of using these or other strategies to manage symptoms or to facilitate movement. The proposed intervention was then introduced, and participants were shown example videos depicting potential actions to be trained (e.g., cleaning glasses). Further discussions centred on identification of actions that would be useful and relevant to include in training, as well as practical issues such as intensity and timing of training and the use of technology.

Participants were advised that any comments made during the focus group could subsequently be removed from the analysis if they so wished. Responses were digitally recorded and transcribed verbatim by an independent transcription service.

2.3. Data Analysis. Data were analysed using thematic analysis, which is a flexible method of identifying and analysing patterns within a dataset [43]. A primarily deductive approach to analysis was taken to identify themes relating to

TABLE 1: Participant demographics and background assessments.

Participant	Sex	Age (years)	Disease duration (years)	Hoehn & Yahr stage	UPDRS motor score	PDQ-8	KVIQ-V	KVIQ-K
1	M	64	2.2	1	26	12.5	17	8
2	F	56	8.5	1	27	40.6	17	13.5
3	M	69	6	2	31	21.9	18.5	19
4	F	63	2.8	3	43	15.6	22.5	18
5	M	73	1	3	63	15.6	14	16
6	M	60	20	3	64	43.8	15	12.5

PDQ-8 = Parkinson's Disease Questionnaire; score given as a percentage (higher scores indicate poorer health status). KVIQ = Kinaesthetic and Visual Imagery Questionnaire (V = visual subscale and K = kinaesthetic subscale); scores out of a maximum of 25.

feasibility and potential target actions, while also allowing for data-driven identification of themes.

The data were coded by the second author (J. Webb) and categories were identified, which were organised into themes. The transcript was then reanalysed by the first author (J. Bek) using the categories and themes identified. Final themes were verified following further discussion within the research team.

3. Results

Motor imagery scores for both visual and kinaesthetic subscales of the KVIQ (Table 1) were within the range previously reported for healthy individuals of a similar age [41], indicating that participants were able to engage in motor imagery and that vividness of imagery was similar to that of healthy older adults.

Analysis revealed five themes, which are described below.

3.1. Theme 1: Experience of Exercise/Physiotherapy and Its Benefits. Participants reported benefits obtained from physiotherapy and exercise that they had previously undertaken, such as gym training.

> *I go to the gym very often...exercise does help.* (P5)

3.2. Theme 2: Use of AO and MI in Everyday Activities

3.2.1. Subtheme 2.1: Action Observation/Imitation. Participants related experiences of using action observation and imitation in the context of exercise classes or in the gym and when walking:

> *I do quite a lot of pilates and yoga classes which are classic examples of imitating somebody else to do the right movements.* (P4)

> *I do find it easier when I'm mimicking walking with [husband] and I tend to walk the same as he does.* (P2)

Participants were also aware of experiencing "automatic" imitation in which observed behaviours and gestures are unconsciously mimicked in social contexts [44]:

> *I do tend to mimic people when I'm talking. I tend to copy their hand movements in socialising.* (P2)

3.2.2. Subtheme 2.2: Motor Imagery. Participants reported using motor imagery in sports and leisure pursuits (racquetball and playing the piano) as well as in more basic movement contexts (getting into bed and walking through doorways):

> *The way I get into bed often is to sit and then spring both my legs up to be along the length of the bed and I guess am thinking quite consciously about how I'm going to do that.* (P3)

> *...the physiotherapist recommended imagining...if I could remember to do it then I could walk straight through a doorway.* (P6)

In addition to the use of MI as a cue to action, participants reported mentally rehearsing activities outside of the immediate context:

> *I took up the piano again...if I'm trying to get to sleep I kind of play through some of my pieces and I think that kind of mental reinforcement definitely helps the physical agility.* (P4)

3.3. Theme 3: Indication of Need for Strategies to Improve Movement

3.3.1. Subtheme 3.1: Interest in Alternative Ways to Manage Symptoms. Participants expressed an interest in methods to help them to improve movement or better manage their symptoms:

> *...spent the first three years resisting taking any drugs, so I was really focusing on movement and exercise to keep me going.* (P4)

> *I'm really interested in ways of managing movement that might allow for a reduction in drugs.* (P6)

> *...with a tool like this, you could have the potential to capture data and develop a numerical score that might be helpful in therapy perhaps.* (P3)

3.3.2. Subtheme 3.2: Use of Compensatory Strategies. Participants reported strategies they had used to compensate for their difficulties in performing everyday tasks:

> *So if my left hand was playing up, I'd sit on it and just practise with my right hand.* (P4)

> *...five finger typing. I long ago reduced to one hand and now even that's getting a bit of a problem. My main solution to that is to talk to the computer and that is very good. I've got a program ...* (P3)

There was also discussion surrounding "*the dilemma...whether you put your energy into practice, or finding alternatives or more convenient and effective methods*" (P4):

> *...brushing your teeth, I found I was holding my brush and moving my head. I have avoided that by getting an electric toothbrush. Perhaps I should have carried on just using a brush.* (P3)

> *...if I do a lot of writing, it is really uncomfortable, but my consultant says to not stop writing, just to keep doing it.* (P1)

3.4. Theme 4: Actions and Aspects of Movement. Participants discussed everyday actions that they had difficulty with and would find useful to train (see Table 2), and it was clear that requirements varied between individuals.

3.4.1. Subtheme 4.1: Everyday Actions. The majority of suggested actions were everyday activities relating to personal care, dressing, work/leisure activities, and household chores. The difficulties participants reported with these actions typically involved fine motor coordination and dexterity:

> *...trying to do things quickly with the mouse buttons, that's awkward.* (P1)

> *...to enhance my ability even just with the one hand to type would be a big help.* (P3)

> *I wear contact lenses...cleaning those is really difficult to put the solution on and rub my two fingers together.* (P1)

> *I can't believe how bad I am at folding laundry...it seems the most difficult thing in the world...* (P4)

Other suggestions indicated the desire to improve more basic mobility tasks, in relation to hypokinesia, (*...very little steps...I could imagine that that could be improved* (P3)) and difficulties with action initiation (*Going upstairs, sometimes you freeze and you just can't get started* (P2)).

3.4.2. Subtheme 4.2: Core Components of Movement. There was also discussion surrounding the value of training specific functional actions versus core movement skills that could be applied more broadly:

> *...what would be interesting to me would be to see whether there's any way of refining core skills so that those skills could then translate into specific contexts...be it brushing teeth or making a cup of tea...the exercises that you do wouldn't necessarily be to do with that but would actually reinforce the skills that you could then apply to whatever the particular task is...* (P4)

> *Having taken up yoga classes, my neck movements have improved enormously and I'm getting the benefit of it when I reverse the car...* (P4)

3.5. Theme 5: Feasibility. This theme encompassed issues pertaining to the feasibility of the proposed intervention, with categories relating to motivation, choice/flexibility, and practical issues.

3.5.1. Subtheme 5.1: Motivation. Comments from all participants indicated that motivation was a key factor in engaging with rehabilitation. In particular, participants wanted to feel that they were progressing in their training:

> *...it's got to be motivating, doing something purely because it will get better, they tell me, or my coach tells me, whatever, would be not enough, I'd want to experience something beneficial to me happening.* (P3)

The potential impact of apathy was also noted:

> *...apathy is a significant feature of Parkinson's...so it's actually harder to sustain things.* (P4)

The need to feel challenged was indicated by some participants:

> *...the actions were so basic and simple that it was hard to feel interested or motivated in them.* (P6)

However, an appropriate level of difficulty was considered important in order to build confidence and maintain engagement in training:

> *...if you can't do something, it's just hopeless because you can't build on it, can you? And if it's too easy, that's hopeless too because there's no reward to it. It's got to be exactly at the right level for the individual.* (P4)

Comments indicated participants' desire to receive feedback on their performance and progress. This might be through noticeable improvement in the trained actions but could also involve a system of awarding scores or points for progress:

> *...to give me the immediate feedback that it is beneficial now, I can clean my teeth better or I can hit the keyboard better or something.* (P3)

> *...you're moving onto the next level or whatever, those sorts of little motivational tricks that are everywhere in computer games now.* (P4)

Corrective feedback was also considered important:

TABLE 2: Everyday actions suggested for inclusion in a home-based training programme.

Work/leisure activities	Household chores	Personal care	Dressing	Mobility
Using computer mouse Typing Writing Separating newspaper pages Folding newspapers	Folding laundry Opening garbage bags/grocery bags Cutting vegetables	Cleaning teeth Shaving Cleaning contact lenses	Putting on sweater/shirt/coat Putting on socks/tights Fastening buttons	Walking (step length) Climbing stairs

> *...if you're not achieving your goals, you need someone to explain what you need to do to try and improve.* (P1)

Motivation was also discussed in relation to the intensity of training. While some participants indicated that they would not be able to commit to the suggested 30 minutes of daily training, others felt that this would be achievable:

> *...getting the motivation to do it every day for half an hour might be difficult.* (P3)

> *I think I'd do it a couple of times a week, otherwise I'd think I'd probably be down to ten minutes a day, I'd love to do it but I can only do ten minutes a day.* (P4)

> *I think personally for me that would be ideal, but not necessarily for somebody else.* (P2)

The importance of social factors in motivation to engage in training was also highlighted, with participants suggesting a group setting or online social support:

> *Personally I prefer to go out to a class and do it, to be interactive with other people.* (P1)

> *...it's rewarding to talk to other likeminded people.* (P2)

> *I think if there was an online group ...something so that you're not doing it in isolation.* (P4)

3.5.2. Subtheme 5.2: Choice and Flexibility. It was considered important for individuals to be able to choose from a broad range of actions:

> *...a package that had the most range of options from very simple to more complex...The more you can build into something, the more likely people are to have a go at part of it, I would think.* (P6)

Comments indicated that the difficulty of a particular action may be variable within an individual from day to day, further emphasising the need for flexibility in training:

> *...sometimes it's easy to manoeuvre a mouse or use a keyboard, other days it's near on impossible.* (P5)

It was also suggested that the proposed intervention could be applied to different settings:

> *It's an additional resource, isn't it, and it can be used by individuals but it can also be used by people supporting people with Parkinson's and through Parkinson's groups. It doesn't have to be just one on one.* (P4)

3.5.3. Subtheme 5.3: Practical Considerations. Possible limitations were identified in terms of age, motor impairment, and the use of technology:

> *I guess it's no good to have an iPad if you can't get into it because your finger isn't...you sort of fail on the first hurdle, don't you?* (P4)

> *...the population with Parkinson's that's older than 70 is huge, and some of them might well be interested in doing something but not as able or as experienced at using technology.* (P6)

However, participants felt that the use of mobile technology would be acceptable and might be particularly useful in certain groups:

> *I'm sure there would be people that would use it and get benefit out of an app on an iPad.* (P1)

> *...something delivered on an iPad would be particularly helpful, I'd have thought, for people in rural areas where there's an issue of transport and mobility.* (P4)

4. Discussion

Analysis of the focus group discussions indicated that people with mild to moderate PD perceived physical activity to be beneficial, as reported previously [35, 45], and were also able to relate positive experiences of using action observation and motor imagery in their daily activities and management of their symptoms.

A need to identify strategies to improve control of movement was expressed. This is consistent with the findings of another recent focus group study, in which the importance of physical approaches to symptom management was reported as an unmet need in the healthcare of people with PD, including access to home activity programmes and management of daily activities [46]. Moreover, the proposed intervention might allow people to continue to perform tasks as they have done previously, instead of finding alternative compensatory strategies.

Potential targets for training were then discussed. Participants reported difficulties in performing a range of everyday actions, which related to symptoms of PD such as bimanual coordination, hypokinesia, and initiation. The heterogeneity of suggested actions indicates variation among individuals with PD in the actions that they find difficult or would value the opportunity to improve. Preferences for training core components of movement or specific tasks also differed between participants. Since some individuals may already be using compensatory strategies for particular tasks, it may be beneficial to offer different options within action observation training (i.e., viewing the task performed using either the original method or the compensatory technique).

Motivation was identified as a key factor in the feasibility of the proposed intervention, consistent with previous findings on patients' views on exercise [35, 45]. Home-based training increases independence and choice for therapy users, as recommended by UK NICE guidelines [47], and independent exercise programmes have previously shown positive effects in PD [48, 49]. However, apathy is a prevalent symptom in PD [50] and its potential impact on adherence to training was considered. Discussions indicated that an appropriate level of difficulty or challenge, monitoring of progress, feedback, and social interaction are all potential contributors to the successful implementation of a user-led home-based intervention. These issues are also of broader relevance in designing interventions for PD and other neurological conditions, and have been identified previously in relation to the development of video-game based therapies [51, 52].

Choice and flexibility were also highlighted as important considerations in the design of home training programmes. Participants expressed the desire to be offered a broad range of actions to train. Personalised action observation therapy, using actions meaningful to the individual, has been found to increase independence in stroke patients [53], and this approach is consistent with Parkinson's UK "personalised treatments" research priority [54]. Quinn et al. [35] have also highlighted the importance of the patient taking an active role in the design of rehabilitation programmes. Symptoms can fluctuate from day to day and also over the course of the day in PD, and training programmes should accommodate this variation in terms of the duration and intensity of practice, which could be selected by the user according to their symptomatic status. Moreover, some users in earlier disease stages may still be in employment or have domestic responsibilities; flexibility is therefore also important in allowing users to adapt their training to fit with their lifestyle.

Finally, practical considerations were highlighted, including the potential difficulty in using mobile technology to deliver training. There is increasing recognition of the value of technology, such as smartphones and tablet PCs, in diagnosis, disease monitoring, and therapy in PD (e.g., [55, 56]). Neurorehabilitation approaches based on video gaming and virtual reality have been implemented successfully in PD [51, 52], and a recent study demonstrated feasibility of a tablet PC-based action observation therapy for stroke patients [57]. However, the present study indicates the importance of considering the effects of age and motor impairment on the use of such technology by some individuals with PD.

Participants' self-reported vividness of MI was similar to that previously found in healthy older adults [41]. This is consistent with other studies showing intact MI in PD [26–28], suggesting that people with PD would be able to engage in MI-based training. However, the proposed intervention may be suitable only for a subset of people with mild to moderate PD who are motivated and able to train at home. AO + MI training may also be best utilised as a tool to complement traditional physiotherapy or group exercise classes, and support from therapists or via a social network may increase uptake of and adherence to training. Although we cannot extrapolate from our findings to patients with more advanced PD, this population may nonetheless also be able to benefit from an AO + MI intervention. Individuals who are not able to physically perform the movements may still be able to practice using AO and MI, but alternative delivery methods might need to be considered.

While providing valuable information to guide the development of an AO + MI intervention for PD, the present study is limited by its small sample size. The participants in the present study were proactive and motivated research volunteers and may thus be unrepresentative of the target population. In addition, although motor imagery ability was intact in the present sample, some individuals with PD may have difficulty in engaging successfully in imagery [26]. Further consultation with carers or family members and healthcare professionals (e.g., physiotherapists and occupational therapists) is also needed to inform intervention development.

5. Conclusions

The focus group indicated that people with mild to moderate PD considered a home-based action observation and motor imagery intervention to be useful and feasible. Key issues in designing home-based interventions were identified, including motivation and choice. The study also highlighted the importance of consulting with user groups in intervention development.

Disclosure

J. Webb worked on this project as part fulfilment of his undergraduate degree in psychology.

Acknowledgments

J. Bek was supported by the Economic and Social Research Council (Grant no. ES/K013564/1). The authors would like to thank Paul Holmes and Sheree McCormick for providing example videos. The authors also thank all the participants for their time and enthusiasm in taking part in this study.

References

[1] S. J. Spaulding, B. Barber, M. Colby, B. Cormack, T. Mick, and M. E. Jenkins, "Cueing and gait improvement among people

with Parkinson's disease: a meta-analysis," *Archives of Physical Medicine and Rehabilitation*, vol. 94, no. 3, pp. 562–570, 2013.

[2] E. E. H. van Wegen, M. A. Hirsch, M. Huiskamp, and G. Kwakkel, "Harnessing cueing training for neuroplasticity in Parkinson disease," *Topics in Geriatric Rehabilitation*, vol. 30, no. 1, pp. 46–57, 2014.

[3] G. Abbruzzese, L. Avanzino, R. Marchese, and E. Pelosin, "Action observation and motor imagery: innovative cognitive tools in the rehabilitation of Parkinson's disease," *Parkinson's Disease*, vol. 2015, Article ID 124214, 9 pages, 2015.

[4] E. Poliakoff, "Representation of action in Parkinson's disease: imagining, observing, and naming actions," *Journal of Neuropsychology*, vol. 7, no. 2, pp. 241–254, 2013.

[5] S. Caspers, K. Zilles, A. R. Laird, and S. B. Eickhoff, "ALE meta-analysis of action observation and imitation in the human brain," *NeuroImage*, vol. 50, no. 3, pp. 1148–1167, 2010.

[6] G. Rizzolatti and C. Sinigaglia, "The functional role of the parieto-frontal mirror circuit: interpretations and misinterpretations," *Nature Reviews Neuroscience*, vol. 11, no. 4, pp. 264–274, 2010.

[7] L. Shmuelof and E. Zohary, "Mirror-image representation of action in the anterior parietal cortex," *Nature Neuroscience*, vol. 11, no. 11, pp. 1267–1269, 2008.

[8] S. L. Small, G. Buccino, and A. Solodkin, "The mirror neuron system and treatment of stroke," *Developmental Psychobiology*, vol. 54, no. 3, pp. 293–310, 2012.

[9] W. S. Anderson and F. A. Lenz, "Review of motor and phantom-related imagery," *NeuroReport*, vol. 22, no. 17, pp. 939–942, 2011.

[10] J. Decety and J. Grèzes, "Neural mechanisms subserving the perception of human actions," *Trends in Cognitive Sciences*, vol. 3, no. 5, pp. 172–178, 1999.

[11] G. Buccino, S. Vogt, A. Ritzl et al., "Neural circuits underlying imitation learning of hand actions: an event-related fMRI study," *Neuron*, vol. 42, no. 2, pp. 323–334, 2004.

[12] D. L. Eaves, L. Haythornthwaite, and S. Vogt, "Motor imagery during action observation modulates automatic imitation effects in rhythmical actions," *Frontiers in Human Neuroscience*, vol. 8, no. 1, article 28, 2014.

[13] K. Stefan, J. Classen, P. Celnik, and L. G. Cohen, "Concurrent action observation modulates practice-induced motor memory formation," *European Journal of Neuroscience*, vol. 27, no. 3, pp. 730–738, 2008.

[14] D. Ertelt, S. Small, A. Solodkin et al., "Action observation has a positive impact on rehabilitation of motor deficits after stroke," *NeuroImage*, vol. 36, no. 2, pp. T164–T173, 2007.

[15] G. Buccino, A. Solodkin, and S. L. Small, "Functions of the mirror neuron system: implications for neurorehabilitation," *Cognitive and Behavioral Neurology*, vol. 19, no. 1, pp. 55–63, 2006.

[16] G. Buccino, "Action observation treatment: a novel tool in neurorehabilitation," *Philosophical Transactions of the Royal Society B: Biological Sciences*, vol. 369, no. 1644, 2014.

[17] K. P. Y. Liu, C. C. H. Chan, R. S. M. Wong et al., "A randomized controlled trial of mental imagery augment generalization of learning in acute poststroke patients," *Stroke*, vol. 40, no. 6, pp. 2222–2225, 2009.

[18] A. Jaywant, T. D. Ellis, S. Roy, C. Lin, S. Neargarder, and A. Cronin-Golomb, "Randomized controlled trial of a home-based action observation intervention to improve walking in Parkinson disease," *Archives of Physical Medicine and Rehabilitation*, vol. 97, no. 5, pp. 665–673, 2016.

[19] E. Pelosin, L. Avanzino, M. Bove, P. Stramesi, A. Nieuwboer, and G. Abbruzzese, "Action observation improves freezing of gait in patients with Parkinson's disease," *Neurorehabilitation and Neural Repair*, vol. 24, no. 8, pp. 746–752, 2010.

[20] E. Pelosin, M. Bove, P. Ruggeri, L. Avanzino, and G. Abbruzzese, "Reduction of bradykinesia of finger movements by a single session of action observation in Parkinson disease," *Neurorehabilitation and Neural Repair*, vol. 27, no. 6, pp. 552–560, 2013.

[21] A. Kikuchi, T. Baba, T. Hasegawa et al., "Improvement of freezing of gait in patients with Parkinson's disease by imagining bicycling," *Case Reports in Neurology*, vol. 6, no. 1, pp. 92–95, 2014.

[22] G. Buccino, R. Gatti, M. C. Giusti et al., "Action observation treatment improves autonomy in daily activities in Parkinson's disease patients: results from a pilot study," *Movement Disorders*, vol. 26, no. 10, pp. 1963–1964, 2011.

[23] R. Tamir, R. Dickstein, and M. Huberman, "Integration of motor imagery and physical practice in group treatment applied to subjects with Parkinson's disease," *Neurorehabilitation and Neural Repair*, vol. 21, no. 1, pp. 68–75, 2007.

[24] C. Bonivento, R. I. Rumiati, E. Biasutti, and G. W. Humphreys, "The role of the basal ganglia in action imitation: neuropsychological evidence from Parkinson's disease patients," *Experimental Brain Research*, vol. 224, no. 2, pp. 211–220, 2013.

[25] R. C. Leiguarda, P. P. Pramstaller, M. Merello, S. Starkstein, A. J. Lees, and C. D. Marsden, "Apraxia in Parkinson's disease, progressive supranuclear palsy, multiple system atrophy and neuroleptic-induced parkinsonism," *Brain*, vol. 120, no. 1, pp. 75–90, 1997.

[26] E. Heremans, P. Feys, A. Nieuwboer et al., "Motor imagery ability in patients with early- and mid-stage Parkinson disease," *Neurorehabilitation and Neural Repair*, vol. 25, no. 2, pp. 168–177, 2011.

[27] K. A. Pickett, D. S. Peterson, and G. M. Earhart, "Motor imagery of gait tasks in individuals with Parkinson disease," *Journal of Parkinson's Disease*, vol. 2, no. 1, pp. 19–22, 2012.

[28] B. F. L. van Nuenen, R. C. Helmich, N. Buenen, B. P. C. van de Warrenburg, B. R. Bloem, and I. Toni, "Compensatory activity in the extrastriate body area of Parkinson's disease patients," *Journal of Neuroscience*, vol. 32, no. 28, pp. 9546–9553, 2012.

[29] S. Thobois, P. F. Dominey, J. Decety et al., "Motor imagery in normal subjects and in asymmetrical Parkinson's disease: a PET study," *Neurology*, vol. 55, no. 7, pp. 996–1002, 2000.

[30] J. Bek, E. Poliakoff, H. Marshall, S. Trueman, and E. Gowen, "Enhancing voluntary imitation through attention and motor imagery," *Experimental Brain Research*, vol. 234, no. 7, pp. 1819–1828, 2016.

[31] K. L. Macuga and S. H. Frey, "Neural representations involved in observed, imagined, and imitated actions are dissociable and hierarchically organized," *NeuroImage*, vol. 59, no. 3, pp. 2798–2807, 2012.

[32] V. Nedelko, T. Hassa, F. Hamzei, M. A. Schoenfeld, and C. Dettmers, "Action imagery combined with action observation activates more corticomotor regions than action observation alone," *Journal of Neurologic Physical Therapy*, vol. 36, no. 4, pp. 182–188, 2012.

[33] M. Villiger, D. Bohli, D. Kiper et al., "Virtual reality-augmented neurorehabilitation improves motor function and reduces neuropathic pain in patients with incomplete spinal cord injury," *Neurorehabilitation and Neural Repair*, vol. 27, no. 8, pp. 675–683, 2013.

[34] S. Vogt, F. Di Rienzo, C. Collet, A. Collins, and A. Guillot, "Multiple roles of motor imagery during action observation," *Frontiers in Human Neuroscience*, vol. 7, article 807, 2013.

[35] L. Quinn, M. Busse, H. Khalil, S. Richardson, A. Rosser, and H. Morris, "Client and therapist views on exercise programmes for early-mid stage Parkinson's disease and Huntington's disease," *Disability and Rehabilitation*, vol. 32, no. 11, pp. 917–928, 2010.

[36] D. R. Young, J. Gittelsohn, J. Charleston, K. Felix-Aaron, and L. J. Appel, "Motivations for exercise and weight loss among African-American women: focus group results and their contribution towards program development," *Ethnicity and Health*, vol. 6, no. 3-4, pp. 227–245, 2001.

[37] M. M. Hoehn and M. D. Yahr, "Parkinsonism: onset, progression, and mortality," *Neurology*, vol. 17, no. 5, pp. 427–442, 1967.

[38] D. L. Morgan and R. A. Krueger, *Planning Focus Groups*, vol. 2, Sage, Thousand Oaks, Calif, USA, 1998.

[39] S. Fahn and R. G. Elton, "Members of the UPDRS development committee: Unified Parkinson's disease rating scale," in *Recent Developments in Parkinson's Disease*, S. Fahn, C. D. Marsden, D. B. Calne, and M. Goldstein, Eds., pp. 153–163, Macmillan Health Care Information, Florham Park, NJ, USA, 1987.

[40] C. Jenkinson, R. Fitzpatrick, V. Peto, R. Greenhall, and N. Hyman, "The PDQ-8: development and validation of a short-form Parkinson's disease questionnaire," *Psychology and Health*, vol. 12, no. 6, pp. 805–814, 1997.

[41] F. Malouin, C. L. Richards, P. L. Jackson, M. F. Lafleur, A. Durand, and J. Doyon, "The Kinesthetic and Visual Imagery Questionnaire (KVIQ) for assessing motor imagery in persons with physical disabilities: A Reliability and Construct Validity Study," *Journal of Neurologic Physical Therapy*, vol. 31, no. 1, pp. 20–29, 2007.

[42] B. Randhawa, S. Harris, and L. A. Boyd, "The kinesthetic and visual imagery questionnaire is a reliable tool for individuals with Parkinson disease," *Journal of Neurologic Physical Therapy*, vol. 34, no. 3, pp. 161–167, 2010.

[43] V. Braun and V. Clarke, "Using thematic analysis in psychology," *Qualitative Research in Psychology*, vol. 3, no. 2, pp. 77–101, 2006.

[44] T. L. Chartrand and J. A. Bargh, "The chameleon effect: the perception-behavior link and social interaction," *Journal of Personality and Social Psychology*, vol. 76, no. 6, pp. 893–910, 1999.

[45] E. Poliakoff, A. J. Galpin, K. McDonald et al., "The effect of gym training on multiple outcomes in Parkinson's disease: a pilot randomised waiting-list controlled trial," *NeuroRehabilitation*, vol. 32, no. 1, pp. 125–134, 2013.

[46] G. Kleiner-Fisman, P. Gryfe, and G. Naglie, "A patient-based needs assessment for living well with Parkinson disease: implementation via nominal group technique," *Parkinson's Disease*, vol. 2013, Article ID 974964, 6 pages, 2013.

[47] National Collaborating Centre for Chronic Conditions, *Parkinson's Disease: National Clinical Guideline for Diagnosis and Management in Primary and Secondary Care*, Royal College of Physicians, London, UK, 2006.

[48] A. Ashburn, L. Fazakarley, C. Ballinger, R. Pickering, L. D. McLellan, and C. Fitton, "A randomised controlled trial of a home based exercise programme to reduce the risk of falling among people with Parkinson's disease," *Journal of Neurology, Neurosurgery and Psychiatry*, vol. 78, no. 7, pp. 678–684, 2007.

[49] V. Lun, N. Pullan, N. Labelle, C. Adams, and O. Suchowersky, "Comparison of the effects of a self-supervised home exercise program with a physiotherapist-supervised exercise program on the motor symptoms of Parkinson's disease," *Movement Disorders*, vol. 20, no. 8, pp. 971–975, 2005.

[50] K. Dujardin and L. Defebvre, "Apathy in Parkinson disease; What are the underlying mechanisms?" *Neurology*, vol. 79, no. 11, pp. 1082–1083, 2012.

[51] J.-F. Esculier, J. Vaudrin, P. Bériault, K. Gagnon, and L. E. Tremblay, "Home-based balance training programme using Wii Fit with balance board for Parkinson's disease: a pilot study," *Journal of Rehabilitation Medicine*, vol. 44, no. 2, pp. 144–150, 2012.

[52] K. Lohse, N. Shirzad, A. Verster, N. Hodges, and H. F. M. Van der Loos, "Video games and rehabilitation: using design principles to enhance engagement in physical therapy," *Journal of Neurologic Physical Therapy*, vol. 37, no. 4, pp. 166–175, 2013.

[53] L. M. Ewan, K. Kinmond, and P. S. Holmes, "An observation-based intervention for stroke rehabilitation: experiences of eight individuals affected by stroke," *Disability and Rehabilitation*, vol. 32, no. 25, pp. 2097–2106, 2010.

[54] K. H. O. Deane, H. Flaherty, D. J. Daley et al., "Priority setting partnership to identify the top 10 research priorities for the management of parkinson's disease," *British Medical Journal*, vol. 4, article e006434, 2015.

[55] J. J. Ferreira, C. Godinho, A. T. Santos et al., "Quantitative home-based assessment of Parkinson's symptoms: the SENSE-PARK feasibility and usability study," *BMC Neurology*, vol. 15, article 89, 2015.

[56] W. Lee, A. Evans, and D. R. Williams, "Validation of a smartphone application measuring bradykinesia in Parkinson's disease," *Movement Disorders*, vol. 30, p. S276, 2015.

[57] S. McCormick and P. Holmes, "See, Imagine, Move—Upper Limb Action Therapy (SIMULATe): iPad-based mental and physical motor (re)learning for stroke recovery," *Stroke*, vol. 47, supplement 1, p. ATP157, 2016.

31

MRI-Guided Focused Ultrasound in Parkinson's Disease

Ilana Schlesinger,[1,2] Alon Sinai,[3] and Menashe Zaaroor[2,3]

[1]*Department of Neurology, Rambam Health Care Campus, Haifa, Israel*
[2]*Technion Faculty of Medicine, Haifa, Israel*
[3]*Department of Neurosurgery, Rambam Health Care Campus, Haifa, Israel*

Correspondence should be addressed to Ilana Schlesinger; i_schles@rambam.health.gov.il

Academic Editor: Amnon Sintov

MRI-guided focused ultrasound is a new technology that enables intracranial ablation. Since lesioning ameliorates some of the symptoms of PD, this technology is being explored as a possible treatment for medication resistant symptoms in PD patients. The purpose of this paper is to review the clinical use and treatment outcomes of PD patients treated to date with this technology.

1. Introduction

Parkinson's disease (PD) is a neurodegenerative disorder characterized by tremor, rigidity, and bradykinesia. Tremor is the most common initial symptom of Parkinson's disease (PD), observed in about 50% of patients at the time of diagnosis [1–3]. The classic PD tremor is the rest tremor that has its greatest amplitude with the limb at rest and transiently disappears with movement but can reemerge with sustained posture. Postural/kinetic tremor is seen in a subset of patients with PD. The pathophysiology of tremor may be different from other PD symptoms which may explain why tremor responds less well to dopaminergic treatments [4]. Tremor-dominant PD is characterized by prominent tremor of one or more limbs with relative bradykinesia and rigidity. The tremor-dominant patients are not only disabled by the tremor itself but also suffer social isolation that further decreases quality of life [5]. A wide range of medications have been used to treat tremor including levodopa, dopamine agonists, anticholinergics, botulinum toxin, clozapine, amantadine, clonazepam, propranolol, and neurontin, but some PD patients have disabling tremor that is refractory to medications. In these patients, neurosurgical intervention is a treatment option.

Another unmet need in PD is treatment of motor fluctuations and dyskinesia that occur as a complication of levodopa therapy [6]. Since all patients with PD will eventually receive levodopa, treating this complication is crucial. Motor complications usually develop within 5 to 10 years of starting this medication [7]. Motor complications are fluctuations between effective control of symptoms, "ON" state, and reemergence of the PD symptoms, "OFF" state. These fluctuating symptoms may be accompanied by involuntary movement called dyskinesias. Though catechol-O-methyltransferase inhibitors [8], dopamine agonists, amantadine, and MAO-B inhibitors improve symptoms in some patients, their effectiveness is limited by declining tolerability with disease progression while complimentary medicine offers only short-term relief of symptoms [9]. Before the introduction of levodopa treatment, thalamotomy and pallidotomy were the mainstay of treatment [10]. Today, neurosurgical intervention, most commonly deep brain stimulation, is proposed, but, though this is an effective treatment, many patients are reluctant to undergo this procedure because of the need to undergo burr holes with insertion of foreign bodies, intracerebral electrodes, and an implanted pulse generator [11–13]. Gamma knife stereotactic radiosurgery is also an option; although effective, it may have delayed serious adverse events [14, 15].

MRI-guided focused ultrasound (MRgFUS) is a new technology that enables intracranial ablation. Since lesioning ameliorates some of the symptoms of PD [16], this technology is being explored as a possible treatment for medication resistant symptoms in PD patients. It has already been approved for the treatment of essential tremor. The purpose of this paper is to review the clinical use and treatment outcomes of PD patients treated with this technology.

2. MRI-Guided Focused Ultrasound

The first to suggest using focused ultrasound beams to treat movement disorders were Fry et al. [17]. In 1958, they reported utilizing four focused ultrasound beams to treat numerous human patients suffering from various movement disorders, in particular Parkinson's disease [18]. In order to focus the beams to the specific brain region at high intensity, they performed craniotomies which eliminate absorption of the rays by the bone, which caused heating of the skull [18, 19]. Today, technological advances allow focusing high intensity ultrasound beams through an intact skull without incisions or burr holes [20, 21]. Advances in MRI technology allow accurate targeting and real-time thermal monitoring using MR thermometry [22], thus providing accurate localization and control of the thermal dose needed for effective ablation [23].

In the MRgFUS procedure, a small brain target is heated with ultrasound rays, a technique called sonication. With this technique, the MRI serves as the surgeon's eyes for targeting the energy and the US rays serve as the surgeon's knife for creating the lesion. These rays heat the tissue, thereby causing thalamotomy since heating any tissue normal or abnormal to 57°C for one second (or an equivalent thermal dose) denatures protein, thus causing 100% cell death. The area of tissue exposed to the temperature and the length of exposure to this heat defines an equivalent thermal dose [24] which determines the extent of the lesion. By focusing the heat to more than one point or by scanning the focus, a volume of tissue can be thermally ablated.

MRgFUS surgery is performed in the MRI suit. The MRI is used for target definition, treatment planning, and intervention guidance with high precision. Simultaneous real-time monitoring of the temperature at the target is achieved with MR thermometry [23], allowing for a gradual procedure that enables lesion effect monitoring at clinically low temperatures when the effects and possible side effects are still presumed to be reversible. Definitive nonreversible thermal ablation is performed only after temporary tremor reduction when the patient reports no adverse effect.

MRgFUS ablation of the thalamus for the relief of tremor was performed by us [25, 26] in a stepwise fashion using ExAblate 2000 (InSightec Inc., Haifa, Israel). In the first stage, sonication is delivered at very low energy to confirm that the sonication focus is in the selected target. This is verified in 3 planes (sagittal, axial, and coronal). When needed, the sonication focus is adjusted. The temperature at this stage typically reaches 41–46°C. The second stage involves sonication with gradually increasing energy to achieve a temporary effect on tremor and to confirm the absence of adverse effects. The target is continuously examined for accuracy according to the planned coordinates and to the patient's clinical and neurological examination including tremor evaluation by drawing spirals, writing, cup holding, and other preoperative known tremor triggering maneuvers. The coordinates are repositioned when necessary according to the clinical status, the patients' feedback, and adverse effects, if any. When no amelioration of tremor is seen, the sonication focus is moved until tremor reduction is achieved taking into account the anatomy of the VIM somatotopic arrangement and its thalamic surrounding nuclei [27, 28]. Typically, temperature at this stage reaches 46–50°C. The third stage, the ablation stage, includes a gradual increase in total energy by either increasing intensity of sonication or by prolonging sonication duration. Sonication is stopped when adequate control of tremor is achieved, with the temperature reaching no more than 60°C. It is possible to repeat the sonication with the maximal energy to verify long lasting effect.

Pallidothalamic tractotomy was performed by Magara et al. [29] in a similar fashion except that at ablative temperatures they first performed a single sonication; but after they concluded that the effect of a single sonication did not persist, they performed multiple sonication with better results, as described below. The exact technique of pallidotomy using MRgFUS has yet to be described in the literature.

A subset of patients have skull features that do not allow enough heating of intracranial structures. This can usually be foreseen by performing a brain CT scan before treatment and calculating a skull density ratio [30]. Low skull density may preclude treatment.

3. MRI-Guided Focused Ultrasound Targets

3.1. Pallidothalamic Tractotomy. The first to report treating PD patients with MRgFUS were Magara et al. [29]. They chose to perform pallidothalamic tractotomy, a target rarely approached with previous lesioning methods. Their rationale was that, in the 1960s, subthalamic lesioning showed symptom relief in PD patients and a histological study they performed led them to believe they were aiming at the thalamic fasciculus. With this target, they reported treating 13 patients (Table 1). They selected patients with refractory symptoms, 9 with tremor predominant PD that experienced severe tremor and 4 with akinetic rigidity with motor fluctuations. In the first four patients, they performed a single sonication at the high temperature which causes ablation. In these patients, beneficial effect did not last and tremor returned within 3 months. Therefore, in the next 9 patients, they performed repeated sonication and reported good results. The validated tool for measuring changes in function, the Unified PD Rating Scale (UPDRS), is reported as the outcome measure, though these authors used a self-modified, not validated, version of the scale. They chose to score mentation, behavior, mood, activity of daily living, and motor complications according to the original UPDRS. But in the motor part of the UPDRS (part III), they declared that they scored only the treated side of the body to a maximal score of 56, while, in the original scale, bilateral signs as well as axial signs are scored to a maximal score of 108. In doing this,

Table 1: Characteristics of Parkinson's disease patients that underwent MRgFUS treatment.

Authors & year	Target	Patients, n	Age, y (range)	Sex, m	Tremor dominant	Levodopa treatment	Disease duration, y (range)
Magara et al. 2014	Pallidothalamic tract	13	64.5 (37–82)	8	9	11	9.7 (3–27)
Schlesinger et al. 2015	Thalamotomy	7	59 (46–74)	6	7	3	5.4 (2.5–10)
Na et al. 2015	Pallidotomy	1	56	0	0	1	12
Zaaroor et al. 2017	Thalamotomy	12*	62.8 (46–75)	11	12	5	7.1 (2–16)

*Of the 12 patients in Zaaroor et al., 7 are the same patients as in Schlesinger et al.

Table 2: Treatment outcomes of Parkinson's disease patients that underwent MRgFUS treatment.

Authors & year	Target	Patients, n	Motor UPDRS (Part II)				Significance
			Pretreatment	Post treatment 3 months	Point reduction	Change (%)	
Magara et al. 2014 Group 1	Pallidothalamic tract	4	18.8*	16.5	2.3	12.2	NA
Magara et al. 2014 Group 2	Pallidothalamic tract	9	18.7*	7.3	11.4	61.0	$p < 0.001$
Schlesinger et al. 2015	Thalamotomy	7	27.0	19.7	7.3	27.0	$p = 0.036$
Na et al. 2015	Pallidotomy	1	10	5	5	50	NA
Zaaroor et al. 2017	Thalamotomy	12**	24.9	13.4***	11.5	46.2	$p = 0.002$

*A modified, not validated version of the motor-UPDRS that scored only the treated side of the body to a maximal score of 56 instead of 108 points in the original scale.
**Of the 12 patients in Zaaroor et al., 7 are the same patients as in Schlesinger et al.
***UPDRS at 6 months.

they scored axial and bilateral symptoms but did not score axial and bilateral signs. They also do not report whether the UPDRS was performed in the ON or OFF state. They report a reduction of UPDRS-motor from 18.8 ± 11.7 at baseline to 16.5 ± 8.2 (2.3 points, 12% relief) at three months after a single sonication at ablative temperature in 4 patients. In 9 patients, they report a reduction in the UPDRS-motor score from 18.7 ± 5.2 at baseline to 7.3 ± 4.5 (11.3 points, 61% relief) at three months $p < 0.001$ after repeated sonication (Table 2). The global symptom relief was reduced by 22.5% and 56.7%, respectively. They reported no adverse event during or after sonication.

The lesion they performed was on target with a mean 3D vector accuracy of 1.0 mm. Lesion volumes for the patients with lasting results was on average of 172 mm^3 in comparison with 83 mm^3 with a single sonication. The temperature at the target on the last sonication ranged between 52°C and 59°C (average 56.2°C). The mean sonication duration was 13 s (range 10–21 s), the maximum acoustic power was 1,200 W, and the maximum applied energy was 20,400 J. They report no target hemorrhages or other untoward tissue reactions.

3.2. Ventral Intermediate Nucleus Thalamotomy. We reported in 2015 our experience with ventral intermediate nucleus thalamotomy (VIM) in 7 medication resistant, tremor predominant PD patients. The VIM was calculated to be located anterior to the posterior commissure, at 25% of the distance from the anterior to the posterior commissure, 14 mm lateral to the anterior-posterior commissural line. In cases where the 3rd ventricle was widened, the initial target was 11.5 mm lateral to the III ventricular wall. In 2016, we reported our experience in 5 additional PD patients [25, 26] (Table 1). Of these 12 PD patients, five received levodopa with motor fluctuations. Tremor stopped in the treated hand in all patients immediately following the treatment. Three patients had essential tremor for many years before they developed PD. UPDRS was examined in the ON state. At one month, UPDRS-motor part decreased from 24.9 ± 8.0 before treatment to 16.4 ± 11.1 (8.5 points, 34.1% relief) after MRgFUS ($p = 0.042$). UPDRS continued to improve over time and was 13.4 ± 9.2 (11.5 points, 46.2% relief) at six months ($p = 0.009$, as compared with baseline) (Table 2). At one month, item 20 and item 21 of the UPDRS (rest and action tremor) decreased from 2.9 ± 1.0 to 0.4 ± 1.0 ($p < 0.001$) and from 3.00 ± 1.2 to 0.6 ± 1.0, respectively, and, at 6 months, to 0.3 ± 0.5 and 0.6 ± 1.1, respectively. PDQ39, a validated quality of life questionnaire used in PD patients, decreased from 38.6 ± 16.8 before treatment to 26.1 ± 7.2 at one month posttreatment ($p = 0.036$) This measure also continued to improve over time and at six months scores reached 20.6 ± 8.8 ($p = 0.008$, as compared with baseline). During follow-up of 6–24 months (mean 11.6 ± 7.2 months, median 12.0 months), tremor reappeared in four of the patients. Two PD patients that suffered from essential tremor for many years before they developed PD were among those had tremor recurrence. In these patients, both rest and kinetic tremor recurred.

Adverse events that transiently occurred during sonication in PD patients included the following: short lasting vertigo ($n = 5$), headache ($n = 4$), dizziness ($n = 3$), nausea ($n = 1$), burning scalp sensation ($n = 1$), and lip paresthesia ($n = 1$). Adverse events that lasted after the procedure included the following: asthenia ($n = 2$), gait ataxia ($n = 1$), unsteady feeling ($n = 1$), unilateral taste disturbances ($n = 1$), and hand ataxia ($n = 1$). No adverse event lasted beyond 3 months. For a complete list of adverse events reported in this paper which also included essential tremor patients, see [26].

Lesions in the planned target were close to spherical with a diameter of 4–9 mm (average, 6.8 ± 1.5 mm). We observed mild edema one day after the procedure with increased edema one week after the procedure. The edema lasted for 3–5 weeks following the procedure. At 3 months, the edema resolved and lesion decreased in size.

The mean maximal temperature at the target was 56.5 ± 2.2°C (range, 55–60°C). Patients underwent on average 21.1 ± 8.3 sonication (range, 14–45) with an average maximal sonication time of 16.2 ± 3.0 seconds (range, 13–24). The mean maximal energy reached was 12,750 ± 4385 Joules (range, 5850–23040).

Recently, Bond et al. [31] reported in abstract form preliminary results of their double-blinded, randomized controlled trial to investigate the effectiveness of MRgFUS thalamotomy in tremor-dominant PD. They found that MRgFUS showed a trend toward improvement in hand tremor and a clinically significant reduction in mean UPDRS. They also noted a significant placebo response. Further information regarding this study is not yet available.

3.3. Pallidotomy. There is one report by Na et al. of lesioning of the globus pallidus interna using MRgFUS [32] (Table 1). They reported their experience in a single woman with severe levodopa in disabling motor fluctuations and severe levodopa-related motor complications. Total UPDRS was 53 at baseline and was reduced to 16 at one month, 14 at 3 months, and 18 at 6 months (37, 39, and 35 points, 69.8%, 73.5%, and 66.0% relief, respectively). The UPDRS-motor part improved from 10 at baseline to 5 at 3 months (Table 2). On MRI, the lesion was distinct one month after treatment and was seen less clearly at 3 months. They did not report adverse events.

On imaging, they observed signal changes consistent with pallidotomy and degree of signal changes was decreased at 3 months.

4. Discussion

MRgFUS is a new emerging treatment for medications resistant symptoms in PD. To date, patients underwent this treatment in order to relieve medication resistant tremor and for disabling motor complications. Significant benefit was seen in most patients with very few transient adverse events.

The target chosen for MRgFUS differed according to the treatment center. Magara et al. chose to lesion the pallidothalamic tract to relieve tremor and dyskinesia [29]. We chose to perform thalamotomy for PD patients with severe tremor [25, 26]. While Na et al. chose to perform pallidotomy in order to ameliorate motor complication [32]. It is not clear which target is most beneficial and whether different targets should be chosen for different symptoms. What makes it hard to compare the targets is the use of different treatment outcome measures. For instance, we used the original motor UPDRS (part III) [25, 26] as our main outcome measure, while Magara et al. [29] used a self-modified UPDRS-motor score, making the scores not comparable. Interestingly, the improvement in the UPDRS-motor scores reported by Magara and by us shows similar improvement (11.3 points in Magara's paper and 11.5 points in our paper), suggesting similar improvement in both treatment targets. More information regarding efficacy and adverse events will be needed in order to answer this question.

Long-term efficacy is also an important issue. Magara et al. reported that, in order to avoid symptom recurrence, repeated ablation at high temperatures at treatment target is needed [29]. This repeated sonication resulted in larger lesions which may account for the better long-term outcome. We reported the longest follow-up of PD patients that underwent MRgFUS [26]. In our experience, 4 of 12 patients had some tremor recurrence. We noted that tremor recurrence was more frequent in patients that suffered from essential tremor for many years before they developed PD. Though we treated only 3 such patients, tremor recurred in 2 of them. This was in comparison to tremor recurrence in 2 of 9 patients with PD with no previous neurological deficit. This observation suggests that MRgFUS may not be the optimal choice in this unique group of patients of PD following essential tremor.

Pallidotomy is a promising target for MRgFUS, but there are unique challenges in treating this target. The first is the technical issue of focusing ultrasound rays to this target because they are at the edge of the treatment area. The second is finding the exact target within the pallidum that will ameliorate symptoms. The third is the proximity of the optic nerve to the globus pallidus internus. To date, it is not clear what will be the best target for treating PD symptoms or whether different targets should be used for different patients. Another question that has yet to be answered is whether bilateral treatments can be performed since currently all treatments are unilateral in order to avoid possibly serious adverse events. Adverse events recently reported in a multicenter trial of focused ultrasound thalamotomy for essential tremor, where most centers had little experience with this technology, included gait disturbances and paresthesias or numbness that persisted after 12 months. Therefore, maybe focused ultrasound thalamotomy should be performed in specialized centers with experience in the procedure [33].

MRgFUS is a new option for PD patients with medication resistant symptoms. It is approved for this indication in Israel, Europe, Korea, and Russia. Further studies are needed in order to better characterize patient selection and treatment targets.

References

[1] D. B. Calne and A. J. Stoessl, "Early Parkinsonism," *Clinical Neuropharmacology*, vol. 9, supplement 2, pp. S3–S8, 1986.

[2] I. Litvan, K. P. Bhatia, D. J. Burn et al., "SIC task force appraisal of clinical diagnostic criteria for parkinsonian disorders," *Movement Disorders*, vol. 18, no. 5, pp. 467–486, 2003.

[3] P. S. Fishman, "Paradoxical aspects of parkinsonian tremor," *Movement Disorders*, vol. 23, no. 2, pp. 168–173, 2008.

[4] R. C. Helmich, M. Hallett, G. Deuschl, I. Toni, and B. R. Bloem, "Cerebral causes and consequences of parkinsonian resting tremor: a tale of two circuits?" *Brain*, vol. 135, no. 11, pp. 3206–3226, 2012.

[5] R. Zimmermann, G. Deuschl, A. Hornig, J. Schulte-Monting, G. Fuchs, and C. H. Lucking, "Tremors in Parkinson's disease: symptom analysis and rating," *Clinical Neuropharmacology*, vol. 17, no. 4, pp. 303–314, 1994.

[6] J. G. Nutt, "Motor fluctuations and dyskinesia in Parkinson's disease," *Parkinsonism and Related Disorders*, vol. 8, no. 2, pp. 101–108, 2001.

[7] J. Jankovic and W. Poewe, "Therapies in Parkinson's disease," *Current Opinion in Neurology*, vol. 25, no. 4, pp. 433–447, 2012.

[8] I. Schlesinger and A. Korczyzn, "Catechol-O-methyl transferase inhibitors in the treatment of Parkinson's disease," in *Parkinson's Disease: Current & Future Therapeutics & Clinical Trials*, N. Gálvez-Jiménez, H. Fernandez, A. Espay, and S. Fox, Eds., Cambridge University Press, Cambridge UK, 2016.

[9] I. Schlesinger, O. Benyakov, I. Erikh, and M. Nassar, "Relaxation guided imagery reduces motor fluctuations in Parkinson's disease," *Journal of Parkinson's Disease*, vol. 4, no. 3, pp. 431–436, 2014.

[10] B. L. Walter and J. L. Vitek, "Surgical treatment for Parkinson's disease," *The Lancet Neurology*, vol. 3, no. 12, pp. 719–728, 2004.

[11] W. M. M. Schuepbach, J. Rau, K. Knudsen et al., "Neurostimulation for Parkinson's disease with early motor complications," *New England Journal of Medicine*, vol. 368, no. 7, pp. 610–622, 2013.

[12] M.-R. Kim, J. Y. Yun, B. Jeon et al., "Patients' reluctance to undergo deep brain stimulation for Parkinson's disease," *Parkinsonism and Related Disorders*, vol. 23, pp. 91–94, 2016.

[13] M. Setiawan, S. Kraft, K. Doig et al., "Referrals for movement disorder surgery: under-representation of females and reasons for refusal," *Canadian Journal of Neurological Sciences*, vol. 33, no. 1, pp. 53–57, 2006.

[14] S.-Y. Lim, M. Hodaie, M. Fallis, Y.-Y. Poon, F. Mazzella, and E. Moro, "Gamma knife thalamotomy for disabling tremor: a blinded evaluation," *Archives of Neurology*, vol. 67, no. 5, pp. 584–588, 2010.

[15] M. S. Okun, N. P. Stover, T. Subramanian et al., "Complications of gamma knife surgery for Parkinson disease," *Archives of Neurology*, vol. 58, no. 12, pp. 1995–2002, 2001.

[16] R. R. Tasker, A. E. Lang, and A. M. Lozano, "Pallidal and thalamic surgery for Parkinson's disease," *Experimental Neurology*, vol. 144, no. 1, pp. 35–40, 1997.

[17] W. J. Fry, W. H. Mosberg Jr., J. W. Barnard, and F. J. Fry, "Production of focal destructive lesions in the central nervous system with ultrasound," *Journal of Neurosurgery*, vol. 11, no. 5, pp. 471–478, 1954.

[18] R. Meyers, W. J. Fry, F. J. Fry, L. L. Dreyer, D. F. Schultz, and R. F. Noyes, "Early experiences with ultrasonic irradiation of the pallidofugal and nigral complexes in hyperkinetic and hypertonic disorders," *Journal of Neurosurgery*, vol. 16, no. 1, pp. 32–54, 1959.

[19] W. J. Fry and R. Meyers, "Ultrasonic method of modifying brain st ructures," *Confinia Neurologica*, vol. 22, pp. 315–327, 1962.

[20] G. T. Clement and K. Hynynen, "A non-invasive method for focusing ultrasound through the human skull," *Physics in Medicine and Biology*, vol. 47, no. 8, pp. 1219–1236, 2002.

[21] J. Sun and K. Hynynen, "The potential of transskull ultrasound therapy and surgery using the maximum available skull surface area," *Journal of the Acoustical Society of America*, vol. 105, no. 4, pp. 2519–2527, 1999.

[22] A. H. Chung, F. A. Jolesz, and K. Hynynen, "Thermal dosimetry of a focused ultrasound beam in vivo by magnetic resonance imaging," *Medical Physics*, vol. 26, no. 9, pp. 2017–2026, 1999.

[23] Y. Ishihara, A. Calderon, H. Watanabe et al., "A precise and fast temperature mapping using water proton chemical shift," *Magnetic Resonance in Medicine*, vol. 34, no. 6, pp. 814–823, 1995.

[24] S. A. Sapareto and W. C. Dewey, "Thermal dose determination in cancer therapy," *International Journal of Radiation Oncology, Biology, Physics*, vol. 10, no. 6, pp. 787–800, 1984.

[25] I. Schlesinger, A. Eran, A. Sinai et al., "MRI guided focused ultrasound thalamotomy for moderate-to-severe tremor in Parkinson's disease," *Parkinson's Disease*, vol. 2015, Article ID 219149, 4 pages, 2015.

[26] M. Zaaroor, A. Sinai, D. Goldsher, A. Eran, M. Nassar, and I. Schlesinger, "Magnetic resonance–guided focused ultrasound thalamotomy for tremor: a report of 30 Parkinson's disease and essential tremor cases," *Journal of Neurosurgery*, 2017.

[27] G. Schaltenbrand and W. Wahren, *Atlas for Stereotaxy of the Human Brain*, Thieme Medical Publishers, Stuttgart, Germany, 1977.

[28] A. R. Rezai, A. G. Machado, M. Deogaonkar, H. Azmi, C. Kubu, and N. M. Boulis, "Surgery for movement disorders," *Neurosurgery*, vol. 62, no. 2, pp. SHC809–SHC838, 2008.

[29] A. Magara, R. Bühler, D. Moser, M. Kowalski, P. Pourtehrani, and D. Jeanmonod, "First experience with MR-guided focused ultrasound in the treatment of Parkinson's disease," *Journal of Therapeutic Ultrasound*, vol. 2, no. 1, article 11, 2014.

[30] W. S. E. Chang, H. H. O. Jung, E. Zadicario et al., "Factors associated with successful magnetic resonance-guided focused ultrasound treatment: efficiency of acoustic energy delivery through the skull," *Journal of Neurosurgery*, vol. 124, no. 2, pp. 411–416, 2016.

[31] A. E. Bond, R. Dallapiazza, D. Huss et al., "A randomized, sham-controlled trial of transcranial magnetic resonance-guided focused ultrasound thalamotomy trial for the treatment of tremor-dominant, idiopathic Parkinson disease," *Neurosurgery*, vol. 63, supplement 1, article 154, 2016.

[32] Y. C. Na, W. S. Chang, H. H. Jung, E. J. Kweon, and J. W. Chang, "Unilateral magnetic resonance-guided focused ultrasound pallidotomy for Parkinson disease," *Neurology*, vol. 85, no. 6, pp. 549–551, 2015.

[33] I. Schlesinger and M. Zaaroor, "A trial of focused ultrasound thalamotomy for essential tremor," *The New England Journal of Medicine*, vol. 375, no. 22, pp. 2201–2203, 2016.

32

The Single Nucleotide Polymorphism rs1014290 of the *SLC2A9* Gene Is Associated with Uric Acid Metabolism in Parkinson's Disease

Jiangfang Miao,[1,2] Jing Liu,[1] Li Xiao,[3] Jiedi Zheng,[1] Chunfeng Liu,[1] Zufu Zhu,[2] Kai Li,[3] and Weifeng Luo[1]

[1]*Jiangsu Key Laboratory of Translational Research and Therapy for Neuro-Psycho-Diseases and The Second Affiliated Hospital of Soochow University, Soochow University, Suzhou, Jiangsu 215021, China*
[2]*Jiangsu Jiangyin People's Hospital, Jiangyin, Jiangsu 214400, China*
[3]*College of Pharmaceutical Science, Soochow University, Suzhou, Jiangsu 215123, China*

Correspondence should be addressed to Kai Li; kaili34@yahoo.com and Weifeng Luo; lwfwxx@126.com

Academic Editor: Anthony Lang

Individuals with Parkinson's disease (PD) have lower uric acid levels than those without PD, and the CC genotype and C minor allele of a single nucleotide polymorphism (SNP), rs1014290 of *SLC2A9*, are associated with lower uric acid levels. We investigated the association of rs1014290 with uric acid metabolism in a cohort of PD cases (220) and controls (110) in a Han Chinese population. Uric acid levels were determined and rs1014290 was assayed using a mutation-sensitive on/off switch technology. PD uric acid levels ($291.65 \pm 76.29\ \mu$mol/L) were significantly lower than the controls ($325.73 \pm 74.23\ \mu$mol/L, $P < 0.001$, t-test). Individuals with rs1014290 TT and CT genotypes had higher uric acid levels, and those with the CC genotype had the lowest uric acid levels among both control and PD cases. The CC genotype and the C minor allele were statistically more frequent in the PD group compared to the control group. Those with the CC genotype had a statistically significant higher risk of PD than those with the TT or TC genotype (odds ratio [OR] = 2.249, 95% confidence interval [CI]: 1.129–4.480, and $P = 0.021$). Thus, SLC2A9 rs1014290 is related to lower uric acid levels in PD patients and can be a risk factor for PD in the Han population.

1. Introduction

Parkinson's disease (PD) is one of the most common neurodegenerative diseases, characterized by the extrapyramidal symptoms of resting tremor, rigidity, bradykinesia, and postural instability. Males have a significantly higher incidence rate of PD, approximately 1.5 times greater than females [1]. Although the etiology of PD remains unclear, it is generally considered to be a combination of complex genetic and environmental factors [2]. Several epidemiological studies suggest that high plasma uric acid levels decrease the risk of developing PD [3, 4], and serum uric acid can be a predictor of clinical and radiographic progression in PD [5].

SLC2A9 is considered to be the most effective urate transporter [6], affecting circulating uric acid levels. The single nucleotide polymorphism (SNP) rs1014290 of the *SLC2A9* gene has been reported to influence the age of onset of PD [7]. Here, through a retrospective case-controlled study, we aimed to identify the correlation between *SLC2A9* SNP rs1014290 and PD pathogenesis and to explore whether this relationship was affected by uric acid metabolism in the Han Chinese population. In all, we aimed to find genotype-endophenotype-exophenotype relationships among rs1014290 in *SLC2A9*, serum uric acid level, and PD in a select Han Chinese subpopulation.

2. Methods

2.1. Participants. A total of 220 patients with sporadic idiopathic PD from the Neurology Department, Second Affiliated Hospital of Soochow University in China, were selected from January 2011 to November 2012. The PD diagnosis was made by neurologists based on criteria consistent with the UK PD Society (UKPDS) Brain Bank criteria [8]. Sporadic idiopathic

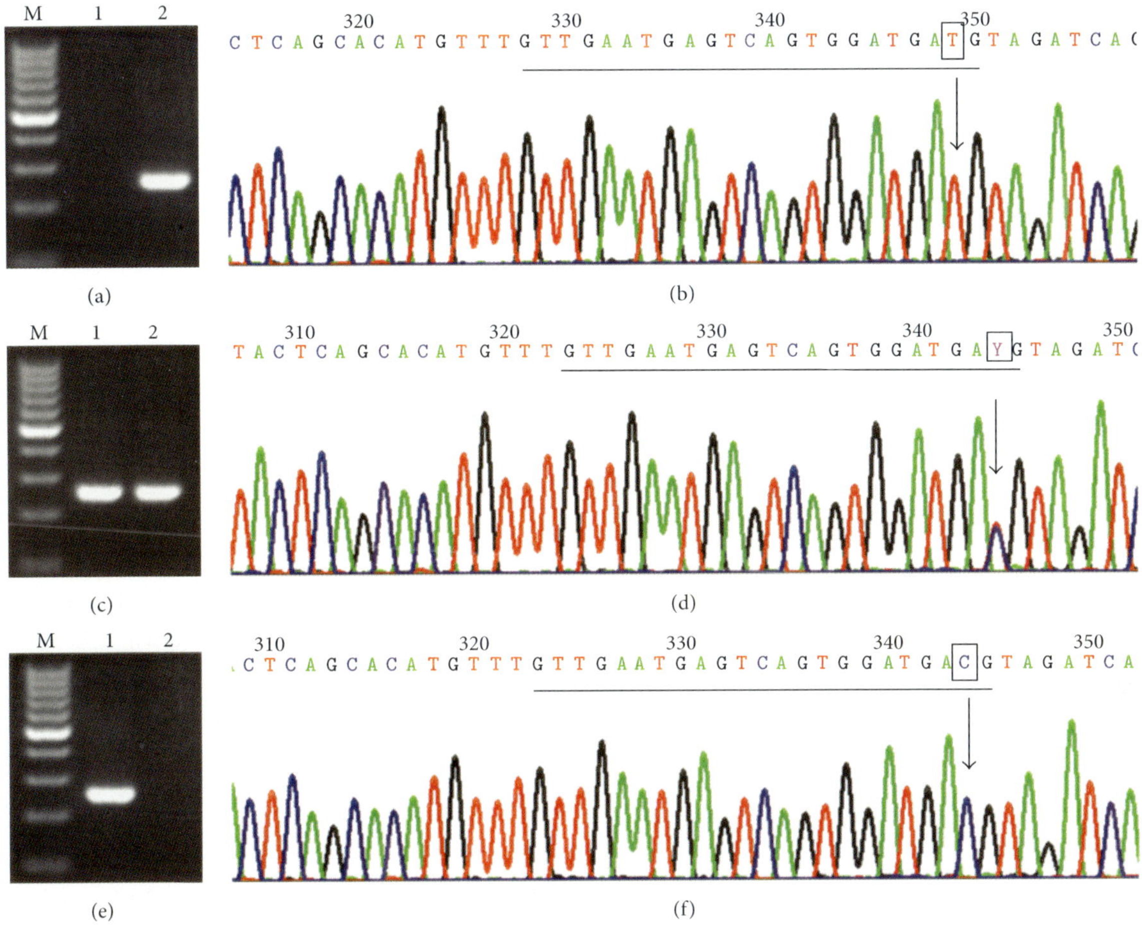

FIGURE 1: Representative illustrations of genotyping data and sequencing chromatography results. PCR product from the C allele template (lane 1) and the amplified fragment from the T allele-specific DNA using the on/off switch (lane 2). (a, c, and e) are the relevant genotypes confirmed by Sanger sequencing. The corresponding genotypes are CC, CT (Y), and TT as indicated with the box. M, marker.

PD is defined as one without a family history of PD. For comparison, 110 unrelated Han healthy controls matched in gender, age, and area of residence were included and investigated by our research group during the PD epidemiological study. All healthy controls were examined by neurologists to rule out neurodegenerative disorders, and detailed clinical data was recorded. And those who had gout and other diseases, such as liver and kidney diseases, were ruled out in all subjects. All subjects provided written informed consent. Ethics approval was obtained from the ethics committee of the Second Affiliated Hospital of Soochow University in China. 4 ml of venous blood was extracted from all subjects in the fasting state, 2 ml for testing serum uric acid levels and 2 ml for gene detection.

2.2. Uric Acid Levels Testing. Uric acid levels were determined using a Beckman Coulter (USA) automatic biochemical analyzer with the original kits at the Second Affiliated Hospital of Soochow University.

2.3. Genotyping. DNA was extracted from peripheral blood using the Magman TM Blood DNA Kit (GenoTheramics, USA) based on magnetic beads. Genotyping for rs1014290 was performed using a new assay employing proofreading PCR technology. We assayed SNP genotyping using a mutation-sensitive on/off switch consisting of 3′ terminal phosphorothioate-modified allele-specific primers and high-fidelity exo+ DNA polymerases. In recent years, this novel technology has been successfully employed in genetic analysis [9–11]. The mutation-sensitive on/off switch eliminates false positive errors and significantly decreases false negatives, which has been demonstrated to have a higher specificity than assays mediated by low-fidelity DNA polymerase. During the assay development stage, Sanger sequencing was used to confirm the proofreading PCR results (Figure 1).

2.4. Statistical Analyses. All statistical analyses were performed using IBM SPSS Statistics 23. The Hardy-Weinberg equilibrium (HWE) of *SLC2A9* rs1014290 for PD patients and controls was verified by Pearson's Chi-Square test, and "deviation" from Hardy-Weinberg is being tested. Allele frequency and genotype frequency between the two groups were compared with Chi-Square test. Uric acid levels were used to compare between the two groups using independent sample t-test. The odds ratio (OR) and 95% confidence interval (CI) were estimated using Chi-Square tests to examine the

TABLE 1: Clinical characteristics of study participants. The mean onset age of PD patients with the rs1014290 CC genotype was lower than that of those with the TT + TC genotype.

Group	PD		P1	Controls		P2
	CC	TT + CT		CC	TT + CT	
Number (M/F)	66 (37/29)	154 (84/70)		17 (8/9)	93 (52/41)	
Age (years)	65.48 ± 9.62	69.22 ± 9.33	0.009	69.59 ± 4.93	69.46 ± 8.72	0.933
Age at onset (years)	59.24 ± 9.77	63.21 ± 9.51	0.005			
Course of disease	6.24 ± 4.00	6.01 ± 4.05	0.699			
UPDRS motor scale	23.21 ± 10.82	23.12 ± 10.88	0.956			
H-Y score	2.00 ± 0.81	2.05 ± 0.86	0.714			

TABLE 2: Frequency of rs1014290 in PD patients and controls in a Han subpopulation. The frequency of the natural CC genotype is significantly higher in PD patients as compared to the controls, and less TT and CT genotypes are observed in PD patients. Analysis of C and T alleles revealed significant differences between groups.

Group	Number	Genotype frequency (%)			P	Allele frequency (%)		P
		TT	CT	CC		T	C	
PD	220	56 (25.5)	98 (44.5)	66 (30.0)	<0.001	210 (47.7)	230 (52.3)	<0.001
Controls	110	33 (30.0)	60 (54.5)	17 (15.5)		126 (57.3)	94 (42.7)	

CC genotype frequency and minor allele frequencies for rs1014290 between PD patients and controls.

3. Results

3.1. Clinical Characteristics of Study Participants. This study included 220 patients with idiopathic PD and 110 unrelated controls, of which 54.5% were male. There was no difference between the mean ages of PD patients (68.10 ± 9.55 years) and those of controls (69.48 ± 8.23 years, $P = 0.175$, t-test). The mean serum uric acid concentration of PD patients (291.65 ± 76.29 μmol/L) tended to be lower than that of the controls (325.73 ± 74.23 μmol/L, $P < 0.001$, t-test) (Table 1).

3.2. The rs1014290 C Allele Genotype Was More Prevalent in the PD Group Compared to the Control Group. The genotype frequencies of the PD group and the control group were in agreement with the HWE (PD: $\chi^2 = 1.318$, $P > 0.05$; controls: $\chi^2 = 0.689$, $P > 0.05$, Pearson Chi-Square test). The minor allele frequency of rs1014290 was 52.0% for the PD group and 42.7% for the control group, which were statistically significant ($\chi^2 = 5.347$, $P = 0.021$, OR = 0.681, and 95% CI = 0.492–0.944, Pearson Chi-Square test) (Table 2). The CC genotype frequencies of rs1014290 were 30.0% for the PD group and 15.5% for the control group ($\chi^2 = 8.242$, $P = 0.004$, OR = 0.427, and 95% CI = 0.236–0.771, Chi-Square test) (Table 2). We then performed multiple factors logistic regression analysis of rs1014290 genotypes on PD risk and found that individuals with the CC genotype had a higher risk of PD than individuals with the TT or TC genotype (OR = 2.189, 95% CI = 1.095–4.376, and $P = 0.027$) (Table 3).

3.3. Clinical Characteristics of PD Patients. The mean onset age of PD patients with the rs1014290 CC genotype (59.24 ± 9.77 years) was lower than that of those with the TT + TC genotype (63.21 ± 9.51 years, $P = 0.005$, t-test). For detailed data of clinical characteristics of PD patients please see Table 1.

3.4. Genotype-Dependent Serum Uric Acid Levels. The mean serum uric acid concentration of individuals with the CC genotype was lower than that of those with the TT and CT genotypes in both the control ($P < 0.001$, t-test) and PD ($P < 0.001$, t-test) groups (Table 4).

4. Discussion

Uric acid is a strong antioxidant in the human body, having a protective effect against oxidative stress and free radical damage, and may slow the progression of many degenerative nervous diseases [12–14]. Uric acid levels in the brain spinal fluid have a linear relationship with levels found in the blood. The protective effect of high levels of uric acid was first reported by Simon and Vanvunakis in 1964 [15]. Thereafter, several epidemiological studies found that high serum uric acid levels were associated with later onset of PD in males or alleviation of the severity of PD in recent years [4, 16, 17]. Genetic engineering technology has been used to dissect the relationship between uric acid levels in the brain and the development of PD [18], and similar data was gleaned from autopsies performed on patients with PD [19]. As all causal genes dissected from PD genetics account for only approximately 5% of PD cases with familial inheritance, confirmation of the large number of modulation genes of PD has several clinical impacts.

SLC2A9 is the most effective one of all uric acid transporters, and *SLC2A9* variants have been shown to influence circulating uric acid levels. SLC2A9's involvement in uric acid metabolism has been documented by both clinical and animal studies [6, 20, 21]. It is proved that the SLC2A9 variant rs3733591 served as an important genetic checkpoint for tophaceous gout and increased uric acid levels from two geographically diverse populations [22]. Various mutations of

TABLE 3: Multiple factors logistic regression analysis of the rs1014290 genotype in *SLC2A9* on the risk of PD*. Individuals with the CC genotype in *SLC2A9* had a higher risk of PD than individuals with the TT or TC genotype.

	B	SE	Wald	*v*	*P*	OR	95% CI	
							Lower	Upper
TT			6.579	2	0.037			
TC	−0.006	0.274	0.000	1	0.983	0.994	0.581	1.702
CC	0.783	0.354	4.909	1	0.027	2.189	1.095	4.376

*Adjusted for age, sex, height, and body weight.

TABLE 4: Average serum uric acid levels in the PD and control groups. Individuals and PD patients carrying the CC genotype had lower uric acid levels as compared to those with the TT and CT genotypes.

Group	Number	UA (μmol/L)		*P*
		TT + CT	CC	
PD	220	303.50 ± 83.62	264.00 ± 45.22	<0.001
Controls	110	334.14 ± 77.50	279.71 ± 18.32	<0.001
P		0.004	0.031	

P values compare individuals with different genotypes within the same group; UA, uric acid.

SLC2A9 were found in hypouricemia patients: Ile118HisfsX27 in a Czech family [23], exon 7 deletion in Ashkenazi Jewish [24], and R380W and R198C in Japanese [25]. Among the large number of genes related to uric acid metabolism, the present study clearly illustrated the close relationship between rs1014290 genotypes in *SLC2A9* and serum uric acid levels; individuals with the TT and CT genotypes have higher uric acid levels, and those with the CC genotype have the lowest uric acid level. This strong relationship between rs1014290 genotypes in *SLC2A9* and uric acid level phenotype was observed in the normal controls of our present study. Furthermore, we found that PD patients with TT and CT genotypes had higher uric acid levels than those with the CC genotype. The genotype-endophenotype relationship of rs1014290 to the serum uric acid level was also observed in the PD group. Our present study demonstrated that the mean serum uric acid concentration of PD patients was lower than that of the controls, which is consistent with our previous study [26]. We found that, compared with the control group, the rs1014290 minor allele and CC genotype frequencies were higher in the PD group. Furthermore, multiple factors logistic regression analysis showed that individuals with the CC genotype had a statistically significant higher risk of PD than individuals with the TT or TC genotype. The present study has established a link between rs1014290 and PD in a relatively large group of Han Chinese. We suggest that this PD phenotype related to the rs1014290 genotype is possibly mediated through the endophenotype of uric acid metabolism.

The mean onset age of PD patients with the CC genotype was relatively low, which confirms that the CC genotype influences the age of onset of PD [7]. Therefore, there is a genotype-phenotype association of *SLC2A9* rs1014290 with PD through uric acid metabolism in Han Chinese. The polymorphism of rs1014290 in *SLC2A9* may be a risk factor for PD in the Han Chinese population.

Uric acid levels of PD patients with TT and CT genotypes were significantly reduced compared to the controls. Low serum uric acid levels in PD patients were associated not only with the polymorphism of rs1014290 in *SLC2A9* loci, but also with other factors. Various SNPs near SLC2A9 have shown to be linked to uric acid level, such as SLC17A1, SLC22A11, and SLC22A12 [27].

Based upon these data, we suggest that SLC2A9 can be used as either a new drug target or a target for gene therapy. In addition to the potential application in the development of new therapies for PD, the confirmed relationship between rs1014290 and PD may also have diagnostic implications. As rs1014290 in *SLC2A9* is only a modulation factor, its value in the diagnosis and prediction of relative risk to a particular individual may be limited. However, when genotyping is combined with measurement of serum uric acid, high risk or susceptible individuals could be identified. In fact, by further including family history, a more informed assessment could be provided. And the study sample of our study was relatively small; we should collect more samples for further analysis, as larger sample sizes would have allowed further subanalyses and conditional analysis of SNPs in moderate-to-high link with rs1014290 near SLC2A9.

5. Conclusions and Future Directions

In conclusion, the present study bridged the divide between genotype, endophenotype, and exophenotype through analysis of rs1014290, serum uric acid level, and incidence of PD. We further confirmed that relatively low uric acid level is a risk factor for PD pathogenesis and that the rs1014290 of *SLC2A9* can be a risk factor for PD in the Han population. The protective effect of high serum uric acid level has been reinforced by our study. As the genotyping assay developed by this study is simple, cost-effective, and extremely reliable, its wide application may be beneficial to PD patients for screening purposes as well as individualized medicine.

Authors' Contributions

Jiangfang Miao and Jing Liu contributed equally to this work.

Acknowledgments

The authors would like to thank Collin Yan for assistance in proofreading this manuscript. This work was supported by Jiangsu Key Laboratory of Translational Research and Therapy for Neuro-Psycho-Diseases (BM2013003), a project funded by the Priority Academic Program Development of Jiangsu Higher Education Institutions, Jiangsu Provincial Special Program of Medical Science (BL2014042), the Guide Project for Suzhou Science and Technology Development Plan (SYSD2014088), the Youth Science and Technology Project of the Health Bureau of Suzhou City (KJXW2014012), the Pre-Research Foundation of the Second Affiliated Hospital of Soochow University (SDFEYQN1407), Suzhou Clinical Key Disease Diagnosis and Treatment Technology Foundation (LCZX201304), the Key Project of Science and Technology Innovation of Soochow University (SZ123819), Suzhou Technology Support Project (SS201112), and the Chinese National 863 Major Grant (no. 2012AA020905).

References

[1] G. F. Wooten, L. J. Currie, V. E. Bovbjerg, J. K. Lee, and J. Patrie, "Are men at greater risk for Parkinson's disease than women?" *Journal of Neurology, Neurosurgery & Psychiatry*, vol. 75, no. 4, pp. 637–639, 2004.

[2] J. L. Eriksen, Z. Wszolek, and L. Petrucelli, "Molecular pathogenesis of Parkinson disease," *Archives of Neurology*, vol. 62, no. 3, pp. 353–357, 2005.

[3] M. K. Kutzing and B. L. Firestein, "Altered uric acid levels and disease states," *Journal of Pharmacology and Experimental Therapeutics*, vol. 324, no. 1, pp. 1–7, 2008.

[4] A. Winquist, K. Steenland, and A. Shankar, "Higher serum uric acid associated with decreased Parkinson's disease prevalence in a large community-based survey," *Movement Disorders*, vol. 25, no. 7, pp. 932–936, 2010.

[5] M. A. Schwarzschild, S. R. Schwid, K. Marek et al., "Serum urate as a predictor of clinical and radiographic progression in Parkinson disease," *Archives of Neurology*, vol. 65, no. 6, pp. 716–723, 2008.

[6] M. J. Caulfield, P. B. Munroe, D. O'Neill et al., "SLC2A9 is a high-capacity urate transporter in humans," *PLoS Medicine*, vol. 5, no. 10, article e197, pp. 1509–1523, 2008.

[7] M. F. Facheris, A. A. Hicks, C. Minelli et al., "Variation in the uric acid transporter gene SLC2A9 and its association with AAO of Parkinson's disease," *Journal of Molecular Neuroscience*, vol. 43, no. 3, pp. 246–250, 2011.

[8] A. J. Hughes, S. E. Daniel, L. Kilford, and A. J. Lees, "Accuracy of clinical diagnosis of idiopathic Parkinson's disease: a clinico-pathological study of 100 cases," *Journal of Neurology Neurosurgery and Psychiatry*, vol. 55, no. 3, pp. 181–184, 1992.

[9] J. Zhang, K. Li, J. R. Pardinas, S. S. Sommer, and K.-T. Yao, "Proofreading genotyping assays mediated by high fidelity exo+ DNA polymerases," *Trends in Biotechnology*, vol. 23, no. 2, pp. 92–96, 2005.

[10] J. Zhang, K. Li, J. R. Pardinas, D. F. Liao, H. J. Li, and X. Zhang, "SNP discrimination through proofreading and OFF-switch of Exo+ polymerase," *Applied Biochemistry and Biotechnology Part B: Molecular Biotechnology*, vol. 27, no. 1, pp. 75–80, 2004.

[11] L. J. Reha-Krantz, "DNA polymerase proofreading: multiple roles maintain genome stability," *Biochimica et Biophysica Acta—Proteins and Proteomics*, vol. 1804, no. 5, pp. 1049–1063, 2010.

[12] M. Rentzos, C. Nikolaou, M. Anagnostouli et al., "Serum uric acid and multiple sclerosis," *Clinical Neurology and Neurosurgery*, vol. 108, no. 6, pp. 527–531, 2006.

[13] T.-S. Kim, C.-U. Pae, S.-J. Yoon et al., "Decreased plasma antioxidants in patients with Alzheimer's disease," *International Journal of Geriatric Psychiatry*, vol. 21, no. 4, pp. 344–348, 2006.

[14] I. Schlesinger and N. Schlesinger, "Uric acid in Parkinson's disease," *Movement Disorders*, vol. 23, no. 12, pp. 1653–1657, 2008.

[15] M. I. Simon and H. Vanvunakis, "The dye-sensitized photooxidation of purine and pyrimidine derivatives," *Archives of Biochemistry and Biophysics*, vol. 105, no. 1, pp. 197–206, 1964.

[16] T. Annanmaki, A. Muuronen, and K. Murros, "Low plasma uric acid level in Parkinson's disease," *Movement Disorders*, vol. 22, no. 8, pp. 1133–1137, 2007.

[17] M. G. Weisskopf, E. O'Reilly, H. Chen, M. A. Schwarzschild, and A. Ascherio, "Plasma urate and risk of Parkinson's disease," *American Journal of Epidemiology*, vol. 166, no. 5, pp. 561–567, 2007.

[18] R. F. Anderson and T. A. Harris, "Dopamine and uric acid act as antioxidants in the repair of DNA radicals: implications in Parkinson's disease," *Free Radical Research*, vol. 37, no. 10, pp. 1131–1136, 2003.

[19] W. H. Church and V. L. Ward, "Uric acid is reduced in the substantia nigra in Parkinson's disease: effect on dopamine oxidation," *Brain Research Bulletin*, vol. 33, no. 4, pp. 419–425, 1994.

[20] A. Döring, C. Gieger, D. Mehta et al., "SLC2A9 influences uric acid concentrations with pronounced sex-specific effects," *Nature Genetics*, vol. 40, no. 4, pp. 430–436, 2008.

[21] V. Vitart, I. Rudan, C. Hayward et al., "SLC2A9 is a newly identified urate transporter influencing serum urate concentration, urate excretion and gout," *Nature Genetics*, vol. 40, no. 4, pp. 437–442, 2008.

[22] H.-P. Tu, C.-J. Chen, S. Tovosia et al., "Associations of a non-synonymous variant in SLC2A9 with gouty arthritis and uric acid levels in Han Chinese subjects and Solomon Islanders," *Annals of the Rheumatic Diseases*, vol. 69, no. 5, pp. 887–890, 2010.

[23] B. Stiburkova, K. Ichida, and I. Sebesta, "Novel homozygous insertion in SLC2A9 gene caused renal hypouricemia," *Molecular Genetics and Metabolism*, vol. 102, no. 4, pp. 430–435, 2011.

[24] D. Dinour, N. K. Gray, S. Campbell et al., "Homozygous SLC2A9 mutations cause severe renal hypouricemia," *Journal of the American Society of Nephrology*, vol. 21, no. 1, pp. 64–72, 2010.

[25] H. Matsuo, T. Chiba, S. Nagamori et al., "Mutations in Glucose Transporter 9 Gene SLC2A9 Cause Renal Hypouricemia," *American Journal of Human Genetics*, vol. 83, no. 6, pp. 744–751, 2008.

Demographic and Clinical Predictors of Trait Impulsivity in Parkinson's Disease Patients

Maddeson Riley,[1,2] Megan Bakeberg,[2,3] Michelle Byrnes,[2,3] Alexa Jefferson,[2] Soumya Ghosh,[2,3] Rick Stell,[2,3] Frank L. Mastaglia,[2,3,4] Dana Hince,[5] and Ryan S. Anderton[1,2,3,5]

[1]*School of Health Sciences, University of Notre Dame Australia, Fremantle, WA, Australia*
[2]*Perron Institute for Neurological and Translational Science, Nedlands, WA, Australia*
[3]*Centre for Neuromuscular and Neurological Disorders, University of Western Australia, Nedlands, WA, Australia*
[4]*Institute of Immunology and Infectious Diseases, Murdoch University, Perth, WA, Australia*
[5]*Institute for Health Research, University of Notre Dame Australia, Fremantle, WA, Australia*

Correspondence should be addressed to Maddeson Riley; maddeson.riley@my.nd.edu.au

Academic Editor: Antonio Pisani

Background. Impulsive behaviour has become increasingly recognised as a neuropsychiatric complication of Parkinson's disease (PD). Thought to be a product of compromised cognitive control, the spectrum of impulsive behaviours in PD ranges from cognitive disinhibition to impulse control disorders (ICDs). *Objective.* At present, there are no indicators for trait impulsivity in PD. The objective of the current study was to identify demographic and clinical predictors of susceptibility to trait impulsivity in a cohort of PD patients. *Methods.* The current study assessed impulsivity using the Barratt Impulsiveness Scale 11 (BIS-11) in a cohort of 87 PD patients. General linear models (GLMs) were used to identify clinical and demographic variables predictive of heightened BIS-11 second-order attentional and nonplanning subscale scores. *Results.* Male gender, no history of smoking, postsecondary education, and heightened disease severity were predictive of increased BIS-11 attentional scores ($p < 0.05$). Similarly, male gender, after secondary education, and disease severity were predictive of increased BIS-11 nonplanning scores ($p < 0.05$). Contrary to previous reports, dopaminergic medication use was not a significant determinant of either BIS-11 subscale scores. *Conclusions.* Several demographic and clinical variables including male gender, no history of past smoking, after secondary education, and elevated disease severity are associated with impulsivity in PD.

1. Introduction

In recent times, a variety of impulsive behaviours, often ranging in severity, have been reported as psychiatric complications associated with Parkinson's disease (PD) [1]. As a construct, impulsivity is broadly defined as the tendency to act prematurely or without foresight, with little regard for the often-negative consequences associated with these actions [2].

Previous studies suggest that PD patients display heightened impulsivity, particularly when taking dopaminergic medication [1, 3]. In addition to this, PD may impair response inhibition, an integral element of impulsivity, with PD patients performing worse on a range of measures of inhibition, including the Stop-Signal Task [4, 5], Go/No-Go [6], and antisaccade [7].

Impulsivity is thought to underlie several psychiatric disorders described in PD, particularly impulse control disorders (ICDs) including pathological gambling, compulsive shopping and eating, and hypersexual behaviours [1, 8, 9]. These behaviours represent extreme manifestations of impulsivity thought to be provoked by dopamine agonist [10] therapy and identified in only 13% of PD patients [11]. Despite the strong association between impulsivity and ICDs, PD patients may display impulsivity even in the absence of an ICD [8, 12]. Additionally, impulsivity represents a significant risk factor for the onset of an ICD, which further suggests that impulsivity in PD can be represented on a spectrum; beginning with mild cognitive and motor disinhibition and eventually manifesting as clinically identifiable ICDs [9].

Previous studies have identified several variables associated with ICDs including male gender [11], cigarette smoking history [11, 13, 14], dopamine agonist use [11, 13], younger age of disease onset [14, 15], a history of drug or alcohol abuse [9, 15], and a novelty-seeking personality [9, 15]. However, there are no current demographic or clinical indicators of future impulsivity in PD. Given the strong association between impulsivity and ICDs in addition with the absence of treatment options for impulsive behaviour, the identification of risk factors for trait impulsivity serves as a valuable clinical tool in optimising the prevention of impulsivity and, in turn, the future onset of ICDs.

As such, the present study characterised a heterogeneous cohort of Western Australian PD patients with the objective of identifying demographic and clinical predictors for the development of trait impulsivity. Trait impulsivity was assessed using the Barratt Impulsiveness Scale 11 (BIS-11), which has been used extensively in PD clinical settings. The BIS-11 is a reliable measure of trait impulsivity, addressing the complexity of impulsivity as a construct with a three-component conceptualization comprising attentional impulsivity (reduced ability to focus on the task at hand and racing thoughts), motor impulsivity (the tendency to act without thinking), and nonplanning impulsivity (lack of future- or fore-thought) [16]. Previous studies have shown adequate internal consistency of BIS-11 second-order attentional and nonplanning subscales with Cronbach's α of 0.74 and 0.72, respectively [17]. However, internal consistency of the BIS-11 second-order Motor subscale is below adequate with a Cronbach's α of 0.59 [17]. Further, the aim of the current study was to assess cognitive domains of impulsivity in PD, rather than motor domains. Therefore, in the current study assessed only subjects BIS-11 attentional and nonplanning scores.

2. Methods

2.1. Subjects. Eighty-seven home-based PD patients (54 males) were sequentially recruited from the Movement Disorders Clinic at the Perron Institute for Neurological and Translational Science (Perth, Australia) between 2008 and 2015. All patients were examined by a movement disorder neurologist prior to inclusion in the study for verification of the diagnosis in accordance with the UK Brain Bank criteria for IPD. All patients were taking levodopa, and 45 patients were on a dopamine agonist (pramipexole, rotigotine, and apomorphine). For medication dosages, LEDD was calculated from patient medication dosages as per the following: LEDD = (regular levodopa dosage) + 0.75 (slow-release levodopa) + 10 (bromocriptine) + 10 (pergolide) + amantadine. Fourteen patients had undergone deep brain stimulation (DBS) therapy. Demographic variables including a history of smoking and patients' level of education were also collected.

2.2. Clinical Assessments and Impulsivity Screening. All clinical assessments were evaluated in the "ON" state. Motor symptoms were evaluated using the MDS-Unified Parkinson's Disease Rating Scale (MDS-UPDRS) Part III and Hoehn and Yahr Scale. In addition, each participant was evaluated by a clinical psychologist and completed a battery of neuropsychological assessments, as previously described [18]. The Mini-Mental State Examination (MMSE) was used to determine patients' cognitive status, with an MMSE score of less than 26 indicating "cognitive impairment" and greater than 26 indicating "normal" cognition. The "Barratt Impulsivity Scale 11" (BIS-11) was employed as a validated self-report questionnaire for screening impulsivity. The BIS-11 consists of 30 questions scored on a four-point scale, with each item corresponding to one of the three BIS-11 second-order subscales. The current study aimed to investigate cognitive domains of trait impulsivity rather than motor impulsivity and therefore only BIS-11 second-order attentional and nonplanning subscale scores are presented. Questions corresponding to these subscales are summarised in Table 1. Overall BIS-11 scores were calculated as the sum of these 30 scores (to yield a score out of 120), with higher scores indicating greater impulsivity. The sum of second-order BIS-11 attentional and nonplanning items was used to calculate patients' BIS-11 second-order subscale scores. BIS-11 second-order attentional and nonplanning scores were scored out of 32 and 44, respectively. During the screening process, patients displaying any signs of an impulse control disorder were invited to seek further consultation with the clinical psychologist.

2.3. Statistical Methods. Data were analysed using IBM-SPSS (v. 24, IBM Corporation). A significant nominal p value of <0.05 was employed. Univariate regression analysis of continuous demographic and clinical variables (MDS-UPDRS III, disease duration, and LEDD) and categorical demographic variables and clinical variables (gender, smoking history, level of education, i.e., secondary school or tertiary education, and cognitive status) was performed in order to determine whether these variables were significantly associated with BIS-11 second-order attentional and nonplanning subscale scores. Level of education was dichotomised into secondary school, referring to participants who reported not progressing past secondary school, and tertiary education, referring to participants who reported entering into a tertiary level of education. Participants who reported entering into a tertiary level of education were considered as having a higher level of education.

General linear models (GLMs) were used to analyse the relationship between variables identified as being significant in the univariate models and the two BIS-II second-order subscales. Variables proposed to be risk factors for the development of impulse control disorders in PD were also included in the GLMs, despite not displaying statistical significance in the univariate models. Variables included in the GLMs were gender, smoking history, dopamine agonist usage, LEDD, DBS history, age at disease onset, disease duration, MDS-UPDRS III scores, cognitive status, and participants' level of education. Nonsignificant variables were removed singularly in order of least significance until the final models were determined.

3. Results

3.1. Cohort Information and Clinical Data. Mean demographic details and the results of clinical assessments are

Table 1: Questions corresponding to BIS-11 second-order attentional and nonplanning domains.

BIS-11 2nd order subscale	Corresponding questions
Attentional impulsivity	5. "I don't pay attention" 6. "I have racing thoughts"' 9. "I concentrate easily" 11. "I squirm at plays or lectures" 20. "I am a steady thinker" 24. "I change hobbies" 26. "I often have extraneous thoughts when thinking" 28. "I am restless at the theatre or lectures"
Nonplanning impulsivity	1. "I plan tasks carefully" 7. "I plan trips well ahead of time" 8. "I am self controlled" 10. "I save regularly" 12. "I am a careful thinker" 13. "I plan for job security" 14. "I say things without thinking" 15. "I like to think about complex problems" 18. "I easily get bored when solving thought problems" 27. "I am more interested in the present than the future" 29. "I like puzzles"

shown in Table 2. The predominantly male cohort ranged in age and disease duration. At the time of the study, a total of 45 participants were medicated with dopamine agonists (DAs), and 14 participants had undergone DBS therapy. When examined according to MMSE score, 70 patients did not display cognitive impairment, and 17 were classified as being cognitively impaired. Overall, the cohort displayed a mean total BIS-11 score of 62.5 (±8.9) and had no prior history of impulsivity, based on information provided during consultation with a clinical psychologist.

Table 2: Baseline clinical characteristics of the PD cohort ($n = 87$) used in this study.

Clinical characteristic	Mean (SD) or n (%)
Gender	
Male	54 (62%)
Female	33 (38%)
Age (years)	62.8 (9.2)
Age of onset (years)	53.3 (10.2)
Disease duration (years)	10.4 (6.8)
Dopamine agonist usage	
Yes	45 (51.7%)
No	42 (48.3%)
LEDD (mg)	671 (389)
Deep brain stimulation	
Yes	14 (16.1%)
No	73 (83.9%)
Smoking history	
Yes	13 (14.9%)
No	74 (85.1%)
Level of education	
Secondary school	58 (66.7%)
Tertiary education	29 (33.3%)
MDS-UPDRS III (motor)	18 (14.2)
Cognitive status	
Cognitively impaired	22 (25.3%)
Not cognitively impaired	65 (74.7%)
BIS-11 scores	
Attentional 2nd order	15.8 (3.7)
Nonplanning 2nd order	24.8 (4.9)
Total score	62.5 (8.9)

3.2. Univariate Association of Demographic and Clinical Variables with Second-Order Attentional and Nonplanning Impulsivity. Univariate regression models revealed selected clinical and demographic variables associated with BIS-11 second-order attentional scores including gender ($p = 0.048$) and MDS-UPDRS III rating ($p = 0.005$). The residuals from these univariate models were normally distributed. The patients' level of education was positively associated with BIS-11 second-order attentional scores; however, this association did not reach statistical significance ($p = 0.076$). BIS-11 second-order nonplanning scores were significantly associated with gender ($p = 0.001$), MDS-UPDRS III rating ($p = 0.001$), and disease duration ($p = 0.003$). While the residual values of the univariate models for MDS-UPDRS III rating and disease duration were normally distributed, those for gender were not.

3.3. Demographic and Clinical Predictors of Second-Order Attentional Impulsivity in Multivariate Models. Multivariate general linear models were fitted to identify demographic and clinical determinants of BIS-11 second-order attentional and nonplanning subscale scores. The residual values for these multivariate models were normally distributed. Dopamine agonist usage, LEDD, DBS surgery, age at onset, disease duration, and cognitive status (cognitively impaired and not cognitively impaired) were found not to be significant predictors of BIS-11 second-order attentional or nonplanning subscale scores. In contrast, being of male gender, no history of smoking, higher level of education, and increased disease severity are predictive of elevated BIS-11 second-order attentional subscale score when entered simultaneously in the model (Table 3). Specifically, male participants were predicted to score 1.8 points higher than female participants ($p = 0.011$).

TABLE 3: Final multivariate model parameter estimates: predictors of BIS-11 second-order attention subscale scores.

Variable	β coefficient	Std. error	p
(Intercept)	12.537	1.3095	0.000
Gender			
Male	1.730	0.7401	0.019
Female	0*	—	—
Smoking history			
Yes	−2.207	1.0318	0.032
No	0*	—	—
Level of education			
Secondary school	0*	—	—
Tertiary education	1.730	0.7581	0.023
MDS-UPDRS III	0.080	0.0253	0.002

*Comparison category set to zero.

The estimated marginal mean (EMM) BIS-11 attentional score for male participants was 15.95 and 14.22 for female participants ($p = 0.019$) (Figure 1). Patients with no smoking history were predicted to score 2.2 points higher than those with a history of smoking ($p = 0.038$), and patients who had pursued tertiary studies were predicted to score 1.7 points higher than those who had attained a secondary level of education ($p = 0.023$) on the BIS-11 second-order attentional subscale. The EMM BIS-11 attentional score for those who undertook a secondary level of education was 14.22 and 15.95 for those who pursued tertiary studies ($p = 0.023$) (Figure 1). In addition to this, for every additional MDS-UPDRS III point, BIS-11 second-order attentional scores were predicted to rise by 0.07 points ($p = 0.003$). For example, a male patient who did not report a history of smoking was predicted to score 2.2 points higher than a female patient who did report a history of smoking.

3.4. Demographic and Clinical Predictors of Second-Order Nonplanning Impulsivity in Multivariate Models. Similarly, multivariate general linear models indicated that being of male gender, greater level of education, and increased disease severity were predictive of elevated BIS-11 second-order nonplanning subscale scores (Table 4). Smoking history was not found to be a significant determinant of nonplanning subscale scores. Specifically, male participants were predicted to score three points higher than female participants ($p = 0.002$). The EMM for BIS-11 nonplanning scores was 26.45 for male participants and 23.09 for female participants ($p = 0.001$). Those who had pursued tertiary education scored two points more than those who had attained a secondary level of education ($p = 0.047$) on the BIS-11 second-order nonplanning subscale. The EMM for BIS-11 nonplanning scores was 23.79 for those who had attained a secondary level of education and 25.76 for those who had pursed tertiary education ($p = 0.047$) (Figure 1). In addition to this, participants were predicted to score 0.1 points higher for every additional MDS-UPDRS III score ($p = 0.001$) on the BIS-11 second-order nonplanning subscale. For example, a patient who obtained an MDS-UPDRS III rating of 50 was predicted to score 3.3 points higher on the BIS-11 second-order nonplanning domain than a patient who obtained an MDS-UPDRS III rating of 20.

4. Discussion

Several risk factors for the onset of ICDs in PD subjects have been identified, including gender [11], smoking history [11, 13, 14], history of drug or alcohol abuse [9, 15], impulsivity [9], and a novelty seeking personality [9, 15]. However, there are no established demographic or clinical indicators for trait impulsivity in PD subjects. In light of the close relationship between trait impulsivity and the development of ICDs, and in conjunction with the absence of treatments for impulsive behaviours, there is a growing need to identify risk factors associated with impulsivity. Our findings suggest that several demographic and clinical variables may underlie impulsive behaviours in PD subjects.

Aligning with previous findings regarding PD-ICD subjects, the current study suggests that being of male gender is a significant risk factor for the development of trait impulsivity [19, 20]. Male subjects displayed significant associations between disease severity and the BIS-11 second-order attentional and nonplanning subscales. Regression analysis revealed that male subjects were predicted to score higher, particularly in the BIS-11 second-order nonplanning subscale, when compared with female subjects. A similar gender-related pattern of impulsive behaviour has been demonstrated in both PD-ICD subjects and the general population. For instance, Kenangil et al. [20] reported that among a cohort of 554 PD patients, 33 had a diagnosed ICD, of which 81% were men. In addition to this, male PD subjects are more likely to develop pathological gambling and hypersexual behaviours than females, with a similar pattern also evident in the general population [11].

This predisposition to developing impulsive behaviours in males may be related to men historically requiring greater stimulation and therefore being more likely to engage in sensation-seeking and impulsive behaviours than females [21]. Studies exploring gender differences in impulsivity have underlined that whilst females display heightened punishment sensitivity and are therefore more likely to avoid danger or risk, males do not exhibit this trait which may underlie the male propensity to partake in risky behaviours and therefore display heightened impulsivity [22]. It is important to note, however, that male PD subjects are less likely to develop compulsive eating and shopping disorders than female PD subjects, thus indicating that the type of impulsive behaviour reported may be gender-specific [11].

To our knowledge, this is the first study to explore the influence of level of education on the development of impulsivity in PD. Given the association between lower education status and accelerated cognitive decline in PD, the current study investigated whether achieving lower level of education (i.e., finishing secondary school and not pursuing tertiary studies) may also be related to elevated trait impulsivity [23]. However, the present study found that pursuing tertiary education and therefore pursuing education after secondary school was a risk factor for elevated BIS-11 second-order attentional and nonplanning scores. Weintraub et al. [11] identified a similar trend in a cohort of 3,090 PD patients, with those diagnosed with an ICD more likely to have more formal education. We suggest that seeking and obtaining

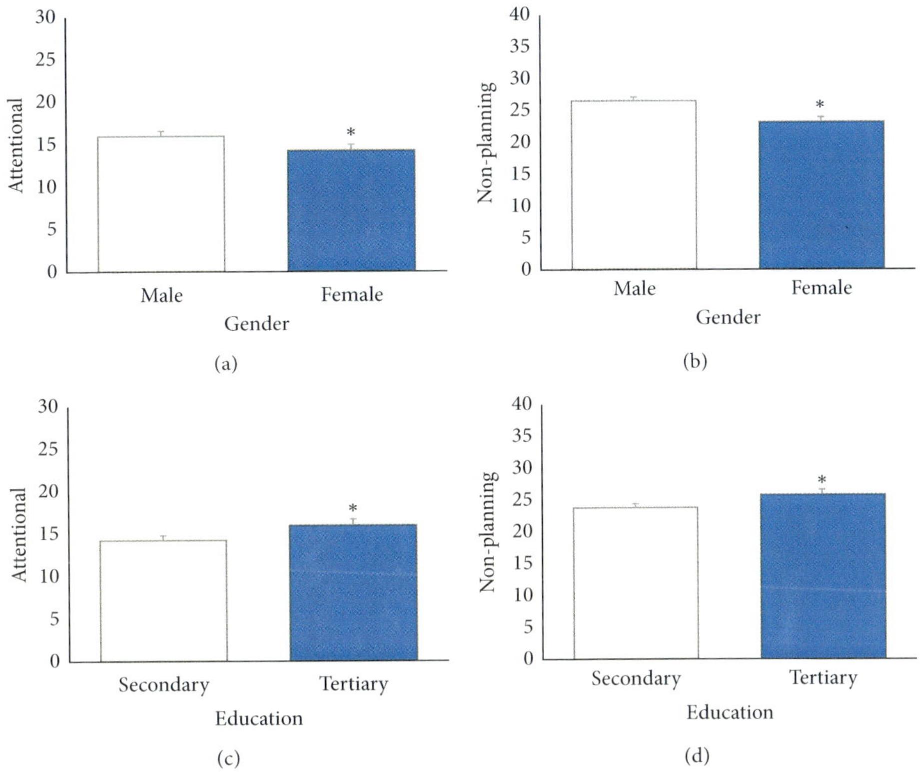

FIGURE 1: Estimated marginal mean (EMM) BIS-11 second-order subscale scores. EMM BIS-11 (a) attentional and (b) nonplanning scores were significantly higher in male subjects. EMM BIS-11 (c) attentional and (d) nonplanning scores were significantly higher in those who had pursued tertiary education when compared with those who had attained a secondary level of education.

further education may reflect distortions in patients' reward processing, an important element of impulsivity, thereby explaining this association between higher education status and trait impulsivity. Neuroimaging studies have demonstrated that PD patients, particularly those taking dopaminergic medication or with a clinically diagnosed ICD, may exhibit blunted reward anticipation and experiencing [24, 25]. In turn, these patients often make riskier choices in order to compensate for this diminished reward response [24, 25]. Although seeking out additional education is not necessarily an inherently risky process, it may nonetheless be related to patients' reduced ability to process and experience reward, possibly leading to dissatisfaction with their current education status and in turn, stimulating patients to pursue further education opportunities with diminished disinhibition.

Heightened disease severity was also a significant determinant of elevated BIS-11 second-order attentional and nonplanning scores in the described cohort, suggesting a relationship between more severe motor symptoms and future trait impulsivity in PD. Indeed, previous studies have discounted disease severity as a risk factor for the development of ICDs in PD subjects. Instead, these studies have underlined an association between motor complications as measured by the MDS-UPDRS IV and the future onset of ICDs, associating this link with elevated dopaminergic loads as a result of dopaminergic medication usage [26, 27]. Despite this, a more recent investigation of impulsivity as a multidimensional rather than unitary construct (i.e., ICD±) has reported a link

TABLE 4: Final multivariate model parameter estimates: predictors of BIS-11 second-order nonplanning subscale scores.

Variable	β coefficient	Std. error	p
(Intercept)	22.154	1.0648	0.000
Gender			
Male	3.366	0.9680	0.001
Female	0*	—	—
Level of education			
Secondary school	0*	—	—
Tertiary education	1.971	0.9936	0.047
MDS-UPDRS III	0.106	0.0328	0.001

*Comparison category set to zero.

between elevated MDS-UPDRS III scores and impulsivity in a cohort of 30 PD patients [6]. In this study, linear regression analysis verified that increased disease severity was significantly associated with impaired performance on a variety of measures of impulsivity including the Frontal Assessment Battery, Stroop test, BIS-11, Stop-Signal Task (SST), Go/No-Go task, and the Cambridge Gambling Task [6]. We propose that the pathophysiological basis underlying this association may be related to deteriorating motor symptoms being reflective of progressive brain atrophy and dopaminergic depletion, which, in turn, has been shown to have implications for performance on a variety of measures of impulsivity and therefore may contribute to the development of impulsive behaviours [6].

Contrary to previous reports, an absence of past smoking was a significant risk factor for elevated BIS-11 second-order nonplanning scores. Although a history of smoking has been associated with the development of ICDs in PD subjects [11, 13], our findings suggest otherwise with regard to impulsivity, indicating an inverse relationship between past smoking and trait impulsivity. However, given only 14 participants reported a history of smoking, this finding is more likely attributed to the small sample size of smokers included in the current cohort, as opposed to the presence of a potential association between smoking history and impulsivity.

A growing body of evidence exists to support the notion that dopamine agonist [10] medication, administered to alleviate the motor symptoms of PD in fact provokes ICDs in PD subjects. DA usage has been associated with a 3.5-fold increased risk of developing an ICD in PD patients [11]. Although the mechanism underlying this association remains unclear, the ability of DAs to stimulate dopamine receptors in the striatal limbic system, an area involved in reward and motivation, may contribute to the development of reward-driven and compulsive behaviours exhibited by PD patients with ICDs [28]. Interestingly, dopaminergic medication was not a significant determinant of trait impulsivity in this PD cohort. Though dopaminergic medication use has been associated with ICDs in PD cohorts, the prevalence of ICDs in only a fraction of PD patients treated with DAs highlights the importance of underlying susceptibility unrelated to dopaminergic medication use in the development of impulsivity [11]. Further, a significant proportion of PD patients have been diagnosed with an ICD before the initiation of any antiparkinsonian treatment, supporting the notion of underlying individual susceptibility to ICDs [8]. Therefore, the current finding further underlines the importance of additional clinical and demographic factors in the onset and development of impulsivity in PD.

5. Limitations

A number of limitations of the current study must be acknowledged. Firstly, the self-report nature of the BIS-11 may introduce a degree of bias in the gathered responses due to patients often being less inclined to report impulsive tendencies. Although the BIS-11 is frequently used as a measure of impulsivity in PD studies, the BIS-11 was not originally designed for use in a PD clinical setting, thereby somewhat limiting the reliability of the BIS-11 second-order scales. As the presence of depression or anxiety was not noted and therefore patients with depression or anxiety were not actively excluded from the current study, the confounding effect of these psychiatric disorders on impulsivity outcomes was not controlled for. In addition to this, patients' cognitive status was determined using an MMSE cutoff score of 26, which may not have accurately identified all patients exhibiting signs of cognitive impairment. Further, available data relating to the level of patient education indicated the commencement of education after secondary school, but did not necessarily provide information on study completion. As such, this study cannot attribute tertiary education attainment to a rise in BIS-11 domain scores, rather the mere pursuit of tertiary education.

6. Conclusion

In conclusion, the current study identified several demographic and clinical indicators of increased trait impulsivity in PD including male gender, heightened disease severity, an absence of past smoking, and higher level of education. The identification of demographic and clinical indicators of trait impulsivity in PD patients may serve as a valuable clinical tool in facilitating the early recognition of impulsivity and determining patients' therapeutic regimen, particularly regarding whether dopaminergic therapy may provoke impulsive behaviours and likely ICDs in the future.

Acknowledgments

The study was funded by grant/research support from the Federal Cooperative Research Centre for Mental Health, the Perron Institute for Neurological and Translational Science, and the University of Notre Dame Australia.

References

[1] L. U. Isaias, C. Siri, R. Cilia, D. De Gaspari, G. Pezzoli, and A. Antonini, "The relationship between impulsivity and impulse control disorders in Parkinson's disease," *Movement Disorders*, vol. 23, no. 3, pp. 411–415, 2008.

[2] J. W. Dalley, B. J. Everitt, and T. W. Robbins, "Impulsivity, compulsivity, and top-down cognitive control," *Neuron*, vol. 69, no. 4, pp. 680–694, 2011.

[3] R. Cools, R. A. Barker, B. J. Sahakian, and T. W. Robbins, "L-Dopa medication remediates cognitive inflexibility, but increases impulsivity in patients with Parkinson's disease," *Neuropsychologia*, vol. 41, no. 11, pp. 1431–1441, 2003.

[4] S. Gauggel, M. Rieger, and T. A. Feghoff, "Inhibition of ongoing responses in patients with Parkinson's disease," *Journal of Neurology, Neurosurgery & Psychiatry*, vol. 75, no. 4, pp. 539–544, 2004.

[5] I. Obeso, L. Wilkinson, E. Casabona et al., "Deficits in inhibitory control and conflict resolution on cognitive and motor tasks in Parkinson's disease," *Experimental Brain Research*, vol. 212, no. 3, pp. 371–384, 2011.

[6] C. Nombela, T. Rittman, T. W. Robbins, and J. B. Rowe, "Multiple modes of impulsivity in Parkinson's disease," *PLoS One*, vol. 9, no. 1, article e85747, 2014.

[7] S. Rivaud-Pechoux, M. Vidailhet, J. P. Brandel, and B. Gaymard, "Mixing pro- and antisaccades in patients with parkinsonian syndromes," *Brain*, vol. 130, no. 1, pp. 256–264, 2007.

[8] A. Antonini, C. Siri, G. Santangelo et al., "Impulsivity and compulsivity in drug-naive patients with Parkinson's disease," *Movement Disorders*, vol. 26, no. 3, pp. 464–468, 2011.

[9] V. Voon, M. Sohr, A. E. Lang et al., "Impulse control disorders in Parkinson disease: a multicenter case-control study," *Annals of Neurology*, vol. 69, no. 6, pp. 986–996, 2011.

[10] S. Y. Jeong and S. David, "Glycosylphosphatidylinositol-anchored ceruloplasmin is required for iron efflux from cells in the central nervous system," *Journal of Biological Chemistry*, vol. 278, no. 29, pp. 27144–27148, 2003.
[11] D. Weintraub, J. Koester, M. N. Potenza et al., "Impulse control disorders in Parkinson disease: a cross-sectional study of 3090 patients," *Archives of Neurology*, vol. 67, no. 5, pp. 589–595, 2010.
[12] A. A. Kehagia, C. R. Housden, R. Regenthal et al., "Targeting impulsivity in Parkinson's disease using atomoxetine," *Brain*, vol. 137, no. 7, pp. 1986–1997, 2014.
[13] G. T. Valenca, P. G. Glass, N. N. Negreiros et al., "Past smoking and current dopamine agonist use show an independent and dose-dependent association with impulse control disorders in Parkinson's disease," *Parkinsonism & Related Disorders*, vol. 19, no. 7, pp. 698–700, 2013.
[14] A. H. Evans, A. D. Lawrence, J. Potts, S. Appel, and A. J. Lees, "Factors influencing susceptibility to compulsive dopaminergic drug use in Parkinson disease," *Neurology*, vol. 65, no. 10, pp. 1570–1574, 2005.
[15] V. Voon, T. Thomsen, J. M. Miyasaki et al., "Factors associated with dopaminergic drug-related pathological gambling in Parkinson disease," *Archives of Neurology*, vol. 64, no. 2, pp. 212–216, 2007.
[16] J. H. Patton, M. S. Stanford, and E. S. Barratt, "Factor structure of the Barratt impulsiveness scale," *Journal of Clinical Psychology*, vol. 51, no. 6, pp. 768–774, 1995.
[17] M. S. Stanford, C. W. Mathias, D. M. Dougherty, S. L. Lake, N. E. Anderson, and J. H. Patton, "Fifty years of the Barratt impulsiveness scale: an update and review," *Personality and Individual Differences*, vol. 47, no. 5, pp. 385–395, 2009.
[18] T. Evans, A. Jefferson, M. Byrnes et al., "Extended "timed up and go" assessment as a clinical indicator of cognitive state in Parkinson's disease," *Journal of the Neurological Sciences*, vol. 375, pp. 86–91, 2017.
[19] R. Anderton, M. Byrnes, A. Jefferson et al., "Sleep disturbance and serum ferritin levels associate with high impulsivity and impulse control disorders in male Parkinson's disease patients," *American Journal of Psychiatry and Neuroscience*, vol. 5, no. 4, p. 45, 2017.
[20] G. Kenangil, S. Ozekmekci, M. Sohtaoglu, and E. Erginoz, "Compulsive behaviors in patients with Parkinson's disease," *Neurologist*, vol. 16, no. 3, pp. 192–195, 2010.
[21] T. L. Waldeck and L. S. Miller, "Gender and impulsivity differences in licit substance use," *Journal of Substance Abuse*, vol. 9, pp. 269–275, 1997.
[22] C. P. Cross, L. T. Copping, and A. Campbell, "Sex differences in impulsivity: a meta-analysis," *Psychological Bulletin*, vol. 137, no. 1, pp. 97–130, 2011.
[23] J. Meireles and J. Massano, "Cognitive impairment and dementia in Parkinson's disease: clinical features, diagnosis, and management," *Frontiers in Neurology*, vol. 3, p. 88, 2012.
[24] J. Riba, U. M. Kramer, M. Heldmann, S. Richter, and T. F. Munte, "Dopamine agonist increases risk taking but blunts reward-related brain activity," *PLoS One*, vol. 3, no. 6, article e2479, 2008.
[25] Z. Ye, A. Hammer, E. Camara, and T. F. Munte, "Pramipexole modulates the neural network of reward anticipation," *Human Brain Mapping*, vol. 32, no. 5, pp. 800–811, 2011.
[26] D. J. Ahearn, K. McDonald, M. Barraclough, and I. Leroi, "An exploration of apathy and impulsivity in Parkinson disease," *Current Gerontology and Geriatrics Research*, vol. 2012, article 390701, 10 pages, 2012.
[27] I. Leroi, M. Andrews, K. McDonald et al., "Apathy and impulse control disorders in Parkinson's disease: a direct comparison," *Parkinsonism & Related Disorders*, vol. 18, no. 2, pp. 198–203, 2012.
[28] A. Hassan, J. H. Bower, N. Kumar et al., "Dopamine agonist-triggered pathological behaviors: surveillance in the PD clinic reveals high frequencies," *Parkinsonism & Related Disorders*, vol. 17, no. 4, pp. 260–264, 2011.

34

Parkinson's Disease and Homocysteine: A Community-Based Study in a Folate and Vitamin B12 Deficient Population

Zhang Wei, Wang Tiandong, Li Yang, Meng Huaxing, Min Guowen, Fang Yalan, and Niu Xiaoyuan

Department of Neurology, First Hospital, Shanxi Medical University, No. 85, Jiefang Nan Street, Yingze District, Taiyuan 030000, China

Correspondence should be addressed to Niu Xiaoyuan; niuxiaoyuan@yeah.net

Academic Editor: Hélio Teive

Background. Homocysteine (Hcy) levels were higher in patients with Parkinson's disease (PD). This could be partially explained by levodopa treatment. Whether untreated PD patients have higher Hcy levels is contradictory. *Methods.* A community-based study was conducted using a two-stage approach for subjects $\geq$ 55 years to find PD patients in 3 towns of Lüliang City. Blood samples were collected. Serum Hcy, folate, and vitamin B12 concentrations were measured. For each untreated PD patient, 5 controls were selected matched with age and sex to evaluate the relationship between Hcy levels and PD. *Results.* Of 6338 eligible residents, 72.7% participated in the study. 31 PD cases were identified. The crude prevalence of PD for people $\geq$ 55 years was 0.67%. Blood samples were collected from 1845 subjects, including 17 untreated PD patients. There was no difference for concentrations of serum Hcy, folate, and vitamin B12 between cases and controls ($P > 0.05$). In univariate and multivariate analysis, there was significant inverse relation between PD and current smoking ($P < 0.05$). No other factor was significant statistically. *Conclusions.* The prevalence of PD was comparable to earlier studies in China. Hyperhomocysteinemia was not a risk factor of PD, as well as folate and vitamin B12 deficiency.

1. Introduction

Parkinson's disease (PD) is the second most common neurodegenerative disease after Alzheimer's disease in the elderly [1]. The estimated number of individuals above age of 50 with PD in the world was between 4.1 and 4.6 million in 2005 [2]. As aging population grows, the number will double to between 8.7 and 9.3 million by 2030 [2]. However, the etiology of PD remains unknown after decades of research. The interracial rates of PD are the same among communities in a common environment [3]. Nevertheless, the prevalence ratios for blacks in different countries varied obviously [4]. Therefore, environmental factors may be more important than genetic factors. Epidemiological studies also indicate that environmental factors, such as cigarettes smoking, are involved in the development of PD [5].

Homocysteine (Hcy) is formed by demethylation of methionine. Hyperhomocysteinemia plays a role in the development of some diseases, such as cardiovascular diseases and neurodegenerative diseases [6–8]. In vitro and in vivo studies indicated that Hcy contribute to the pathogenesis of mesencephalic dopaminergic neuronal death occurring in PD [9]. However, available data from clinical studies were contradictory [9]. Hcy levels were 30% higher in PD patients compared to controls [10]. This could be partially explained by regular treatment of levodopa [11]. Investigating the Hcy levels of naive PD patients may give some clues on the causal relationship between Hcy and PD.

The population living in Lüliang City, Shanxi Province, China, had inadequate folate and vitamin B12 intake [12] which may lead to high prevalence of hyperhomocysteinemia [13]. Meanwhile, because of low Development and Life Index [14], we presumed that most PD patients were undiagnosed and untreated. Thus, it was a proper area to research the relationship between Hcy and PD. In addition, there was no study regarding the prevalence of PD in rural North China. Similar studies were performed in large cities, such as Beijing and Shanghai, and areas around them in China before.

Aim of this study was bifold: (1) to find PD patients and estimate the prevalence of PD in Lüliang City; (2) to examine whether untreated PD patients had higher Hcy levels and the association between hyperhomocysteinemia and PD risk by case-control method.

2. Methods

2.1. Population Description. The study was performed in Lüliang City, Shanxi Province, China. Lüliang, a mountainous region, is located in the midwest of Shanxi Province which is an underdeveloped area of China. There are approximately 3,720,000 inhabitants, 80% of whom live in rural areas. 148 rural towns belong to Lüliang City, which can be divided into three categories (North, Center, and South) by orientation. Three townships (Kangcheng, Gaojiagou, and Caijiaya) from all three categories were selected as the target populations because of good cooperation of local governments. There was no tap water supply in the 3 towns and people all drank well water there.

2.2. Eligibility Criteria. We obtained a census list for 2012 from the household registry department of each town. The study was restricted to residents at age of 55 years or older (birth before 1958-01-01). Residents living in a Lüliang City residence less than 2 months per year were excluded from the study.

2.3. General Study Design. The study was performed from August 2012 to December 2012. A free medical consultation in local village health clinics was conducted to improve participation. About 10 days before the survey information on the opportunity to participate was published in local communities via leaflets and posters. Community workers contacted the residents via telephone calls or house visits one or two days before the evaluation to notify them of the time and place of examination. All respondents gave their written informed consent.

A two-stage community-based survey design was employed to detect PD patients. In the first stage, trained interviewers (doctors and senior clinical medical students) administrated a screening questionnaire [15] for PD in local health clinics. Demographic and medical information was also collected, including smoking, tea drinking, and alcohol drinking habits. If targeted residents did not appear in the local health clinics, interviewers visited their house once to administrate the questionnaire. Residents not at home during home visits were considered to have dropped out of the study. The questionnaire contains 9 questions. Residents who responded positively to at least 2 of the 9 questions were selected for the second stage. Sensitivity of the questionnaire was measured in a sample of 47 patients affected by PD; specificity was investigated in 217 outpatients free of parkinsonism. The sensitivity was 97.9% and the specificity was 73.7%. For reducing the false negative rate, subjects who gave positive answers to the question "Do your arms or legs shake?" entered into the second stage as well. We also asked the residents regarding whether levodopa was took and PD was diagnosed before, and subjects giving a positive answer of either question entered into the second stage.

In stage 2, a structured clinical workup comprising the Unified PD Rating Scale [16], a neurologic examination, and standardized history taking, was used to establish the diagnosis of parkinsonism and the classification of parkinsonism. Neurologists from First Hospital, Shanxi Medical University, performed the examinations in local health clinics or at home. Diagnosis of parkinsonism required the presence of bradykinesia and at least one of the following: muscular rigidity, rest tremor, or postural instability [17]. PD was diagnosed according to the United Kingdom Parkinson's Disease Society Brain Bank clinical diagnostic criteria [17]. The staging of PD was assigned according to the Hoehn and Yahr scale [18]. Non-PD parkinsonism including vascular parkinsonism, drug-induced parkinsonism, multiple system atrophy, progressive supranuclear palsy, and other parkinsonism types was diagnosed according to descriptions published previously [19].

Blood samples were collected from subjects who agreed. Approximate 10 mL venous fasting blood samples were obtained from subjects who appeared in the local village health clinics in the early morning hours after a 12 h fast by trained nurses in the field. For PD patients who could not come to the field, the fasting blood samples were collected at home. The serum samples were separated within 30 min of collection by centrifugation (4°C, 20 min, at 2000 RPM) in the field or at home and transported in a cooler to the First Hospital, Shanxi Medical University, Taiyuan, China, where the samples were stored at −70°C until analyzed. Serum total homocysteine (Hcy), folate, and vitamin B12 were measured at the First Hospital, Shanxi Medical University, Taiyuan, China. Hcy was measured by an enzyme cycling method using a Beckman UniCel DxC 800 Synchron Clinical System Analyzer (Beckman Coulter, Inc.). Serum folate and vitamin B12 were measured simultaneously by a radioassay kit (MP Biomedical, Inc.).

Among subjects with blood samples collected, for each untreated PD patient, 5 controls were selected matched with age (±2 years) and sex randomly.

2.4. Statistics. For case-control study, current smokers were defined as subjects who smoked during investigation or quitted smoking for less than 3 months. Current alcohol drinkers were defined similarly. Serum Hcy, folate, and vitamin B12 were categorized into binary variable according to the medians.

Prevalence rates were calculated for PD and expressed as percentages. The 95% confidence intervals (CI) were obtained. In addition, prevalence rates standardized to the age composition of the 2010 China census were also calculated. Linear-by-linear association chi-square test was used to test significance of linear relationship between prevalence and age. Differences between categorical variables were calculated using Pearson's chi-square test. Student's t-test or Mann-Whitney U test was used to compare continuous variables depending on the distribution types. Univariate logistic regression was used to estimate the odds ratios (ORs) and 95% CI for PD. Multivariate logistic regression was used

Table 1: Age and sex distribution of the targeted population, participants and participation rates.

Age, years	Targeted population, n			Participants, n			Participation rates, %		
	Men	Women	Total	Men	Women	Total	Men	Women	Total
55–64	1600	1607	3207	1128	1198	2326	70.5	74.5	72.5
65–74	905	949	1854	679	741	1420	75.0	78.1	76.6
75–84	563	559	1122	401	366	767	71.2	65.5	68.4
≥85	75	80	155	42	50	92	56.0	62.5	59.4
Total	3143	3195	6338	2250	2355	4605	71.6	73.7	72.7

to analyse all the risk factors. A P value < 0.05 was considered to be statistically significant. Data were analysed using the Statistical Package for Social Sciences (SPSS) software (version 13.0) and EpiCalc 2000.

3. Results

There were 6338 eligible residents living in the three towns in Lüliang City. Of these, 4605 (72.7%) were screened in stage 1. Age and sex distribution for the target population, participants, and participation rates in this study is presented in Table 1. Of the 4605 who were screened, 367 (7.97%) were suspected to have parkinsonism and entered stage 2. In stage 2, 22 (6.0%) cases could not be traced. Of the 345 (94.0%) subjects clinically evaluated by the neurologists, 37 were diagnosed with parkinsonism. Of the subjects with parkinsonism, 31 (83.8%) had PD, 1 (2.7%) had drug-induced parkinsonism, 1 (2.7%) had progressive supranuclear palsy, and 4 (10.81%) had vascular parkinsonism.

Among 31 PD patients, 30 (96.8%) were newly identified and did not receive treatment of levodopa. The other one had been diagnosed with PD and treated with Madopar for 3 years. 20 patients were males and 11 were females. The mean age at onset of PD was 70.37 ± 10.07 years. The mean duration of disease was 3.31 ± 2.95 years. All 31 patients with PD had two or more cardinal signs of parkinsonism; 24 (77.4%) had three or more signs; 8 (25.8%) had all four. In PD cases, 31 (100%) had bradykinesia, 27 (87.1%) had resting tremor, 26 (83.9%) had rigidity, and 10 (32.3%) had impaired postural reflexes. Regarding the Hoehn and Yahr scale, there were 8 (25.8%) patients in stage I, 13 (41.9%) in stage II, 8 (25.8%) in stage III, 1 (3.2%) in stage IV, and 1 (3.2%) in stage V.

The crude prevalence of PD for people aged 55 years or older was estimated to be 0.67% (95% CI 0.46–0.96). The age-standardized prevalence for people aged 55 years or older was 0.67% after being adjusted to the 2010 China census. The age- and sex-specific prevalence of PD is shown in Table 2. The prevalence of PD increased with advancing age (P = 0.00). There was no significant difference for PD prevalence between men and women (P = 0.08).

Blood samples were collected from 1845 subjects, including 17 untreated PD patients. Prevalence of hyperhomocysteinemia, low folate levels, and low vitamin B12 levels was high [20]. For each untreated PD patient, 5 controls were selected matched with age (±2 years) and sex. General characteristics of cases and controls are presented in Table 3. There was no difference for concentrations of serum Hcy, folate, and vitamin B12 between cases and controls (P = 0.341; P = 0.396; P = 0.696, resp.). Untreated PD patients had lower prevalence of current smoking (P = 0.005). The prevalence of current alcohol drinking, tea drinking, and pesticide exposure was not different significantly between cases and controls (P = 0.119; P = 0.586; P = 0.586, resp.)

Table 2: Age-specific and sex-specific prevalence of Parkinson's disease.

Age, years	Men		Women		Total	
	n	%	n	%	n	%
55–64	4	0.35	4	0.33	8	0.34
65–74	3	0.44	5	0.67	8	0.56
75–84	11	2.74	1	0.27	12	1.56
≥85	2	4.76	1	2.00	3	3.26
All ages (≥55)	20	0.89	11	0.47	31	0.67

In univariate analysis there was significant inverse relation between PD and current smoking (Table 4). Current smokers were found to be less likely to have PD (OR = 0.212; 95% CI 0.067–0.674; P = 0.009). High homocysteine levels (P = 0.070), low folate levels (P = 0.427), low vitamin B12 levels (P = 0.427), current alcohol drinking (P = 0.999), tea drinking (P = 0.999), and pesticide exposure (P = 0.999) were found not to have a significant relation with Parkinson's disease in this population. In multivariate analysis, similar results were obtained (Table 4).

4. Discussion

In China, the most widely accepted prevalence study on PD was conducted in Beijing, Xian, and Shanghai, which were the largest cities of China [21]. However, regional development differences were obvious in China [14]. In addition, environmental factors were important in the pathogenesis of PD. The present population had different characteristics from those in large cities, such as high prevalence of hyperhomocysteinemia. Investigating the prevalence in this area was necessary.

This study employed a two-stage community-based design to estimate the prevalence rate of PD in a Chinese population, which was popular in epidemiological studies on PD [19, 22, 23]. The differences among those studies were chiefly regarding how to screen PD in stage 1 and we utilized a questionnaire with high sensitivity (97.9%) to perform it. The questionnaire also showed high sensitivity (100%) in community-based study [24]. There was a low chance to miss PD patients in stage 1 in our study. A total of 31 cases were ascertained to have PD, which generated a crude

TABLE 3: General characteristics of cases and controls.

Variables	n (%) or medians (25th–75th percentile)		P value
	Cases $n = 17$	Control $n = 85$	
Age, years	72.0 (62–80)	72.0 (62–78)	0.989
Sex (%)			
Male	11 (64.7)	55 (64.7)	1
Female	6 (35.3)	30 (35.3)	
Town			
Kangcheng	4 (23.5)	32 (37.6)	0.330
Gaojiagou	5 (29.4)	28 (32.9)	
Caijiaya	8 (47.1)	25 (29.4)	
Serum tHcy, μmmol/L	27.45 (19.70–32.81)	20.71 (14.50–31.50)	0.341
≤22.175	5 (29.4)	46 (54.1)	0.063
>22.175	12 (70.6)	39 (45.9)	
Serum folate, nmol/L	6.92 (4.83–11.13)	7.50 (5.55–13.49)	0.396
≤7.375	10 (58.8)	41 (48.2)	0.425
>7.375	7 (41.2)	44 (51.8)	
Serum vitamin B12, pmol/L	132.45 (95.06–198.84)	149.64 (89.79–195.94)	0.696
≤147.295	10 (58.8)	41 (48.2)	0.425
>147.295	7 (41.2)	44 (51.8)	
Current smoking (%)			
Yes	10 (58.8)	74 (87.1)	0.005
No	7 (41.2)	11 (12.9)	
Current alcohol drinking (%)			
Yes	0 (0)	14 (16.5)	0.119
No	17 (100)	71 (83.5)	
Tea drinking (%)			
Yes	0 (0)	6 (7.1)	0.586
No	17 (100)	79 (92.9)	
Pesticide exposure (%)			
Yes	0 (0)	6 (7.1)	0.586
No	17 (100)	79 (92.9)	

TABLE 4: Univariate and multivariate analysis for the association between PD and possible risk factors.

Factors	Univariate results		Multivariate results	
	OR (95% CI)	P value	Adjusted OR (95% CI)	P value
Serum tHcy concentrations				
≤22.175	1		1	
>22.175	2.831 (0.917–8.738)	0.070	3.013 (0.785–11.560)	0.108
Serum folate concentrations				
≤7.375	1		1	
>7.375	0.652 (0.227–1.874)	0.427	0.627 (0.172–2.286)	0.480
Serum vitamin B12 concentrations				
≤147.295	1		1	
>147.295	0.652 (0.227–1.874)	0.427	0.312 (0.059–1.642)	0.169
Current smoking				
Yes	0.212 (0.067–0.674)	0.009	0.138 (0.034–0.561)	0.001
No	1		1	

prevalence rate of 0.67% for people aged 55 years or older. The result was comparable to earlier studies conducted in Chinese populations in Kinmen, Taiwan (0.587%, ≥50 years) [25], Ilan county, Taiwan (0.368%, ≥40 years) [19], and Beijing, Xian, and Shanghai, China (1%, ≥55 years) [21]. The prevalence of PD in the present population increased with age, which was in line with the previous studies [19, 25].

Hcy employs multiple neurotoxic mechanisms that have been associated with the pathogenesis of neurodegenerative disorders [9]. Among subjects with blood samples in the present study, most (72.1%) had hyperhomocysteinemia. Several studies regarding hyperhomocysteinemia were conducted in China. Compared to the study of Wang et al. in East China (10.5 μmmol/L, 45–75 years) [13], our study revealed a higher Hcy mean (24.6 μmmol/L) [20]. Hao et al. also showed lower Hcy medians (8.8 μmmol/L for South China and 11.4 μmmol/L for North China) [26] than ours (19.3 μmmol/L) [20]. However, the prevalence of PD in this area was not higher than that on behalf of China (1%, ≥55 years) [21], which indicated that Hcy may be not involved in the pathogenesis of PD.

Several studies found elevated plasma Hcy levels in PD patients treated with levodopa [27–29]. Because of the influence of levodopa, naive PD patients were proper cases for the investigation of the true relationship between Hcy and PD. Some studies had evaluated Hcy levels in untreated PD patients before and the results were contradictory [30, 31]. Small sample sizes (range 15–30) might account for the divergence. A meta-analysis including 6 studies found that there was no significant difference in plasma Hcy levels between untreated patients and healthy controls [32]. In the present study, most PD cases (96.8%) were firstly diagnosed and did not receive treatment, which could be partially interpreted by low development degree of local area. There was no difference for Hcy, folate, and vitamin B12 levels between untreated PD cases and controls in this population. Our results were in accord with the meta-analysis. In univariate and multivariate analysis, hyperhomocysteinemia was not a risk factor of PD, as well as folate and vitamin B12 deficiency. Current smoking was found to be a protective factor for PD, which was widely accepted [33, 34]. The above results indicated that Hcy did not play an important role in the pathogenesis of PD. In cohort studies, intake of folate or vitamin B12 was also not related to the risk of Parkinson's disease [35, 36].

Our study had limitations. There were only 17 untreated PD cases in the case-control study and this could lead to bias. Patients from epidemiological study had common background and were more appropriate for case-control study than cases from hospitals. However, the epidemiological study was costly and hard to expand sample sizes. Nevertheless, our results were generally consistent with the previous studies [32, 35, 36] and credible.

5. Conclusions

The prevalence of PD was comparable to earlier studies conducted in Chinese populations and increased with age. There was no difference for Hcy, folate, and vitamin B12 levels between untreated PD cases and controls. Hyperhomocysteinemia was not a risk factor of PD, as well as folate and vitamin B12 deficiency. Hcy did not play an important role in the pathogenesis of PD.

Authors' Contributions

Zhang Wei and Wang Tiandong contributed equally to this work.

Acknowledgments

The authors are grateful to all of the participants and families in this study. The study was completed with the help of local government and township health centers. Gao Shengwei, Hou Zhizong, Liu Tingting, Gao Bianfang, Zhang Yuting, Wang Juan, Dong Hai, Wang Li, and other senior medical students worked as volunteers in this study.

References

[1] K. Wirdefeldt, H.-O. Adami, P. Cole, D. Trichopoulos, and J. Mandel, "Epidemiology and etiology of Parkinson's disease: a review of the evidence," *European Journal of Epidemiology*, vol. 26, supplement 1, pp. S1–S58, 2011.

[2] E. R. Dorsey, R. Constantinescu, J. P. Thompson et al., "Projected number of people with Parkinson disease in the most populous nations, 2005 through 2030," *Neurology*, vol. 68, no. 5, pp. 384–386, 2007.

[3] L. C. S. Tan, N. Venketasubramanian, C. Y. Hong et al., "Prevalence of Parkinson disease in Singapore: Chinese vs Malays vs Indians," *Neurology*, vol. 62, no. 11, pp. 1999–2004, 2004.

[4] B. S. Schoenberg, B. O. Osuntokun, A. O. G. Adeuja et al., "Comparison of the prevalence of Parkinson's disease in black populations in the rural United States and in rural Nigeria: door-to-door community studies," *Neurology*, vol. 38, no. 4, pp. 645–646, 1988.

[5] H. Checkoway and L. M. Nelson, "Epidemiologic approaches to the study of Parkinson's disease etiology," *Epidemiology*, vol. 10, no. 3, pp. 327–336, 1999.

[6] R. Clarke, L. Daly, K. Robinson et al., "Hyperhomocysteinemia: an independent risk factor for vascular disease," *The New England Journal of Medicine*, vol. 324, no. 17, pp. 1149–1155, 1991.

[7] R. Clarke, A. D. Smith, K. A. Jobst, H. Refsum, L. Sutton, and P. M. Ueland, "Folate, vitamin B12, and serum total homocysteine levels in confirmed Alzheimer disease," *Archives of Neurology*, vol. 55, no. 11, pp. 1449–1455, 1998.

[8] N. K. Kim, B. O. Choi, W. S. Jung, Y. J. Choi, and K. G. Choi, "Hyperhomocysteinemia as an independent risk factor for silent brain infarction," *Neurology*, vol. 61, no. 11, pp. 1595–1599, 2003.

[9] S. Zoccolella, C. dell'Aquila, L. M. Specchio, G. Logroscino, and P. Lamberti, "Elevated homocysteine levels in Parkinson's

disease: is there anything besides L-dopa treatment?" *Current Medicinal Chemistry*, vol. 17, no. 3, pp. 213–221, 2010.

[10] E. F. dos Santos, E. N. B. Busanello, A. Miglioranza et al., "Evidence that folic acid deficiency is a major determinant of hyperhomocysteinemia in Parkinson's disease," *Metabolic Brain Disease*, vol. 24, no. 2, pp. 257–269, 2009.

[11] F. Blandini, R. Fancellu, E. Martignoni et al., "Plasma homocysteine and L-DOPA metabolism in patients with Parkinson disease," *Clinical Chemistry*, vol. 47, no. 6, pp. 1102–1104, 2001.

[12] B. Wang, J. Huo, J. Huang, and J. Sun, "Total diet study on certain nutrients in Shanxi regions with a high incidence of birth defects," *Wei Sheng Yan Jiu*, vol. 37, no. 6, pp. 702–706, 2008.

[13] Y. Wang, X. Li, X. Qin et al., "Prevalence of hyperhomocysteinaemia and its major determinants in rural Chinese hypertensive patients aged 45–75 years," *British Journal of Nutrition*, vol. 109, no. 7, pp. 1284–1293, 2013.

[14] *Reginal Development and Life Index Reports of 2011*, National Bureau of Statistics of China, Beijing, China, 2013, http://www.stats.gov.cn/tjsj/zxfb/201412/t20141231_661933.html.

[15] Z. Wei, N. Xiaoyuan, G. Shengwei, H. Zhizong, L. Jiyuan, and L. Yang, "Evaluation of a screening questionnaire for Parkinson's disease in a Chinese population," *Journal of Clinical Neuroscience*, vol. 21, no. 2, pp. 278–281, 2014.

[16] S. Fahn and R. L. Elton, *Recent Developments in Parkinson's Disease*, vol. 2, MacMillan Healthcare Information, Florham Park, NJ, USA, 1987.

[17] A. J. Hughes, S. E. Daniel, L. Kilford, and A. J. Lees, "Accuracy of clinical diagnosis of idiopathic Parkinson's disease: a clinico-pathological study of 100 cases," *Journal of Neurology, Neurosurgery & Psychiatry*, vol. 55, no. 3, pp. 181–184, 1992.

[18] M. M. Hoehn and M. D. Yahr, "Parkinsonism: onset, progression, and mortality," *Neurology*, vol. 17, no. 5, pp. 427–442, 1967.

[19] R. C. Chen, S. F. Chang, C. L. Su et al., "Prevalence, incidence, and mortality of PD: a door-to-door survey in Ilan County, Taiwan," *Neurology*, vol. 57, no. 9, pp. 1679–1686, 2001.

[20] W. Zhang, Y. Li, T. D. Wang et al., "Nutritional status of the elderly in rural North China: a cross-sectional study," *Journal of Nutrition, Health and Aging*, vol. 18, no. 8, pp. 730–736, 2014.

[21] Z.-X. Zhang, G. C. Roman, Z. Hong et al., "Parkinson's disease in China: prevalence in Beijing, Xian, and Shanghai," *The Lancet*, vol. 365, no. 9459, pp. 595–597, 2005.

[22] M. C. de Rijk, C. Tzourio, M. M. Breteler et al., "Prevalence of parkinsonism and Parkinson's disease in Europe: the EUROPARKINSON Collaborative study. European Community Concerted Action on the Epidemiology of Parkinson's disease," *Journal of Neurology, Neurosurgery & Psychiatry*, vol. 62, no. 1, pp. 10–15, 1997.

[23] J. Benito-León, F. Bermejo-Pareja, J. Rodríguez, J.-A. Molina, R. Gabriel, and J.-M. Morales, "Prevalence of PD and other types of parkinsonism in three elderly populations of central Spain," *Movement Disorders*, vol. 18, no. 3, pp. 267–274, 2003.

[24] M. T. Barbosa, P. Caramelli, D. P. Maia et al., "Parkinsonism and Parkinson's disease in the elderly: a community-based survey in Brazil (the Bambuí Study)," *Movement Disorders*, vol. 21, no. 6, pp. 800–808, 2006.

[25] S.-J. Wang, J.-L. Fuh, E. L. Teng et al., "A door-to-door survey of Parkinson's disease in a Chinese population in kinmen," *Archives of Neurology*, vol. 53, no. 1, pp. 66–71, 1996.

[26] L. Hao, J. Ma, J. Zhu et al., "High prevalence of hyperhomocysteinemia in Chinese adults is associated with low folate, vitamin B-12, and vitamin B-6 status," *Journal of Nutrition*, vol. 137, no. 2, pp. 407–413, 2007.

[27] S. Özkan, Ö. Colak, C. Kutlu, M. Ertan, and Ö. Alatas, "Plasma homocysteine levels in pergolide-treated Parkinson disease patients," *Clinical Neuropharmacology*, vol. 27, no. 4, pp. 163–165, 2004.

[28] T. Müller, B. Werne, B. Fowler, and W. Kuhn, "Nigral endothelial dysfunction, homocysteine, and Parkinson's disease," *The Lancet*, vol. 354, no. 9173, pp. 126–127, 1999.

[29] S. Zoccolella, P. Lamberti, E. Armenise et al., "Plasma homocysteine levels in Parkinson's disease: role of antiparkinsonian medications," *Parkinsonism and Related Disorders*, vol. 11, no. 2, pp. 131–133, 2005.

[30] D. Religa, K. Czyzewski, M. Styczynska et al., "Hyperhomocysteinemia and methylenetetrahydrofolate reductase polymorphism in patients with Parkinson's disease," *Neuroscience Letters*, vol. 404, no. 1-2, pp. 56–60, 2006.

[31] Z. Todorović, E. Džoljić, I. Novaković et al., "Homocysteine serum levels and MTHFR C677T genotype in patients with Parkinson's disease, with and without levodopa therapy," *Journal of the Neurological Sciences*, vol. 248, no. 1-2, pp. 56–61, 2006.

[32] X.-W. Hu, S.-M. Qin, D. Li, L.-F. Hu, and C.-F. Liu, "Elevated homocysteine levels in levodopa-treated idiopathic Parkinson's disease: a meta-analysis," *Acta Neurologica Scandinavica*, vol. 128, no. 2, pp. 73–82, 2013.

[33] A. Grandinetti, D. M. Morens, D. Reed, and D. MacEachern, "Prospective study of cigarette smoking and the risk of developing idiopathic Parkinson's disease," *American Journal of Epidemiology*, vol. 139, no. 12, pp. 1129–1138, 1994.

[34] J. M. Gorell, B. A. Rybicki, C. C. Johnson, and E. L. Peterson, "Smoking and Parkinson's disease: a dose-response relationship," *Neurology*, vol. 52, no. 1, pp. 115–119, 1999.

[35] H. Chen, S. M. Zhang, M. A. Schwarzschild et al., "Folate intake and risk of Parkinson's disease," *American Journal of Epidemiology*, vol. 160, no. 4, pp. 368–375, 2004.

[36] L. M. L. de Lau, P. J. Koudstaal, J. C. M. Witteman, A. Hofman, and M. M. B. Breteler, "Dietary folate, vitamin B12, and vitamin B6 and the risk of Parkinson disease," *Neurology*, vol. 67, no. 2, pp. 315–318, 2006.

Permissions

All chapters in this book were first published in PD, by Hindawi Publishing Corporation; hereby published with permission under the Creative Commons Attribution License or equivalent. Every chapter published in this book has been scrutinized by our experts. Their significance has been extensively debated. The topics covered herein carry significant findings which will fuel the growth of the discipline. They may even be implemented as practical applications or may be referred to as a beginning point for another development.

The contributors of this book come from diverse backgrounds, making this book a truly international effort. This book will bring forth new frontiers with its revolutionizing research information and detailed analysis of the nascent developments around the world.

We would like to thank all the contributing authors for lending their expertise to make the book truly unique. They have played a crucial role in the development of this book. Without their invaluable contributions this book wouldn't have been possible. They have made vital efforts to compile up to date information on the varied aspects of this subject to make this book a valuable addition to the collection of many professionals and students.

This book was conceptualized with the vision of imparting up-to-date information and advanced data in this field. To ensure the same, a matchless editorial board was set up. Every individual on the board went through rigorous rounds of assessment to prove their worth. After which they invested a large part of their time researching and compiling the most relevant data for our readers.

The editorial board has been involved in producing this book since its inception. They have spent rigorous hours researching and exploring the diverse topics which have resulted in the successful publishing of this book. They have passed on their knowledge of decades through this book. To expedite this challenging task, the publisher supported the team at every step. A small team of assistant editors was also appointed to further simplify the editing procedure and attain best results for the readers.

Apart from the editorial board, the designing team has also invested a significant amount of their time in understanding the subject and creating the most relevant covers. They scrutinized every image to scout for the most suitable representation of the subject and create an appropriate cover for the book.

The publishing team has been an ardent support to the editorial, designing and production team. Their endless efforts to recruit the best for this project, has resulted in the accomplishment of this book. They are a veteran in the field of academics and their pool of knowledge is as vast as their experience in printing. Their expertise and guidance has proved useful at every step. Their uncompromising quality standards have made this book an exceptional effort. Their encouragement from time to time has been an inspiration for everyone.

The publisher and the editorial board hope that this book will prove to be a valuable piece of knowledge for researchers, students, practitioners and scholars across the globe.

List of Contributors

Jie Zhang, Yan Xing and Xiuli Ma
Aviation General Hospital, China Medical University, Beijing 10023, China

Liqun Feng
Anzhen Hospital, Capital Medical University, Beijing 10029, China

Stefano Gambardella, Rosangela Ferese, Simona Scala, Francesca Biagioni, Nicola Modugno, Francesco Fabbiano, Diego Centonze and Stefano Ruggieri
IRCCS Neuromed, Pozzilli, Italy

Stefania Zampatti
IRCCS Neuromed, Pozzilli, Italy
Molecular Genetics Laboratory UILDM, Santa Lucia Foundation, Rome, Italy

Francesco Fornai
IRCCS Neuromed, Pozzilli, Italy
Department of Translational Research and New Technologies in Medicine and Surgery, University of Pisa, Pisa, Italy

Stefania Carboni
Molecular Genetics Laboratory UILDM, Santa Lucia Foundation, Rome, Italy

Giardina Emiliano
Molecular Genetics Laboratory UILDM, Santa Lucia Foundation, Rome, Italy
Department of Biomedicine and Prevention, University of Rome "Tor Vergata", Rome, Italy

C. Buhmann and E. Lehmann
Department of Neurology, University Medical Center Hamburg-Eppendorf, Martinistrasse 52, 20246 Hamburg, Germany

D. Jungnickel
Department of Social Sciences, University of Hamburg, Allende-Platz 1, 20146 Hamburg, Germany

Nilgul Yardimci
Neurology Department, Minasera Aldan Hospital, Ahmet Taner Kislali Mah. 2741, Street No. 2 Cayyolu, Ankara, Turkey

Ozlem Cemeroglu and Hasim Cakirbay
Physical Medicine and Rehabilitation Department, Medical Park Ankara Hospital, Kentkoop Mah., Kentkoop Parkici Yolu, Yenimahalle, Ankara, Turkey

Eda Ozturk
Biostatistics Department, Medicine Faculty, Hacettepe University, Hacettepe Mah., 06230 Ankara, Turkey

Gülsüm Gürlü, Esra Fahin and Saliha Bozkurt
Physical Medicine and Rehabilitation Department, Medicine Faculty, Turgut Ozal University, Alparslan Turkes Cad. No. 57, Emek, 06510 Ankara, Turkey

Tugba Cengiz and Gulderen Karali
Neurology Department, Medicine Faculty, Turgut Ozal University, Alparslan Turkes Cad. No. 57, Emek, 06510 Ankara, Turkey

Atilla Elhan
Neurology Department, Medicine Faculty, Gazi University, Emniyet, Yenimahalle, 06560 Ankara, Turkey

Dustin Anderson, Grayson Beecher and Fang Ba
Department of Medicine, University of Alberta, Edmonton, AB, Canada T6G 2G3

Murat Gultekin, Ayse Caglar Sarılar, Ayten Ekinci and Meral Mirza
Department of Neurology, Erciyes University School of Medicine, Kayseri, Turkey

Gozde Erturk
Department of Biostatistics, Erciyes University School of Medicine, Kayseri, Turkey

Kathrin Badstuebner and Immo Weber
Department of Neurology, University of Rostock, Rostock, Germany

Ulrike Gimsa
Institute of Behavioural Physiology, Leibniz Institute for Farm Animal Biology, Dummerstorf, Germany

Armin Tuchscherer
Institute of Genetics and Biometry, Leibniz Institute for Farm Animal Biology, Dummerstorf, Germany

Jan Gimsa
Chair of Biophysics, University of Rostock, Rostock, Germany

Erik L. Friesen and Mitch L. De Snoo
Krembil Research Institute, Toronto Western Hospital, University Health Network, 60 Leonard Avenue, Toronto, ON, Canada

Department of Laboratory Medicine and Pathobiology, University of Toronto, 1 King's College Circle, Toronto, ON, Canada

Suneil K. Kalia
Krembil Research Institute, Toronto Western Hospital, University Health Network, 60 Leonard Avenue, Toronto, ON, Canada
Department of Laboratory Medicine and Pathobiology, University of Toronto, 1 King's College Circle, Toronto, ON, Canada
Division of Neurosurgery, Department of Surgery, University of Toronto, 149 College Street, Toronto, ON, Canada

Lorraine V. Kalia
Krembil Research Institute, TorontoWestern Hospital, University Health Network, 60 Leonard Avenue, Toronto, ON, Canada
Department of Laboratory Medicine and Pathobiology, University of Toronto, 1 King's College Circle, Toronto, ON, Canada
Morton and Gloria Shulman Movement Disorders Clinic and The Edmond J. Safra Program in Parkinson's Disease, Division of Neurology, Department of Medicine, Toronto Western Hospital, University Health Network, 399 Bathurst Street, Toronto, ON, Canada
Division of Neurology, Department of Medicine and Tanz Centre for Research in Neurodegenerative Diseases, University of Toronto, 190 Elizabeth Street, Toronto, ON, Canada

Luckshi Rajendran
Faculty of Medicine, University of British Columbia, 317-2194 Health Sciences Mall, Vancouver, BC, Canada

Marcelo Rezende Young Blood and Carlos Henrique Ferreira Camargo
Neurology Service, Hospital Universitário, State University of Ponta Grossa, Ponta Grossa, PR, Brazil

Marcelo Machado Ferro
Neuropsychopharmacology Laboratory, State University of Ponta Grossa, Ponta Grossa, PR, Brazil

Renato Puppi Munhoz
Movement Disorders Centre, Toronto Western Hospital, University of Toronto, Toronto, ON, Canada

Hélio Afonso Ghizoni Teive
4Movement Disorders Unit, Neurology Service, Internal Medicine Department, Hospital de Clínicas, Federal University of Paraná, Curitiba, PR, Brazil

Ingrid Åström and Peter Hagell
The PRO-CARE Group, Faculty of Health Science, Kristianstad University, Kristianstad, Sweden
Department of Health Sciences, Lund University, Lund, Sweden

Catharina Sjödahl Hammarlund
The PRO-CARE Group, Faculty of Health Science, Kristianstad University, Kristianstad, Sweden
Department of Health Sciences, Lund University, Lund, Sweden

Albert Westergren
The PRO-CARE Group, Faculty of Health Science, Kristianstad University, Kristianstad, Sweden
The Research Platform for Collaboration for Health, Faculty of Health Science, Kristianstad University, Kristianstad, Sweden

Anna-Karin Edberg
The Research Platform for Collaboration for Health, Faculty of Health Science, Kristianstad University, Kristianstad, Sweden

Yanna Ren
Department of Psychology, Medical Humanities College, Guiyang University of Chinese Medicine, Guiyang 550025, China
Cognitive Neuroscience Laboratory, Graduate School of Natural Science and Technology, Okayama University, Okayama 7008530, Japan

Fengxia Wu, Jiajia Yang, Satoshi Takahashi and Yoshimichi Ejima
Cognitive Neuroscience Laboratory, Graduate School of Natural Science and Technology, Okayama University, Okayama 7008530, Japan

Jinglong Wu
Cognitive Neuroscience Laboratory, Graduate School of Natural Science and Technology, Okayama University, Okayama 7008530, Japan
Intelligent Robotics Institute, Beijing Institute of Technology, Beijing 100081, China
Shenzhen Institute of Neuroscience, Shenzhen 518057, China

Keisuke Suzuki and Koichi Hirata
Department of Neurology, Dokkyo Medical University, Tochigi 3210293, Japan

Weiping Yang
Department of Psychology, Hubei University, Wuhan 430062, China

Yanling Ren
Department of Light and Chemical Engineering, Guizhou Light Industry Technical College, Guiyang 550025, China

Y. N. Zhang
School of Computer Science and Technology, Beijing Institute of Technology, Beijing 100081, China
College of Computer Science and Information Engineering, Tianjin University of Science and Technology, Tianjin 300222, China

Fan Lou, Xiaoguang Luo and Yan Ren
Department of Neurology, First Affiliated Hospital of China Medical University, Shenyang, Liaoning, China

Ming Li
Department of Neurology, The Fourth Affiliated Hospital of China Medical University, Shenyang, Liaoning, China

Andreas Waldner
Department of Neurological Rehabilitation, Private Clinic Villa Melitta, Via Col di Lana 6, 39100 Bolzano, Italy

Sarah Dassati
Department of Neurological Rehabilitation, Private Clinic Villa Melitta, Via Col di Lana 6, 39100 Bolzano, Italy
Division of Molecular Biology, Biocenter, Innsbruck Medical University, Innrain 80-82, 6020 Innsbruck, Austria

Bernhard Redl
Division of Molecular Biology, Biocenter, Innsbruck Medical University, Innrain 80-82, 6020 Innsbruck, Austria

Nicola Smania and Marialuisa Gandolfi
Neuromotor and Cognitive Neurorehabilitation Research Centre (CRRNC), Department of Neurosciences, Biomedicine and Movement Sciences, University of Verona UOC Neurorehabilitation—AOUI Verona, University Hospital, P.le L.A. Scuro 10, 37134 Verona, Italy

Artur Schumacher-Schuh
Postgraduate Program in Medical Sciences, Universidade Federal do Rio Grande do Sul, Porto Alegre, RS, Brazil

Carlos E. Mantese
Postgraduate Program in Medical Sciences, Universidade Federal do Rio Grande do Sul, Porto Alegre, RS, Brazil
Mãe de Deus Hospital, Porto Alegre, RS, Brazil

Carlos R. M. Rieder
Postgraduate Program in Medical Sciences, Universidade Federal do Rio Grande do Sul, Porto Alegre, RS, Brazil
Universidade Federal de Ciˆencias da Sa´ude de Porto Alegre (UFCSPA), Porto Alegre, RS, Brazil
Hospital de Cl´ınicas de Porto Alegre (HCPA), Porto Alegre, RS, Brazil

Jiang Huang and Guoxu Xu
Department of Ophthalmology, Second Affiliated Hospital of Soochow University, Suzhou, China

Yi Li and Jianjiang Xiao
Department of Ophthalmology, Huashan Hospital North, Fudan University, Shanghai, China

Qin Zhang, Guanhui Wu and Weifeng Luo
Department of Neurology, Second Affiliated Hospital of Soochow University, Suzhou, China

Tong Liu
Institute of Neuroscience, Soochow University, Suzhou, China

Péter Kincses, Kázmér Karádi, Ádám Feldmann, Tibor Szolcsányi, Árpád Csathó and János Kállai
Institute of Behavioral Sciences, University of P´ecs, P´ecs 7624, Hungary

Norbert Kovács, Zsuzsanna Aschermann and Sámuel Komoly
Clinical Center, Department of Neurology, University of Pécs, Pécs 7623, Hungary

Krisztina Dorn
Pediatric Clinic, Clinical Center, University of P´ecs, P´ecs 7623, Hungary

Tatsuya Ueno, Haruo Nishijima, Yukihisa Funamizu, Tomoya Kon, Rie Haga, Akira Arai, Chieko Suzuki, Jin-ichi Nunomura, Masayuki Baba and Masahiko Tomiyama
Department of Neurology, Aomori Prefectural Central Hospital, Aomori, Japan

Megumi Sasaki
Department of Rehabilitation, Aomori Prefectural Central Hospital, Aomori, Japan

Marina Maffoni, Anna Giardini and Antonia Pierobon
Psychology Unit, Istituti Clinici Scientifici Maugeri, IRCCS Montescano (PV), Pavia, Italy

Davide Ferrazzoli and Giuseppe Frazzitta
Parkinson's Disease and Brain Injury Rehabilitation Department, Moriggia-Pelascini Hospital, Gravedona ed Uniti, Italy

Annelise Ayres and Geraldo Pereira Jotz
Postgraduate Program in Health Sciences, Universidade Federal de Ciências da Saúde de Porto Alegre, Porto Alegre, RS, Brazil

Carlos R. M. Rieder
Postgraduate Program in Medical Sciences, Universidade Federal do Rio Grande do Sul, Porto Alegre, RS, Brazil
Department of Neurology and Postgraduate Program in Rehabilitation, Universidade Federal de Ciências da Saúde de Porto Alegre (UFCSPA), Porto Alegre, RS, Brazil

Maira Rozenfeld Olchik
Department of Surgery and Orthopaedics, Universidade Federal do Rio Grande do Sul, Porto Alegre, RS, Brazil

Xun Zhou and Qian Xu
Department of Neurology, Xiangya Hospital, Central South University, Changsha, Hunan 410008, China

Yuan Zhang
Department of Neurology, Xiangya Hospital, Central South University, Changsha, Hunan 410008, China
Department of Geriatrics, Xiangya Hospital, Central South University, Changsha, Hunan 410008, China

Xinxiang Yan
Department of Neurology, Xiangya Hospital, Central South University, Changsha, Hunan 410008, China
National Clinical Research Center for Geriatric Diseases, Changsha, Hunan 410078, China
Key Laboratory of Hunan Province in Neurodegenerative Disorders, Central South University, Changsha, Hunan 410008, China

Jifeng Guo and Beisha Tang
Department of Neurology, Xiangya Hospital, Central South University, Changsha, Hunan 410008, China
National Clinical Research Center for Geriatric Diseases, Changsha, Hunan 410078, China
Key Laboratory of Hunan Province in Neurodegenerative Disorders, Central South University, Changsha, Hunan 410008, China
State Key Laboratory of Medical Genetics, Changsha, Hunan 410078, China

Qiying Sun
Department of Geriatrics, Xiangya Hospital, Central South University, Changsha, Hunan 410008, China
National Clinical Research Center for Geriatric Diseases, Changsha, Hunan 410078, China
Key Laboratory of Hunan Province in Neurodegenerative Disorders, Central South University, Changsha, Hunan 410008, China

Minhan Yi
State Key Laboratory of Medical Genetics, Changsha, Hunan 410078, China
Institute of Information Security and Big Data, Central South University, Changsha, Hunan 410083, China

Benxu Cheng, Pinki Anand, Feroz Akhtar and Virginia L. Scofield
Regional Academic Health Center, School of Medicine, University of Texas Rio Grande Valley, Edinburg, TX, USA

Anxiu Kuang
Department of Biology, University of Texas Rio Grande Valley, Edinburg, TX, USA

Jing Hui Yang, Ya Qun Wang, You Gen Cheng and Xiao Zhen Feng
Department of Rehabilitation Medicine, Tongde Hospital of Zhejiang Province, Hangzhou, China

Sai Qing Ye
Department of Rehabilitation Medicine, West China Hospital of Sichuan University, Chengdu, China

Yu Chen
Wuxi Tongren International Rehabilitation Hospital, Wuxi, China

Seyed-Mohammad Fereshtehnejad
Department of Neurology and Neurosurgery, McGill University, Montreal, QC, Canada
Division of Clinical Geriatrics, Department of Neurobiology, Care Sciences, and Society (NVS), Karolinska Institutet, Stockholm, Sweden

Örjan Skogar
Division of Clinical Geriatrics, Department of Neurobiology, Care Sciences, and Society (NVS), Karolinska Institutet, Stockholm, Sweden
FUTURUM, Academy for Health and Care, Jönköping, Sweden

Johan Lökk
Division of Clinical Geriatrics, Department of Neurobiology, Care Sciences, and Society (NVS), Karolinska Institutet, Stockholm, Sweden
Department of Geriatric Medicine, Karolinska University Hospital, Stockholm, Sweden

Giulia Di Lazzaro, Tommaso Schirinzi, Maria Pia Giambrone, Maria Giuseppina Palmieri, Camilla Rocchi, Nicola Biagio Mercuri and Antonio Pisani
Department of Systems Medicine, University of Rome Tor Vergata, Rome, Italy
Fondazione Santa Lucia IRCCS, Rome, Italy

Roberta Di Mauro and Stefano Di Girolamo
Department of Otorhinolaryngology, University of Rome Tor Vergata, Rome, Italy

Michele Tinazzi
Department of Neuroscience, Biomedicine and Movement Sciences, University of Verona, Verona, Italy

U. Hidding, A. Horn, C. Buhmann, C. Gerloff and M. Pötter-Nerger
Department of Neurology, University Medical Center Hamburg-Eppendorf, 20246 Hamburg, Germany

A. Gulberti
Department of Neurology, University Medical Center Hamburg-Eppendorf, 20246 Hamburg, Germany
Department of Neurophysiology and Pathophysiology, University Medical Center Hamburg-Eppendorf, 20246 Hamburg, Germany

A. K. Engel and C. K. E. Moll
Department of Neurophysiology and Pathophysiology, University Medical Center Hamburg-Eppendorf, 20246 Hamburg, Germany

W. Hamel, J. A. Koeppen and M. Westphal
Department of Neurosurgery, University Medical Center Hamburg-Eppendorf, 20246 Hamburg, Germany

D. Weiss
Department for Neurodegenerative Diseases and Hertie Institute for Clinical Brain Research, University of Tübingen, 72076 Tübingen, Germany

François D. H. Gould Andrew Gross and Rebecca Z. German
Department of Anatomy and Neurobiology, Northeast Ohio Medical University, Rootstown, OH, USA

Jason R. Richardson
Department of Pharmaceutical Science, Northeast Ohio Medical University, Rootstown, OH, USA

Guotao Liu, Yanping Zhang, Xiuquan Du and Chenchu Xu
School of Computer Science and Technology, Anhui University, Hefei 230601, China

Zhenghui Hu
Center for Optics and Optoelectronics Research, College of Science, Zhejiang University of Technology, Pingfeng Campus, Liuhe Road 288, Xihu District, Hangzhou 310023, China

Wanqing Wu
Shenzhen Institutes of Advanced Technology, Chinese Academy of Sciences, Shenzhen 518055, China

Xiangyang Wang
Anhui Electrical Engineering Professional Technique College, Hefei 230051, China

Shuo Li
Department of Medical Imaging, Schulich School of Medicine and Dentistry, University of Western Ontario, 1151 Richmond St, London, ON, Canada

Luiz Felipe Vasconcellos, João Santos Pereira and Mariana Spitz
Movement Disorders Unit, Neurology Service, Pedro Ernesto University Hospital, State University of Rio de Janeiro, Rio de Janeiro, RJ, Brazil

Marcelo Adachi
Radiology Department, Hospital Central da Polícia Militar, Rio de Janeiro, RJ, Brazil

Denise Greca, Manuela Cruz, Ana Lara Malak and Helenice Charchat-Fichman
Psychology Department, Pontifical Catholic University of Rio de Janeiro (PUC-Rio), Rio de Janeiro, RJ, Brazil

Judith Bek, Jordan Webb, Emma Gowen and Ellen Poliakoff
University of Manchester, Manchester, UK

Stefan Vogt and Trevor J. Crawford
Lancaster University, Lancaster, UK

Matthew S. Sullivan
Manchester Metropolitan University, Manchester, UK

Ilana Schlesinger
Department of Neurology, Rambam Health Care Campus, Haifa, Israel
Technion Faculty of Medicine, Haifa, Israel

Menashe Zaaroor
Technion Faculty of Medicine, Haifa, Israel
Department of Neurosurgery, Rambam Health Care Campus, Haifa, Israel

Alon Sinai
Department of Neurosurgery, Rambam Health Care Campus, Haifa, Israel

Jing Liu, Jiedi Zheng, Chunfeng Liu and Weifeng Luo
Jiangsu Key Laboratory of Translational Research andTherapy for Neuro-Psycho-Diseases and The Second Affiliated Hospital of Soochow University, Soochow University, Suzhou, Jiangsu 215021, China

Jiangfang Miao
Jiangsu Key Laboratory of Translational Research andTherapy for Neuro-Psycho-Diseases and The Second Affiliated Hospital of Soochow University, Soochow University, Suzhou, Jiangsu 215021, China
Jiangsu Jiangyin People's Hospital, Jiangyin, Jiangsu 214400, China

Zufu Zhu
Jiangsu Jiangyin People's Hospital, Jiangyin, Jiangsu 214400, China

Li Xiao and Kai Li
College of Pharmaceutical Science, Soochow University, Suzhou, Jiangsu 215123, China

Maddeson Riley
School of Health Sciences, University of Notre Dame Australia, Fremantle, WA, Australia
Perron Institute for Neurological and Translational Science, Nedlands, WA, Australia

Ryan S. Anderton
School of Health Sciences, University of Notre Dame Australia, Fremantle, WA, Australia
Perron Institute for Neurological and Translational Science, Nedlands, WA, Australia
Centre for Neuromuscular and Neurological Disorders, University of Western Australia, Nedlands, WA, Australia
Institute for Health Research, University of Notre Dame Australia, Fremantle, WA, Australia

Alexa Jefferson
Perron Institute for Neurological and Translational Science, Nedlands, WA, Australia

Megan Bakeberg, Michelle Byrnes, Soumya Ghosh and Rick Stell
Perron Institute for Neurological and Translational Science, Nedlands, WA, Australia
Centre for Neuromuscular and Neurological Disorders, University of Western Australia, Nedlands, WA, Australia

Frank L. Mastaglia
Perron Institute for Neurological and Translational Science, Nedlands, WA, Australia
Centre for Neuromuscular and Neurological Disorders, University of Western Australia, Nedlands, WA, Australia
Institute of Immunology and Infectious Diseases, Murdoch University, Perth, WA, Australia

Dana Hince
Institute for Health Research, University of Notre Dame Australia, Fremantle, WA, Australia

Zhang Wei, Wang Tiandong, Li Yang, Meng Huaxing, Min Guowen, Fang Yalan and Niu Xiaoyuan
Department of Neurology, First Hospital, Shanxi Medical University, No. 85, Jiefang Nan Street, Yingze District, Taiyuan 030000, China

Index

S

T

U

V